Nutrition Research Methodologies

The Nutrition Society Textbook Series

Clinical Nutrition, 2nd Edition
Edited by Elia, Ljungquist, Stratton and Lanham-New
December 2012
ISBN : 978-1-4051-6810-6

Sport and Exercise Nutrition
Edited by Lanham-New, Stear, Shirreffs and Collins
October 2011
ISBN : 978-1-4443-3468-5

Nutrition and Metabolism, 2nd Edition
Edited by Lanham-New, MacDonald and Roche
November 2010
ISBN: 978-1-4051-6808-3

Introduction to Human Nutrition, 2nd Edition
Edited by Gibney, Lanham-New, Cassidy and Vorster
March 2009
ISBN : 978-1-4051-6807-6

Public Health Nutrition
Edited by Gibney, Margetts, Kearney and Arab
November 2004
ISBN: 978-0-632-05627-9

Nutrition Research Methodologies

Edited on behalf of The Nutrition Society by

Professor Julie A Lovegrove

Hugh Sinclair Unit of Human Nutrition and Institute
for Cardiovascular and Metabolic Research
Department of Food and Nutritional Sciences
University of Reading
UK

Associate Professor Leanne Hodson

Oxford Centre for Diabetes, Endocrinology & Metabolism
Radcliffe Department of Medicine
University of Oxford
UK

Professor Sangita Sharma

Centennial Professor, Endowed Chair in Aboriginal Health, Professor
of Aboriginal & Global Health Research, Aboriginal and Global Health
Research Group, Department of Medicine, Faculty of Medicine & Dentistry
University of Alberta
Canada

Editor-in-Chief

Professor Susan A Lanham-New

Department of Nutritional Sciences, School of Biosciences
and Medicine, Faculty of Health and Medical Sciences
University of Surrey
UK

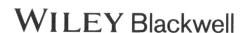

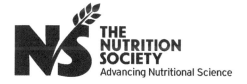

Registered Office
John Wiley & Sons, Ltd, The Atrium, Southern Gate, Chichester, West Sussex, PO19 8SQ, UK

Editorial Offices
9600 Garsington Road, Oxford, OX4 2DQ, UK
The Atrium, Southern Gate, Chichester, West Sussex, PO19 8SQ, UK
1606 Golden Aspen Drive, Suites 103 and 104, Ames, Iowa 50010, USA

For details of our global editorial offices, for customer services and for information about how to apply for permission to reuse the copyright material in this book please see our website at www.wiley.com/wiley-blackwell

Library of Congress Cataloging-in-Publication Data

Nutrition research methodologies / [edited by] Julie Lovegrove, Sangita Sharma, Leanne Hodson.
    p. ; cm. – (The Nutrition Society textbook series)
  Includes bibliographical references and index.
  ISBN 978-1-118-55467-8 (pbk.)
I. Lovegrove, Julie, editor.   II. Sharma, Sangita (Professor in aboriginal and global health research), editor.
III. Hodson, Leanne, editor.   IV. Series: Human nutrition textbook series.
  [DNLM: 1. Biomedical Research–methods.   2. Nutritional Physiological Phenomena.   3. Models, Biological.
4. Research Design. QU 145]
  R850
  610.72′4–dc23
                                    2014037007

A catalogue record for this book is available from the British Library.

Cover image: Courtesy of iStockphoto/skystardream
Cover design by Mark Lee (www.hisandhersdesign.co.uk)

Set in 9.5/11pt Minion by SPi Publisher Services, Pondicherry, India

1   2015

Contents

Contributors

Dr Les Bluck
MRC Human Nutrition Research
UK

Marc-Jeroen Bogaardt
Wageningen University
and Research Centre
Netherlands

Professor Kathleen M Botham
The Royal Veterinary College
UK

Dr Lorraine Brennan
University College Dublin
Ireland

Dr Barbara Burlingame
Food and Agriculture Organization of the
United Nations
Italy

Professor Judith Buttriss
British Nutrition Foundation
UK

Professor Janet Cade
University of Leeds
UK

Dr U Ruth Charrondiere
Food and Agriculture Organization of the
United Nations
Italy

Dr Baukje de Roos
University of Aberdeen
UK

Dr Moira Dean
Queen's University Belfast
UK

Dr Barbara A Fielding
University of Surrey
UK

Dr Heinz Freisling
International Agency for Research
on Cancer
France

Associate Professor Leanne Hodson
University of Oxford
UK

Dr Peter Hollman
Wageningen University
Netherlands

Graham Horgan
Biomathematics and Statistics Scotland
UK

Dr Jayne Hutchinson
University of York
UK

Dr Inge Huybrechts
International Agency for Research on Cancer
France

Dr Anne-Kathrin Illner
International Agency for Research on Cancer
France

Professor Alan A Jackson
University of Southampton
UK

Dr Fariba Kolahdooz
University of Alberta
Canada

Dr Gunter G C Kuhnle
University of Reading
UK

Professor Liisa Lähteenmäki
Aarhus University
Denmark

Professor Susan A Lanham-New
University of Surrey
UK

Professor Julie A Lovegrove
University of Reading
UK

Professor John C Mathers
Human Nutrition Research Centre
Newcastle University
UK

Dr Maria J Maynard
Leeds Beckett University
UK

Dr Michelle C McKinley
Queen's University Belfast
UK

Professor Anne Marie Minihane
University of East Anglia
UK

Dr Melissa J Morine
The Microsoft Research–University of Trento Centre
for Computational Systems Biology (COSBI)
Italy

Dr Peter Murgatroyd
NIHR/Wellcome Trust Clinical Research Facility,
Cambridge
UK

Professor Chris C Patterson
Queen's University Belfast
UK

Professor Corrado Priami
The Microsoft Research–University of Trento Centre
for Computational Systems Biology (COSBI)
Italy

Professor Monique M Raats
University of Surrey
UK

Professor Helen M Roche
University College Dublin
Ireland

Professor Andrew M Salter
University of Nottingham
UK

Professor Sangita Sharma
University of Alberta
Canada

Dr Nadia Slimani
International Agency for Research on Cancer
France

Professor Margot Umpleby
University of Surrey
UK

Professor Pieter van't Veer
Wageningen University
Netherlands

Dr Christian Viertler
Medical University of Graz
Austria

Laura Watson
NIHR/Wellcome Trust Clinical
Research Facility,
Cambridge
UK

Professor Robert W Welch
University of Ulster
UK

Professor Klaas R Westerterp
Maastricht University
Netherlands

Professor Martin Wiseman
University of Southampton
UK

Professor Jayne V Woodside
Queen's University Belfast
UK

Dr Stephen A Wootton
University of Southampton
UK

Professor Kurt Zatloukal
Medical University of Graz
Austria

Series Foreword

The Nutrition Society was first established in 1941, as a result of a group of leading physiologists, biochemists and medical scientists recognising that the emerging discipline of Nutrition would benefit from its own specific Learned Society. This was very much driven by concerns about the nutritional status of the UK population during World War II. The Nutrition Society's mission was, and still firmly remains, '*To advance the scientific study of nutrition and its application to the maintenance of human and animal health*'. The Society is the largest Learned Society for Nutritional Sciences in Europe and has over 2900 members worldwide. More details about the Society and how to become a member can be found by visiting the Society's website at www.nutritionsociety.org.

The Society's first journal, *The Proceedings of the Nutrition Society*, published in 1944, records the scientific presentations made to the Society. Shortly afterwards, in 1947, the *British Journal of Nutrition* was established to provide a medium for the publication of primary research on all aspects of human and animal nutrition by scientists from around the world. Recognising the needs of students and their teachers for authoritative reviews on topical issues in nutrition, the Society began publishing *Nutrition Research Reviews* in 1988. The journal *Public Health Nutrition*, the first international journal dedicated to this important and growing area, was subsequently launched in 1998. The Society is constantly evolving and has most recently launched the *Journal of Nutritional Science*. This is an international, peer-reviewed, online-only, open access journal.

The Nutrition Society Textbook Series, first established by Professor Michael Gibney (University College Dublin) in 1998 and now under the direction of the second Editor-in-Chief, Professor Susan Lanham-New (University of Surrey), continues to be an extraordinarily successful venture for the Society. This series of human nutrition textbooks is designed for use worldwide and this has been achieved by translating the series into many different languages, including Spanish, Greek and Portuguese. The sales of the five current textbooks (more than 55,000 copies) are a tribute to the value placed on the textbooks both in the UK and worldwide as a core educational tool.

Nutrition Research Methodologies is an outstanding sixth textbook to add to the series. The Editorial Team, led by Professor Julie Lovegrove (University of Reading), provides the reader with a complete outline of key nutrition methodologies – from basic and applied statistics, to the fundamentals of measuring dietary intake and nutritional status in individuals and populations, to the application of some of the newest techniques in nutritional sciences, including the 'omic' techniques. The textbook is an absolute must-read for students, nutritionists, dieticians, medics, nursing staff and other allied health professionals involved in the science of nutrition.

It gives me great pleasure to write the Foreword for this first edition of *Nutrition Research Methodologies*. I know from my time as the first Chairman of the UK Food Standards Agency how important high-quality nutrition science is for underpinning sound policies, both in the UK and worldwide. This textbook brings together science and the practical application of methodologies in nutrition and is a most valuable resource to all those working in the field.

Professor Lord John Krebs Kt
MA DPHIL FRS FMedSci
Principal, Jesus College,
University of Oxford

Preface

The sixth book in Nutrition Society's Textbook Series has arrived! I am absolutely delighted to introduce *Nutrition Research Methodologies* (NRM), which I do, as Editor-in-Chief (E-i-C), with great pride and with tremendous honour. The NRM Editorial team has worked tirelessly to produce this book focusing on new and established Research Methods in Nutritional Sciences. We first started the planning of the Textbook in 2011; what a joy to see the Lovegrove *et al* NRM first edition (1e) in print after so much hard work!

Nutrition Research Methodologies 1e has been led superbly by Professor Julie Lovegrove (Hugh Sinclair Professor of Nutrition, University of Reading) as Senior Editor of the book and her Editorial Team in the name of Associate Professor Leanne Hodson (University of Oxford) and Professor Sangita Sharma (Unversity of Alberta). They have planned out meticulously the details of the chapters and managed to secure the world-leaders in the field to contribute key chapters. How indebted we are to all the contributors for making the book such a comprehensive review of nutritional sciences methods.

NRM 1e is intended for those with an interest in nutritional science whether they are nutritionists, food scientists, dietitians, medics, nursing staff or other allied health professionals. We hope that both undergraduate and postgraduate students will find the book of great help with their respective studies.

NRM 1e is comprised of a total 20 chapters; commencing with the purpose and implications of research in nutrition in general and aspects concerning study design (Chapters 1–3). Assessment of dietary intake, food composition and biomarkers of intake are covered in Chapters 4–6, and this is followed by an in-depth review of more applied aspects of methodology spanning Chapters 7–17. Particular highlights include chapters on Data Analysis, Biobanks, Epigenetics, Nutrient-Gene Interactions, Food-Related Behaviour and Stable Isotopes (Chapters 7–17). The book closes with chapters covering Animal and Cellular Models in Nutrition research (Chapters 18–19) and the Translation of Nutrition Research (Chapter 20). It is particularly special for us that the first chapter of NRM 1e is written Professor Alan Jackson CBE, Director of the only NIHR Biomedical Research Centre in Nutrition (University of Southampton) and first Chair of the UK's Scientific Advisory Committee on Nutrition (SACN; 2000 to 2010).

We are extremely honoured that the Foreword for NRM 1e has been written by Professor Lord John Krebs, Principal, Jesus College, University of Oxford and our first Chairman of the UK Food Standards Agency. It gives us great confidence in this Textbook to have such a seal of approval from Lord Krebs and our sincerest of thanks indeed for his support of NRM 1e.

The first and second textbooks in the Series: *Introduction to Human Nutrition* (IHN) and *Nutrition & Metabolism* (N&M) are now out in 2nd Edition and sales continue to go extremely well, with third Editions under-preparation. We are currently working on the 2nd Edition of the third textbook in the Series, *Public Health Nutrition* (PHN) led by Professor Judy Buttriss (British Nutrition Foundation) and which will be published in 2016. This will be a very special 75th Anniversary year in the Society's history. Sales of Professor Marinos Elia *et al*'s *Clinical Nutrition* 2nd Edition (CN 2e - fourth textbook) continue to sell apace and our fifth textbook in the Series, *Sport and Exercise Nutrition* 1st Edition (SEN 1e) have surpassed all expectations. We are most grateful to Professor Richard Budgett OBE, Chief Medical Officer for the London 2012 Olympic and Paralympic Games and now CMO at the International Olympic Committee (IOC) based in Lausanne, Switzerland and Dame Sally Davies , Chief Medical Officer (CMO) for England, and the UK Government's Principal Medical Adviser for their respective enthusiasm, support and most generous Forewords in SEN 1e and CN 2e respectively.

The Society is most grateful to the textbook publishers, Wiley-Blackwell for their continued help with the production of the textbook and in particular, Hayley Wood, Madeleine Hurd, and James Schultz. We would also like to thank Sandeep Kumar from SPi Publisher Services for his great help with NRM 1e finalisation and Fariba Kolahdooz (Unversity of Alberta) for her tremendous work on the preparation of the NRM 1e's Glossary. In addition, many grateful thanks to Professor Lisa Roberts, Dean of the Faculty of Health and Medical Sciences and Professor David Blackbourn FSB, Head of the School of Bioscience and Medicine, University of Surrey for their respective great encouragement of the Textbook Series production.

Sincerest of thanks indeed to the Nutrition Society past-President, Professor Sean J.J. Strain (University of Ulster) and current-President, Professor Catherine Geissler (King's College London) for their belief in the Textbook Series and to past-Honorary Publications Officer, Professor David Bender (University College London), and present-Honorary Publications Officer Professor Paul Trayhurn (University of Liverpool) for being such a tremendous sounding boards for the Textbook Series. I am hugely grateful for their wise counsel. Thanks indeed also to Sharon Hui (past-Assistant Editor, NS Textbook Series) for her important contribution to the development of the Series.

Finally, the Series is indebted to the forward thinking focus that Professor Michael Gibney (University College Dublin) had at that time of the Textbook Series development. It remains a great privilege for me to follow in his footsteps as the second E-i-C.

It is my absolute wish that you will find the textbook a great resource of information ....enjoy!

With my warmest of wishes

Professor Susan A Lanham-New FAfNFSB
E-i-C, Nutrition Society Textbook Series and Head,
Department of Nutritional Sciences
School of Biosciences and Medicine,
Faculty of Health and Medical Sciences
University of Surrey

About the Companion Website

This book is accompanied by a companion website:

www.wiley.com/go/lovegrove/nutritionresearch

The website includes:

- Powerpoints of all figures from the book for downloading
- Multiple choice questions
- Short answer questions
- Essay titles

1

Nature, Purpose and Implications of Research in Nutrition

Alan A Jackson, Stephen A Wootton and Martin Wiseman

NIHR Southampton Biomedical Research Centre, University of Southampton

---

A fundamental feature of life: The needs for survival

The subject of nutrition concerns the nature of foods and food nutrients and the needs of humans and animals for these substances.

Metabolism is the name given to the sum of the chemical and physical processes continuously going on in the living organism.

(Lloyd, McDonald and Crampton 1959)

1.1 Introduction: The defining characteristic

The enabling science for nutritional investigation embraces many disciplines, including mathematics, physics, chemistry, biochemistry, physiology, physical and mental development, disease prevention, clinical care, food production, food processing, food marketing, consumer behaviour and choice, social relations, micro- and macroeconomics, policy and planning. This invites the important question of whether nutrition is a discrete discipline in its own right. If these threads are to be brought together to make a whole, then it is important to be clear about the particular or defining characteristic of that whole that represents nutrition research. This requires an agreed conceptual framework based on fundamental principles. These principles underlie every aspect of nutrition and should be explicitly acknowledged and taken into account at all times.

By the end of this chapter you should be able to recognise that:

- Nutrition is a demand-led process, the study of which draws on many disciplines to understand how energy

and nutrients are made available to the cells of the body to enable function.

- By its nature nutrition is integrative and complex, because it relates to how cells, tissues and the body are organised, as well as how people organise themselves in society, to ensure ongoing availability of a sufficient and appropriate mix of energy and nutrients.
- This complexity comes about because of the nature of two major systems and their interaction: the (internal) metabolic system of the body, and the (external) system through which food is acquired from the environment.
- Each system in its own right is inherently complex and their interaction adds an additional level of complexity, thus each system requires explicit investigation of how the component parts act in concert to satisfy the demand.
- Diet plays a pivotal role in these processes, but is only part of the story. The dietary intake is the ultimate source of energy and nutrients for the body, but in addition cells and tissues satisfy their needs for nutrients through integrated processes involving endogenous formation of nutrients, mobilisation of nutrients from structural and functional pools and the availability of nutrients as products of the gut microbiome.
- Research in nutrition requires a focus on a particular aspect of these complex interactions, but that focus needs to be interpreted as an integral part of the wider whole.

Therefore, research in nutrition can be seen at one level as quite simple, but at another as increasingly complex. The diet contains many components, some of which are necessary for metabolism (nutrients), others which have biological activity but are not metabolically essential or

---

may be toxic, and still others which cannot be utilised. Consumption of too little, or of too much, of the nutrients themselves can have adverse effects in terms of deficiency or toxicity, respectively. Thus, there is a preferred range of consumption for each nutrient. Extreme changes in any one aspect of nutritional exposure can induce dramatic and readily measurable change. More modest variability within the usual or preferred range of consumption also has effects, but these may be more subtle and less immediately obvious, as the integrated system operates to maintain an assured and balanced supply of nutrients to the cells of the body.

This chapter outlines some of the fundamental principles of nutrition, how they contribute to building and maintaining the complex systems that represent the function of the body, and how the systems through which food is extracted from the environment can and do exert influence on this. The principles outlined here act as a foundation on which it is possible to consider different aspects of nutrition research methodology. At the same time, we highlight specific limitations of our conceptual understanding that need to be addressed.

1.2 Simplicity to complexity

The nature of nutritional science

We live, survive and thrive in a world of almost infinite variety and complexity. Like other living organisms, we are able to do this by maintaining a constant internal environment. Maintaining this constancy requires the behaviour of all cells, tissues and organs, which maintain structure and function and protect against challenge from the external environment, to be integrated and regulated. The integrity of the body depends on the complex interaction of physical and chemical processes that together characterise metabolism. This is supported by energy derived from the oxidation of macronutrients contained in food. These chemical reactions take place within an aqueous environment, so water is the major constituent of individual cells and the body as a whole. Hence, a fundamental feature of life is that we have to draw continually from the environment around us the oxygen, water and food that we require to stay alive. These are dynamic processes operating within a dynamic system and they are fundamental to the maintenance of health at all ages.

From the time of conception, normal growth and development through childhood to adulthood create a demand for energy and nutrients and depend on their availability, as well as on the body's ability to perform the processes of normal metabolism that allow it to utilise them. Healthy infancy, childhood, adolescence and pregnancy are characterised by a positive energy and nutrient balance, with ordered net tissue deposition leading to increased capability in both structure and function. Health in adulthood is generally represented by an energy and nutrient balance, with constant height and weight and similar body composition over extended periods of time, consistent with physical, mental, intellectual and social function.

By its nature, nutrition is an integrative discipline. A core feature of nutritional science is the exploration of how chemicals, most of which comprise the substance of other living organisms, are drawn from the environment to provide the energy, substrates and co-factors needed to support and enable life. Nutrition occupies the space between the food we eat and the health we enjoy. Its core is the endogenous environment, including the colonic microbiome, where a varied and inconstant intake is transformed into a constant and appropriate supply for normal function. Nutrition is by nature multifaceted, embracing a wide spectrum of biological and other human experience.

Any individual's needs vary with age, gender, physiological state, lifestyle and behaviour, as well as in comparison to other individuals. At the same time, the foods we consume are also very varied. This contrasts with the relative constancy of the internal environment within and among individuals. Such constancy is enabled through regulatory processes and assured through adaptive mechanisms. There is a need to organise our understanding, and our approach to scientific investigation, more effectively to determine more clearly the nature of our nutritional demands and how they might be adequately met across all contexts.

Maintaining integrity – the science of nutrition

The cell is the basic unit of all life. The maintenance of cellular integrity ensures integrated organ and tissue function, keeping intact the body's defences with appropriate inflammatory and immune responses. An intrinsic feature of health is the ability to cope with a changing environment associated with the usual challenges of everyday life, and unusual stresses from time to time, as well as the ability to recover. The stresses may be biological, such as infections with bacteria or viruses, or physical trauma; behavioural or psychological, as with smoking, alcohol, inactivity or poor mental health; or social, as associated with poverty, deprivation or lack of personal control. The ability to maintain the internal environment is called homeostasis; the ability to cope with external stresses, allostasis. The summary of all the internal and external stresses that tax the ability of the organism to maintain constancy represents the allostatic load. The ability of the organism to adapt – to accommodate changes in the internal and external environment – is fundamental to survival and is central to the achievement of homeostasis and allostasis. For this to be achieved in the face of the uncertain nature, extent, severity and duration of changes in the internal or external environment requires a reserve capability that can be drawn on as required, and that is known as resilience. Thus, the nutritional integrity of the organism requires the ability to maintain the usual function, but is intimately linked to the adaptive responses. An insufficient intake of food or a poor-quality diet constrain the adaptive responses, leading to loss of resilience and vulnerability to both internal and external perturbations and hence susceptibility to ill-health.

The balance and amount of energy and nutrients needed depend on this range of experiences with which the healthy body copes as a matter of course. The underlying objective of nutrition research is to understand the needs of individuals, groups and populations for energy and nutrients, and how these might best be met from dietary intake and through other processes.

Structured organisation

How can we manage this complexity, which extends from the molecular, through the cellular, to tissues and whole organisms interacting to maintain the body's function in different environmental contexts? One helpful way of conceptualising the complexity is to consider it as the interaction of two systems, with the whole body as the point of interaction. One system is within the body: its regulated biochemical, physiological and metabolic processes, which maintain the integrity of the system as a whole. However, the body itself is part of a wider social system with even higher levels of organisation within family and community, which incorporate complex social systems and interactions operating at national and global levels. Nutritional science in its broadest sense embraces the way in which each of the systems is organised and functions, but also the way in which they interact. Nutritional science seeks to understand how to ensure the ongoing availability of an adequate diet, in terms of quantity and quality of the pattern of foods consumed, to meet the needs of every individual in the population.

As with all systems, these relationships are dynamic and have multiple regulatory feedback loops. Think of riding a bicycle. It is easy to maintain control so long as the bicycle is in a dynamic state, moving forwards, but it becomes particularly challenging if the bicycle is stationary. The challenges for research in nutrition are to understand how

the many relationships are held in dynamic tension, within and between levels of organisation; to be able to comprehend, measure and manage these relationships; and to be aware of the preferred point of equipoise to achieve a dynamic equilibrium for the component parts and the system(s) as a whole.

Simplified models have been developed to describe, measure and help understand this process. One of the best known is the UNICEF framework, which characterises the different levels of organisation that have to be considered in relation to the factors leading to ill-health and their interplay: proximal, intermediate and distal. This type of model is of value in helping to conceptualise the relationships. The bigger challenge is to quantify the dynamics within and across different levels of organisation. Central to this task is the ability to make valid measurements of the critical factors, and their interactions, and in particular the demand for energy and nutrients in relation to what is available, the supply.

1.3 Structure and function: Appreciating complexity

The individual as an organised system

Understanding the synthetic or integrative nature of nutrition presupposes knowledge and understanding of the component parts. While life starts with a single fertilised egg, ultimately each individual exists as an organised dynamic system, as a body that has boundaries in relation to the outside world. The dynamism within the system creates demands for energy and nutrients on an ongoing basis, which have to be satisfied and are 'topped up' intermittently, most obviously from the dietary intake. Foods represent the vehicle through which energy and nutrients are drawn from the environment. The heart of nutritional science is determining the energy and nutrients that are required to maintain the integrity of the organism, which are formally articulated as the Dietary Reference Values (DRVs), Recommended Daily Allowances (RDAs) or Population Reference Intakes (PRIs).

A major challenge within nutritional science is the inherent variability of many of the factors involved. Ultimately, molecular interactions enable cellular structure, function, replication, terminal differentiation and apoptosis. There are higher levels of complexity for organs and tissues and their interactions. From conception, through fetal life, infancy and childhood to adulthood, growth is based on the acquisition of energy and nutrients as tissues (structure), accompanied by the refinement of function with maturation. Increases in organ size lead to greater functional competence. Enhanced intellectual capability enables progressively increasing efficiency in the processes through which food is made available, thereby creating the space and time for individuals and groups to engage in wider creativity, exploration and discovery.

The demand

The dynamic state at every level of organisation is a reflection of continuing turnover and exchange. The cellular and physiological environment is maintained within relatively narrow limits by integrated metabolic regulation. Any individual's dietary intake is inherently variable from day to day, as is their physical activity. DRVs are captured as references: amounts that need to be taken in the diet to maintain health in otherwise healthy people. Their determination recognises the obvious physiological variability associated with age, sex, growth, maturation, pregnancy, lactation and different levels of physical activity. While it allows for environmental protection, it does not consider the effects imposed by infection, trauma or other exceptional stresses, the demands of recovering from such a challenge, or the need to repair the system subsequently. Nor can the values for individual nutrients take account of potentially simultaneous variations in other essential nutrients. Ongoing cellular replication is a critical feature of the usual environmental protection, for the maintenance of external boundaries (skin) and internal mucosal boundaries (gut, respiratory tract, bladder), as well as immune surveillance and continuing protection. All of these create demands.

In terms of energy, the body's ongoing demand under standardised resting conditions represents the basal metabolic rate. The demand comprises three major functions: membrane transport (especially brain and nervous tissue), macromolecular turnover (especially liver and muscle) and internal mechanical work (cardiac, respiratory, gastrointestinal and so on). These are continuous processes and the energetic need is met through the oxidation of macromolecules (protein, lipid and carbohydrate) drawn from the availability within the body itself. This resource is intermittently replenished through dietary intake, which for active individuals is exquisitely well regulated so that energy expenditure is matched by energy intake. The availability of macromolecules for oxidation is a regulated process ensuring that the pattern of macronutrients oxidised exactly matches that taken in the diet, which achieves balance and constancy of weight and body composition.

Meeting the demand (supply)

Food (in)security is the term that has been adopted to characterise a country's food supply status. Its use has evolved and it is now applied to the situation of individual countries, communities or even households; conceptually it can also be applied to individuals. A related but separate term is nutrition security, which similarly has been applied at different levels of organisation. The purpose of both is to capture as a simple, single statement the extent to which food and/or nutritional needs are adequately provided for in terms of dietary supply. Availability is considered, but this in itself is not enough, because the food also has to be acceptable and accessible for consumption. Although the degree of food security is important for different groupings, it is ultimately a summary of the adequacy of provision, availability and consumption at the level of the individual.

Food security consists of two elements, one quantitative and the other qualitative. The quantitative element is a statement of the extent to which food supply adequately meets nutritional needs. The qualitative element embraces the extent to which the pattern of nutrients available from the diet meets an individual's pattern of demands.

For all practical purposes, the quantitative aspect of the diet is determined by the amount of food that has to be consumed to satisfy an individual's energy needs. The maintenance energy needs are determined by that individual's basal energy needs (the basal metabolic rate or BMR) and the level of physical activity. The energy expenditure from most forms of physical activity is proportionate to the BMR, which varies with height, weight, sex, age, maturity and physiological state (pregnancy and lactation). The energy needs are met from the oxidation of amino acids, lipids and carbohydrates, in the same proportions as they are present in the diet. The quality of the diet is determined by the mix of foods and their nutrient composition; that is, the proportions of amino acids, lipids, carbohydrates, minerals, vitamins, trace elements and water.

In general terms, those who are less physically active expend less energy and need less food to meet their requirements. However, if less food is consumed, then the intake of all nutrients is likely to be less. Therefore, if a diet is marginal in any nutrient, that potential limitation is likely to become obvious sooner or more readily in those who are less active (unless they are eating more food than they need). This is one problem for subsistence societies where the quality of the diet might be poor. At the higher levels of physical activity associated with rural life, food consumption is likely to be higher to meet the higher energy requirements, so whatever diet is usually consumed is more likely to meet the needs for nutrients. With urbanisation, decreased energy expenditure and a reduction in the need for food consumption to meet the requirements for energy, any nutrient limitation in the diet is more likely to become exposed.

Similar considerations are likely to prevail in the sick, where illness is associated with reduced activity and energy expenditure, lower energy requirements and decreased food consumption. Illness or stresses such as infection or inflammation have an important effect on the relationship between energy requirements and food intake. The ability to cope with an allostatic load is associated with a stress response, manifest as increased activity of the hypothalamo-pituitary-adrenal and sympathetic nervous systems, and associated glucocorticoid and catecholamine responses. With more severe degrees of stress, there are increasingly obvious metabolic effects: loss of appetite, altered metabolic demands by the tissues, an acute phase response associated with altered delivery of nutrients to tissues, and an unbalanced increase in losses of nutrients from the body (breakdown of tissues and specific nutrient losses in their own right). The magnitude of these responses is related to the magnitude of the allostatic load, and the ability to cope through adaptive responses. One important consequence is that for those on a diet of marginal quality before the imposition of the stress, the ability of the same diet to match the pattern of nutrient needs during and beyond the stress is likely to be impaired. Full and adequate recovery will require a better-quality diet. The period of convalescence may also need to be extended to allow for full recovery from illness or stress.

What this discussion makes clear is that assessment of the adequacy of diet in terms of quality and quantity has to be contextualised to the living conditions and lifestyles of individuals and groups. Although general statements can be made about these needs, the idea that a single 'prescription' will be fit for purpose under all circumstances is unlikely to hold. One objective of nutrition research is to gain a better understanding of the nature of the supply that best fits the demands under any particular circumstance, and to characterise diets that adequately meet that purpose. The objective of the profession of nutrition is to understand how to apply that generic and specific knowledge from one context or individual to another.

Failing to meet the demand

The demands for nutrients and energy are very variable, and the diets that can meet those demands also vary widely. When the demands are adequately satisfied by diet, the result is health. If the supply fails to meet the demands over an extended period, then ultimately ill-health will be the consequence. The period of time over which this becomes obvious may be very variable, depending on the particular circumstances, from minutes and hours to months or years. In practice, the imbalance between demand and supply will in due course lead to an alteration in the partitioning of nutrients to different tissues and/or functions. This is most simply identified as changes or progressive alterations in the structure of the body. Body shape, size and composition are the simplest summary articulation of the adequacy of the diet to meet the body's needs over extended periods. Thus, the simplest routine measures of the shape and size of the body, height and weight, are summary statements of the historical adequacy of the diet to meet an individual's needs. The relationship between height and weight, relative to reference norms, is the basis for all anthropometric markers of nutritional status that are used in individuals and in populations to mark well-being, risk and outcome. Measures of body habitus in structural terms are also closely related to the functional capabilities of the body. Thus, measures of body shape and size are used to indicate functional state in broad terms, but may be severely limited in this regard at the extremes or important critical times (see later in this chapter).

Ultimately, the foods we consume provide the components from which all of the needs of the body are met. Some of these are derived directly from the chemicals contained in the food, or made available to the body from the food following digestion and absorption. Others are made within the body from the chemicals contained in the food to meet the specific needs of the body. The pathways for the endogenous formation of compounds can be tightly regulated. Other components are made available to the body from the microbiome in the intestinal tract; again, this process may be regulated, controlled or influenced directly by the needs of the body itself. People consume widely different diets, without regard to their composition in terms of energy and nutrients, and the body's regulated metabolic processes modify the pattern ultimately available within the system.

The energy and nutrients required by the body are made available in stages. Following digestion in the gastrointestinal tract, simpler compounds become available for the body to absorb. Protein is needed in the diet, but as a source of amino acids rather than as the native protein. It is only available in a useful form when the individual amino acids contained within the dietary protein have been released by digestion and incorporated into the amino acid pool of the body itself. Similar considerations apply to all macromolecules. One aspect of dietary quality is the extent to which the pattern of simpler molecules generated following digestion matches the body's pattern of need, or the extent to which further metabolic inter-conversion might be required to meet this pattern more effectively. Ultimately, the energy needs of the body are met through the oxidation of macromolecules. As balance is maintained, the energy released is derived from a similar pattern of macromolecules to that taken in the diet. The actual processes associated with the achievement of balance for lipid, protein and carbohydrate are still unclear, but are absolutely dependent on the dynamic processes of turnover that enable regulation.

For individual nutrients, achieving balance, or regulation of the body pool, may be achieved in very different ways. For monovalent cations such as sodium or potassium, absorption is virtually complete, and regulation is predominantly at the level of excretion through the kidney. At the other extreme, for a divalent cation such as iron, regulation of the amount in the body is almost entirely at the level of absorption. Thus, it is not appropriate to expect to increase the body content simply by adding more to the diet, without an appreciation of the factors that regulate absorption and excretion. For other divalent cations such as calcium, the control is more complex, with regulation both at the level of absorption and at that of excretion, as well as elaborate controls on the endogenous interchange between different body compartments and tissues. It is possible to identify general classes of nutrient handling, related to the chemical, physical and biological function of individual nutrients. The important consideration is that regulated absorption and excretion contribute to matching the availability of nutrients to the body's needs.

An intake that is inadequate to meet the needs of the body constrains function, leading to problems associated with deficiency. An intake that is in excess of needs has to be disposed of or excreted in a safe form, and if the capacity to do this is exceeded then the excess that cannot be excreted represents a metabolic stress in its own right. For energy and each nutrient there is a range of intake that meets the needs of the body without the risk of either inadequacy or excess, and this is associated with health and minimal, or no, stress. One important overriding protection is the change in appetite in relation to the adequacy of the diet in meeting the body's needs. One consequence of a deficiency in the diet of a specific nutrient is eventually loss of appetite. Being presented with a poor-quality diet is often associated with loss of appetite, and this combination can lead to metabolic disequilibrium, and ultimately death. This has resulted in the identification of an important fundamental principle in nutrition: limiting nutrients.

Limiting nutrients

The idea of limiting nutrients was first defined in 1840 by J. von Liebig, who stated that the rate of growth of a plant, the size to which it grows and its overall health depend on the amount of the scarcest of its essential nutrients that is available to it. This concept has now been broadened into a general model of limiting factors for all organisms, including the limiting effects of excesses of chemical nutrients and other environmental factors. The identification of limiting nutrients has been the important basis for the determination of nutrient requirements, and for the classification of nutrients in the diet as essential (indispensable) or non-essential (dispensable). Replenishment of the diet with the nutrient that is lacking immediately reverses the constraint, leading to improvement in appetite and return of normal structure, function and behaviour.

The great success of nutrition research over the past 100 years has been to gain a better determination of the body's needs for energy under a range of circumstances, and of the absolute requirements for individual nutrients and their relative proportions. One powerful approach was to determine the effect on the body when a single nutrient was excluded from the diet. It was possible to determine that for many components, their absence from the diet, or their presence in limited, inadequate amounts, led to adverse consequences. The more obvious extreme responses were seen within a very short period of the poor-quality diet being consumed, with loss of appetite, reduction in weight and altered body composition. Examples here would be the dietarily indispensable amino acids. At the other extreme, for some nutrients of which there was a significant store, such as vitamins A or B12, changes might not become manifest for weeks or months. For others, such as iron, copper or magnesium, dietary inadequacy might be ameliorated in the short term by adaptation. Tissue reserves were drawn on, albeit at a functional cost, and the metabolic cost only became obvious over extended periods of time. The ability and ease with which the need for any individual nutrient could be determined vary across this wide spectrum of response, and hence the approach used differed accordingly.

Thus, the lack of availability of energy or any single nutrient can act to limit function, either as a substrate or as a specific co-factor. This can lead to some complex interactions. For example, there is an important and well-established interaction between the energy and protein content of the diet. At marginal levels of protein imbalance, an increase in energy intake will re-establish nitrogen balance; at marginal levels of energy imbalance, an increase in protein intake may re-establish energy balance. This general relationship applies to all nutrients under what is known as Kleiber's law: if the energetic efficiency of a diet is improved by the addition of a single nutrient, that nutrient was limiting in the diet. For diets of poor quality that are deficient in a particular nutrient, growing animals consume a greater amount to maintain an equivalent rate of weight gain. Addition of the deficient nutrient improves the efficiency with which energy is utilised from the diet. These nutrient–energy interactions can also be demonstrated for nutrient–nutrient interactions. This is why a reference such as the DRV is defined as the amount required to maintain health in otherwise healthy individuals, *on the assumption that* the requirements for energy and all other nutrients have been met.

If a diet lacking a sufficient amount of an individual nutrient is consumed in excess of the needs for energy, some of the excess may lead to thermogenesis and be lost as heat, but more usually it is deposited as tissue. As a nutrient limitation is likely to constrain lean tissue deposition, the likelihood is that the excess energy will be retained as adipose tissue.

Endogenous formation: Proteins and amino acids, building blocks and regulators

Dietarily indispensable components may be organic or inorganic. Inorganic ions or molecules, such as potassium, sodium, chloride, iron and zinc, have to be provided pre-formed in the diet, although they may be an intrinsic part of an organic molecule. The indispensable nutrients derived from organic molecules might be expected historically to have been found in normal diets in amounts adequate to meet metabolic needs, as throughout evolution there can have been no selective advantage in maintaining the pathways for their formation, and loss of these pathways did not incur any survival cost.

Dietarily non-essential, dispensable components may not need to be provided pre-formed in the diet, but they are nevertheless an absolute requirement for normal metabolism. It may be that they can be omitted from the usual diet without incurring any obvious cost in the short or longer term, and examples of this would be non-essential amino acids (dispensable amino acids) or longer-chain polyunsaturated fatty acids. The ability to omit them from the diet without any consequence requires that their precursors are available in sufficient amounts, either from the diet or from metabolic exchange. However, such precursors may be required by the body in amounts much greater than can usually be provided in the diet. In addition, they are often the building blocks for special compounds required in large amounts or they perform important regulatory roles in the body, for example fatty acids to form stable and healthy cell membranes, or the amino acid precursors for DNA and RNA synthesis. Although the capability to make these molecules may exist, the capacity to do so is potentially limited, therefore if the demand is particularly high, it may not be possible to make a sufficient quantity. Under these circumstances these nutrients become 'conditionally essential' in the diet.

The metabolic pathways through which dispensable nutrients are formed within the body are often protected, in order to ensure the capability to support vital processes and to protect cellular integrity. For this reason, it may not be easy to expose a dietary limitation. The extent of this buffering capability in terms of availability is one important aspect of resilience. The buffering may be achieved by trading one important process for another, for instance stunting in the face of inflammation or infection. The pathways that enable the endogenous formation of these nutrients are usually critically dependent on the availability of many other micronutrients, and hence their metabolic availability may be especially vulnerable in poor-quality diets. Limitations in the formation or availability of these nutrients might only be exposed by a stress test.

Thus, dietarily indispensable nutrients have to be provided pre-formed in the diet; dietarily dispensable nutrients do not have to be provided pre-formed in the diet, but the pathways for their endogenous formation must be intact and have the capacity to meet the need. For conditionally indispensable nutrients, the demands can under some circumstances exceed the capacity for endogenous formation. There has been an assumption that the ability to meet the nutrient needs of the body is determined only by the dietary intake and the capacity for endogenous metabolic formation. It is increasingly clear, however, that a significant contribution to meeting the nutrient needs of any individual might be derived from the metabolic activity of the microbiome.

Microbiome

Many species of bacteria have evolved and adapted to live and grow in the human intestine. The microbiome of the gut contains 300–500 different species of bacteria, and the number of microbial cells within the gut lumen is about 10 times greater than the number of eukaryotic cells in the human body. In humans, most bacteria exist in the colon and terminal ileum, but in other animals, such as ruminants or rodents (and other animals that practise refection), there are substantial populations in other parts of the gut. The microbiome and the organisms that comprise it represent an ecosystem in its own right, with complex metabolic interactions within the ecosystem and with the host itself.

It is increasingly clear that cross-talk between the organisms, both metabolically and genetically, plays an important role in maintaining the viability and resilience of both the microbiome and the host. There is energy and nutrient exchange within the ecosystem and hence the ability to make nutrients that can be made available to the host. The presence of this exchange is clearly demonstrated by the dependence of ruminants on a viable and supportive rumen activity. The extent to which this happens in humans is less clear, either for macronutrients or for micronutrients. However, it is clear that it does occur for water and minerals such as potassium, sodium, calcium and magnesium, chloride, vitamins such as vitamin K, and to some extent B vitamins and nitrogen balance. There are other complex interactions, such as the microbial fermentation of non-absorbed carbohydrate ('dietary fibre') to short-chain fatty acids, with direct effects on gut function and more widely on metabolism.

What is undoubted is that the activity of the microbiome is responsive to the nutritional state of the host and can make available nutrients that otherwise would be limiting if dependence for all nutrients was on simple dietary provision, or the host metabolism alone. Thus, it is not clear to what extent variability in an individual's ability to meet a suitable pattern for their own metabolic needs is enabled through a responsive metabolism of the resident microbiome. Indirect evidence suggests that this contribution can be substantial under certain circumstances, and is critical for nitrogen balance.

1.4 The integrated system

Normal growth and development

Growth is an ordered and structured process characterised by increasing tissue mass, complexity, organisation and maturation. Growth is often captured simply as changes in height, weight, relative body proportions and body composition. More refined changes associated with maturation may be captured as bone age or the timing of critical events such as puberty. Nevertheless, even the most sophisticated of these articulations are pale reflections of the complex, regulated processes taking place. The nature and timing of these processes are determined by genetic endowment, and by modified genetic expression related to epigenetic change. They are also regulated by a sophisticated interplay of the hormonal environment. However, ultimately all of them depend on the availability of sufficient energy and an appropriate pattern of nutrients at the appropriate time to enable net tissue deposition of a suitable composition.

The WHO (World Health Organization) growth standards have been developed out of the experience of the growth of normal children from around the world. They show that children grow similarly across all societies given an equal chance of a healthy and a nutritious environment before pregnancy, in the peri-conceptual period and during pregnancy, infancy and childhood. Any constraint on growth reflects adverse environmental conditions. There is a measure of innate variability,

but this is small compared with the marked differences associated with environments of different quality. Failure of growth, marked either as wasting or stunting, is associated with functional consequences for every tissue and organ. The growth constraint results in a limitation in acquired functional capacity. It may be sufficiently small to require a stress test to demonstrate its extent, but more significant insults express themselves as readily demonstrable limitations of function, for any system of the body. At early ages these constraints are potentially reversible, but this plasticity is lost progressively with age. In practice, the loss of capacity represents a reduction in the extent of reserves and a decrease in resilience. The decrease in resilience represents greater vulnerability, or loss of allostatic capability, and hence greater susceptibility to all environmental challenges. For any individual with reduced resilience, ill-health is more likely to express itself at an earlier stage or more aggressively for the same environmental challenge. Growth takes place in a craniocaudal direction and, when subject to constraint, the brain tends to be protected at the expense of other organs. Hence, the capacity of the other tissues to support and protect brain function will be determined by the extent to which their own nutritional environment during earlier life has been enabled or constrained.

Adaptation

The ability to maintain function in the face of widely different dietary or other environmental exposures is brought about through a series of processes characterised as adaptation. This is how the body achieves a functionality that is fit for purpose in the particular context. One important characteristic of adaptation is that the processes that change in response to the altered context are reversible. The system reverts to its former state given a return to the previous environment, such as the development of polycythaemia at altitude. These adaptive processes enable and protect vital functions. The ability to respond appropriately is the hallmark of resilience, but it carries a cost, in terms of both energy and nutrients. If the supply of energy and nutrients is not matched to the demand over a period of time, the most obvious consequence is a change in body weight.

Weight loss is a consequence of the body having to meet its energy needs from the oxidation of macronutrients derived from tissues without adequate dietary replenishment. To an extent all tissues lose some mass, but the brunt is borne by muscle and fat. Less obvious is the accompanying compromise in function, with the reserve capacity that represents resilience being sacrificed at an early stage. This loss of capacity applies to all functions to a greater or lesser extent and leads both to increased vulnerability to external challenge and to impaired capability to achieve and maintain homeostasis. This process is known as *reductive adaptation* and is the basis for a greatly increased risk of morbidity and mortality in under-nourished individuals and populations.

At the other extreme, the consistent consumption of a diet that provides energy in excess of needs leads to an increase in weight and body mass. This is most obviously seen as increased adiposity, but there is also an increase in the mechanical and metabolic machinery required to support the increased mass, which can be characterised as *expansive adaptation*.

When the dietary intake of energy and nutrients exceeds requirements, the body responds to reduce the metabolic and physiological burden and avoid toxicity. In the short term, balance may be achieved by lowering intake, reducing absorption or increasing excretion in the urine. The extent to which balance is achieved depends on the magnitude and nature of the excess, but is usually associated with increased metabolic work or a re-prioritisation of metabolism, representing both a challenge and a cost to the system. For example, balance in the face of an excess amino acid intake is achieved through transamination, deamination with increased urea formation and excretion. In the same way, for those inorganic elements where the availability is regulated at the level of absorption – such as calcium and iron – increased faecal excretion will be associated with changes in the local environment within the bowel that may alter the colonic microbiome, change the biophysical properties of the bowel content (e.g. soap formation with calcium salts) or directly increase the potential oxidant load on cells of the gut (e.g. iron).

The capacity to accommodate excess macronutrient intake is limited. In the immediate postprandial period when the rate at which exogenous nutrients appear in the circulation exceeds their clearance and assimilation, normal physiological regulation and control are compromised, with consequent changes in nutrient partitioning, blood pressure and haemostatic responses. This poor metabolic control, or lack of ability to cope with excess, marks an increased vulnerability to disease. Over longer periods, with continued excess, as the capacity of the adaptive responses is exceeded there is increasing dysregulation, loss of resilience and increased vulnerability. This state is marked by increasing weight and fatness, increasing deposition of fat centrally and ectopically within muscles and viscera, elevated concentrations of circulating nutrients and hormones, in both the fasted and postprandial states, chronic inflammation and impaired haemostatic and vascular function, and abnormalities in lipid, amino acid and glucose metabolism. Together, these processes mark expansive adaptation that enables survival, but at the cost of reduced resilience.

Diagnostic criteria based on these features (increased waist circumference and poor metabolic control) have been used clinically to identify and treat those with increasing risk of cardiometabolic disease (e.g. 'metabolic syndrome').

The challenge is to gain a better understanding of the underlying pathophysiology and the innate and modifiable factors that contribute to variability in the capacity to accommodate excess. Accumulation of fat within the abdomen as visceral adipose tissue is sometimes, but not always, associated with inflammation. Some individuals may be overweight but have good metabolic control and a lower risk of morbidity and mortality. This may be attributed to better integration and control of the metabolism through a limited number of processes that are very sensitive to the availability of specific micronutrients, especially vitamins, which act as co-factors in the regulation of endocrine control, inflammation and immune competence. Poor micronutrient status in the face of excess macronutrient intake acts as an additional stressor and may explain some of the variability in metabolic dysregulation and associated morbidity in the overweight and obese. Importantly, the ability to maintain metabolic control is linked directly to physical activity and metabolic processes within skeletal muscle. Improved control may be enabled through the disposal of energy via contraction; through the endogenous provision of substrates for metabolism synthesised within and exported from muscle; and through the release of regulatory peptides or myokines that act systemically to influence metabolism in other tissues. The capacity of muscle to contribute to whole-body metabolism may be determined by the mass of skeletal muscle (e.g. organ size), the level of metabolic activity within muscle associated with being physically active, or both. There is a need for a more complete appreciation of the nutritional factors that determine the integration and control of metabolism, and their variation from person to person.

The individual: A component of society as an organised system

The challenge for all societies is to enable and ensure a consistent supply of food to meet the needs of all individuals. This depends on a series of complex interactions, which can be characterised as a food-acquisition system. There is seasonal variation in the quantity, quality and diversity of food available, though in modern societies this is buffered by national, international and global activities of food production and movement. For traditional societies the wider environment and climate play a more dominant role and the degree of resilience is likely to be reduced. The interplay of these factors has a significant role in the development of social and cultural behaviours, the relationship with religious practice and many aspects of how societies are organised. A period of poor nutrition can have an immediate effect on the risk of ill-health or death, and families use a range of mechanisms to protect themselves. However, the cost of employing protective behaviours might have an impact on the entire family for long periods of time, and may even have inter-generational consequences.

By definition, successful societies have managed to secure regular access to food of adequate quality and quantity. The cuisine and traditional food practices have evolved based on accumulated experience and wisdom, determined ultimately by survival and being fit for purpose. These experiences are deeply ingrained in all cultures as patterns of food preparation and consumption. With the monetisation of food and its use as a commodity, these relationships change, so that the processes of food production have become divorced from the practices of food preparation and consumption. Progress in food production, processing techniques and technologies has enabled great efficiencies of land use, preservation, storage and transport over large distances. One consequence of this has been a substantial reduction in the diversity of the diet, however. Reduced diversity leads to a significant risk of a reduced quality of diet because of a greater difficulty in ensuring a match for the varied needs within the population.

Our perceptions of diet quality are directly related to our understanding of nutrient requirements, which are themselves imperfect. The simple observation that obesity is now an increasingly common problem, which appears to evade all attempts at prevention and effective treatment, makes it clear that we do not have adequate control of these relationships. In practice, the most direct way of determining how well the provision from the diet matches needs is to explore the relationship between diet and either markers of risk for ill-health, the development of disease itself or death. This is classic nutritional epidemiology.

The most useful summary statement of an individual's historical and current nutritional status is offered by height, and weight in relation to height, captured as weight for length or height in childhood, or Body Mass Index (BMI) in adulthood. Both a lower and a higher BMI are associated with increased mortality, leading to a U- or J-shaped relationship between BMI and mortality. Increased mortality for people who are relatively lighter is associated with death from chronic lung disease, and for those who are relatively heavier with death from cardiovascular disease, type 2 diabetes and some cancers. A preferred range exists within which risk of ill-health and death is the least. There is a similar U-shaped relationship for the relationship between height and mortality.

Shortness is associated with death from cardiovascular disease, and tallness with death from some cancers. These are population statements of risk, but clearly lightness, heaviness, shortness and tallness have important nutritional correlates over the life course.

More complex relationships can be drawn in terms of body composition, body proportions, growth patterns and the timing of maturation, but the underlying importance lies in the fact that cumulative nutritional experience throughout life leads to differences in nutritional partitioning to organs and tissues. These underlying biological processes are linked to susceptibility to ill-health and mortality, although the mechanisms through which these linkages operate are not yet clear. Importantly, what is not known is the extent to which the associations are causally related, either directly or indirectly, or how far they are simply indicative of common underlying factors. Bringing clarity to these relationships through a more insightful understanding of the underlying mechanisms is one very important challenge for nutritional research. This requires an understanding of the nature of the interactions and complexities of each system in its own right at the different levels of organisation, as well as the ability to integrate this knowledge effectively across those different levels.

1.5 Developing nutritional research

Nutritional research embraces factors operating at all levels of organisation, but it also requires the ability to synthesise understanding between the different levels of organisation and across disciplinary boundaries. To achieve this, clarity and consistent use of language are required to enable communication, together with standardised and quality-assured approaches to measurement to facilitate synthesis and interpretation. In this sense, as an integrative science, nutrition represents the meeting place for many different interests and disciplines. Although there has been progress in enabling this exchange, modern technologies offer very significant new opportunities. It is therefore imperative to ensure that commonality of purpose and understanding among the different disciplines are achieved rapidly. For this to happen, nutrition research needs to build on its components to achieve a better understanding of the systems themselves, and of the interactions of both their individual parts and the systems with each other.

These investigative activities can and do take place at different levels of complexity, but accessing any one level, or the interaction between the levels, is challenging. It has not yet been offered in any standard way or with consistency. This has led to problems in carrying out nutritional research that is of high quality and of value in a coordinated way across a range of sectors and activities. The development of 'toolboxes' that are fit for specific purposes should enable and facilitate better and more effective investigation.

Toolboxes

Nutritional science has two defining characteristics: the ability to determine the requirements for energy and nutrients (the nutritional demand); and the ability to determine the extent to which the demand has been met (the nutritional state or status). The assessment of nutritional state, at the level of the cell, the organ, the whole body or the population in humans, animals or plants, is an area of research specific to nutrition and there are specific 'tools' that are used to make an assessment. Most simply, the assessment can be captured in three dimensions: what you eat (a statement about food, diet and feeding behaviour), what you are (capturing the size, shape and composition of the body) and what you can do (the functional competence expressed in terms of biochemical and physiological measures of micronutrient status, performance and functional capacity, and level of physical activity). Each dimension is important, but each in isolation is insufficient to describe nutritional status completely. Therefore, any 'toolbox' needs to include a measure of all three dimensions. There are many different measurement instruments available and the choice among them depends on the specific nature of the question to be addressed and the time, funds and expertise required to quality assure their use.

The level of complexity and sophistication of the toolbox need to be appropriate and proportionate to the question being addressed. For an entry-level toolbox, the tools should be immediately accessible, require the least physical resource and be least likely to impose on volunteers and staff engaged in the study. The information gained will be limited in both amount and utility, but should be sufficient to offer a broad categorisation of nutritional state and to determine whether there has been a change in that state. Detailed information will not be provided on all aspects of dietary exposure, body composition or micronutrient status. At this level, intake may be assessed using short questionnaires on reported appetite or the extent to which eating behaviour is consistent with current dietary guidance (e.g. healthy eating score or index) or dietetic plan. This will indicate the need for further assessment or intervention. Body size and shape may be assessed by simple anthropometry (stature, weight and girth – both current and change), while functional capacity can be assessed using short questionnaires that capture reported activity behaviour (levels of activity or sedentary behaviour) or well-being.

More detailed assessment would require more advanced tools such as a food frequency questionnaire or a multiple pass 24-hour recall questionnaire to describe either the dietary pattern or quantitative measures of reported energy and nutrient intake; bioelectrical impedance analysis or skinfold thickness measurement for assessment of body composition; and measures of muscle function, exercise capacity or conventional biochemistry to assess micronutrient status as a marker of functional state. Greater depth of understanding can be acquired with more advanced analytical techniques characterising patterns of consumption, or taking a multi-compartment approach to the determination of body composition. Isotopic probes can also be used to investigate the flux through metabolic pathways and the function of different physiological systems. It is now possible to take a life systems view combining all measures within an 'omics' approach to provide summative statements on the phenome or metabolome.

Increasing sophistication is associated with increasing cost and invasiveness. Irrespective of the level of complexity of the toolbox, confidence in the measures and their interpretation can only be achieved where measurements are taken in accordance with national governance requirements and conducted within a quality assurance framework. For all measures, there is a need to be able to demonstrate the validity and performance characteristics of all equipment. The individuals making the measurements also need to be appropriately trained using standardised operating procedures (SOPs) and to be demonstrably competent in using objective measures of accuracy, validity and standardisation.

Nutritional research of the future will have to embrace all aspects of the reductionist science that has powered and enabled such remarkable progress in the past, but it will also have to develop much more refined capabilities for synthesising the knowledge gained. This will ensure a better understanding of the systems involved, how they might be regulated, and the interventions that are most likely to achieve change that leads to longer life with better health.

1.6 Conclusion

For research in nutrition to be of great benefit, it needs to provide a base of evidence to improve health promotion, disease prevention and clinical care, drawing on understanding from science to improve practice. A central feature of this activity would be the ability to characterise reliably the nutritional phenotype, its determinants and variability, and to intervene to maintain or improve the phenotype at individual, group and population levels. Achieving this requires an understanding of the determinants of at least three major systems and how they articulate to enable better health. These three systems are the social systems that embrace the social determinants of health; the lifestyle systems that contribute and determine individual behaviours and how they relate to health; and the whole-body human biological system, its regulation and integration.

Nutrition research has to draw on the widest range of approaches and methods available to achieve a better understanding of how the body is enabled to meet its requirements for energy and nutrients. The methods are rich and varied and each gives a perspective on particular aspects of a system. These different perspectives then have to be interpreted and understood in the context of the system as a whole. Integrating understanding within and between systems is not always carried out in a consistent way, and data have not always been collected with a view to facilitating this integration. By their very nature, each of the systems is dynamic, with exchange, turnover, regulation and control representing the hallmarks of achieving stability and healthy function. There are fundamental principles underlying these exchanges and interactions, and consistency of language, together with quality assured measurements, should enable greater coherence in integration within and across different levels of organisation. Within each area of investigation there are also aspects that are inherently variable, such as dietary intake and physical activity, therefore their value can only be determined in the context of the extent to which they better enable the body to meet its inherently variable requirements. Ultimately, nutrition revolves around what the body can do for itself to meet its cellular and metabolic needs, and how this can best be supported through the regular consumption of a sufficient diet of appropriate quality.

This chapter has considered how understanding can be organised to enable better scientific investigation and to comprehend more clearly the nature of nutritional demands, how they might be measured and how they might be adequately met across all contexts. One of the most important objectives of nutrition research is to gain greater knowledge of the nature of the supply that best fits the demands under any particular circumstance. In turn, the objective of the profession of nutrition is to understand how to apply that generic and specific knowledge from one context or individual to another.

Reference

Lloyd, L.E., McDonald, B.E. and Crampton E.W. (1959) *Fundamentals of Nutrition*, W.H. Freeman & Co, San Francisco, CA.

2
Study Design: Population-Based Studies

Janet Cade[1] and Jayne Hutchinson[2]

[1]*University of Leeds*
[2]*University of York*

Key messages

- Ecological studies may be the first step in generating hypotheses concerning diet and disease relationships, but they are limited by the 'ecological fallacy'. This occurs when relationships that are observed for groups are assumed to hold for individuals.
- In population studies the researcher has no control over the exposure of interest (the diet).
- Confounding of diet–disease relationships is a possibility in observational studies; relationships seen between diet and disease can change considerably when confounders are included. Confounders are variables that affect both the exposure (diet) and the outcome (disease).
- Cross-sectional studies measure exposure and disease at the same point in time and so cause and effect cannot be determined.
- Case-control studies are subject to recall bias due to problems in reporting past diet.
- Cohort studies are often large, long-term studies in which recall bias is avoided if exposure data is collected before outcome data. However, they are expensive and not particularly useful for rare diseases.

2.1 Introduction

This chapter will discuss population-based, observational studies. The methods used are based on epidemiological approaches; epidemiology is the study of diseases in populations. The key consideration in population-based studies is that the researcher has no control over the exposure of interest (e.g. diet). Study types include ecological, case-control and cohort studies. They are useful for generating hypotheses and exploring associations between diet and health outcomes. These study designs can help to build up evidence to support a suggested effect of a particular dietary factor on a certain disease, but they cannot categorically show cause-and-effect association, which is required for proof of a link between a dietary factor and a disease. Since these methods do not use randomisation to select participants, they are more prone to bias than are randomised controlled trials (RCTs). Bias is a systematic error resulting in an estimated association between exposure and outcome that deviates from the true association in a direction that depends on the nature of the systematic error. Selection bias can result in systematic differences between characteristics of participants in different exposure or outcome groups within a study, which can lead to confounding of the results. Non-response bias at the start of a study and non-random attrition (dropping out of participants) during a study are other forms of selection bias. Recall bias and social desirability reporting bias are forms of measurement bias; the systematic differences in recall and reporting between exposure or outcome groups who have dissimilar characteristics can lead to confounding of the results.

Confounding variables can provide alternative explanations for an apparent association between a dietary exposure and a disease/health outcome in observational studies. Confounders are associated with both the exposure of interest (diet) and the outcome variable (disease), but are not on the causal pathway between exposure and outcome. Confounders can be dealt with in a number of ways depending on the study design: during the design of the study by matching or by restricting study members; or

Nutrition Research Methodologies, First Edition. Edited by Julie A Lovegrove, Leanne Hodson, Sangita Sharma and Susan A Lanham-New.
© 2015 John Wiley & Sons, Ltd. Published 2015 by John Wiley & Sons, Ltd.
Companion Website: www.wiley.com/go/nutritionsociety

through data analysis by stratification (e.g. age stand-ardisation), restriction or adjustment in regression mod-els. Most analyses of disease risk control for age, since disease risk increases with age and age is often associated with dietary intake. Confounders are discussed further in Section 2.6.

This chapter will consider ways to minimise problems. However, its overall aim is to provide an overview of dif-ferent methods used in observational epidemiology.

2.2 Ecological studies

The focus of this type of study is on characterising popu-lation groups rather than on linking individuals' expo-sures to health outcomes. Ecological studies of diet and health explore associations between population or group indicators of diet or nutritional status and population or group indices of health status. Two population-based measures are needed for this type of study, one for the exposure of interest (the diet) and the other for the health outcome (the disease). The individuals in the popula-tions used to describe the dietary exposure may or may not be the same as those providing data for health out-comes. In nutritional epidemiology, ecological studies have predominantly been used to explore geographical or temporal relationships between diet and health: for example, exploring country differences in dietary intakes and health, or comparing changes in diet in populations over time.

There are occasions when ecological studies may be the only feasible research method available to explore the association between diet and disease. This would occur when exposure data are not available at the individual level, such as for fluoride in drinking water.

Methods

In the simplest study, two population-based measures are required, one for the exposure of interest and the other for the health outcome.

Indices of dietary intake
Estimates of population dietary intake can be made from survey data collected for the purpose of the study in a population or from pre-existing dietary data, which will be less costly although it may not sufficiently reflect consumption.

National food supply
An important source of internationally available food data comes from the Food and Agriculture Organization (FAO) food balance sheets, available at http://faostat3.

fao.org/faostat-gateway/go/to/home/E. These provide a comprehensive picture of the pattern of a country's food supply for a particular time point. For each food item, they show the total quantity produced and imported and link this to utilisation, including export, amounts fed to livestock and used for seed, and losses during storage and transport. From this the amount of each food avail-able for human consumption can be estimated. This type of data has been used to assess trends in dietary intakes; however, it may overestimate dietary intakes (Pomerleau, Lock and McKee 2003).

Household budget surveys
These studies collect data on food availability at a house-hold level. Participants record food purchases and other food coming into the home. This type of data is used to generate consumer price indices, which are used as measures of inflation. A household expenditure survey, now called the Living Costs and Food Survey, has been conducted annually in the UK since 1957, making it a useful tool for monitoring changes in family food behav-iour over time.

Individual survey data
Nutrition and health population-based surveys were used to estimate mean fruit and vegetable intake for the Global Burden of Disease study (Lim *et al.* 2012). Ecological analysis has been undertaken using diet and health infor-mation collected from a range of European countries included in the European Prospective Investigation into Cancer (EPIC) cohort study.

Indices of health outcomes
Routine measures of mortality and morbidity
Measures of mortality or morbidity at a national level are usually available through government reports or World Health Organization (WHO) publications. National mor-tality data and Global Burden of Disease data can all be found here: http://www.who.int/healthinfo/statistics/en/

A classic example

Ecological studies are generally the first step in exploring whether there is a differential distribution of disease among people with different risk profiles. For example, ecological comparisons showed that economically devel-oped countries with a higher intake of dietary fat had much higher coronary heart disease (CHD) rates than countries with lower dietary fat consumption. This evi-dence was based on an early study analysing diets from groups of men in seven different countries (Keys *et al.* 1986); see Figure 2.1. These results have been challenged over the years because of difficulties in characterising the

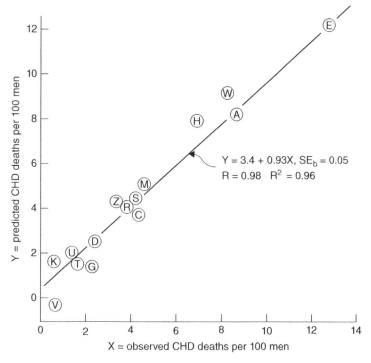

Figure 2.1 Observed 15-year death rates per 100 men compared with death rates from coronary heart disease (CHD) predicted from the multiple regression of the ratio of monounsaturated to saturated fatty acids in the diet, adjusting for age, body mass index, systolic blood pressure, serum cholesterol, and number of cigarettes smoked daily in the Seven Countries Study. Keys, A. *et al.* (1986) The diet and 15-year death rate in the Seven Countries Study, *American Journal of Epidemiology*, **124** (6), 903–915, by permission of Oxford University Press.

dietary intakes of the different country populations. Other types of study are needed to show causation.

A recent example

Diet features very strongly as a risk factor for top adverse health outcomes in the recently published Global Burden of Disease Study 2010 (Lim *et al.* 2012); see Figure 2.2. This study used published and unpublished secondary sources of data to calculate the relationships between 67 different risk factors in 21 regions and linked them with deaths or disease burden for each region between 1990 and 2010. Out of the top 20 leading risk factors contributing to the burden of disease in 2010, 6 are dietary factors (diet low in fruit, nuts and seeds, whole grains, vegetables, seafood and omega-3 fatty acids, and high in sodium) and another 7 are directly linked to diet (high blood pressure, high body mass index, high fasting plasma glucose, childhood underweight, iron deficiency, suboptimal breastfeeding and high total cholesterol). An ecological approach was employed to link risk factors to disease outcomes, using data collected via different epidemiological methods. The data do not directly link individual exposures to risk factors with the diseases of interest. Limitations include variable quality of exposure data across countries and the possibility of residual confounding (see Section 2.6), meaning that some associations could be the result of other factors that have not been considered or taken into account in the analysis.

Analysis of ecological data

The most straightforward analysis would be the calculation of a correlation coefficient between the exposure of interest and the outcome. This is a measure of the strength and direction of the linear relationship between two different continuous variables, for example energy intake and body mass index. The correlation coefficient, denoted by 'r', can have values between +1 (a perfect positive linear relationship) and −1 (a perfect inverse linear relationship). A value of 0 indicates no linear relationship between the two variables. An ecological analysis of 21 wealthy countries (Pickett *et al.* 2005) found that income inequality was positively correlated with the percentage of obese men (r = 0.48, p = 0.03). The relationship was even stronger for obese women in these countries, with a positive correlation coefficient of 0.62 (p = 0.003).

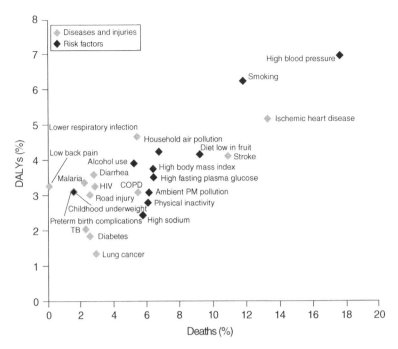

Figure 2.2 The 10 leading diseases and injuries and 10 leading risk factors based on percentage of global deaths and disability-adjusted life years (DALYs), 2010. http://www.healthmetricsandevaluation.org/gbd/publications/policy-report/global-burden-disease-generating-evidence-guiding-policy.

Further analysis of ecological studies could include multiple regression modelling to estimate the magnitude of associations, taking into account other factors of relevance that may otherwise confound the analysis. Confounding factors may include age and other lifestyle factors. Regression modelling can be undertaken using continuous variables as the dependent variable or outcome, such as height or weight. In this case linear regression modelling would be undertaken. When the outcome is categorical or dichotomous, such as the presence or absence of a disease, then logistic regression is appropriate. A study of routine data from South Australia used logistic regression analysis to assess factors that might affect food security, a dichotomised outcome (Foley *et al.* 2010). Food insecurity was highest in households with low levels of education or limited capacity to save money, and in Aboriginal households and those with three or more children.

Problems with ecological analyses

The 'ecological fallacy' is the major trap for the unsuspecting researcher. This occurs when relationships that are observed for groups are assumed to hold for individuals. For example, ecological analysis has shown that countries with more fat in the diet have higher rates of breast cancer, suggesting that women who eat fatty foods would be more likely to develop breast cancer. This assumption is only weakly supported by case-control and cohort data. Correlations found in ecological analyses may be due to confounding by other related factors that have not been controlled for, some of which may be difficult to measure at the population level. Age standardisation often needs to be undertaken, since countries may have very different age profiles. This process adjusts disease rates to a standard population, allowing comparisons to occur. When disease rates are age standardised, any differences in the rates over time or between geographical areas will not simply reflect variations in the age structure of the populations. This is important when looking at disease rates because some conditions, such as cancer, can predominantly affect the elderly. So if rates are not age standardised, a higher disease rate in one country may simply reflect the fact that it has a greater proportion of older people. Additionally, the quality of diagnostic data can differ widely between countries and over time.

2.3 Cross-sectional studies

A cross-sectional survey is a type of observational or descriptive study. The information in this type of survey represents a snapshot about the population at one point in time and it is not possible to determine whether the exposure and the outcome are causally related. Cross-sectional surveys are also known as prevalence surveys, since they can be used to estimate the prevalence of disease in a population. The prevalence is the number of cases of a disease in the population at a particular point in time usually expressed as a rate.

A recent example

A cross-sectional analysis of data from older people in the Singapore Longitudinal Ageing Study found that higher measures of fasting homocysteine and low folate were negatively associated with measures of performance-oriented mobility and activities of daily living (Ng *et al.* 2012). Although these results are suggestive of a relationship in the direction of poorer nutrition to poorer physical function in older people, it is not possible to claim causality, primarily because temporal relationships between exposure and disease were not examined. It is equally plausible that older people with poorer physical functioning have a poorer diet and therefore a worse nutritional status. In order to prove cause-and-effect relationships a different type of study, a randomised controlled trial, would be needed.

Methods

Describing population characteristics

The major nutrition survey conducted in the UK is the National Diet and Nutrition Survey (NDNS). It is a rolling programme that began in 2008 and collects nationally representative dietary data from 1000 individuals per year aged 18 months and over from private households. The National Health and Nutrition Examination Survey (NHANES) is a major rolling programme of survey data collection in the USA that began in the early 1960s. About 5000 individuals are surveyed each year. The sample is selected to represent the US population of all ages. To produce reliable statistics, NHANES over-samples people 60 and older, African Americans, Asians and Hispanics.

There are two major aspects of national nutrition surveys that are important with respect to data collection: cost and organisation. Data should be as *nationally representative* as possible and also be as *accurate and complete* as possible (Stephen *et al.* 2013). In the NDNS, national representation in terms of age, gender and region is achieved by randomly selecting postcodes and addresses from the UK population as a whole (Figure 2.3).

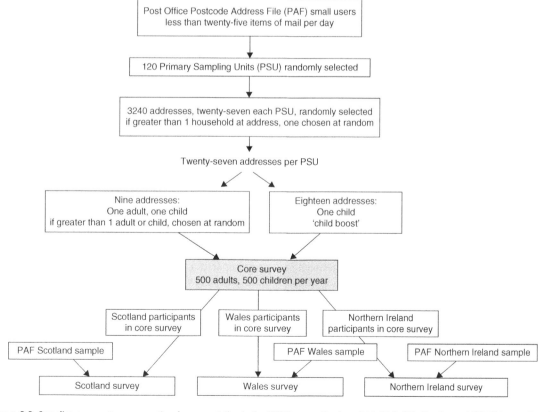

Figure 2.3 Sampling process to ensure national representation in the NDNS survey. Stephen, A.M., Mak, T.N., Fitt, E. *et al.* (2013) Innovations in national nutrition surveys, *Proceedings of the Nutrition Society*, **72** (1), 77–88. Reproduced with permission of Cambridge University Press.

The NDNS currently uses the four-day estimated diary to assess diet. This is a compromise between detail and respondent burden. Respondent burden is particularly important to consider in large-scale surveys of this kind. A high level of low-energy reporting has been found in a previous national survey of older British adults that used four-day weighed diaries, which was considered to be a result of the weighed intake method and reluctance to report consumption of unhealthy food.

Three large cross-sectional data sets from the USA, including NHANES, were used to explore causes of changing energy intake in children from 1977 to 2010. Changes in the number of eating/drinking occasions per day and portion size per eating occasion were the major contributors to changes in total energy intake per day (Duffey and Popkin 2013).

Prevalence surveys

Demographic and Health Surveys (DHS) are nationally representative household surveys that provide data for a wide range of monitoring and impact evaluation indicators in the areas of population, health and nutrition. More than 300 surveys have been conducted in over 90 countries, and survey data and results can be found at http://www.measuredhs.com/. Among the nutrition topics included and reported is the prevalence of anaemia in children and women, as well as the percentage breast fed and anthropometric indicators. High response rates, national coverage, interviewer training and standardised data-collection procedures across countries as well as consistent content over time enable comparisons to be made across populations cross-sectionally and temporally (Corsi et al. 2012).

Migrant studies

Cross-sectional analyses of migrants, comparing populations migrating from rural to urban areas or migrating between countries, have been undertaken to explore the associations between genetic background and environmental exposures in relation to risk of disease. Rural–urban migrants experience rapid environmental changes associated with urbanisation, enabling epidemiological transitions to be examined. Changes seen in migrants over relatively short time periods may therefore provide insights into wider population health changes. The Indian Migration Study (Bowen et al. 2011) explored the impact of migration to urban areas on dietary patterns, comparing migrants with their rural siblings. Migrant and urban participants reported up to 80% higher fruit and vegetable intake than rural participants (p = 0.001) and up to 35% higher sugar intake (p = 0.001). Meat and dairy intake were higher in migrant and urban participants than in rural participants (p = 0.001); see Figure 2.4.

Analysis of cross-sectional data

As with ecological analyses, cross-sectional data can be analysed using correlations between exposures and outcomes. In addition, regression modelling can be used to explore the influence of one continuous variable on another, while taking into account potential confounding factors.

Problems with cross-sectional studies

The main disadvantage of cross-sectional studies is that, since the exposure and disease or outcome are measured at the same time, it is not possible to say which is cause and which is effect. For example, an analysis of questionnaire data recording women's use of vitamin C supplements and irritable bowel syndrome (IBS; Hutchinson et al. 2011) could not be certain whether the supplementary vitamin C had been taken to prevent or manage symptoms of disorders or whether vitamin C had caused them, due to the cross-sectional nature of the data. Associations observed with IBS could have been due to abdominal pain and diarrhoea caused by taking large doses of vitamin C. However, since the associations occurred at any dose of vitamin C, rather than at high doses specifically, a plausible explanation is that very health-conscious women who take supplements may also be prone to anxiety, which might cause IBS.

Others have suggested that using cross-sectional datasets like NHANES to draw conclusions about short-lived environmental chemicals and chronic complex diseases is inappropriate since a one-off snapshot of intakes cannot adequately characterise the relevant exposures. Furthermore, snapshots may be inadequate at capturing exposure detail from people with acute fatal diseases who have a short illness between diagnosis and death, for example pancreatic cancer.

2.4 Case-control studies

In case-control studies, people with a disease (cases) are compared to people without the disease (controls). Both groups have past exposure to the dietary factors of interest measured and they are compared to estimate the risk of disease associated with the risk factor. Case-control studies are quicker to conduct and cheaper than longer-term, larger-scale cohort studies; they are also useful for rare conditions. This study design potentially leads to greater statistical power as well as rapid and cost-effective management of the study. However, challenges arise with regard to the choice of appropriate controls and obtaining an unbiased measure of previous dietary exposure.

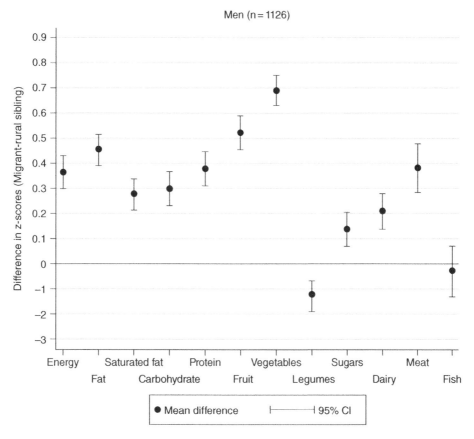

Figure 2.4 Differences in food intake z-scores between migrant and rural siblings in India. Bowen, L. *et al.* (2011) Dietary intake and rural-urban migration in India: a cross-sectional study, *PLoS One,* **6** (6), e14822.

Example case-control study

INTERHEART is one of the largest case-control studies that has been undertaken. It was designed to assess the importance of risk factors for coronary heart disease worldwide and 15 152 cases and 14 820 controls were enrolled from 52 countries, representing all inhabited continents. Specific objectives were to determine the strength of associations between various risk factors and acute myocardial infarction in the overall study population and to ascertain if this association varied by geographical region, ethnic origin, sex or age. Daily fruit and vegetable intake was found to reduce risk with an odds ratio of 0.70 (95% confidence interval [CI] 0.64 to 0.77). This means that people who ate fruit and vegetables every day had a 30% reduced risk of acute myocardial infarction compared to people who did not eat fruit and vegetables every day (Yusuf *et al.* 2004). Obesity doubled the risk, with an odds ratio of 2.24 (95% CI 2.06–2.45).

Methods

The research question to be studied needs to be formulated in order to ensure that the best population is chosen with an adequate supply of cases and suitable controls. In the study population there should also be a diversity of exposure to the dietary risk factors being studied. This is particularly important, since the error associated with dietary measurements tends to obscure potential associations with disease. If those in the study population are all similar with regard to dietary behaviour and the range of food or nutrient intakes is small from the lowest to highest values, it will be difficult to demonstrate an effect of the food or nutrient on the risk of disease due to measurement error. This may be larger than the real differences in intakes between cases and controls.

Selection of cases

The study population must be large enough with a high enough incidence of the disease of interest to provide enough cases over the course of the study. Cases may be incident or newly diagnosed during the recruitment period. Prevalent, either existing or fatal, cases are sometimes used as an alternative to incident cases, since they may be more common and easier to find. However, associations made with prevalent or fatal cases need to be interpreted carefully, since the effect of the diet might be on survival rather than on the development of the disease. For example, if a case-control study found that vitamin D status was associated with an increased risk of pancreatic cancer mortality, this effect might not have occurred because vitamin D actually increases the risk of the disease. It could also be that lower vitamin D is associated with a higher cure rate or longer survival once a tumour is present.

Cases can be identified from hospital or general practice records or alternatively from case-finding in the general population. Using cases from hospitals or general practice would lead to missing undiagnosed people from the general population. Factors that determined earlier diagnosis might also be linked to differences in diet: for example, people who consult their doctor more frequently than others might also eat more healthily. If this is the case, then spurious associations could arise when studying only newly diagnosed patients.

The specificity of diagnosis is also important in the selection of cases. For example, it may be important to know the particular type of stomach cancer being linked to dietary behaviour, since different cancer types may have a different relationship. Intake of fruit and vegetables has been associated with an overall decreased risk of gastric cancer, but dietary intake seems to have a clearer effect on the intestinal type of stomach cancer compared to diffuse types.

Selection of controls

Selection of controls is one of the most difficult aspects of establishing a case-control study, as it is prone to bias. Controls should be selected from the same population, or one that represents the source population from which cases were drawn. Not only does this help to balance confounders between case and control groups, it is also important that selection of controls is independent of exposure status and is representative of the source population in terms of exposure. For instance, if cases are selected from screening clinics, then controls should also be selected from these clinics to avoid self-selection bias, since those attending clinics are likely to be more health conscious than the general population and may eat more healthily. They may also be in a specific age range or genetically more at risk than the general population, depending on the type of clinic. When cases are selected from hospitals, other than via screening clinics, then the selection is less straightforward. Patients with other diseases can be used as controls. Ideally, both cases and

controls should be blind to the purpose of the study to avoid explanations for the disease under study being provided through their responses to the questionnaire. Additionally, selection of controls with a range of diseases may reduce the bias relating to exposure. Alternatively, controls can be selected from the general population, whose exposure may be more representative of the population at risk of becoming cases. Nevertheless, bias can occur because of differences between responders and non-responders.

More than one control from the study can be matched to each case to increase the power to detect associations. Cases and controls can be matched on variables such as age and sex, which are often related to disease and exposure. The use of siblings as controls can be useful, since shared genetic, socio-economic and environmental factors can be controlled for that otherwise may be difficult to measure or define. However, over-matching causing selection bias or reduced efficiency to detect associations should be avoided. This occurs when a factor is used to match cases and controls that is not a confounder of the exposure–disease association. For example, if a case-control study of fat intake in relation to type 2 diabetes matched cases and controls on body mass index (BMI), this could be considered over-matching, since BMI is on the causal pathway between fat intake and diabetes development. So by matching cases and controls on this factor, it will not be possible to assess the effect of fat intake on the risk of developing the condition. Variables used for matching cannot be studied in the analysis. Individual matching is expensive and time-consuming; alternatively group matching, also called frequency matching, can be used, which is a form of stratified sampling. For instance, the control group could be selected to have the same proportion of women as the case group, and the same distribution of ages stratified into age ranges.

Measurement of dietary exposure

A particular challenge for case-control studies is identifying the past dietary behaviour that will be relevant to the disease process. A disease may have a long pre-clinical phase and so the relevant exposure to diet may have occurred many years before diagnosis. People find it difficult to report past diet accurately and answers to questions on dietary behaviour in the past are strongly influenced by current eating patterns. If cases have changed their diets as a result of the disease process, then this will lead to error. Changes in diet are quite likely in diseases such as cancer or renal problems, which can affect appetite. Ideally, cases should be identified before they become symptomatic, thus reducing the risk of behaviour change as a result of the disease. This is only really possible using screening clinics to identify cases, such as from the breast-screening programme to identify women with very early-stage breast cancer. Due to the potential for dietary behaviour change occurring in cases, the main method of collecting dietary information in case-control studies would be using food frequency questionnaires, which usually assess intake over the previous 12 months rather than current intake, which may have been affected by the disease.

Nested case-control studies

A nested case-control study can be developed from a cohort study; a subset of non-cases (controls) from the cohort are compared to the incident cases. Controls are selected for each case by matching on factors such as age. Usually, the exposure of interest (diet) is only measured among the cases and the selected controls. This design may be used when the exposure of interest is difficult or expensive to obtain, such as with coding food diaries or when the outcome is rare. By making use of data previously collected from a large cohort study, the time and cost of beginning a new case-control study are avoided. In addition, by only measuring the diet in as many participants as are necessary, the cost and effort of exposure assessment are reduced. Furthermore, since the dietary information was collected prior to disease incidence, the impact of recall bias on the exposure is reduced.

For example, a nested case-control study of dietary fibre intake and colorectal cancer risk was conducted using seven UK cohort studies, which included 579 case patients who developed colorectal cancer and 1996 matched control subjects. Dietary data obtained from four- to seven-day food diaries was used to calculate the odds ratios for colorectal, colon and rectal cancers with the use of conditional logistic regression models that adjusted for relevant covariates. The multivariable-adjusted odds ratio of colorectal cancer for the highest versus the lowest quintile of fibre intake density was 0.66 (95% CI 0.45–0.96), suggesting a protective effect (Dahm *et al.* 2010).

Analysis of case-control data

The main measure of association that is calculated from a case-control study is the odds ratio (OR). This is a measure of association between an exposure and an outcome. The OR evaluates whether the odds of a certain event or outcome are the same for two groups. Specifically, the OR measures the ratio of the odds that an event or result will occur to the odds of the event not happening. The OR represents the odds that an outcome (disease of interest) will occur given a particular exposure (dietary factor of interest), compared to the odds of the outcome occurring in the absence of that exposure. Typically the data consist of counts for each of a set of conditions and outcomes. By creating a 2×2 table (Table 2.1) the OR is a simple statistic to calculate: $[OR = (a \times d)/(b \times c)]$.

Table 2.1 Distribution of exposure in unmatched case-control studies.

	Cases	Control
Exposed to diet factor	a	b
Unexposed to diet factor	c	d

Matched studies use a different approach to calculate the OR, making use of the number of case-control pairs. If controls have been matched to cases, then a special type of logistic regression, conditional logistic regression, is used for the analysis. This means that controls are only compared to cases within the same matched set.

Confounding factors can be taken into account by using a logistic regression model. This will give an estimated OR and associated confidence intervals that are adjusted for the confounders included.

Odds ratios are also used in the analysis of nested case-control studies. Controls can be selected from the cohort to match cases depending on the date of their baseline intake measurement so that follow-up times are comparable; this deals with the varying recruitment dates within a whole cohort.

Problems with case-control studies

The two main areas of concern with case-control studies are dietary measurement error due to recall bias, and choice of controls. Both of these are discussed in the relevant sections earlier in this chapter.

The impact of recall bias on the results of case-control studies can be seen particularly in systematic reviews of the relationship between diet and disease where both case-control and cohort studies have been included. For example, Figure 2.5 shows that results from case-control studies exploring salt intake and risk of stomach cancer have a fivefold increased risk of stomach cancer per additional serving of salty foods per day; this is in comparison with data from cohort studies that show a much more modest and non-statistically significant increased risk. These differences may well be due, at least in part, to the impact of dietary recall bias in the case-control studies.

2.5 Prospective longitudinal studies

In a prospective longitudinal study (also known as a follow-up or cohort study), individuals are followed up over a period of time and disease or health outcomes are identified during the follow-up period. Individuals should be free of the disease being investigated at the start of the study (if not, they should be excluded from the analysis).

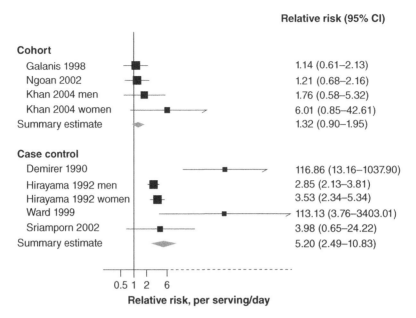

Relative risk (95% CI)

Cohort
Galanis 1998   1.14 (0.61–2.13)
Ngoan 2002   1.21 (0.68–2.16)
Khan 2004 men   1.76 (0.58–5.32)
Khan 2004 women   6.01 (0.85–42.61)
Summary estimate   1.32 (0.90–1.95)

Case control
Demirer 1990   116.86 (13.16–1037.90)
Hirayama 1992 men   2.85 (2.13–3.81)
Hirayama 1992 women 3.53 (2.34–5.34)
Ward 1999   113.13 (3.76–3403.01)
Sriamporn 2002   3.98 (0.65–24.22)
Summary estimate   5.20 (2.49–10.83)

0.5 1 2   6
Relative risk, per serving/day

Figure 2.5 Salty/salted foods and stomach cancer risk. Results from a systematic review. This material has been reproduced from the 2007 WCRF/AICR Report *Food, Nutrition, Physical Activity and the Prevention of Cancer: a Global Perspective*.

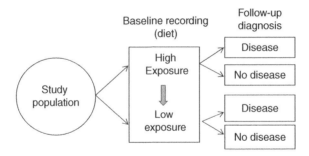

Figure 2.6 Flow chart of a cohort study.

Baseline data on nutritional and lifestyle exposures of interest that may be associated with the disease/health outcome are collected for all individuals (Figure 2.6).

In contrast to case-control studies, where systematic differences in reporting of exposures could occur between those with and those without the disease, recall bias associated with the outcome is avoided in prospective studies since exposure data is collected before the outcome data. In general, prospective studies are also less likely to be subject to the selection bias mentioned earlier in this chapter. Additional advantages are that cohort data can be used to study a wide range of disease and health outcomes, and by careful selection of individuals uncommon exposures or specific dietary patterns can be studied (e.g. vegetarian or Mediterranean diet). A well-designed cohort, for which a variety of

exposures and confounders have been gathered, can also be used at a later date to test new hypotheses. A wider intake range of exposures can be gathered in cohorts compared to case-control or RCT studies, thus allowing useful dose–response relationships between exposure and outcome to be examined. Unlike cross-sectional studies, the time relationship between exposure and disease can be determined in longitudinal studies, therefore results can elucidate aetiology and may provide some evidence for causality if biases are minimised.

Examples

Using a cohort of 2635 pregnant women recruited between 8 and 12 weeks of pregnancy, caffeine intake during pregnancy was found to be associated with an increased risk of fetal growth restriction (CARE Study Group 2008). Habitual caffeine intake from all potential sources from 4 weeks before pregnancy and during pregnancy was measured using a validated questionnaire. Details of potential confounders such as smoking, alcohol intake, maternal height and weight and ethnicity were also gathered using this questionnaire and adjusted for in the analysis. The association was found to be stronger in women with faster caffeine clearance compared to slower clearance; the caffeine half-life (the proxy for clearance) was determined by measuring caffeine in saliva (CARE Study Group 2008).

Much larger cohorts, such as the European Prospective Investigation into Cancer and Nutrition (EPIC) cohort, have been established and followed up over many years to investigate associations between dietary intake and a range of cancers and other chronic diseases in the general population. EPIC includes over 500,000 people recruited in 10 European countries: Denmark, France, Germany, Greece, Italy, the Netherlands, Norway, Spain, Sweden and the UK. There are two UK studies in the EPIC group, EPIC-Norfolk and EPIC-Oxford, which recruited over 23 000 and 65 000 people respectively and have used food frequency questionnaires (FFQs) and food diaries to gather dietary intake data (http://epic.iarc.fr/). Blood samples from individuals have also been taken, from which concentrations of nutrients and hormones have been measured and used in analyses to investigate the relationship between diet and chronic diseases. In Epic-Norfolk, plasma ascorbic acid was inversely associated with cancer mortality in men but not women. Pooling the individuals from all or a number of EPIC studies increases the power to detect associations.

Methods

Selection of the study population

First, it is important to define the population from which the study sample (that is, the study population) is to be drawn and to which the results need to be generalised. This should also be undertaken for other types of observational studies. Ideally, a sampling frame needs to be compiled or sourced. This is a list of population members from which the study sample can be selected. If the exposure of interest is common, for instance fruit and vegetable intake, then the study sample can be selected from the general population using electoral registers, school registers or list of patients in general practices. EPIC-Norfolk, for instance, recruited people registered with 35 Norfolk GPs. In order for the findings of the sample to be generalisable to the population from which it is drawn, a large number of individuals need to be randomly selected from the sampling frame. Nevertheless, even for very large cohorts, random selection from

subsets of the sampling frame stratified by age, gender, socio-economic status (SES) or other important factors may be necessary to ensure representativeness in these factors, as proposed for the UK Biobank (http://www.ukbiobank.ac.uk/). In this cohort, 500 000 people aged 40–69 from across the UK were recruited from National Health Service (NHS) registers held centrally.

Alternatively, individuals can be randomly selected from geographical clusters within the sampling frame (e.g. schools, GPs). Cluster sampling has advantages of cost and convenience in recruitment, but it is not truly random and similar characteristics of people living within one cluster may affect the results. Such effects may be reduced by increasing the number of clusters and selecting areas to include a range of known influencing characteristics, such as SES. Additionally, it may be necessary to weight the clusters in the analysis in order for the results to be representative of the proportions of individuals in the population rather than the proportion in the sample.

Incompleteness of the sampling frame also needs to be acknowledged, since hard-to-reach individuals such as the homeless or travellers are unlikely to be found on registers. Furthermore, the recruitment of pregnant women during their first trimester from antenatal clinics may miss women who attend their first clinic late in their pregnancy and who are often from lower SES.

If the exposure is not particularly common, for instance a vegetarian diet, then the study population can be selected based on their exposure to ensure that sufficient individuals with this exposure are included. The UK Women's Cohort Study (UKWCS) was established to compare vegetarians, fish eaters and red meat eaters. All eligible women who replied to an initial World Cancer Research Fund (WCRF) survey and stated that they were vegetarian or that they did not eat red meat were selected to take part in the cohort (Cade *et al.* 2004). However, only a proportion of the red meat–eating majority was invited to participate and a method of selection that was likely to avoid bias was used: for each vegetarian the next non-vegetarian in the list aged within 10 years was selected. Alternatively, vegetarians could be targeted more directly, as undertaken by the EPIC-Oxford study, which mailed members of the Vegetarian Society of the UK. Similarly, Seventh-Day Adventists, who usually follow a vegetarian diet, were recruited directly in studies established in California, USA, the Netherlands and other countries. Additionally, the UK Biobank may contain sufficient vegetarians to power analyses. Individuals participating completed an online 24-hour diet recall questionnaire that asked whether they routinely followed a vegetarian diet.

Power calculations utilising statistical packages are needed to determine the size of cohort required based on estimates such as the overall risk of the outcome in the population, the ratio of unexposed to exposed individuals in the population and the follow-up time.

Smaller nested case-control studies can be established within large cohorts. Nevertheless, care is needed to avoid bias in the selection of the controls and cases, as outlined earlier.

Measurement of dietary exposures

Usually diet is measured only at baseline (the start of the cohort study). An assumption in longitudinal studies is that eating habits remain relatively stable before and after baseline data collection. However, this may not always be the case due to changes in dietary fashion and advice. To overcome this, some cohorts have undertaken additional wave collections of dietary exposures at a number of follow-up time points, although this adds to the study resource requirements, as well as leading to losses to follow-up and complexities of analysis. Although dietary intake between assessment points would be unknown, an average may be used for analysis, or respondents may be categorised for instance as 'always', 'sometimes' or 'never' within specified intake ranges at assessment. Similarly, the effect of intermittent supplement use (at least one but not all assessment points) and more consistent use (at all assessment points) could be compared in the analyses to never reporting use. Alternatively, questions relating to supplement use may be worded to obtain information on length of use as well as type, dose and numbers taken.

Although the disease outcome is collected prospectively in longitudinal studies, there is an element of retrospective recall of exposure data with the use of some instruments, such as FFQs and diet histories. FFQs usually obtain estimated average intake relating to the previous 12 months. More current and detailed, but short-term, dietary intake may be gathered by 24-hour recalls or by diary over a period of four to seven days. However, transferring information from paper-based diaries to electronic format requires substantially more time and resources in large-scale cohort studies. Resource requirements can be reduced by creating a much smaller nested case-control study within a large cohort or a number of cohort studies such as the UK Dietary Cohort Consortium, which was used to explore the relationship between breast cancer risk and vitamin C intake from both diet and supplements (Hutchinson *et al.* 2012).

Analysis of cohort data

Cohort studies allow us to measure disease incidence, since we have a healthy population who are followed up over time and the rate of new disease development (incidence) can be calculated. If the follow-up times for all the individuals in the cohort are similar, then relative risk ratios can be estimated. For instance, in birth cohorts the relative risk of an outcome in the offspring at a specified age in relation to specified intake during pregnancy can be calculated. The relative risk is the cumulative incidence in the exposed group compared to the cumulative incidence in the unexposed group. However, since it is important to adjust for potential confounders in all risk analyses of cohort data, multiple regression analysis is most often undertaken. If the outcome is continuous, then multiple linear regression can be used, but if the outcome is dichotomous, then logistic regression should be carried out.

In the CARE study, multiple linear regression analysis was used to estimate the reduction in birth weight with higher caffeine intake after adjustment for various factors. However, logistic regression was used to estimate the odds of giving birth to a baby with fetal growth restriction (birth weight < 10th centile after accounting for maternal factors) depending on caffeine intake during pregnancy. In nutritional epidemiology, intake is usually split into quartiles or quintiles for reporting estimates with confidence intervals; in this study, intake of < 100 mg/day was compared to intake groups of 100–199, 200–299 and ≥ 300 mg/day. Dose–response relationships, which can provide some evidence of causality, were found in testing for trends using intake as a continuous exposure and, as commonly done, p values for these were reported. Additionally, the risk of fetal growth restriction was plotted against increasing caffeine intake using fractional polynominal regression, a more advanced statistical technique. This showed a linear dose–response relationship with no threshold effects.

If follow-up times differ substantially between individuals in the cohort, then the total person-time at risk is needed to calculate hazard ratios (rate ratios) in time-to-event analysis (also called survival analysis, even when the event is a disease incidence and not a death). This method is useful when recruitment takes place over a number of years. Person-years at risk is calculated for each individual as the time from the measurement of dietary intake at their baseline date until disease incidence or the censor date or the individual was lost to follow-up. Cox regression (also known as proportional hazards regression) is one method of time-to-event analysis. Individuals known to have the outcome at the set-up of the cohort should be excluded from all risk analyses. This is one of the main analysis methods used in the EPIC and UKWCS cohorts mentioned earlier.

One of the biggest issues with the reliability of the results in cohort studies is confounding, which is explained in Section 2.6. The selection of confounders used for adjustment in an analysis of cohorts and other observational studies may appear to be more of an art than a science, since it often requires subjective decision-making. Univariate analyses should be undertaken to determine associations between the potential confounders and the outcome and then between the potential confounders and the dietary exposure. Variables that are significantly associated with both should be considered for adjustment. Variables that do not meet this criterion in the study but where there is strong prior evidence of confounding from previous studies should also be considered for inclusion for adjustment. Visual methods, for instance creating diagrams called directed acyclic graphs (DAGs), can help clarify the direction of the effects of variables to help identify which may or may not be potential confounders (Greenland, Pearl and Robins 1999). Variables that appear to be on the causal pathway between the dietary exposure and the outcome should not be included, since controlling for these mediators would attenuate associations between exposure and outcome. Finally, over-adjustment can occur if too many confounders are included, particularly if they are collinear; that is, they are strongly correlated. This can lead to associations being missed where they may really exist.

Another way of controlling for a confounder in cohort studies, other than through multiple regression, is by restricting the analysis to those individuals who are not affected by the confounder. For instance, the majority of studies exploring associations between nutrient intake and disease have only measured intake from diet, and have not included the nutrient intake from supplements, which are commonly consumed in the Western world. Furthermore, some studies that have gathered supplement data have not obtained the strength dosage of supplements. To avoid supplement intake being a confounder, all supplement users could be excluded from an analysis, if this basic information is provided. These results could then be compared to results prior to exclusions.

Problems with longitudinal studies

Longitudinal studies are very time-consuming and expensive. Since only a small percentage of individuals may develop the outcome by the end of the follow-up period, very large sample sizes as well as long follow-up periods are needed to detect a significant result if an association exists. Sample size calculations are recommended prior to the creation of the cohort and also prior to analyses. Additionally, as seen in later chapters, the methods for collecting and electronically capturing exposures are very time-consuming for the individual and the research team. Nevertheless, new technologies such as the 'My Meal Mate' (MMM) mobile smartphone application and the online 24-hour recalls 'ASA24' and 'myfood24' are being developed to improve accuracy and reduce data-capture resource requirements. Since participants may find these methods less burdensome,

they may be willing to provide extra days of consumption to classify their intake more appropriately compared to traditional methods.

In particular, cohorts are an inefficient or impractical method of studying relatively rare outcomes such as pancreatic cancer, since a large number of individuals would be needed to find a significant association, if one existed. Nevertheless, this may be partially overcome in cohort studies by undertaking a meta-analysis of results from a number of studies, or, better still, by pooling individual data for analysis from a number of cohort studies.

Due to long follow-up periods, substantial numbers of individuals may drop out during this time (attrition). If the outcomes for these individuals cannot be determined and these losses to follow-up are related to both the exposure and the outcome, then this differential loss to follow-up produces a form of selection bias. Multiple methods of contact and surveillance may reduce losses to follow-up. Since health workers and civil servants are usually more easily traced than the general population, cohorts have been established using these study populations, for instance the Whitehall Study (Marmot and Brunner 2005) and the Nurse's Health Study (Zhang et al. 1999). In countries such as the UK and USA, losses to follow-up for some outcomes can now be mainly overcome, and therefore the quality of cohort studies increased, by obtaining outcome data from national and regional registries, for example for cancer and heart disease outcomes, rather than by direct contact with the individual. Consent to obtain this information must be obtained from individuals at the start of the study. Although selection bias by researchers is less of a problem in cohorts than in case-control studies, self-selection – that is, the type of person who volunteers for participation in cohorts – can create selection bias.

Despite efforts to control for confounders in analyses, residual confounding may remain and may account for some of the significant though unknowingly spurious results that are published. Nevertheless, on the whole, cohort results usually provide better support for aetiological suggestions than other observational studies, since they have fewer methodological limitations.

2.6 Confounding

In observational studies, confounders must be taken into account because they can influence the estimated size, direction and/or significance of association between the dietary factor of interest and the disease outcome. As mentioned in the introduction to this chapter, potential confounders are variables that may be associated with both the exposure of interest (diet) and the outcome variable (disease), but are not on the causal pathway

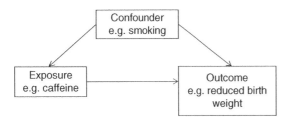

Figure 2.7 An example of confounding.

between exposure and outcome. A confounder can provide an alternative explanation for an apparent association between a dietary exposure and a disease/health outcome. For instance, a positive association between increased coffee consumption and reduced birth weight could be explained by higher smoking levels, because it is well established that smoking during pregnancy is associated with reduced birth weight, and smoking has also been associated with increased coffee consumption (this relationship is illustrated in Figure 2.7). In the Caffeine and Reproductive Health (CARE) study, smoking status was adjusted for as a confounder in multiple regression analyses to produce results showing associations between maternal coffee drinking and fetal birth weight independent of smoking status (CARE Study Group 2008).

Confounding variables need to be identified, measured and controlled for in analyses. Depending on the study design, confounders can be dealt with during the design of the study by matching or by restricting study members; and through data analysis by stratification (e.g. age standardisation), by restriction or by adjustment in regression models.

Even after controlling for measured confounders, some residual confounding may remain. However, in general, confounding variables can often be measured more accurately than dietary variables, and therefore any significant associations with health outcomes found in unadjusted analyses often disappear or are greatly attenuated after adjustment for confounders. This may be due to genuine confounding; alternatively, true dietary associations may be masked by confounders because these dietary exposures are measured less accurately.

Although confounding is less likely in RCTs because covariates are randomly distributed between interventions, nutritional interventions for RCTs may not be feasible or may present their own problems. Individuals may not be willing to be randomised to a diet for the number of years that would be necessary to cause substantial alterations in disease risk. Furthermore, unlike drug interventions where the accessibility of drugs is restricted and amounts provided are known, nutritional interventions can never be completely controlled. For instance, vitamin supplements as an active intervention

can be easily obtained by study individuals, meaning that supplement intake can also happen in the control group; furthermore, additional supplement intake can easily occur in the intervention group. Due to the limitations of RCTs in nutrition research, results of observational studies remain useful for exploring the role of nutritional exposures in the causation of disease, despite confounding and other weaknesses.

2.7 Conclusion

Population-based observational studies use epidemiological techniques to explore associations between diet and health outcomes. Ecological and cross-sectional studies are useful first steps in generating hypotheses; however, they cannot be used to test aetiological theories due to methodological limitations. Case-control studies are useful for studying diet and disease relationships, but they present problems in the choice of appropriate controls and recall of past diet. Cohort studies allow more rigorous testing of diet–disease relationships than other approaches. All of these methods are potentially influenced by confounding factors, variables that may be associated with both the exposure of interest (diet) and the outcome (disease).

References and further reading

Bowen, L., Ebrahim, S., De Stavola, B. *et al.* (2011) Dietary intake and rural-urban migration in India: a cross-sectional study. *PLoS One*, **6** (6), e14822.

Cade, J.E., Burley, V.J., Greenwood, D.C.; The UKWCS Steering Group (2004) The UK Women's Cohort Study: Comparison of vegetarians, fish-eaters and meat-eaters. *Public Health Nutrition*, **7** (7), 871–878.

CARE Study Group (2008) Maternal caffeine intake during pregnancy and risk of fetal growth restriction: A large prospective observational study. *British Medical Journal*, **337**, a2332.

Corsi, D.J., Neuman, M., Finlay, J.E. and Subramanian, S. (2012) Demographic and health surveys: A profile. *International Journal of Epidemiology*, **41** (6), 1602–1613.

Dahm, C.C., Keogh, R.H., Spencer, E.A. *et al.* (2010) Dietary fiber and colorectal cancer risk: A nested case-control study using food diaries. *Journal of the National Cancer Institute*, **102** (9), 614–626.

Duffey, K.J. and Popkin, B.M. (2013) Causes of increased energy intake among children in the U.S., 1977–2010. *American Journal of Preventive Medicine*, **44** (2), e1–8.

Foley, W., Ward, P., Carter, P. *et al.* (2010) An ecological analysis of factors associated with food insecurity in South Australia, 2002–7. *Public Health Nutrition*, **13** (2), 215–221.

Greenland, S., Pearl, J. and Robins, J.M. (1999) Causal diagrams for epidemiologic research. *Epidemiology*, **10** (1), 37–48.

Hutchinson, J., Burley, V.J., Greenwood, D.C. *et al.* (2011) High-dose vitamin C supplement use is associated with self-reported histories of breast cancer and other illnesses in the UK Women's Cohort Study. *Public Health Nutrition*, **14** (5), 768–777.

Hutchinson, J., Lentjes, M., Greenwood, D. *et al.* (2012) Vitamin C intake from diary recordings and risk of breast cancer in the UK Dietary Cohort Consortium. *European Journal of Clinical Nutrition*, **66** (5), 561–568.

Keys, A., Menotti, A., Karvonen, M.J. *et al.* (1986) The diet and 15-year death rate in the Seven Countries Study. *American Journal of Epidemiology*, **124** (6), 903–915.

Lim, S.S., Vos, T., Flaxman, A.D. *et al.* (2012) A comparative risk assessment of burden of disease and injury attributable to 67 risk factors and risk factor clusters in 21 regions, 1990–2010: A systematic analysis for the Global Burden of Disease Study 2010. *Lancet*, **380** (9859): 2224–2260.

Marmot, M. and Brunner, E. (2005) Cohort profile: The Whitehall II Study. *International Journal of Epidemiology*, **34** (2), 251–256.

Ng, T.P., Aung, K.C., Feng, L. *et al.* (2012) Homocysteine, folate, vitamin B-12, and physical function in older adults: Cross-sectional findings from the Singapore Longitudinal Ageing Study. *American Journal of Clinical Nutrition*, **96** (6), 1362–1368.

Pickett, K.E., Kelly, S., Brunner, E. *et al.* (2005) Wider income gaps, wider waistbands? An ecological study of obesity and income inequality. *Journal of Epidemiology and Community Health*, **59** (8), 670–674.

Pomerleau, J., Lock, K. and McKee, M. (2003) Discrepancies between ecological and individual data on fruit and vegetable consumption in fifteen countries. *British Journal of Nutrition*, **89** (6), 827–834.

Stephen, A.M., Mak, T.N., Fitt, E. *et al.* (2013) Innovations in national nutrition surveys. *Proceedings of the Nutrition Society*, **72** (1), 77–88.

Yusuf, S., Hawken, S., Ounpuu, S. *et al.* (2004) Effect of potentially modifiable risk factors associated with myocardial infarction in 52 countries (the INTERHEART study): Case-control study. *Lancet*, **364** (9438), 937–952.

Zhang, S., Hunter, D.J., Forman, M.R. *et al.* (1999) Dietary carotenoids and vitamins A, C, and E and risk of breast cancer. *Journal of the National Cancer Institute*, **91** (6), 547–556.

3
Study Design: Intervention Studies

Jayne V Woodside,[1] Robert W Welch,[2] Chris C Patterson[1] and Michelle C McKinley[1]

[1] Centre for Public Health, Queen's University Belfast
[2] Northern Ireland Centre for Food and Health, School of Biomedical Sciences, University of Ulster

Key messages

- Substantial evidence links nutrition to the improvement of physiological function and/or the reduction of the risk of major chronic diseases.
- Intervention studies fulfil an important role in establishing the link between nutrition and improvements in health as, if well designed, they may allow the testing of causality.
- Nutrition intervention studies can range in type from a double-blind, randomised, placebo-controlled, nutrient supplementation study through to a community-based lifestyle intervention, or a population-based fortification project.
- Nutrition intervention studies can range in duration, from short-term studies assessing acute postprandial effects of specific dietary modifications through to long-term interventions running over many months or years that examine change in risk markers or incidence of disease.

- The study design process should include careful consideration of the hypothesis, duration, intervention, amount and mode of delivery, control and blinding, primary and secondary outcome measures (including assessment of background diet), statistical power, eligibility criteria, data-collection methodology and ways of measuring and encouraging compliance.
- Advice from a statistician during both study design and statistical analysis is recommended.
- Local ethical approval and research governance procedures must be followed, and intervention studies registered on a publicly accessible database before recruitment commences. Any potential conflicts of interest, for example when funding has come from the food industry, should be declared.

3.1 Introduction

There is substantial evidence linking dietary factors to the primary and secondary prevention of major chronic diseases such as heart disease, diabetes and certain cancers, as well as the improvement of physiological function and the maintenance of adequate nutritional status.

Although observational studies (see Chapter 2) can demonstrate an association between a particular nutrient, food or diet and a functional or disease-related endpoint, causality cannot be demonstrated using such study designs. To demonstrate cause and effect requires an intervention study in which consumption of a nutrient, food or diet is altered in a controlled way and the effect on selected outcomes is measured. Intervention studies are higher up the hierarchy of scientific evidence than observational studies, although a combination of different study designs is usually utilised to develop a comprehensive evidence base for a link between consumption of a particular food or nutrient and a health-related outcome. Observational studies often generate hypotheses, which can be tested more rigorously in an intervention study.

This chapter will examine the different types of intervention study and then outline some of the key factors to consider when planning such studies. It includes intervention study design when the focus of interest is a particular nutrient, whole food, food group or whole diet, and also discusses nutrient supplementation studies.

3.2 Intervention study types

Intervention studies should be hypothesis driven and have a strong evidence basis. Intervention study designs can range from a short-term study, where the immediate

Nutrition Research Methodologies, First Edition. Edited by Julie A Lovegrove, Leanne Hodson, Sangita Sharma and Susan A Lanham-New.
© 2015 John Wiley & Sons, Ltd. Published 2015 by John Wiley & Sons, Ltd.
Companion Website: www.wiley.com/go/nutritionsociety

effect of the intervention (consumed once) is measured over minutes to hours (for example, postprandial, or post-meal, studies), through to long-term studies that evaluate the effects of the intervention over a period of weeks, months or years. The study setting can also vary, from those in free-living populations through to studies conducted entirely in purpose-built research facilities such as metabolic suites, or within clinical facilities such as metabolic wards. The main study designs are outlined in this section.

Pilot studies

Different definitions exist for a pilot study (sometimes the terms 'feasibility study' or 'exploratory study' are also used interchangeably), but they are generally regarded as studies that are implemented on a small scale in order to test whether all the study processes operate as anticipated before undertaking a full-scale trial. There are many different reasons for performing pilot studies: for example, they are often undertaken in order to assess how realistic it would be to conduct a full-scale trial, to test recruitment procedures in a defined population, to develop and test research instruments, to develop and test a novel intervention (e.g. to evaluate food matrix issues or to ascertain dose or amount to be consumed), to identify logistical challenges in implementing a full-scale trial and to convince funding bodies that such a trial is worth funding. These studies can also provide data on the distribution/variability and timescale of outcome responses, which can be used for power calculations in subsequent definitive studies. Pilot studies vary in design and may test all, or only some, aspects of a full-scale study. They may be single-arm (before and after) studies with no control group, and these can be a cost- and time-effective way of assessing potential effects, but only as a forerunner to controlled studies. Pilot studies add to the totality of evidence, but on their own cannot determine the effect of intervention.

In general, data from pilot studies should be reported in descriptive terms and caution should be exercised when interpreting any statistical tests of significance, which will typically lack power. Publishing pilot data provides important insights and information that can be used by other researchers and represents an important element of good study design, particularly for complex interventions. Whole-diet or broader lifestyle interventions, including diet, may be considered 'complex interventions', and should be developed according to the UK Medical Research Council's guidelines on developing and evaluating complex interventions. Development of interventions according to these guidelines will involve the use of qualitative research methods (see Chapter 10).

Randomised controlled trials: Parallel and cross-over

Once these early studies have been completed, studies with greater rigour, in which participants are randomised to study groups, will test the hypothesis that the nutrient, food or diet will alter the selected outcome measures. Usually a series of studies will be conducted, with later studies extending the work as the evidence accrues. Examples include increasing the range of populations studied, using new and/or longer-term outcome measures, assessing the minimum effective amount (or 'dose') to be consumed, and evaluating different forms of presentation or delivery of the nutrient or food.

In any controlled study, in addition to measuring outcomes in participants receiving the active nutrient, food or dietary intervention, the same outcome measurements will be collected in a control group. The inclusion of a control group, which may receive either a placebo or no intervention, allows control outcomes to be compared with intervention outcomes and therefore increases confidence that changes observed during the study are directly attributable to the intervention. Without a control group, it is inappropriate to make cause-and-effect statements about an intervention, as other factors may be responsible for the effects observed. For example, if a study is conducted over several months without a control group, it is possible that any changes observed are attributable to normal seasonal changes rather than the intervention itself. As well as allowing seasonal variations to be taken into account, having a control group also means that the 'placebo effect' can be assessed. In some cases, just taking a supplement or eating in a different way is enough to make an individual feel 'better' to some extent, and this is particularly relevant when dealing with more subjective outcomes such as quality-of-life scales.

Two basic randomised controlled trial (RCT) study designs are encountered: *parallel group studies* and *cross-over studies*. The key features of these study designs are illustrated in Figure 3.1. In parallel group studies, each participant receives only one of the nutrition interventions (e.g. product A or B, or low intake or high intake) under study. Comparisons between groups must therefore be made on a between-participant basis. However, in some studies it may be feasible to use a different design in which participants receive more than one intervention. In cross-over studies, participants receive all interventions under comparison and the design specifies the order of interventions. This has the advantage that comparisons between interventions can be made on a within-participant basis, with a consequent improvement in the precision of comparisons and therefore in the power of the study, and a reduction in the required sample size. In such designs, participants act as their own controls. In a

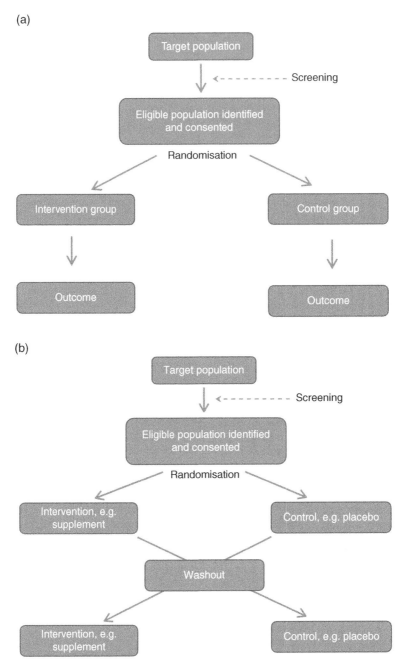

Figure 3.1 Study design for parallel and cross-over RCTs. Acute studies can follow either of these general designs, but durations will be markedly shorter. (a) Parallel group randomised controlled trial flowchart; (b) Cross-over randomised controlled trial flowchart.

cross-over design for two interventions, the participants are allocated to two groups that receive interventions in a different order. Assessments are performed at the end of each intervention period, although in some cross-over studies baseline measurements may also be taken at the start of each intervention period. Depending on the intervention and outcome measure, a washout period may be required between intervention periods to avoid contamination or carry-over effects; that is, the effect of an intervention given in one treatment period extending into the following treatment period(s). A run-in period may also be desirable in advance so as to minimise order effects. During this period participants may be asked to avoid certain foods. A Latin square design may be used, where appropriate, to extend cross-over studies to more than two interventions. However, since participants receive all interventions, increasing the number of interventions will extend the study duration and so may add to the participant drop-out rate.

For studies that require longer-term interventions, parallel studies are usually preferred, because of their shorter overall time frame. Furthermore, parallel studies are essential where a washout period may be ineffective at returning outcome measures to baseline, for example in certain tests of cognitive function. Parallel studies are also required where intentionally returning to baseline may be unethical, for example if body weight or bone mineral density is the outcome measures. Parallel studies are least suited to outcomes that show large inter-participant variation. Cross-over studies are favoured where participant availability may be restricted and in very short-term studies, for example postprandial studies to evaluate glycaemic responses or effects on satiety and short-term energy intakes. However, they are adversely affected by dropouts and necessitate a more complex analysis methodology.

The choice of study design will depend on these considerations, but also on the time frame, the availability of other resources such as cost, the level of financial support and research staff time available, and the potential roles of confounding factors, such as seasonal variations. Using cost as an example to be considered, the sample size for cross-over studies will be smaller, and the time frame for recruitment therefore shortened, but the overall time frame will be longer than for a parallel trial, as participants need to complete both intervention and control arms with an appropriate washout period. The effect of these differences on cost would have to be estimated for each individual study.

Other less commonly used types of RCT include the *factorial design* (in which all possible combinations of two or more interventions are tested, therefore permitting the evaluation of intervention interactions) and the *cluster randomised design* (in which the unit of randomisation is not the individual but a cluster of individuals defined, for example, by family, school class or primary care group). Further guidance on these designs is available in statistical texts on clinical trials.

Quasi-experimental studies

Like RCTs, quasi-experimental studies are designed to estimate the impact of an intervention on a group of participants. Although they can be similar to RCTs in design, they lack one or more key features of a true experiment; most commonly the element of random assignment to the intervention or control group is absent and sometimes the control group is lacking altogether.

Quasi-experimental studies are often used in public health, for example community food-based interventions. They are easier, quicker and cheaper to implement than RCTs and so require less forward planning and a shorter lead-in time. In some situations quasi-experimental studies are the only viable option, as it may not be ethical to have a control group that does not receive any intervention, for example in the provision of vitamins to infants. Some public health interventions, by necessity or for practical reasons, need to be rolled out quickly and on a wide scale, which excludes the incorporation of a control group. Quasi-experimental studies can provide valuable information about the potential usefulness of an intervention, but their internal validity (i.e. their ability to establish causality) will be compromised compared to the RCT design and this limitation must be appreciated when interpreting their results.

There are many different variations of quasi-experimental studies, but two frequently encountered designs are:

- *A before-and-after study without a control group.* In this case, data are collected on the endpoint of interest before and after an intervention takes place, but there is no control group for comparison and so it is not possible to be certain that any differences that have occurred between the start and end of the study are directly attributable to the intervention. It is possible that something else happened between the before and after measurements that influenced the results, or it is possible that completion of the pre-test assessments influenced completion of the post-test assessments, if non-objective data-collection methods such as questionnaires were used. For example, an intensive education intervention to reduce fat intake in a group of overweight participants took place over a six-month period and, at the same time, a public health campaign targeting fat intake was launched. Without a control group it would not be possible to say whether changes in fat intake that took place during the study were attributable to the intensive education intervention or to the public health campaign.

- *A before-and-after study with a non-equivalent groups design*. In this type of study, one group of individuals is recruited and assigned to the intervention and another group of participants is chosen to act as the control group. Since the groups are not created through random assignment, they may not be similar (or equivalent) in all key aspects at the start of the study and this may affect the outcome of the study and thus its internal validity; that is, its ability to conclude that the intervention was causally related to the study outcome. For example, in a study examining the effects of a dietary intervention on total cholesterol, if participants are not randomly assigned to the intervention or the control group at study outset, it is possible that participants in the intervention group may have lower total cholesterol concentrations and a healthier diet at the start of the study compared to the control group. In this case, the intervention group would be unlikely to benefit as much from the intervention as the control group, thus the non-equivalence of the groups at the start of the study would bias the results towards the null hypothesis.

Population-based fortification studies

Food fortification is defined by the World Health Organization (WHO) as 'the practice of deliberately increasing the content of an essential micronutrient, i.e. vitamins and minerals (including trace elements) in a food, irrespective of whether the nutrients were originally in the food before processing or not, so as to improve the nutritional quality of the food supply and to provide a public health benefit with minimal risk to health'.

Food manufacturers can fortify foods on a voluntary basis, in line with government legislation, meaning that the individual can make a choice about whether to purchase such foods or not. An example of this would be fortification of ready-to-eat cereals. In contrast, population-based food-fortification programmes are sometimes implemented as part of public health policy to correct dietary deficiencies (e.g. iodised salt to prevent iodine deficiency) or enhance the status of a micronutrient to a level that will prevent specific undesirable health outcomes (e.g. fortification of flour with folic acid to prevent neural tube defects). Population-based fortification programmes require careful planning and consideration of a wide range of background scientific data before commencement, including the following:

- Examination of high-quality data on the dietary intake (usual food intake and dietary patterns) and nutritional status of the population, including age- and sex-specific subgroups, in order to inform decisions about the most appropriate food vehicle for fortification and

to allow modelling of dietary exposure in relation to tolerable upper limits as part of the overall risk-assessment process.
- Calculation of the dose and most appropriate form of micronutrient to add based on: data from efficacy and effectiveness trials; the food vehicle chosen; the bioavailability of the nutrient in question when delivered in the food matrix; and findings from risk-assessment modelling.

Furthermore, careful monitoring for undesirable consequences (e.g. over-exposure in certain population subgroups resulting in toxic side effects) as well as desirable effects (improved population micronutrient status, reducing the incidence of the targeted adverse health outcome) of the fortification programme in the short, medium and long term is paramount and should be carefully planned before programme implementation.

3.3 Considerations when planning intervention studies

The major factors involved in the planning, conducting and reporting of intervention studies are identified in Table 3.1, which uses a similar structure to that in the Consolidated Standards of Reporting Trials (CONSORT) checklist for clinical trials. An expanded discussion of these factors appears in this section. These factors will be most relevant for RCTs, as described above, but some factors will also apply to intervention studies in general.

Table 3.2 gives some examples, from peer-reviewed journals, of the different study designs described in Section 3.2. Some published studies, particularly earlier ones, do not give clearly stated null hypotheses based on a single primary outcome measure. In these cases, the null hypotheses in Table 3.2 have been inferred from the hypotheses, aims or objectives given in the paper. The distinction between null hypotheses and alternate hypotheses is outlined later in this section. Achieving a study design that fully satisfies all the considerations described here may be constrained in practice by a number of factors, which include practical and logistical issues and the availability of resources, eligible participants and appropriate outcome measures. Thus, the purpose of Table 3.2 is to illustrate the range of types of study design that have been used, rather than to provide examples that may be considered to satisfy fully all the considerations described.

Hypothesis

The primary hypothesis, which is tested statistically, should be framed as a null hypothesis, which states that there is no difference between the tested intervention

Table 3.1 Factors to consider and recommended standards for human intervention trials evaluating health benefits of nutrients, foods and diets. Modified from Welch *et al.* (2011) and Woodside *et al.* (2013).

Phase	Factor	Recommended standard
Design	Hypothesis	Clear hypothesis
	Study design	Appropriate design, randomised where possible
	Duration	Appropriate to design, intervention and outcome measures
	Intervention	Test and control interventions suitably matched
	Amount	Appropriate to outcome measures and to practical usage
	Outcome assessment	Define primary outcome and method of measurement
		Define all secondary outcomes and methods of measurement
	Eligibility criteria	Define all eligibility criteria
	Statistical considerations	
	Randomisation	Use randomised design; ensure appropriate allocation, sequence generation and concealment
	Blinding	Ensure double blinding if feasible, single blinding if not
	Size of study	Conduct power calculation based on primary outcome measure
Conduct	Study protocol	
	Ethical approval and trial registration	Obtain approval, register trial, comply with Declaration of Helsinki
	Recruitment	Define recruitment strategy and process, including settings and dates
	Data collection	Define relevant measures, select suitable methods for assessment, collection and analysis
	– Demographics, lifestyle, background health status and diet, and diet changes	
	– Adverse events and unintended effects	Use suitable methods to record and respond appropriately
	Compliance	Define acceptable level, strive to maximise, assess
Analysis and interpretation	Statistical analysis	Devise appropriate analysis methods, based on study design and outcome measures
	Discussion and interpretation	Consider study limitations and generalisability of findings
	Conclusions	Relate directly to hypothesis, study design, intervention and participants

and the control (see Table 3.2). If the statistical test rejects the null hypothesis, then the alternative hypothesis is accepted, indicating that there is a difference between the two interventions. The primary hypothesis to be tested directly influences all aspects of the study, including the study design and duration, the eligibility criteria, the amount of food or nutrient that will be provided and the nature of the control group. The hypothesis should be based on a thorough review of the available evidence. This review should not only encompass other intervention studies, but also consider epidemiological, animal and *in vitro* studies. Where possible, all available evidence should be reviewed systematically and an assessment of safety and potential risks should be carried out. The primary outcome measure should be clearly defined and must relate to the primary hypothesis.

Duration

The study duration must be long enough to allow changes in the primary outcome measure and will be determined by data from previous intervention studies and from knowledge of the underlying physiology and

biochemistry, for instance relevant tissue-turnover rates. The duration must also relate to the timescale of the hypothesis, which may address acute effects (e.g. glycaemic response or increased alertness) or longer-term outcomes. Thus, no standard can be set for duration, but the aim should be to set the shortest feasible duration for ethical reasons, to conserve resources and to avoid participant fatigue leading to non-compliance or withdrawal. In some cases, post-study follow-up measures are desirable to evaluate persistence or other longer-term effects, although such follow-up can add significantly to study costs.

Intervention nutrient, food or diet

The intervention will be the nutrient, food or diet under investigation. Consideration must be given, however, to the intended use of the intervention, and the study design should take this into account. For example, if it is intended that a food should be consumed as part of a mixed meal, once a day, then the study design should be testing that pattern of consumption and details of frequency and timing of ingestion reported. If a particular food is the

Table 3.2 Examples of the different study designs that have been used in human nutrition intervention studies published in peer-reviewed journals.

Exploratory, feasibility or pilot studies

Null hypothesis	Duration	Intervention	Control	Main outcome measures	Participant and eligibility criteria	Randomisation	Blinding	Source
Phytoestrogen supplementation does not increase urinary phytoestrogen metabolite excretion or a range of biochemical biomarkers	One day and one week	80 mg mixed phytoestrogen supplement per day	None	Phytoestrogen metabolites, lipids, antioxidant status, DNA damage, insulin status	10 healthy women	No	No	Woodside *et al.* (2006)
A low-carbohydrate, ketogenic diet has no effect on glycaemia and medication use in free-living overweight and obese patients with type 2 diabetes	16 weeks	Low-carbohydrate, ketogenic diet	None; before vs after intervention	Haemoglobin A1c, glucose, insulin, medication use	28 men and women with Type 2 diabetes, 35–75 years; body mass index (BMI) > 25 kg/m^2	No	No	Yancy *et al.* (2005)
A self-monitoring weight-management smartphone app is neither acceptable nor feasible as a standalone weight loss intervention	6 months	Smartphone self-monitoring app	No control per se; similar self-monitoring information to smartphone app group delivered via a website or paper diary	Feasibility and acceptability (adherence to the trial and adherence to the intervention); secondary measures – anthropometry	128 overweight (BMI > 27 kg/m^2) men and women aged 18–65 years	Yes	Researchers carrying out anthropometry assessments blinded to group allocation	Carter *et al.* (2013)
Modified citrus pectin (MCP) does not increase prostate-specific antigen doubling time	One year	14.4g MCP taken as 6 capsules 3 times per day with water or juice	None; before vs after intervention	Prostate-specific antigen doubling time (PSADT)	Men with prostate cancer after localised treatment (n=13)	No; non-randomised	No	Guess *et al.* (2006)

Randomised controlled trials – parallel design

Consumption of wheat aleurone does not increase plasma betaine or affect related biomarkers	4 weeks	Ready-to-eat cereals and bread providing 27 g wheat aleurone/day	Ready-to-eat cereals and bread balanced for macronutrients and fibre	Plasma betaine, choline, B vitamins, homocysteine, LDL-cholesterol	80 men and women at risk of metabolic syndrome (45–65 years; BMI ≥25 kg/m²)	Yes	Single (participant blinded)	Price et al. (2010)
Consumption of nuts does not increase antioxidant status in participants who may have impaired antioxidant status	8 weeks	Habitual diet + cashew or walnuts (20% of daily energy intake)	Prudent control diet; energy adjusted to maintain body weight	Antioxidant status	68 men and women with diagnosed metabolic syndrome according to NCEP ATP III criteria	Yes	No	Davis et al. (2007)
Consumption of whey peptides with in vitro ACE-inhibitory properties does not decrease blood pressure	12 weeks	125 ml milk drink per day with whey peptides	125 ml milk drink per day without whey peptides	Blood pressure, selected inflammatory markers, insulin, glucose	54 patients with mild hypertension not receiving ACE inhibitors or angiotensin II receptor blockers	Yes	Double	Lee et al. (2007)
Probiotics do not prevent gestational diabetes in high-risk pregnant women	16 weeks' gestation to delivery	Probiotic capsule – 1 x 10⁹ cfu each of Lactobacillus rhamnosus GG and Bifidobacterium lactis BB-12 per capsule	Placebo capsule	Diagnosis of gestational diabetes	540 women recruited at 14–16 weeks' gestation (singleton pregnancy) with BMI >25.0 kg/m²	Yes	Double	Dekker Nitert et al. (2013)
Isoflavone-enriched foods do not affect bone mineral density or hormone status	One year	110 mg isoflavones per day in biscuits and bars	Isoflavone-free biscuits and bars identical in composition, taste and appearance	Bone mineral density, panel of hormones, bone biomarkers, lipids and routine clinical chemistry profile	300 women, Caucasian, menopausal for 12–60 months, non-osteoporotic	Yes	Double	Brink et al. (2008)
Beta-carotene supplementation does not reduce risk of malignant neoplasms and cardiovascular disease	12 years	50 mg beta-carotene supplement in capsules on alternate days	Placebo capsules on alternate days	Malignant neoplasms, cardiovascular disease incidence or overall mortality	22 071 male physicians, 40–84 years; 11% current and 39% former smokers BMI 22–29 kg/m²	Yes	Double	Hennekens et al. (1996)

(Continued)

Table 3.2 (*Continued*)

Null hypothesis	Duration	Intervention	Control	Main outcome measures	Participant and eligibility criteria	Randomisation	Blinding	Source
The Mediterranean Diet has no effect on primary cardiovascular disease prevention	Median follow-up 4.8 years	Dietitian-led advice to follow a Mediterranean diet plus provision of key foods (either 1 l extra-virgin olive oil/week or 30 g mixed nuts/day)	Control diet (advice to reduce dietary fat; similar frequency and intensity of dietary advice as intervention groups)	Primary endpoint: composite of myocardial infarction, stroke and death from CVD	7447 men (aged 55–80 years) and women (aged 60–80 years) with no CVD, but who either had diabetes or at least three CVD risk factors	Yes	No (endpoint confirmation conducted blind)	Estruch *et al.* (2013)

Randomised controlled trials – cross-over design

Null hypothesis	Duration	Intervention	Control	Main outcome measures	Participant and eligibility criteria	Randomisation	Blinding	Source
Food and energy intake during ad libitum ingestion of pasta, rice or potato with a meal does not affect food and energy intakes, or insulin and ghrelin levels	One day	Ad libitum intake of meals with pasta, rice or potatoes.	No control per se; a comparison of potatoes, rice or pasta	Food intake (g), energy intake, satiety and hunger feelings, blood insulin, ghrelin and glucose	11 participants with no signs and symptoms of an acute or chronic disease or taking medication; no family history of diabetes mellitus	Yes	No	Erdmann *et al.* (2007)
Availability of different-sized food portions does not affect food and energy intake sensations in normal-weight and overweight adults over four consecutive days under fully residential conditions	4 days	Provision of standard or large portions of the same foods and beverages in a residential setting	No control per se; a comparison of standard and large portions	Food intake (g) and energy intake	44 men and women; 18–65 years; BMI 18·5–30 kg/m²; non-smokers; omnivores; apparently healthy	Yes	Single (participant blinded)	Kelly *et al.* (2009)
Cocoa flavanols from cocoa do not affect dermal microcirculation	One day	100 ml cocoa drink with high flavanol content	100 ml cocoa drink with low flavanol content	Skin microcirculation – blood flow and velocity measured by echo Doppler	10 healthy women, non-smoking and non sunbathing	Yes	Not reported	Neukam *et al.* (2007)

Quasi-experimental studies

Before and after study

Cooking classes will not improve the dietary intake of people with type 2 diabetes	Four weekly cooking classes – each 3 hours' duration	Series of cooking classes for people with type 2 diabetes and their family members held in community locations including schools, churches and senior centres	No	Change in dietary intake (energy, macronutrients, sodium) assessed using three-day food records completed prior to attending cooking school and one month after completing the classes	Type 2 diabetes	n/a – no control group	No	Archuleta *et al.* (2012)

Non-equivalent groups design

Provision of a new food hypermarket in a 'food-retail deficit' community in Glasgow will not increase food availability or have a positive effect on fruit and vegetable consumption, self-reported or psychological health	10 months	Natural experiment – opening of a new food hypermarket in one area of Glasgow	A matched 'comparison' community in Glasgow	Before and after questionnaire assessment of fruit and vegetable consumption, self-reported and psychological health; data for the intervention community compared with data for the 'comparison' community	Intervention community and 'comparison' community were 5 km apart; postal questionnaires distributed to a random selection of households (by postcode) in each community two months before the new hypermarket opened and again 10 months after	No	No	Cummins *et al.* (2005)

intervention being tested, then investigators need to decide whether participants will substitute the test food for habitual foods, whether the test foods will be added to their usual diets, or whether some sort of food-exchange model can be implemented with participants, as each of these scenarios will be answering a slightly different research question. This section outlines some factors to consider when planning the intervention.

Amount consumed

The dose of a nutrient or other component, or the amount of the food to be consumed, will depend on a number of factors (e.g. previous data, underlying physiology, food matrix, palatability and bioavailability). However, the amount to be consumed should be close to that intended for practical use. Furthermore, it is important to test and document the amount of the nutrient or food that is provided, for example by directly measuring the amount of a particular nutrient present in a supplement capsule.

Control group intervention

The control is a food, nutrient, substance or product that does not provide the component that is being tested, and its composition should also be analytically documented. The control should be matched for sensory characteristics and taken in the same way as the test intervention. A control is relatively easy to achieve in supplementation studies using pills or similar preparations by producing a placebo preparation. However, in studies of foods or whole diets, it is more difficult, and perhaps impossible, to develop a control intervention identical to the test intervention but not containing the active component(s) under study. Blinding may not be possible for many foods where the intervention is easily identifiable by both trial participants and researchers, as may be the case with some minimally processed foods such as fruit or vegetables, and some manufactured consumer foods such as cereal products. However, some degree of blinding may be made possible by the use of suitable packaging that conceals products from the researchers and study participants. If the aim is to use a single food group, such as fruit or nuts, then the formulation of a control food is impossible and instead the control arm would receive either no food or a smaller number of portions of the food being studied; this may have effects on other aspects of diet and behaviour. For whole-diet interventions, for example the Mediterranean Diet, it is usual to measure self-reported adherence to that diet using a previously developed scoring scheme, with control groups not receiving the dietary advice and therefore being less adherent to the whole-diet pattern and consequently attaining lower scores. Further guidance on attaining an ideal control is available in other published literature, but is likely to vary depending on the type of intervention being tested.

Outcome measures

All intervention studies will assess outcome measures and will compare these between intervention and control groups, if a control group features in the study design. Most studies will have a range of outcome measures, but the study should be powered based on the pre-specified primary outcome measure, as stated in the hypothesis, and the sample size calculated using that outcome measure (see the discussion of size of study later in this chapter). Similarly, if an outcome is assessed at several time points over the course of the study, either a single time point or a single summary measure of results at several time points should be pre-specified as the primary outcome measure. All outcome measures, whether primary or secondary, should be stated and defined in the study protocol.

It is essential that the outcome measure is of biological relevance. In some cases the outcome measure is clearly relevant, as it is a direct, objective measure of the impact on nutritional intake or status (e.g. energy intake or nutrient concentration in plasma – see Chapters 4, 6, 11 and 12) or intended health effect (e.g. body weight, or diagnosis of a disease or muscle strength). Subjective measures are also used, such as feelings of health, appetite or fatigue; in these cases, it is important to use validated instruments if these are available. When the effect cannot be measured directly, indirect or surrogate factors such as biological markers or risk factors are used to reflect a functional, physiological or biochemical characteristic associated with a disease, or as a predictor of the later development of the disease. Examples include glycated haemoglobin as an indicator of long-term hyperglycaemia and risk of type 2 diabetes complications, plasma LDL-cholesterol as a measure of cardiovascular disease risk, bone mineral density as a measure of osteoporosis risk, complex metabolomic or proteomic profiles as markers of function and disease risk, and the presence of adenomatous colon polyps as an early indicator of colon cancer. Most indirect outcome measures are chosen because they reflect consensus guidelines or are commonly used by experts in the area. For example, detailed guidelines have been proposed for particular outcomes such as the assessment of glycaemic responses or satiety. However, very few markers have been assessed and validated by expert consensus in terms of their specificity, variability, limitations and applicability to a range of population groups.

Methodological aspects

An effort should be made to standardise all outcome measure assessments and reduce measurement error as far as possible (e.g. by standardising measurement protocols, training observers and averaging several measurements rather than using a single measurement), especially if measurement errors are known to be large. Where possible, the researcher assessing study outcomes should be blinded to the intervention assignment.

Analytical variability

Laboratory analytical methods should be precise, accurate, sensitive and specific, and these performance characteristics should be recorded in a file of standard operating procedures (SOPs) or similar-quality record documents for the study. Intra-laboratory analytical variability should be minimised by using automated equipment to analyse samples in duplicate or triplicate, in batches that represent the range of interventions, participants and sampling times, with suitable internal and external standards and participation in quality assurance programmes. Ideally, all samples from a study should be analysed at the same time, and all samples from an individual participant in one run, but this may be precluded by degradation in storage, even at low temperatures. Biomarkers that have high methodological variability will often require a larger number of trial participants to give the study adequate power.

Biological variability

Biological variability arises from many factors (e.g. genetic background, circadian rhythm, seasonal differences, menstrual cycle) and may introduce systematic bias. Thus, it is important to understand the factors underlying this variability for the biomarkers, and to take samples or adapt the study design accordingly.

Biologically meaningful changes

Although a trial may find a statistically significant change in an outcome measure, such a response does not necessarily mean that the intervention will be effective in terms of producing a discernible health benefit or risk reduction in the target group. Thus, the size of the change and its potential biological, clinical or public health significance should also be considered when performing the sample size calculation (see later in this chapter).

Selection of participants: Eligibility criteria

Eligibility criteria, which often include age, gender, health and disease status, are functional, physiological or clinical characteristics or demographic variables used to define the study population. Eligibility criteria may also include lifestyle factors, such as smoking habit or level of physical activity, and dietary factors such as low fibre intake or the consumption of restricted diets. Eligibility criteria can be presented as inclusion and exclusion criteria.

Eligibility criteria should describe participants adequately, so that the results can be appropriately interpreted in terms of their generalisability. Eligibility criteria should also be selected with the target population for the

test intervention, as well as the hypothesis and outcome measures, in mind. Inter-participant variation may be reduced by using stricter eligibility criteria to select a more homogenous group of participants for the study. However, this approach also has the disadvantage of restricting the target population and consequently will limit the generalisability of the findings. Children and women of childbearing age will need to be excluded from any studies that may have an adverse effect on normal growth and development or have teratogenic potential.

It is important to define eligibility criteria using objective quantitative descriptors wherever possible. For example, many nutrition interventions use 'apparently healthy' participants. Health may be evaluated by using a questionnaire on medical history and surgical events, or this may be extended to a physical examination and screening of blood and urine. 'Health' may merely refer to the absence of diagnosed disease, or to a specific aspect such as a healthy blood pressure, and in such cases the criteria can be very specific and may follow official guidelines. However, 'apparently healthy' may also include a healthy lifestyle, which could be assessed using questionnaires, for example for physical activity, dietary habits, smoking, alcohol and medication use.

Statistical considerations

Randomisation

Randomisation is the allocation of participants to interventions using a random process such as the toss of a coin. It ensures that the investigator does not bias the study outcome by influencing the intervention to which a participant is allocated. The main advantage of random allocation is that it will produce study groups that are comparable with respect to both known and unknown factors that could influence the outcome measure. That is, it ensures that potential confounding factors are equally distributed between groups. Consequently, it increases the internal validity of the study, meaning that any observed difference in the responses of the two intervention groups is likely to be due to the effects of the intervention. Randomisation helps to ensure that the comparison of interventions is fair (by eliminating selection bias) and that the statistical analysis is valid.

To allocate individual participants to intervention groups, random number generation (either from tables or more usually by computer) is often used. However, it is advisable to ensure that approximately equal numbers of participants are assigned to each group by using a restricted (or block) randomisation, in which participants are divided into blocks within which equal numbers of allocations are made to each intervention. To avoid any possible predictability of the allocations at the end of a block, it is advisable to vary the block size. It is often desirable to stratify participants into subgroups defined by important variables such as age, gender and ethnicity that could influence the response to intervention. A restricted randomisation is then conducted within each subgroup. Stratification will generally result in more comparable study groups and can also reduce variability in the response measure when incorporated into the statistical analysis. Minimisation, a technique that minimises imbalance between the participants in the intervention groups over a number of variables simultaneously, may offer a more practical approach than stratification on multiple variables.

Concealment of the intervention allocations

CONSORT highlights the importance of detailing who generated the study randomisation schedule, who allocated participants and what steps were taken to conceal the allocation in order to minimise bias, subconscious or otherwise. Successful randomisation should result in an unpredictable allocation sequence (i.e. the researcher will not be able to predict to which group the next participants will be assigned) and adequate concealment of the allocation sequences until the participant is made aware of their group assignment. In a multicentre trial, a telephone randomisation procedure can be implemented to safeguard the allocation sequence. For a small, single-centre trial, a simple way to eliminate any possible bias of this sort is to implement randomisation using sealed envelopes. In this process, the random intervention allocations are concealed in sequentially numbered, opaque, sealed envelopes, prepared by a researcher who is not involved in the recruitment or allocation of participants. Only after a participant has given consent, been enrolled in the study and the envelope endorsed with the participant's name should the seal be broken to reveal to which intervention the participant has been allocated. This process ensures that knowledge of forthcoming assignments is not available to researchers and shields the allocation sequence until assignment occurs.

Blinding

The assessment of study outcomes may be influenced by knowledge of which intervention was received, particularly for subjective outcomes. Such bias can be avoided by using blinded assessment. If neither assessor nor participant knows which intervention the participant received, then the study is double blind. If the participant knows but the assessor does not (or vice versa), then the study is single blind. Blinding should also be carried through into laboratory determinations and statistical analysis. The time of unblinding, which is usually after the freezing of the database (i.e. when all data entry for the study is completed and the study database has been checked and finalised), should be documented in the study report and may be mentioned in any subsequent document.

Where possible, and particularly for food products, the effectiveness of blinding should be assessed at the end of the study and commented on in the study report. This can be achieved by the use of a simple questionnaire asking participants which product (test or control) they thought they were consuming.

Size of study (power calculation)

It is essential to estimate the number of participants required for the study. A study that is too small is likely to fail to detect important differences between interventions, while one that is too large may needlessly waste resources and would be unethical. In certain circumstances trials may be designed to be analysed after every participant's result becomes available (sequential design) or after pre-specified numbers of participants' results become available (group sequential designs). These designs are ethically appealing because they ensure that inferior interventions are quickly identified, so minimising the numbers receiving them. However, even when such early termination is feasible it is not always advisable, since it can lead to intervention effects being estimated with poor precision.

The usual methods for sample size estimation require specification of the magnitude of the smallest meaningful difference in the outcome variable. The study must be sufficiently large to have acceptable power to detect this difference as statistically significant, and must take into account possible non-compliance and the anticipated drop-out rate. Information about the degree of variability in the outcome is also required and may come from previous published or unpublished data, or from a pilot or exploratory study specifically performed for the purpose (discussed earlier in this chapter). A multicentre study may be necessary if the study is too large to be performed in a single centre. Statisticians are key members of research teams and it is recommended they are involved at an early stage, not only in study size calculation but also in planning the design and analysis of the study.

Ethical approval and study registration

Researchers should determine the appropriate local ethical approval and research governance procedures required for their study, and seek these approvals before the study commences. While not all nutrition research may be classified as medical research, it is recommended that researchers adhere to the World Medical Association's Helsinki Declaration. One of its recommendations is that every clinical trial (including human nutrition intervention studies) must be registered in a publicly accessible database before recruitment of the first participant. Such registration, with accompanying protocol details, is intended to reduce the consequences of non-publication of studies (for example, repetition of negative studies), of selective reporting of outcomes and of reporting per protocol (PP) rather than intention to treat (ITT) analyses (see on the discussion of statistical analysis later I this chapter). The WHO has stated that 'the registration of all interventional trials is a scientific, ethical and moral responsibility', while the International Committee of Medical Journal Editors only considers trials for publication if they are registered before enrolment of their first participant. The academic view is that a priori trial registration is essential for ethical research in humans.

Recruitment and participant flow

The study protocol should state the methods by which participants will be recruited, and details of the recruitment process should be carefully described, with details of numbers of participants approached, screened, recruited and completing, and reasons noted for non-recruitment (ineligibility, lack of willingness to participate) and non-completion. Informed consent should be obtained. When reporting the study, this information is best summarised in a participant flow diagram, such as that suggested by CONSORT (as illustrated in Figure 3.2).

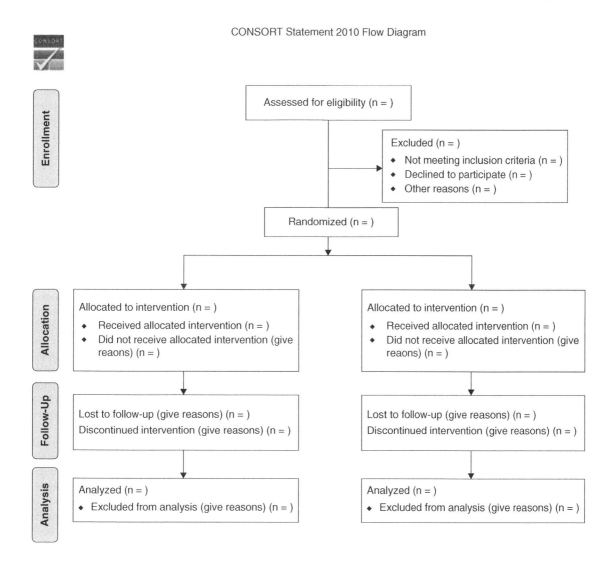

CONSORT Statement 2010 Flow Diagram

For more information, visit www.consort-statement.org.

Figure 3.2 Flow diagram of the progress through the phases of a parallel randomised trial of two groups. Schulz, K.F., Altman, D.G. and Moher, D. (2010) CONSORT 2010 Statement: Updated guidelines for reporting parallel group randomised trials. *British Medical Journal*, **340**, c332.

Data collection

Data should be collected using a standardised case report form. Participants should be assigned a unique study number at the start of the study, and all their data should then be held under that study number. That is, no participant-identifiable information should be held by the researchers, other than a single sheet where the study number is linked to the participant contact details. All data, both paper and computer-based, should be kept securely and all data collection conducted in line with the required local ethical and research governance regulations.

Background diet and change in diet during intervention

The nature of the participants' background diet may be one of the eligibility criteria. Regardless of this, and particularly in longer-term studies, it is important to collect background dietary information in order to characterise the participants' habitual diet in terms of nutrient intake, food consumption and overall dietary pattern. Diet should also be assessed during longer-term interventions in order to detect changes in it over time that may potentially confound the results of the study. Such an assessment will be particularly important when the intervention is with whole foods or whole diets, where the control arm is more difficult to design and define, and where blinding is not possible. Where a nutritional supplement is being tested against a placebo, randomisation has been performed and double blinding has been possible, any dietary changes over the course of the intervention period would be expected to be equally distributed between the intervention and control groups. However, with food or whole-diet interventions where participant blinding is impossible, dietary changes will differ between intervention and control groups, and full dietary assessment is particularly important to establish, for example, how a particular food or food group has been incorporated into the overall diet; whether other foods have been displaced as a result of the intervention; and the impact that has had on overall diet quality and nutrient intake. For some outcome measures that are affected by body weight, such as insulin resistance, assessment of the impact of a dietary change ideally requires body weight to be maintained over the course of the intervention, and therefore intervention and control diets will have to be carefully energy matched and weight monitored during the intervention period.

A number of dietary assessment methodologies are available, including retrospective tools such as a food frequency questionnaire or diet history, and prospective methods such as a food diary or weighed food record (see Chapter 4). However, dietary intake assessment methods are subject to misreporting. In order to check the reliability of dietary data, reported energy intakes should be compared with the estimated energy requirement for each participant and compared to established cut-offs for under- or over-estimating energy intake. This is particularly important if these assessments are being used as a way of monitoring compliance.

Background health status and lifestyle, and changes in health status and lifestyle during intervention

In addition to their possible role as eligibility criteria, it is also important to characterise the study population in terms of demographic background, health status and lifestyle behaviours, in order to allow appropriate interpretation and generalisation of the results. Examples include age, gender, level of medication use, years of formal education, socio-economic status, physical activity and smoking habit. The monitoring of health status and lifestyle behaviours should also be carried out in the course of longer-term studies to assess potential between-group differences, which may confound outcome measures.

Adverse events

An adverse event (AE) is any unfavourable and unintended sign (including an abnormal laboratory finding), symptom or disease temporally associated with the use of an intervention, whether or not it is considered to be related to the intervention. Recording AEs is of major importance in pharmaceutical studies, allowing a risk–benefit analysis. Hence, there is an abundance of guidelines for the management of AEs in the clinical study setting (e.g. European Medicines Agency; International Conference on Harmonisation of Technical Requirements for Registration of Pharmaceuticals for Human Use; US Department of Health and Human Services, Food and Drug Administration). There are no guidelines for nutrition intervention studies, given that these studies involve testing foods, supplements or ingredients in participants that are usually apparently healthy. However, the formal recording of AEs is required for good practice in nutrition research.

It is generally regarded as good practice to record all AEs, no matter how trivial, in a participant's file. In the case of nutrition studies, AEs are likely to be very minor in nature, for example mild nausea or minor gastrointestinal discomfort. Such occurrences may be the result of changes in dietary pattern or consumption of unfamiliar products and will often lessen over time as the body adjusts to the dietary changes. These minor events are sometimes known as unintended effects (to use recent CONSORT terminology). Their recording is desirable and important in human nutrition interventions, as it contributes to data on the tolerability of the product.

Some of these minor occurrences will be anticipated by investigators; if so, questionnaires should be used to provide quantifiable data, employing standardised formats where available, for example to assess gastrointestinal effects such as bloating or flatulence. Data should be collected at baseline and at suitable intervals during the study to assess onset and time course. Time, intervention and group effects should be tested statistically and, if significant, potential influence on compliance, withdrawal and outcome measures should be considered.

Any serious or unexpected adverse events that are encountered, whether or not they appear to be related to the intervention, should be reported immediately to the lead researcher, the relevant research ethics committee, the sponsor and other relevant regulatory bodies for review and appropriate management.

Compliance

Any deviations from protocol can affect the validity and relevance of an intervention study. Low levels of participant compliance in nutrition studies decrease the power to detect effects on specified endpoints, result in false negative findings, and ultimately mean that the study is unable to provide evidence to support or refute a potentially beneficial effect of the intervention. Poor compliance in a particular subgroup will also reduce the generalisability of the results and has implications for wide-scale implementation of the intervention. When compliance is very different between allocated groups, this may be because acceptability of the interventions differs. Therefore, a nutrition intervention study should aim to have measures in place to maximise and assess compliance.

Methods to encourage and measure compliance

The choice of compliance assessment methods will depend on study design, duration and intervention type. In acute or postprandial studies, the intervention is usually consumed only once, or a limited number of times, under supervision, and thus compliance is not usually an issue. However, maintaining compliance throughout longer-term studies is very important and may employ one of the strategies discussed here. Consumption under supervision throughout the dietary intervention will maximise compliance; however, this has resource implications, as it will require the use of a special nutrition facility and an intensive level of research staffing (observations may last a few hours, be at meal times only or extend to residential studies lasting several days or weeks). The complete provision of intervention supplements or food or diets for consumption in a free-living situation is a more commonly used approach and par-

ticipants would be asked to return any unconsumed items. However, in this case an assumption is made that all unreturned items have been consumed, which may not be the case. In addition to providing intervention foods, maintaining regular contact with participants is key to achieving good compliance, as it allows any issues to be identified and dealt with at an early stage. Furthermore, informing participants that compliance will be measured is likely, in itself, to improve adherence to the dietary intervention. Dietary records, such as food diaries or diet recall methods, can be used to measure compliance, but such self-reported intake data are predisposed to errors (see earlier in this chapter). Thus, the assessment of tissue biomarkers as independent and objective measures of compliance is preferred when possible (e.g. serum selenium or fatty acid composition of erythrocyte membranes; see Chapter 8).

Acceptable levels of compliance

Acceptable levels of compliance for human nutrition studies have rarely been stated and are difficult to comment on definitively (see later in this chapter for discussion of how compliance will affect statistical analysis). A decision about the statistical analysis approach will be partly influenced by whether studies are designed as tests of efficacy (biological effect) or effectiveness (with the potential to modify outcome in a real-life situation), as the former studies will be more focused on maximising compliance. Making a decision on an acceptable level of compliance relies on an accurate, objective assessment of compliance being available. A priori decisions should be made regarding the acceptable level of compliance for inclusion in a PP analysis. For example, in a supplement study a level of consuming more than 80% of the supplements provided might be specified as an indicator of good compliance.

Statistical analysis

There are a number of statistics books that cover the basics of randomised intervention trial methodology, both in the design and analysis phases. It is good practice to include a statistical analysis plan that specifies the statistical methods to be used in the trial protocol. The hypotheses to be tested for both primary and secondary outcomes (including whether they are one-sided or two-sided) and the significance level to be employed should be clearly stated.

Rationale for using statistical methodology

In common with other research in medicine and the biological sciences, the differences between groups that the investigator wishes to identify in a nutrition study are usually masked by several types of variation (inter- and intra-participant variation, measurement error and so on); strategies to minimise these have been outlined earlier in this chapter.

These errors mean that there is a need for the results of a study to be assessed objectively using appropriate statistical methodology. This section describes the basic statistical concepts necessary for the analysis of nutrition intervention studies. Although tests of hypotheses play a key role here, it is worth emphasising that the calculation of confidence intervals for intervention effects can often be more informative.

In general, statistical techniques require an assumption that the group under study may be considered to be a random sample from a target population about which inferences are to be made. In practice, there would be considerable practical difficulties in mounting an intervention study on a truly random sample from a target population, and usually a convenience sample such as a group of healthy volunteers or patients attending a hospital out-patient clinic will be studied. The investigator should be particularly cautious in any extrapolation of findings beyond the population from which the study sample was drawn. It is also worth emphasising that statistical methods will only take account of sampling error (i.e. variation arising from the process of sampling); they cannot quantify the extent of biases attributable to nonrandom sampling, particularly bias that may be introduced through losses to follow-up.

Preliminary steps in data analysis
Before attempting any formal statistical comparisons, it is important to visualise the data with histograms and scatter diagrams to examine the shapes of distributions, to check for outliers and to establish the nature of any relationships between variables.

Suitable descriptive statistics should also be presented to characterise the participants under study, and an indispensable step is to construct a table of participant characteristics by group. For quantitative variables, this should include both measures of location and measures of dispersion, typically the mean and standard deviation for roughly symmetrically distributed variables or the median and interquartile range for variables whose distribution is heavily skewed. For categorical variables, both frequencies and percentages should be included in this table. In an adequately randomised study it is not usually considered necessary to perform statistical tests on these baseline group characteristics, since any differences observed between groups must be due to chance.

Hypothesis tests for comparing groups
Along with the study design, the scale of measurement of the response variable is of fundamental importance in deciding which statistical analysis techniques to use.

Here we provide a brief description of statistical techniques suitable for simple randomisation studies.

Parametric methods
For a study using a parallel groups design and an interval scale response variable (e.g. weight or blood pressure), the independent samples t-test will be used to compare two groups and one-way analysis of variance to compare three or more groups. For the two-period cross-over study, a refinement of the paired t-test is available, suggested by Hills and Armitage (2004), which takes account of the variability attributable to period effects and provides a test for carryover. If baseline values of a response variable are available, then changes in the variable during the intervention may be calculated and used in the analysis. However, if the baseline response values are not highly correlated with the final response values, then it can be more beneficial to analyse the final value in an analysis of covariance with the initial value considered as the covariate. For studies that take more than two serial measurements of response variables, the derivation of a summary measure such as a slope or area under the curve may permit the application of straightforward statistical techniques and avoid the need for more complex methods for correlated responses. Intervention effects, often expressed as means or differences in means, should be estimated along with their associated 95% confidence intervals.

Non-parametric methods
For ordinal scale outcomes non-parametric methods are typically employed, with the Mann–Whitney U test used to compare two groups, and Kruskal–Wallis one-way analysis of variance of ranks to compare three or more groups. However, these techniques focus on hypothesis testing, and confidence limits associated with them are not widely available. Non-parametric methods may also be useful for analysing interval scale variables for which the assumptions necessary for parametric methods are in doubt. Particularly in small studies, the assumption of normality in the distribution of the response variable is important. However, in such situations it may be possible to avoid resorting to non-parametric methods by transforming the data (often using a logarithmic transformation to reduce the degree of positive skew) prior to applying a parametric method.

Contingency table methods
For nominal scale (or unordered categorical) outcome variables, analysis is performed using chi-squared tests for contingency tables or Fisher's exact probability test where numbers are small. Confidence intervals for proportions, for differences in proportions, for odds ratios or for risk ratios may also be useful for characterising intervention effects.

If information on covariates is available, then it may be incorporated into an analysis of covariance to improve the precision of comparisons between intervention groups for an interval scale response. The technique does assume that there is a linear relationship between the response and the covariate in each group and that the linear relationships are parallel in the groups, assumptions that should be checked prior to using the method. It may also be useful in adjusting for chance imbalances between the intervention groups on factors relevant to the response. For a two-category response variable, logistic regression analysis may be employed in a similar way.

The interpretation of analyses involving more than two intervention groups may be complicated by the multiplicity of statistical tests. If the aim of an analysis is restricted to making only a small number of pre-specified comparisons between groups, as stated in the study protocol, then multiple testing is less of an issue. However, tests of hypotheses other than these (e.g. hypotheses formulated after looking at the results) require a more conservative approach in the statistical analysis to limit the risk of false positive findings. A similar issue arises in the interpretation of tests on multiple response variables. Ideally investigators should nominate the primary outcome measure in the study protocol. Other responses may still be analysed, but a stricter significance level may be appropriate to safeguard against false positive findings.

A recent development in nutrition research has been to use genomics, proteomics and metabolomics approaches as endpoints in nutrition intervention studies (see Chapter 13). Such studies often have multiple endpoints and no prior hypotheses, which raises similar statistical issues. If the multiple endpoints are independent, then a simple Bonferroni correction is sufficient to control the risk of type 1 error, with a significance level set not at the α level but at the α/k level, where k is the number of endpoints. An alternative approach, which retains more power than the Bonferroni correction and is more suited to microarray work, is to control the false discovery rate; that is, the expected proportion of false positives among the results that are declared significant. For dependent endpoints, comparisons are better performed by a permutation test. This involves comparing the largest test statistic obtained in the analyses of the various endpoints, not with a standard distribution (such as the t distribution or chi-squared distribution), but instead with its permutation distribution, obtained by calculating the largest test statistic in every possible random relabelling of the groups (or at least in a very large random sample of them).

Intention to treat or per protocol
An important issue in the analysis of interventions is to decide how protocol deviations should be handled.

Usually the most relevant comparison of interventions will include all randomised participants who began the intervention, and the analysis will be conducted on an 'intention to treat' (ITT) principle. In an ITT analysis, once participants have been randomised to intervention groups, all available results are analysed in the groups to which they were allocated, regardless of whether or not the participants complied with the intervention. In nutrition studies there is often interest in examining response in the subset of participants who showed the best, or different levels of, compliance with the intervention (for a discussion of adequate levels of compliance see earlier in this chapter) and a 'per protocol' (PP) analysis may then be more relevant, even though this approach has a greater potential for introducing bias into the comparison of interventions.

Interpretation

The interpretation of study findings, and the discussion section of a resulting publication, should include a consideration of the study limitations, including any potential sources of bias (for example imbalance in baseline characteristics), imprecision (in outcome assessments) or an acknowledgement of the possibility of spurious statistically significant findings arising from multiple comparisons. The generalisability of the study findings should also be considered and limitations acknowledged. Conclusions should be confirmed and justified by the accompanying data. The conclusions should relate directly to the hypothesis, to the intervention at the dose or amount consumed, and to the population included in the study. Conclusions about secondary outcome measures should be stated as such and interpreted appropriately.

Roles and responsibilities of the research team

Complex issues arise because of potential conflicts of interest and scientific bias, particularly when research funding may come from the food industry. Many journals now require statements of the roles and responsibilities of all members of the research team, including the funders or sponsors, and declarations of any potential conflicts of interest. This should be standard practice when publishing any intervention study.

3.4 Conclusion

Intervention studies are a vital part of nutrition research, as if well designed they allow the testing of causality. Nutrition intervention studies vary considerably in study design and duration, but there are a number of key design factors that must be considered when planning such a study, including the research question or hypothesis; duration; the intervention nutrient, food or diet; the intervention dose or amount; the control arm and blinding of the control; the primary and secondary outcome measures (including assessment of background diet); eligibility criteria; data-collection methodology; and measuring and encouraging compliance. Early involvement of a statistician in the study team to guide on both study design and statistical analysis is crucial. Local ethical approval and research governance procedures must be followed, and intervention studies registered before recruitment starts on a publicly accessible database. Finally, when reporting the results of the intervention, interpretation should be appropriate and any potential conflicts of interest, for example when funding has come from the food industry, should be declared.

Acknowledgements

JVW, RWW and CCP were members of the Expert Group on Guidelines for Human Intervention Studies to Scientifically Substantiate Claims on Foods, which was a working group of the ILSI Europe Functional Foods Task Force, and acknowledge the discussions of that group, which led to a scientific publication (listed in the references) and was the basis of the guidance presented here.

References and further reading

Archuleta, M., Vanleeuwen, D., Halderson, K. *et al.* (2012) Cooking schools improve nutrient intake patterns of people with type 2 diabetes. *Journal of Nutrition Education and Behavior*, **44** (4), 319–325.

Blundell, J., de Graaf, C., Hulshof, T. *et al.* (2010) Appetite control: Methodological aspects of the evaluation of foods. *Obesity Reviews*, **11** (3), 251–270.

Bonell, C.P., Hargreaves, J., Cousens, S. *et al.* (2011) Alternatives to randomisation in the evaluation of public health interventions: Design challenges and solutions. *Journal of Epidemiology and Community Health*, **65**, 582–587.

Brink, E., Coxam, V., Robins, S. *et al.* (2008) Long-term consumption of isoflavone-enriched foods does not affect bone mineral density, bone metabolism, or hormonal status in early postmenopausal women: A randomized, double-blind, placebo controlled study. *American Journal of Clinical Nutrition*, **87**, 761–770.

Brouns, F., Bjorck, I., Frayn, K.N. *et al.* (2005) Glycaemic index methodology. *Nutrition Research Reviews*, **18** (1), 145–171.

Carter, M.C., Burley, V.J., Nykjaer, C. and Cade, J.E. (2013) Adherence to a smartphone application for weight loss compared to website and paper diary: Pilot randomised controlled trial. *Journal of Medical Internet Research*, **15** (4), e32.

Craig, P., Dieppe, P., Macintyre, S. *et al.* (2008) Developing and evaluating complex interventions: The new Medical Research Council guidance. *British Medical Journal*, **337**, a1655.

Cummins, S., Petticrew, M., Higgins, C. *et al.* (2005) Large scale food retailing as an intervention for diet and health: Quasi-experimental evaluation of a natural experiment. *Journal of Epidemiology and Community Health*, **59**, 1035–1040.

Davis, P.A., Vasu, V.T., Gohil, K. *et al.* (2007) The effects of high walnut and cashew nut diets on the antioxidant status of subjects with metabolic syndrome. *European Journal of Nutrition*, **46**, 155–164.

Dekker Nitert M., Barrett1, H.L., Foxcroft, K. *et al.* (2013) SPRING: An RCT study of probiotics in the prevention of gestational diabetes mellitus in overweight and obese women. *BMC Pregnancy and Childbirth*, **13**, 50.

Erdmann, J., Hebeisen, Y., Lippl, F. et al. (2007) Food intake and plasma ghrelin response during potato-, rice- and pasta-rich meals. *European Journal of Nutrition*, **46**, 196–203.

Estruch, R., Ros, E., Salas-Salvadó, J. et al. (2013) Primary prevention of cardiovascular disease with a Mediterranean diet. *New England Journal of Medicine*, **368**, 1279–1290.

European Medicines Agency (1995) *Note for Guidance on Clinical Safety Data Management: Definitions and Standards for Expedited Reporting* (CPMP/ICH/377/95), http://www.ema.europa.eu/docs/en_GB/document_library/Scientific_guideline/2009/09/WC500002749.pdf (accessed October 2013).

Friedman, L.M., Furberg, C.D. and DeMets, D.L. (2010) *Fundamentals of Clinical Trials*, 4th edn. Springer, New York.

Guess, B.W., Scholz, M.C. and Strum, S.B. (2006) Modified citrus pectin (MCP) increases the prostate-specific antigen doubling time in men with prostate cancer: A phase II pilot study. *Prostate Cancer and Prostatic Diseases*, **6**, 301–304.

Hennekens, C.H., Buring, J.E., Manson, J.E. *et al.* (1996) Lack of effect of long-term supplementation with beta carotene on the incidence of malignant neoplasms and cardiovascular disease. *New England Journal of Medicine*, **334**, 1145–1149.

Hills, M. and Armitage, P. (2004) The two-period cross-over clinical trial. *British Journal of Clinical Pharmacology*, **58**, S703–S716.

International Committee of Medical Journal Editors (n.d.) *Clinical Trial Registration*. http://www.icmje.org/recommendations/browse/publishing-and-editorial-issues/clinical-trial-registration.html (accessed June 2014).

Kelly, M.T., Wallace, J.M.W., Robson, P.J. *et al.* (2009) Increased portion size leads to a sustained increase in energy intake over 4 d in normal-weight and overweight men and women. *British Journal of Nutrition*, **102**, 470–477.

Lee, Y.M., Skurk, T., Hennig, M. and Hauner, H. (2007) Effect of a milk drink supplemented with whey peptides on blood pressure in patients with mild hypertension. *European Journal of Nutrition*, **46**, 21–27.

Machin, D. and Fayers, P. (2010) *Randomized Clinical Trials: Design, Practice and Reporting*. Wiley-Blackwell, Chichester.

Matthews, J.N., Altman, D.G., Campbell, M.J. *et al.* (1990) Analysis of serial measurements in medical research. *British Medical Journal*, **300**, 230–235.

Moher, D., Hopewell, S., Schulz, K.F. *et al.* (2010) CONSORT 2010 Explanation and Elaboration: Updated guidelines for reporting parallel group randomised trials. *British Medical Journal*, **340**, c869.

Neukam, K., Stahl, W., Tronnier, H. *et al.* (2007) Consumption of flavanol-rich cocoa acutely increases microcirculation in human skin. *European Journal of Nutrition*, **46**, 53–56.

Peace, K.E. and Chen, D. (2011) *Clinical Trial Methodology*. Chapman & Hall/CRC, Boca Raton, FL.

Piantadosi, S. (2005) *Clinical Trials: A Methodological Perspective*, 2nd edn. John Wiley & Sons, Inc, Hoboken, NJ.

Pocock, S.J. (1983) *Clinical Trials: A Practical Approach*. John Wiley & Sons Ltd, Chichester.

Price, R.K., Keaveney, E.M., Hamill, L.L. *et al.* (2010) Consumption of wheat aleurone-rich foods increases fasting plasma betaine and modestly decreases fasting homocysteine and LDL-cholesterol in adults. *Journal of Nutrition*, **140**, 2153–2157.

Schulz, K.F., Altman, D.G. and Moher, D. (2010) CONSORT 2010 Statement: Updated guidelines for reporting parallel group randomised trials. *British Medical Journal*, **340**, c332.

Welch, R.W., Antoine, J.-M., Berta, J.-L. *et al.* (2011) Guidelines for the design, conduct and reporting of human intervention studies to evaluate the health benefits of foods. *British Journal of Nutrition*, **106**, S2–S15.

Woodside, J.V., Campbell, M.J., Denholm, E.E. *et al.* (2006) Short-term phytoestrogen supplementation alters insulin-like growth factor profile but not lipid or antioxidant status. Journal of Nutritional Biochemistry, **17**, 211–215.

Woodside, J.V., Koletzko, B.V., Patterson, C.C. and Welch, R.W. (2013) Scientific standards for human intervention trials evaluating the health benefits of foods and their application to infants, children and adolescents. *World Review of Nutrition and Dietetics*, **108**, 18–31.

World Medical Association (2008) *Declaration of Helsinki – Ethical Principles for Medical Research Involving Human Subjects*, http://www.wma.net/en/30publications/10policies/b3/index.html (accessed October 2013).

Yancy, W.S. Jr, Foy, M., Chalecki, A.M. *et al.* (2005) A low-carbohydrate, ketogenic diet to treat type 2 diabetes. *Nutrition and Metabolism*, **2**, 34.

4
Methods to Determine Dietary Intake

Nadia Slimani, Heinz Freisling, Anne-Kathrin Illner and Inge Huybrechts

International Agency for Research on Cancer, France

Key messages

- We are living through major nutritional, methodological and technological transitions that raise new challenges and new opportunities to measure, monitor and compare dietary intakes.
- Different traditional dietary intake assessment methods are being used in various study settings. Each method has its unique features with its strengths and limitations.
- Dietary methodologies should benefit from new technologies. However, a clear distinction should be made between (new) dietary methodologies and (new) technologies. While existing dietary methodologies are relatively limited, the increasing development of different new technologies might confuse users' evaluation of their respective features and challenge the choices made.

- Dietary methodologies are prone to measurement errors, which should be carefully evaluated and minimised as much as possible.
- Dietary patterns aim to combine a large number of correlated dietary variables, estimated at the food, nutrient and/or related biomarker levels, into fewer independent (uncorrelated) components (i.e. patterns).
- Frontline nutritional research increasingly favours the use of integrated approaches to measure dietary intake. This includes (repeated) open-ended dietary methods (24-hour dietary recalls or food records) complemented by a food propensity questionnaire (for infrequently consumed foods) and biological markers (including metabolomics).

4.1 Challenges to assessing and monitoring dietary intake

Among the different environmental and lifestyle risk factors, diet is one of the most complex exposures to investigate in relation to some diseases. Indeed, diet is a universal exposure consumed in infinite combinations of foods and recipes, with large variations within and between individuals and over the whole life span. In addition, the several thousand chemicals (including contaminants) present in the diet may have complex synergistic or antagonistic bioactive effects. As a consequence, it makes it difficult to disentangle individual chemical and nutrient effects as well as to remove confounding completely when investigating diet–disease relationships and their underlying biological mechanisms. Diet may also have strong social, religious and psychological features that have impacts on study and questionnaire designs, logistics and ultimately the individual's dietary intakes.

The 'nutrition transition', characterised by a moving away from traditional diets towards more Western diets (rich in energy, fats, salt and sugar), is consistently observed with accelerated phenomena worldwide. This is another major challenge in measuring, monitoring and investigating diet and its associations with diseases, particularly cancer and cardiovascular disease. Indeed, cancer is a multiphasic and multifactorial disease, often occurring late in life. However, the lifelong cumulated risks might be affected by different (early) 'exposure windows', which are difficult to evaluate through single (or limited) repeated dietary measurements collected in nutritional epidemiology. Furthermore, the food frequency questionnaire (FFQ) assessment method predominantly used in large study settings has been repeatedly challenged with respect to its validity and reliability for measuring individual dietary intake. As a consequence, nutritional research has increasingly favoured approaches integrating traditional and more innovative measurements of dietary exposure (including biological and

Nutrition Research Methodologies, First Edition. Edited by Julie A Lovegrove, Leanne Hodson, Sangita Sharma and Susan A Lanham-New.
© 2015 John Wiley & Sons, Ltd. Published 2015 by John Wiley & Sons, Ltd.
Companion Website: www.wiley.com/go/nutritionsociety

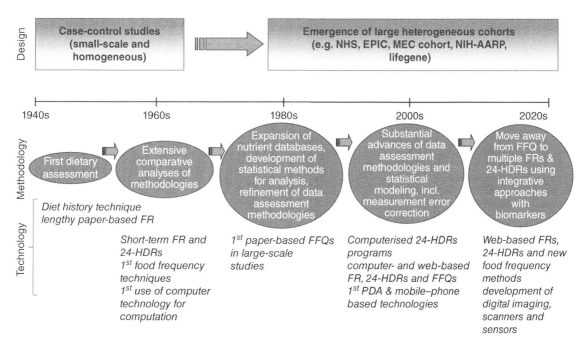

Figure 4.1 Evolution of design, methodology and technology in dietary assessment.

metabolite – intermediate or surrogate – markers) to improve the individual and population mean intakes and distribution.

This chapter reflects the major methodological and technological transitions in measuring individual dietary intake that have occurred over the last two to three decades by reporting both traditional and more innovative dietary assessment methodologies (or technologies), including combined approaches (Figure 4.1). A better understanding of their respective strengths and limitations as well as their comprehensive integration should pave the way for a more holistic and reliable estimation of individual (or population) dietary exposure, as an essential prerequisite for cost-effective and front-line nutritional research and monitoring.

4.2 Traditional dietary assessment methods

Dietary assessment methodologies can be classified according to different criteria, including the *duration of the period of registration* (short-term versus long-term dietary assessment methods) and the *time frame of the data collected* (e.g. past/retro versus current/prospective dietary intake assessment). Although the dietary assessment methods described in this chapter do not use any arbitrary categorisation, these notions are important to have in mind when evaluating and selecting the most appropriate dietary assessment method according to the study-specific aims and designs, as well as the logistical conditions and constraints. In this section, the dietary assessment methods and their respective strengths and weaknesses will be described in turn. The main results are summarised in Table 4.1 to facilitate comparison.

Description of methodologies

Observation methods

When using the observation method to assess participants' dietary intake, fieldworkers visit homes or school canteens to observe meal times and record dietary intake. Observation is an objective method to assess dietary intake, although in practice it can only be done in settings such as canteens or school dinner halls and for discrete time periods. However, new and existing technologies like cameras also allow the observation of subjects' dietary intake in different settings (see Section 4.3).

An important strength of the observation method is the fact that it provides an objective assessment of dietary intake. However, this method is highly intensive for researchers and is therefore expensive. When not performed covertly, the observation may alter individuals' usual eating patterns. Furthermore, this method is not feasible for obtaining habitual dietary data at either a group or an individual level. Observation of dietary intake is most commonly undertaken as a reference method for validating other dietary assessment methods.

Table 4.1 Traditional dietary assessment methods (comparison of important characteristics, errors and potential for standardisation).

	Food records	24-hour dietary recall	FFQ	Diet history	Screener
Type of information available					
Detailed information about foods/recipes	x	x		x	
Not detailed information about food groups			x		x
Scope of information sought					
Total diet	x	x	x	x	
Specific components					x
Time frame of single administration					
Short term (e.g. yesterday, today)	x	x		x	x
Long term (e.g. last month, last year)			x	x	x
Adaptable to diet in distant past					
Yes			x	x	x
No	x	x			
Cognitive requirements					
Measurement or estimated recording of foods and drinks as they are consumed	x				
Memories of recent consumption		x		x	x
Ability to make judgements of long-term diet			x	x	x
Potential for reactivity					
Low		x	x	x	x
High	x				
Time required to complete					
Low			x		x
High	x	x	(x)*	x	
Respondent burden					
Low		x	x		x
High	x			x	
Investigator cost					
Low			x		x
High	x	x		x	
Affecting food choices					
Yes	x				
No		x	x	x	x
Possibility for automated data entry					
Yes	x	x	x	x	x
No					
Literacy required#					
Yes	x		x	x	x
No		x			
Usable for retrospective data collection					
Yes			x	x	x
No	x	x			
Potential for standardisation					
High potential	x	x			
Low potential			x	x	x
Error					
Systematic under-reporting of intake	x	x	x	?	x
Systematic over-reporting of intake			x (detailed FFQ)		
Person-specific biases associated with gender, obesity etc.	x	x	x		x

*high amount of time required to complete very detailed FFQs.
#depending on administration method (e.g. interview versus self-administration).

(a)

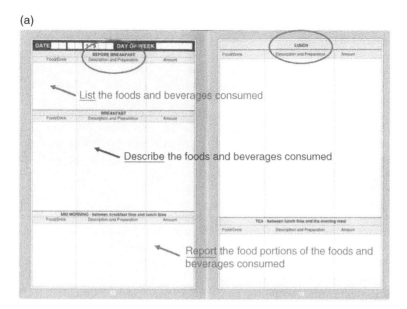

List the foods and beverages consumed

Describe the foods and beverages consumed

Report the food portions of the foods and beverages consumed

(b)

Breakfast   Place: (at home) / outdoor[1]

Product group	Food item	Brand name and/description	Quantity	Coding (for dietician)
Breakfast cereals E.g. muesli, cornflakes				
Bread E.g. cereal bread toast, ...	Cereal bread	Large, round bread	2 slices of the middle	
Sandwich filling E.g. cheese, jam, bacon, ...	Gouda cheese, Strawberry jam	Ripe gounda cheese, materne light jam	1 slice (10−10 cm) 1 teaspoon	
Fat E.g. low-fat spread, margarine, butter	Margarine	Becel, control	1 teaspoon per slice of bread	
Drinks E.g. water, milk, fruit juice, soft-drinks, ...	Orange juice Milk	Freshly squeezed Skimmed milk	1 orange 1 beaker	
Other foods E.g. egg, yoghurt, fruit, porridge, ...				

Figure 4.2 Food diaries. (a) Example of a food diary from the UK EPIC study. (b) Example of a Belgian food diary.

Food diary or food record methods

The food record or food diary (Figure 4.2) is an open-ended method that requires that the subject (or observer) reports all foods and beverages consumed at the time of consumption, to minimise reliance on memory. These records can be kept over one or more days and portion sizes may be determined by weighing or by estimating volumes (e.g. using visual aids like pictures, food models or food packets). In some situations, only those foods of particular study interest are recorded. For example, to estimate the intake of a certain food component (e.g. cholesterol, which is found in animal products only), food records might be limited to meat, poultry, fish, eggs or dairy products. However, if total energy intake or total diet estimates are required, the food record must include all foods and beverages consumed. Food records are generally completed by the subjects themselves using paper-based or more innovative (web/IT) technological supports (see Section 4.3), though in some situations a proxy might be employed (e.g. for children, the elderly or when literacy is too limited). To complete a food record, each respondent must be trained in the level of detail required to describe adequately the foods and portion sizes consumed, including the name of the food (brand name if possible), preparation methods, recipes for food mixtures and portion sizes. Reviewing the food records with the participants right after data collection is desirable in order to capture adequate detail.

The most important strength of the food record is its level of detail, given its open-ended nature and the fact that it refers to the current diet (i.e. dietary intake estimated at time of consumption). In addition, the report of actually consumed foods contributes to increasing the accuracy of portion sizes. As this method does not require recall of foods eaten, there is no memory problem. However, participants who keep food records sometimes delay recording their intakes for several hours or days, in which case they rely on memory. The most important disadvantages of the food record are its high investigator cost and respondent burden and the fact that it might affect the respondents' eating behaviour (subjects might change their eating behaviour due to the recording). Extensive respondent training and motivation are required and several repeated days are needed to capture individuals' usual intake. The intake often tends to be under-reported and the number of food items regularly decreases with time. Drop-out increases with the number of daily records requested, and the fact that literacy and high respondent motivation and compliance are required may lead to a non-representative sample and subsequent non-response bias.

The food record is often used in dietary programmes, as writing down all food and drinks consumed could enhance self-monitoring for weight control or other behaviour change (see Section 4.3). Furthermore, multiple food records (usually between three and seven days) are often used as a reference method in relative validation studies (e.g. for validating FFQs).

24-hour dietary recall methods

The 24-hour dietary recall method (Figure 4.3) is an open-ended method asking the respondent to remember and report all the foods and beverages consumed in the preceding 24 hours or over the previous day. The recall is often structured (e.g. per meal occasion), using specific probes and cognitive processes, to help respondents recall their diet. Probing is especially useful in collecting the necessary details, such as how foods were prepared. The recall typically is conducted by interview (in person or by telephone), either using a paper-and-pencil form or through computer-assisted interview. However, self-administered electronic forms of administration have also recently become available (see Section 4.3). When the recall is interviewer administered, well-trained interviewers are crucial. However, non-nutritionists with sufficient training on foods and recipes available in the study region and in interview techniques can be cost-effective.

Important strengths of the 24-hour dietary recall method are its relatively low respondent burden and the fact that it does not affect respondents' eating behaviour. This method is appropriate for most population groups, which reduces the potential for non-response bias and facilitates comparisons between populations. Another advantage is the fact that portion sizes are being recalled for all foods and beverages (using different quantification means), allowing estimation of individual intake. Disadvantages of the 24-hour dietary recall method are its high investigator cost (when interviewer administered) and the fact that repeated measurements are needed to capture individuals' usual intake (see also the section on food records earlier in this chapter). Furthermore, the fact that 24-hour dietary recall relies on subjects' short-term memory should also be considered as a relative disadvantage compared to food records (but not FFQs). In addition, socially desirable answers could introduce some recall bias during the a 24-hour dietary recall interview. As for food records, a 24-hour dietary recall tends also to under-report individual intakes.

Two repeated 24-hour dietary recall interviews are often used in large-scale dietary monitoring surveys, because of the low respondent burden and high level of standardisation. Furthermore, this method has also been applied as a reference calibration method in large-scale surveys to estimate population mean intake and correct for the measurement error of less accurate methods (e.g. FFQs).

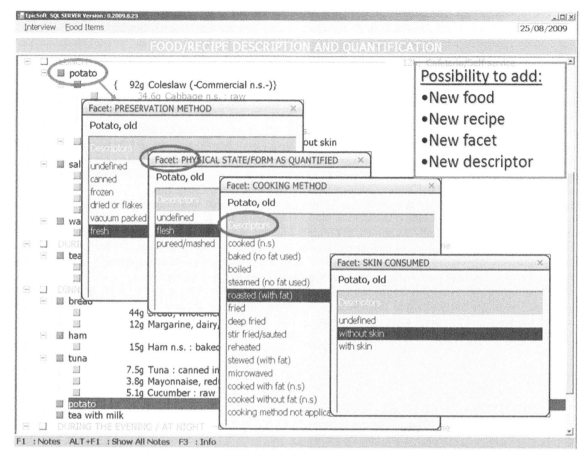

Figure 4.3 Food descriptions in the standardised EPIC-Soft 24-hour dietary recall method. (EPIC-Soft has since been renamed GloboDiet.)

Diet history methods

In 1947, Burke developed a dietary history interview and attempted to assess an individual's usual diet. This original dietary history interview included 24-hour dietary recall, a menu recorded for 3 days and a checklist of foods consumed over the preceding month. This checklist consisted of a detailed listing of the types of foods and beverages commonly consumed at each eating occasion over a defined time period, most often a 'typical' week. A trained interviewer probed for the respondent's customary pattern of food intake on each day of the typical week. The reference time frame could also be the past month or the past several months, or might reflect seasonal differences if the time frame was the past year. This checklist was the forerunner of the more structured dietary questionnaires in use today (e.g. FFQs, described below). A highly skilled and trained professional is needed for both the interview and the processing of the information.

An important strength of the diet history is that it assesses the individual subject's usual intake while not affecting eating behaviour. This method is very detailed, which means that information on the total diet can be obtained.

An important disadvantage of this detailed method is its high respondent and investigator burden. It is a difficult cognitive task for respondents to recall their usual individual intake and the estimation of usual portion sizes remains a challenge.

Due to its significant respondent and investigator burden and high costs, the dietary history is seldom applied in current or recent dietary surveys.

Food frequency questionnaire (FFQ) methods

The basic *food frequency questionnaire* (FFQ) consists of two components: a closed food list and a frequency response section for subjects to report how often each food (e.g. banana) or food group (e.g. fruit) was eaten. For each item on the food list, the respondent is asked to estimate the frequency of consumption based on open or specified frequency categories, which indicate the number of times the food is usually consumed per day, week, month or year. The number and/or types of food items and frequency categories may vary according to the study objectives and designs. Brief FFQs may focus on one or several specific nutrients. FFQs generally include between 50 and 150 (mostly generic) food items.

Different types of FFQ are usually considered: *non-quantitative* (alternatively called qualitative), *semi-quantitative* or completely *quantitative FFQs*. Non-quantitative questionnaires do not specify any portion sizes (standard portions derived from other study populations or data sets might be added afterwards), whereas semi-quantified instruments provide a combination of individual or typical/standard portion sizes to estimate food quantities (standard portions are part of the food item line). A quantitative FFQ allows the respondent to indicate any amount of food typically consumed. FFQs are commonly used to rank individuals by intake of selected foods or nutrients. Although FFQs are not designed for estimating absolute nutrient intakes, the method is often used for estimating average intake of those nutrients that have large day-to-day variability and for which there are relatively few significant food sources (e.g. alcohol, vitamin A and vitamin C).

Some FFQs also include questions regarding usual food preparation methods, trimming of meats and identification of the brand of certain types of foods, such as margarines or ready-to-eat cereals.

FFQs are generally self-administered (see Figure 4.4), but may also be interviewer administered. Proxies can be used to complete the FFQ in particular situations (e.g. for children, elderly, hospitalised patients and so on).

The most important strengths of the FFQ are its low investigator burden and cost and the fact that it does not affect the respondent's eating behaviour. Furthermore, it has the advantage that usual individual intake is being requested (over a long time frame), which avoids the need for repeated measurements. The completion of an FFQ remains a difficult cognitive task for respondents and this should be considered as an important limitation of this dietary intake assessment method. Usual portion sizes are difficult to estimate precisely and the intake estimates may be misreported.

Because of its low respondent burden and rather reduced cost (compared to more detailed methods like food records or 24-hour recalls), the FFQ is often the method of choice for large-scale dietary studies

(a)

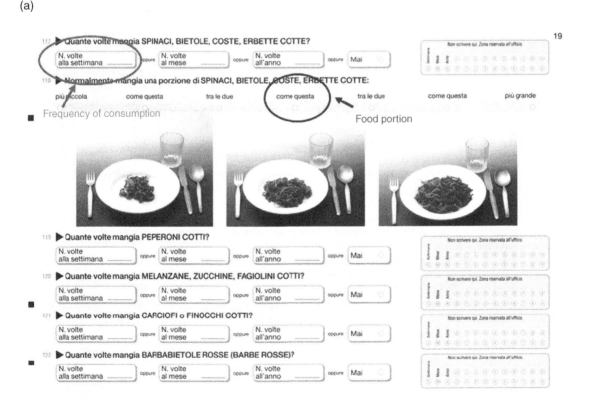

Figure 4.4 Self-reported FFQs. (a) A self-reported FFQ from the Italy EPIC study.

(b)

Food groups	How often do you consume the following product?	And what is the average portion per day?	Example portion sizes	Which type do you usually use?
Coffee	○ Never or less than once a month ○ 1–3 days per month ○ 1 day per week ○ 2–4 days per week ○ 5–6 days per week ● Every day	● 200 mL or less ○ Between 200–400 mL ○ Between 400–600 mL ○ 600 mL or more	*1 cup: 125 mL* *1 beaker: 225 mL*	● With caffeine ○ With reduced caffeine ○ Without caffeine
Tea	○ Never or less than once a month ○ 1–3 days per month ○ 1 day per week ○ 2–4 days per week ○ 5–6 days per week ● Every day	● 200 mL or less ○ Between 200–400 mL ○ Between 400–600 mL ○ 600 mL or more	*1 cup: 125 mL* *1 beaker: 225 mL*	○ Regular english tea ○ Green tea ● Herbal tea

Food groups	**How often** Does your child consume the following products?	And what is **the average** portion per day?	Example portion sizes
Water (*tap water, bottled water,...*)	○ Never or less than once per month ○ 1–3 days per month ○ 1 day per week ○ 2–4 days per week ○ 5–6 days per week ○ every day	○ 200 ml or less ○ Between 200 and 400 ml ○ Between 400 and 600 ml ○ 600 ml or more	*1 glass = 150 ml* *1 beaker = 150 ml*
Coffee and tea without sugar	○ Never or less than once per month ○ 1–3 days per month ○ 1 day pet week ○ 2–4 days per week ○ 5–6 days per week ○ every day	○ 200 ml or less ○ Between 200 and 400 ml ○ Between 400 and 600 ml ○ 600 ml or more	*1 cup= 125 ml* *1 beaker = 225 ml*
Coffee and tea with sugar	○ Never or less than once per month ○ 1–3 days per month ○ 1 day pet week ○ 2–4 days per week ○ 5–6 days per week ○ every day	○ 200 ml or less ○ Between 200 and 400 ml ○ Between 400 and 600 ml ○ 600 ml or more	*1 cup= 125 ml* *1 beaker = 225 ml*

Figure 4.4 (*Continued*) (b) An example of a Belgian FFQ.

investigating subjects' usual/habitual dietary intake, for instance large-scale cohort or intervention studies. However, its limited accuracy for assessing usual individual intakes increasingly means that complementary or alternative approaches are required (see Section 4.3).

Screeners or brief dietary assessment methods

In a variety of settings, comprehensive dietary assessments are not necessary or practical, for instance in studies where diet is not the main focus or is only considered as a covariate, as in health interview surveys. This has led to the development of diverse brief dietary assessment instruments, often called 'screeners', aiming to measure a limited number of foods and/or nutrients. Short questionnaires are often used to assess the intake of particular food items like fruit and vegetables in surveillance and intervention research. As mentioned in the previous section, complete FFQs typically contain between 50 and 150 food items to capture the range of foods contributing to the many nutrients in the diet. If an investigator is interested only in estimating the intake of a single nutrient or food group, however, then fewer foods need to be assessed. Often, only 15 to 30 foods might be required to account for most of the intake of a particular nutrient.

The most important strengths of brief instruments or screeners are their low respondent burden and low investigator cost. Screeners generally assess usual individual (specific food group) intakes, though often only for a limited number of food items (e.g. fruit and vegetables). Like other retrospective dietary assessment instruments (e.g. FFQs), they do not affect the subject's eating behaviour. The disadvantages of these brief instruments are very similar to those reported for FFQs, namely a difficult cognitive task for the respondent and a challenge to quantify usual portion sizes. Furthermore, screeners often only assess a limited number of nutrients/foods.

These brief instruments may have utility in clinical settings or in situations where health promotion and health education are the goals. They can also be used to examine relationships between some specific aspects of diet and other exposures, as in the National Health Interview Survey. Finally, some groups use short screeners to evaluate the effectiveness of policy initiatives.

Specific tools for dietary supplement intake assessments

Dietary supplements contribute to the total intakes of some nutrients, such as calcium, magnesium, iron and vitamins C, D and E. Failure to include these nutrient sources would lead to a serious underestimation of intakes. Therefore, dietary supplement information is increasingly collected via the traditional dietary intake assessment methods described above. However, precise information on product names and brand names as well as related quantities consumed (e.g. number and frequency of consumption of pills, drops, tablets) is required to assess accurately the nutrient intakes derived from dietary supplements. Furthermore, many formulations are now available over the internet and validation of the nutrient content can be difficult. Another method applicable to supplements but not to foods is the use of pill inventories, which are widely employed in obtaining information about other medications. For some supplements, inferences about use can be made from blood or urine biomarkers, if available, although they provide only qualitative rather than quantitative information.

Because most of the methods for assessing the intake of dietary supplements are similar to (or part of) those used for assessing dietary intake, they have the same strengths and limitations as the other methods mentioned in this chapter.

Main applications of traditional dietary assessment methods

The choice of the most appropriate dietary assessment method depends on many factors and requires careful consideration. The following questions should be answered in selecting the method that will best meet the study objectives:

- Is information needed about foods, nutrients, other food components (e.g. bioactive components) and/or specific dietary behaviours and which items are of primary interest according to the research question?
- Is the focus of the research question on the group or individual data level and are absolute or relative intake estimates required?
- What are the population characteristics (age, sex, education, literacy, cultural diversity, motivation) and the time frame of interest?
- What level of accuracy and precision is needed?
- What are the available resources, including money, logistical conditions and constraints, interview time, staff and food composition data (if nutrients are to be calculated)?

Based on the answers to these questions, one can decide on the most appropriate dietary intake assessment method to be used for the particular study design and conditions.

Although these traditional methods are also used in *clinical settings*, the methods to be employed depend on the clinical conditions, which go beyond the scope of this chapter.

In *epidemiological settings*, at least three important study designs can be considered: cross-sectional/monitoring surveys, case-control studies and cohort studies. Any of the dietary instruments discussed in this chapter can be used in cross-sectional studies. Some of the instruments, such as 24-hour dietary recall, are appropriate when the study purpose requires detailed and reliable quantitative estimates of intake, and frequently as a substitute for food-weighted or recorded methods. In addition, the 24-hour dietary recall method has the advantage that it does not require literacy, which in large-scale surveys increases the number of respondents, including those of lower socio-economic status. Other instruments, such as FFQs or behavioural indicators, are appropriate when qualitative estimates are sufficient for ranking individuals according to their (low, medium or high) level of consumption, for example frequency of consuming soda/fizzy drinks.

For case-control studies, the period of interest for dietary exposure could be either the recent past (e.g. the year before diagnosis) or the distant past (e.g. 10 years ago or in childhood). Because information about diet before the onset of disease is needed, dietary assessment methods that focus on current behaviour, such as food diaries or 24-hour dietary recalls, are not useful in retrospective studies. The food frequency (and diet history) methods are well suited for assessing past diet and are therefore the only viable choices for case-control (retrospective) studies (unless more accurate information from the past is available, as for instance in nested cohort case-control studies). However, the accuracy of such distant past dietary intake estimations is lower than for recent dietary intake assessment methods (e.g. food diaries or 24-hour dietary recalls) due to the significance of recall bias.

In cohort studies or prospective dietary studies, dietary intake and/or status are measured at baseline, when study subjects are free of diseases, and are then related to later incidence of disease. A broad assessment of diet is usually desirable in prospective studies because many dietary exposures and many (intermediate) disease endpoints will ultimately be investigated and areas of interest may not even be recognised at the beginning of a cohort study. In order to relate diet at baseline to the eventual occurrence of disease, a measure is needed of the usual intake of foods by study subjects. Multiple 24-hour dietary recalls or food records, diet histories and food frequency methods have all been used effectively in prospective studies. Cost and logistical issues tend to favour food frequency methods because many prospective studies require thousands of respondents. However, because of concern about significant measurement error and attenuation attributed to the FFQ, other approaches are being considered (see Section 4.3). Incorporating emerging technological advances in administering dietary records, such as using mobile phones, increases the

feasibility of such approaches in prospective studies (again, see Section 4.3). If an FFQ is used in a cohort, it is desirable to include multiple recalls or records in subsamples of the population (preferably before beginning the study) to design the FFQ in the best way and to calibrate it (see Section 4.4).

Measurement in *public health settings* of the effects of nutrition promotion and education requires a valid measure of change from baseline to the conclusion of the intervention period. Researchers have found that dietary records and scheduled 24-hour dietary recalls were associated with changed eating behaviour during the recording days. However, because of resource constraints, large intervention studies have often relied on less precise measures of diet, including FFQs and brief instruments.

The choice of the most optimal dietary intake assessment method to be used also frequently depends on the population characteristics, for instance the age group (diaries are often used for children, while 24-hour dietary recalls are recommended for adults). FFQs and screeners have been applied in all age groups, although proxy reported in certain population groups (e.g. in children). Furthermore, a better understanding of various instruments' strengths and weaknesses has led to the creative blending of approaches, with the goal of maximising the strengths of each instrument. For example, a record-assisted 24-hour dietary recall has been used in several studies with children. The children keep notes of what they have eaten and then use these notes as memory prompts in a later 24-hour dietary recall.

4.3 Innovative dietary assessment methods and technologies

Description of innovative dietary assessment methods and technologies

Innovation in dietary assessment includes two basic conceptual notions: *new methodologies,* substantially different approaches for collecting dietary information (e.g. integrating and combining different types of self-reports, or self-reports and biomarkers; see Section 4.6) versus *new technologies,* related to the way in which dietary data are collected, handled and disseminated or exchanged. In particular, the growing prominence of internet and telecommunication technologies has allowed for a rapid evolution in ways of assessing and processing dietary intakes that has previously not been possible. The use of new technologies to collect and process dietary data is especially but not exclusively promising for children, adolescents and younger adults who are familiar with such technologies in their daily lives. Since the early

2000s, innovative technologies reported in the literature have included both technically advanced approaches to traditional (self-report) methods (e.g. web-based FFQs) and technically new devices integrating objective measurement features (e.g. digital imaging for portion size estimation). It is therefore sometimes difficult to disentangle from the innovative technologies what are methodological features of the dietary assessment methods (see Section 4.2) and what are actually new approaches to assessing and processing dietary intake. This misconception contributes to obscuring the understanding and proper evaluation and use of the new technologies.

Table 4.2 gives an overview of the six main groups of innovative technologies that show promise for improving, complementing or replacing the traditional dietary assessment methods, including a description of their group-specific technology-related strengths and weaknesses. The examples provided reflect the different existing variants of the same technology and the currently ongoing developments of such new tools for different purposes and populations. The classification applied is rough and requires regular revisions to reflect the extremely dynamic development of new dietary technologies. The main technological groups can have overlapping technological features, which are highlighted.

Validity and reproducibility of innovative dietary assessment methods and technologies

Research to investigate the validity and reproducibility of innovative technologies is crucial, but science-based evidence is still missing. Well-designed validation studies that include biomarkers are lacking for most of the technology groups, particularly for personal digital assistant technologies, mobile phone–based technologies and technically new 24-hour dietary recalls. Moreover, the bias inherent in self-reported dietary data by individuals (that is, individual and population bias, such as BMI, socio-economic position and so on) remains a problem that even innovative technologies may not eradicate completely.

Available studies suggest that the validity of individual dietary intake as reported on personal digital assistant technologies may be low to moderate. The validity of mobile phone–based technologies is less well studied. Complete technology validation studies have only been undertaken on the well-known Wellnavi instrument. By contrast, several studies have been done to assess the validity and reproducibility of interactive computer-based and web-based technologies. In particular, technically advanced FFQs and other dietary questionnaires have been compared with more established or traditional dietary assessment methods, for example 24-hour dietary recalls or food records. The correlation between the innovative and traditional approaches for most foods and nutrients is in the range of 0.4 to 0.7. In addition, the comparisons of web-based FFQ and traditional paper-based FFQs to various reference methods yielded similar correlations, indicating that the underlying methodology of innovative and traditional FFQs is unchanged by the technology. So far, a limited number of studies have assessed the relative validity of 24-hour dietary recall developed by the use of interactive computer- and web-based technologies. One recent study assessed the criterion validity of the Automated Self-administered 24-hour Recall (ASA24) through a feeding design and found somewhat better performance relative to true intakes for matches, exclusions, and intrusions in the interviewer-administered Automated Multiple-Pass Method. Furthermore, accurate portion-size estimation appears to depend on the technical presentation on the screen. Most studies on camera- and tape recorder–based technologies have integrated a validation component. Studies on camera-based technologies showed moderate to good relative validity against traditional food records and observation methods.

Application of innovative dietary assessment methods and technologies

Innovative technologies are used for dietary assessment in clinical and epidemiological settings as well as in public health settings for nutrition promotion and education. Although there is no rulebook with regard to selecting an innovative dietary assessment technology for a specific context, considerations depend on the study's objectives, its target population and the financial resources available.

In *clinical settings*, innovative technologies are applied for determining a person's dietary adequacy or risk and for purposes of treatment or counselling. In particular, handheld technologies that only capture data on current intake (e.g. personal digital assistant or mobile phone technologies) showed their usefulness in helping patients to self-monitor current diet and/or make good dietary decisions. Much of the published literature focuses on chronic disease management, particularly obesity, type 2 diabetes and chronic kidney dysfunction. In addition, web-based technologies are widely applied for weight loss/management trials.

In *epidemiological settings*, innovative technologies are applied for assessing a person's usual dietary intake. The primary applied advanced methods are interactive computer-based and web-based technologies that aim to address the methodological challenges faced in nutritional epidemiology. In this context, the recent scientific preference for using repeated short-term methods in combination with dietary questionnaires (and biomarkers of intake, discussed later in this chapter) is reflected by the development of several web-based 24-hour dietary recall and dietary questionnaires (see Section 4.6). Web-based technologies are also the method of choice for assessing diet in some newly established large epidemiological

Table 4.2 Description of technologies with potential for improving, complementing or replacing the traditional dietary assessment methodologies. Reproduced from Illner, A.K., Freisling, H., Boeing, H. *et al.* (2012) Review and evaluation of innovative technologies for measuring diet in nutritional epidemiology. *International Journal of Epidemiology*, **41** (4), 1187–1203, by permission of Oxford University Press.

	Description	Common assessment procedure and technology-related strengths and weaknesses	Examples in the literature with variable assessment procedures**
Technologies with potential for improving, complementing and/or replacing traditional food record methodology			
Personal digital assistant technologies*	Hand-held computers that integrate computing and networking features using stylus and/or keyboard for input	The participant is asked to record dietary intake right after consumption, by selecting food items from a drop-down menu of foods and beverages. Amount consumed is estimated by portion size estimation aids. Data is uploaded and matched with food composition databases. • **Strengths:** facilitated real-time data collection, entry and coding; capacity to capture open-ended text; integration of data quality algorithms and easy data transfer to a PC; often good respondent acceptance and possibility for standardised and/or repeated measurements. • **Weaknesses:** substantial initial costs of equipment and software purchases, though cost savings can be achieved with the removal of data-entry costs and data coding; requires respondent training; use of PDA technologies can result in changes in current eating behaviour.	Beasely *et al.* (2005) Yon *et al.* (2006) Fowles *et al.* (2008) Fukuo *et al.* (2009) McClung *et al.* (2009)
Mobile phone–based technologies*	Portable electronic telecommunication devices connected to wireless communication network	The participant is asked to record dietary intake at eating events, by capturing digital images and/or voice records with a mobile phone. Data are transmitted by SIM card. • **Strengths:** widely available way of data collection, user-friendly and suitable for low-literacy subjects; provision of open-ended dietary data, if they are coupled with digital image-assisted assessment; advanced data-quality control due to real-time and often memory-independent assessment. • **Weaknesses:** high method-development and data-processing effort, e.g. for image analysis and volume estimation; time-consuming training for data managers and respondents (e.g. with regard to power management as the data-storage capacity is limited).	Six *et al.* (2010) (Mobilephone Food record/mpFR) Weiss *et al.* (2010) (Mobile Food Intake Visualisation and VoiceRecogniser/FIV*R*) Kristal, A. (Dietary Data Recordersystem/DDRS)
Camera- and tape recorder–based technologies	Devices that capture images and/or write voice records onto a tape that are then encoded	Food selection and plate waste are visually or verbally recorded. Trained observers review images on a computer screen by comparing them to reference portions of known food quantities or analysing taped records. Estimates are manually entered into databases. • **Strengths:** fast, cheap, robust and non-repetitive data collection; suitable methods for subjects with memory impairment and for parent-assisted dietary assessment in children. The frequency rate of omitted or forgotten food items can be reduced. • **Weaknesses:** recording can affect food choices and under-reporting and/or result in reduced food consumption. Camera- and tape recorder–based technologies provide only a snapshot of food consumed and multiple measurements are needed.	Lindquist *et al.* (2000) Williamson *et al.* (2004) Higgins *et al.* (2009) Dahl Lassen *et al.* (2010)

(Continued)

Table 4.2 (*Continued*)

	Description	Common assessment procedure and technology-related strengths and weaknesses	Examples in the literature with variable assessment procedures**

Technologies with potential for improving, complementing and/or replacing traditional FFQ and 24-hour dietary recall methodologies

| Interactive computer-based technologies* | Programmable machines with hardware and software components | The participant is asked to report dietary intake during a specified period in the recent and distant past, using computer software with multimedia attributes. Data is directly transferred into electronic databases.
• **Strengths:** data consistency and completeness through technical mean, such as skip patterns, plausibility and range checks; reduced organisational study constraints and costs (excluding costs for software development), particularly for larger study populations.
• **Weaknesses:** Many interactive computer-based technologies are designed as technically advanced FFQs, diet histories or 24-HDRs, suggesting similar methodology-associated measurement errors (listed in Sections 4.1 and 4.2); literacy, access to a computer and computer skills are required, which can be attributable to selection and response bias. | 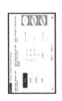 Zoellner *et al.* (2005)
Heath *et al.* (2005)
Wong *et al.* (2008)
Murtaugh *et al.* (2010)
Baranowski *et al.* (2010) (Food Intake Recording Software System/ FIRSST)
Vereeken *et al.* (2005) |
| Web-based technologies* | Internet-connected tools that shift applications and software from the computer desktop to websites that users access online with their browser | The participant reports short- or long-term dietary intake, using web-based data-collection systems. Data is processed in real time.
• **Strengths:** advantageous to reach larger samples and culturally different and geographically dispersed groups; can be completed at any time and location and allow for facilitated repeated measurements; cost- and time-effectiveness due to direct transfer of complete data to the study centre; easily adaptable (e.g. to other languages, to different dietary assessment methodologies).
• **Weaknesses:** Similar to computer-based technologies, methodology-associated measurement errors can be introduced; additional reporting and memory bias due to self-completion difficulties of more complex web-based dietary methods, such as 24-HDRs (e.g. resulting from limited nutritional knowledge, difficulties in quantifying portion sizes, reduced level of open-ended food choices); literacy and computer and internet skills are required. | Boeckner *et al.* (2002)
Matthys *et al.* (2007)
Subar *et al.* (2007) (ASA24)
Beasely *et al.* (2009)
Arab *et al.* (2010)
Touvier *et al.* (2011) |

Other technology groups

| Scan- and sensor-based technologies | Tools that read and digitise data by passing through a scanner or sensor | Subjects scan purchased food item barcodes or wear sensors that automatically record measures of biological movements related to eating activities.
• **Strengths:** objective measurements of features related to food consumption (e.g. automatically captured images); low respondent burden.
• **Weaknesses:** substantial instrument development costs (for sensor-based technologies); data processing requires specific scan/sensor hardware and processing algorithms (e.g. for images); possible narrow camera field of view and insufficient battery life of devices. | Lambert *et al.* (2005)
Amft *et al.* (2009)
Sun *et al.* (2010) (eButton)
Jia W, Chen H-C, Yue Y *et al.* (2014) |

*May have overlapping technological features.
**From the first to the most recent.

studies, as practical and cost-effective approaches for dietary assessment (e.g. the Oxford WebQ within the framework of the UK Biobank study).

In *public health settings* for nutrition promotion and education, innovative technologies are applied for both changing a person's usual diet towards a healthier diet and transferring nutritional knowledge. Web-based technologies, sometimes supported by social networking sites like Facebook, Twitter and Snapchat as well as interactive computer-based technologies, are prominent research approaches to improving nutritional behaviour and conducting intervention programmes. In addition, the continuing growth of mobile phone–based technology use has offered high potential to transfer nutritional knowledge, particularly in adolescents, but also in middle-aged people.

4.4 Measurement errors in dietary intake

The main goal in dietary assessment is to estimate the usual intake, which is the long-term average intake of food or nutrients of a given individual or population. This long-term average intake or usual intake is a key concept in dietary monitoring and nutritional epidemiology. Depending on the study objectives, the time frame of interest, which should be captured by the usual intake, can be as much as one year or even decades.

The usual intake is not directly observable, but can be estimated from self-reported 'actual' (or acute) intakes. With short-term instruments, repeated measurements on each individual of a given population sample need to be collected to estimate the usual intake. For example, for dietary monitoring, two (non-consecutive) repeated 24-hour dietary recalls per individual are sufficient to estimate the usual population mean and distribution. However, more repeated 24-hour dietary recalls are required to estimate the usual individual mean intake, depending on the food or nutrient of interest. In contrast, a single administration of a long-term instrument, such as a diet history questionnaire or FFQ, may aim to capture individual usual intakes directly, at least to rank individuals according to their intake within a study population for diet–disease evaluations.

However, estimation of the usual intake is challenging, since all methods to measure dietary intake (or any other exposure) are affected by several types of measurement error. Measurement error can be broadly defined as a deviation from the true value – from either the true mean, the true variation or both – and can be assessed by calculating the sample mean and the variation around the mean, expressed by the variance (or standard deviation). Measurement error can be categorised into *random errors* and *systematic errors*. Both types of error can occur at two levels: the *individual level* (within-person) and *group or population level* (between-person).

Random within-person error

An individual's dietary intake varies randomly around his or her usual mean intake, which is referred to as the 'day-to-day-variation' and reflects the true daily variability in a person's eating habits. This daily variability is pronounced in foods that are infrequently consumed (e.g. liver or other offal) or in nutrients that are found in a few food sources only (e.g. vitamin A in high concentration in liver and other offal). In addition, variation around the usual mean intake may result from random measurement errors at the individual level due to instrumental errors. An example is given by errors in portion size estimation, where respondents may randomly under- or overestimate their dietary intake.

The sum of these two sources of variation, day-to-day variation and instrumental errors, is referred to as the *random within-person error* (or random within-person variation); the two sources cannot and usually do not need to be separated in practice (Figure 4.5).

Random between-person error

Between-person variation can be expressed by the difference between an individual's usual intake and the population's usual intake; in Figure 4.5 this is shown as the difference between person A's and person B's usual intakes (solid lines) from the true usual intake of the population (dashed line).

The random within-person error leads to the random between-person error at population level:

$$\sigma^2_{observed} = \sigma^2_{true} + \sigma^2_{within}$$

$\sigma^2_{observed}$ = observed variation (SD); σ^2_{true} = true variation; σ^2_{within} = random within-person error

Overall, random within-person error or variation will not affect the mean intake of a population, because these types of errors will cancel out provided that the sample size is large enough (large enough sample sizes in national dietary surveys usually comprise ~2000 participants or more); an overestimated or high intake of a given food/nutrient will be balanced by an underestimated or low intake of the same food/nutrient on subsequent measurements/days. However, random within-person error contributes to, and thus inflates, the observed between-person variation (or variation at group level). Therefore, the observed SD of a population is larger than the true SD, which should reflect true differences/variation in intake between individuals only (Figure 4.6).

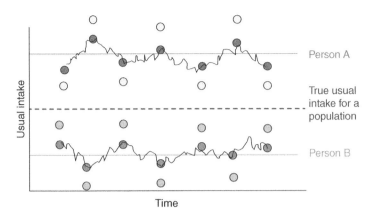

Figure 4.5 Within-person and between-person variation. For persons A and B, the dark-coloured dots represent their day-to-day variation in intake and the light-coloured dots represent their measured intake; taken together these represent within-person variation or random within-person error. Between-person variation is represented by the difference between person A's and person B's usual intake and the population's usual intake. Adapted from NHANES Dietary Web Tutorial (http://www.cdc.gov/nchs/tutorials/Dietary/Advanced/ModelUsualIntake/index.htm).

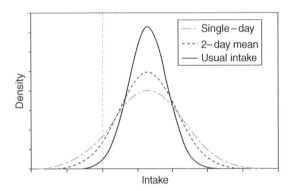

Figure 4.6 Hypothetical distribution of usual intake of a nutrient or a food with no between-person random error (black solid line), contrasted with the estimated distribution from a single or 2-day mean short-term dietary assessment instrument (e.g. 24-hour recall) containing between-person random error (dashed lines). The vertical dashed line represents a hypothetical cut-off of interest (e.g. dietary recommendation). Adapted from NHANES Dietary Web Tutorial (http://www.cdc.gov/nchs/tutorials/Dietary/Advanced/ModelUsualIntake/index.htm).

The main consequences of random between-person errors (i.e. inflated SD) are that the proportion of the population below or above a certain cut-off point (e.g. nutrient recommendation) is over- or underestimated; and, furthermore, the strength of an association between a dietary intake and a health outcome is biased, usually towards no effect (attenuated).

Systematic within-person errors

In addition to the random within-person error, individuals may also systematically under- or overestimate their true food intake (consciously and subconsciously). This

is referred to as a *systematic within-person error* and is defined as the difference between observed and true (long-term average) intake.

Systematic within-person errors can take three forms:

- A systematic error that applies to all individuals equally, for example caused by systematic errors in food composition tables or in picture books for portion size estimation; this error is referred to as *systematic additive error/bias*.
- A systematic error that is proportional to the level of individual intake, for example individuals with higher intakes under-report relatively more than individuals with lower intakes; this error is referred to as *intake-related bias* or multiplicative bias.
- A systematic error that differs between individuals according to specific characteristics such as age, sex, education or other unmeasured characteristics; for example obese people tend to underestimate their food intake more than non-obese people, different interviewers conduct interviews (and differ in the way interviews are done); this error is referred to as *person-specific bias*.

Systematic between-person errors

If systematic within-person errors occur non-randomly between individuals, these errors can lead to systematic errors at population level (i.e. systematic between-person errors). As a consequence, the observed mean intake of a given population will be incorrect and either over- or underestimated; this applies to all three forms of systematic error as described above with the exception of person-specific bias. At the group level, these errors can cancel each other out, in which case this error would not contribute to systematic between-person errors. However, this type of error contributes to the observed variation and affects the true intake distribution, so that the observed SD will be further inflated:

$$\sigma^2_{observed} = \sigma^2_{true} + \sigma^2_{within} + \sigma^2_{person\text{-}specific}$$

In practice, all three forms of systematic within-person error tend to be present simultaneously, so that both the population mean intake and its SD are measured with error. This can be summarised by the formula:

$$Q_{ij} = b_0 + b_1 T_i + r_i + e_{ij}$$

where Q = instrument; T = true intake; i = person; j = day; b_0 = additive bias; b_1 = multiplicative bias; r_i = person-specific bias; e_{ij} = random (within-person) error excluding person-specific bias.

In the case of systematic between-person errors, the mean dietary intake of a population is biased (i.e. the observed population mean differs from the true mean). As a consequence, the proportion of the population below or above a certain cut-off point – for example, of a dietary recommendation – is biased. However, diet–health associations are not necessarily biased (i.e. correlation or regression coefficients are unaffected by systematic errors, provided that no person-specific bias is present).

How to reduce measurement errors at the data-collection stage

Random errors

- Repeat measurements for each individual and take the average; the number of repeated measurements depends on the objectives of a given study.
- Standardise measurements, for example through written guidelines (operations manual), training of all people involved in the study, careful selection and standardisation of measurement tools, standardisation of questionnaires, use of computer software. Furthermore, all interviewers should be knowledgeable and trained about foods available in the marketplace and about preparation practices, including prevalent regional or ethnic foods.

Systematic errors

- Apply the same principles as for random errors regarding the standardisation of measurements.
- Use the best available measurement tools or techniques (depending on feasibility).
- Use calibrated measurement tools.
- Perform unobtrusive measurements (e.g. neutral interview techniques).

- Use 'blinding', where the study objectives are unknown to the participants (although be aware that this may not always be possible; for more information see Chapter 3).

Evaluating measurement errors in dietary intake

After considering all possible and feasible measurement error-reduction techniques, dietary intake measurements (like any measurement) can still contain substantial error. It is thus also important to quantify the overall magnitude of both random and systematic errors in evaluation studies, ideally before a selected dietary assessment instrument/method is applied in the main study. Evaluation includes reproducibility and validation studies.

Reproducibility studies address random errors and investigate the consistency of dietary intake measurements on more than one administration to the same person at different times and under similar conditions. Reproducibility can be quantified in several ways. Often coefficients of variation of differences within individuals are calculated to provide a measure for *precision*. Correlation coefficients can be computed to quantify the consistency of ranking of individuals on two or more occasions (i.e. to distinguish between individuals), which is referred to as *reliability*.

Validation studies address systematic errors and investigate the degree to which a method accurately measures the diet variable that it was designed to measure – that is, the true value over a specified period of time. For example, a valid 24-hour dietary recall would be a complete and accurate record of all food and drink consumed on the day preceding the recall. Depending on a study's objective, validity refers to the accuracy of a population's mean intake, of an individual's usual intake or of ranking of individuals. Validity can be assessed by comparing the main instrument with a superior reference measure. In theory, such a reference measure is free of systematic errors (i.e. unbiased for true intake at population level and no multiplicative error) and random errors are uncorrelated to true intake and to the errors of the main instrument. However, in dietary assessment only a few ideal reference measures are currently available: doubly labelled water for energy intake, 24-hour urinary nitrogen excretion for protein intake, and 24-hour urinary potassium excretion for potassium intake. The lack of a perfect reference method also indicates a continued need to search for better gold standards.

Furthermore, there should be an examination of how the measurement errors affect the results of the study. The outcomes of evaluation studies can subsequently be considered in the interpretation of the study results (e.g. whether the results are under- or overestimating the true value) and used to (partially) correct the observed results of the main study for dietary measurement errors.

Correcting random and systematic measurement errors at the stage of data analysis

Depending on the study objectives, it will often be necessary to correct for measurement errors using statistical approaches.

Linear regression calibration

With a technique referred to as linear regression calibration, random errors, in the form of within-person random error, and systematic errors, in the form of additive and multiplicative bias, can be at least partially corrected for or mitigated. However, *calibration studies* are needed to supply the best predictors of the true usual intake.

In a calibration study, ideally on a subsample of the full cohort or the main study, diet is measured with a superior method – a so-called reference instrument – where the reference instrument should have the same properties as in the validation studies described above. For practical reasons, non-ideal reference measures are often used: 24-hour dietary recalls or food records (see earlier in this chapter). Although it has been shown that 24-hour dietary recalls are less biased than, for example, FFQs, they have been shown to be biased for true intake and to have errors that are correlated with true intake and with the errors of an FFQ. However, it is still preferable to mitigate the effect of measurement errors in a main instrument (e.g. FFQs) with a non-optimal reference measure (e.g. 24-hour dietary recall).

Regression calibration involves two steps (regressions):

- Regress the dietary intake as measured with the reference instrument (superior method) on the main instrument to get the prediction equation (expected values from the superior method) or, alternatively, the so-called attenuation coefficient.
- Regress the health outcome on the prediction equation or divide the risk estimate by the attenuation coefficient; or in other words, recalculate the association between dietary intake and health outcome using the expected values from the reference instrument.

The mean intake of the main instrument can be replaced by the predicted values from the reference instrument and thus the mean intake of the population recalculated – that is, the calibrated mean intake (partially) corrected for measurement error. However, it is important to keep in mind that the measurement error correction is incomplete as long as a non-ideal reference method is used as a reference instrument.

Energy adjustment

Energy adjustment is another way to mitigate the effect of measurement errors. In validation studies, correlation coefficients between dietary intakes of the test instrument (e.g. FFQ) and reference instrument (e.g. biomarker) improve after energy adjustment, which is mostly due to reduced measurement error. A possible explanation is that errors for energy and nutrient intake are correlated and they tend to cancel each other out in the energy-adjusted nutrient intake. The nutrient density method (i.e. nutrient/total energy) is most commonly used, but other methods exist (e.g. nutrient residuals).

Removing within-person variation

Finally, if the interest is in estimating intake distributions of the usual intake at population level, then statistical techniques can be used to remove/reduce the within-person errors (day-to-day variation), leaving only the between-person variation. This is particularly needed in dietary monitoring, where short-term instruments such as 24-hour dietary recalls are the method of choice, in order to estimate the proportion of a population below or above a given dietary recommendation or cut-off point. Basic approaches rely on simple analysis of variance to separate within- from between-person variation and remove the within-person variation. Newer approaches involve additional steps such as normalising transformations, back transformations of varying complexity and the use of empirical distributions. Several methods have been developed in the last few years and there is also a wide range of software solutions available (see Section 4.6).

All approaches require an estimate of the within-person variation for the food group or nutrient of interest in order to separate it from the between-person variation. A prerequisite to calculating the within-person variation is that at least one repeated day of intake data (e.g. repeated 24-hour recalls) has been collected in at least a subsample of the study population. A less favourable approach is to borrow estimates of within-person variation from another study population with similar dietary habits. The magnitude of the within-person variation in relation to the between-person variation not only differs across foods or nutrients, but also across countries, ages, sex and other factors. For example, milk might be consumed on a daily basis among preschool children while not necessarily among adults, leading to higher within-person variability among adults than among children. Differences in the availability of foods by days of the week or season also affect the day-to-day variation (within-person variation) of dietary intake. For example, if citrus fruits (a good source of vitamin C) are mostly consumed during one season, then the within-person variation of vitamin C will be high. Seasonal variation is usually more pronounced for foods than for nutrients and less for total energy intake. For these reasons, it is recommended that a dietary survey covers all seasons at population level, with at least one repeated day of intake data as mentioned above. Generally, the intake of most nutrients varies more within individuals (from day to day) than between individuals. The higher the within-person variation for a given nutrient, the poorer the estimate of an individual's usual intake, for example, if only a single 24-hour dietary recall was available. In contrast, long-term instruments such as an FFQ measure usual intakes over a longer time period (e.g. the previous 12 months), which results in a low within-person variation. Therefore, a separation of within- and between-person variation is usually not needed for long-term instruments. However, it has to be kept in mind that long-term instruments are usually more prone to systematic errors.

4.5 Multivariate analyses of dietary intake

Dietary patterns

Dietary patterns – also referred to as eating patterns or food patterns – were defined in 1982 by Schwerin and co-workers as 'distinct and discrete patterns of consuming foods in different combinations'. The goal of dietary pattern analysis is to summarise a large number of correlated dietary variables, estimated at the food level, but more recently also at the nutrient and/or related biomarker levels, into fewer independent (uncorrelated) components without much loss of information. These patterns are thought to be easier to analyse as compared with a multitude of (individual) foods or food constituents, such as nutrients and other chemicals, and to allow inferences to be drawn to the total diet. In the last three decades, various approaches to derive dietary patterns have evolved and continue to develop. The main methods that have already been frequently applied in nutritional research are described in more detail in this section.

Methods to derive dietary patterns

Dietary patterns are not directly observable or measurable. Statistically, they can be referred to as latent (unobserved) variables. Three main techniques for computing dietary patterns in multivariate analyses can be distinguished (Figure 4.7): hypothesis-oriented (a priori) methods; exploratory (a posteriori) methods; and hybrid methods combining a priori and a posteriori techniques.

Hypothesis-oriented (a priori) methods

Dietary patterns that are defined according to some a priori criteria for a healthy diet (i.e. a hypothesis-oriented approach) are referred to as *diet quality indices* or scores. Such indices can be based on pre-existing dietary recommendations for the general population or specific population subgroups (e.g. food plate, food guide pyramid); guidelines for the prevention of a specific disease (e.g. WCRF [World Cancer Research Fund]/AICR [American Institute for Cancer Research] recommendations for cancer prevention); or dietary habits known to be healthy (e.g. Mediterranean diet). Indices are usually composed of foods, nutrients or a combination of both. Some indices also incorporate measures for dietary diversity or moderation. Diet quality indices that incorporate non-dietary components such as physical activity, body fatness or smoking are usually referred to as *healthy lifestyle indices*. Depending to which degree a given dietary recommendation is met or not, a specific score is assigned and then summed up to the overall index. For example, the Healthy Eating Index (HEI) has ten components consisting of dietary recommendations for five food groups, four nutrients and a component for dietary variety. For each component, individuals receive a score ranging from 0 to 10. If a recommendation is fully met, a score of 10 is given, and this score declines proportionally depending on the degree to which the recommendation is met. The underlying measurement of index items can be quantitative food/nutrient intake, frequency of food intake or a count of reported food groups from short- (e.g. 24-hour dietary recalls) or long-term dietary assessment instruments (e.g. FFQs). However, it is

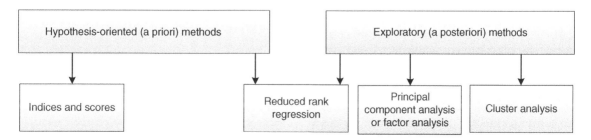

Figure 4.7 Main methods to derive dietary patterns in nutritional research. Adapted from Schulze, M.B. and Hoffmann, K. (2006) Methodological approaches to study dietary patterns in relation to risk of coronary heart disease and stroke. *British Journal of Nutrition*, **95**, 860–869.

important to consider that the dietary data used should be appropriate for the purpose of a given index (e.g. to evaluate the usual diet).

Exploratory (a posteriori) methods

Dietary patterns can also be empirically derived (a posteriori) from the collected dietary data using different statistical techniques. *Factor analysis* (FA) or *principal component analysis* (PCA) aggregates specific foods (groups) or nutrients into a limited number of patterns (factors/components) based on the degree to which these dietary variables are inter-correlated. Individual scores are then computed from each retained component as the sum of products of the observed variables multiplied by weights proportional to the loadings (i.e. linear combinations). The retained patterns or components account for the largest part of the total variation of the underlying dietary variables between individuals. With *cluster analysis*, individuals with similar diets, rather than dietary variables, are aggregated into relatively similar non-overlapping subgroups (clusters). Individuals within a given cluster share similar dietary intakes. The *treelet transform* method is a third empirical approach that produces sparse factors (i.e. foods with zero loadings are ignored to compute patterns) in combination with a cluster tree to visualise related groups of foods or nutrients, and this produces easily interpretable patterns. Input dietary variables for all exploratory methods can be foods, food groups, nutrients or combinations expressed in weight, servings or frequency of consumption as assessed with dietary assessment instruments that provide usual intakes (e.g. FFQs), but also biological markers or (food) metabolites. The patterns are usually labelled according to the highest factor loadings or specific combinations of foods and/or nutrients.

Hybrid methods combining a priori and a posteriori approaches

More recently, methods such as *reduced rank regression* (RRR) or *partial least squares regression* (PLS) have been developed that bridge the gap between a priori and a posteriori approaches. These methods identify dietary patterns by considering a priori information to predict another set of correlated response variables, typically intermediate markers (biomarkers) of disease or nutrient intakes. Biological pathways from the diet to a disease outcome are taken into account by identifying dietary patterns associated with biomarkers of a specific disease. *Decision tree analysis* identifies subgroups of a population whose members share dietary characteristics that influence (intermediate markers of) disease. They can be seen as hybrid methods, because the identified patterns depend on a priori knowledge to select the biomarkers/ nutrients and the empirical correlation structure in the dietary data. Similar to exploratory methods, input

dietary variables can be foods, food groups, nutrients or combinations expressed in weight, servings or frequency of consumption as assessed with dietary assessment instruments that provide usual intakes (e.g. FFQs). In addition, the hybrid approaches require response variables, which need to be continuous variables, such as biomarker levels. The patterns can be labelled according to characteristic pattern combinations of foods or predicted response variables.

Strengths and limitations of dietary pattern approaches

In general, all of the three methods, a priori, a posteriori and hybrid, have their specific advantages and disadvantages that need to be considered when choosing one or the other. In this respect, it is essential that the derived dietary patterns are evaluated in terms of reproducibility and validity. Comparisons of different methodologies are also recommended. The main strengths and limitations of each of the three methods are shown in Table 4.3.

Dietary patterns (*multivariate analyses*) are considered complementary to the traditional single food or nutrient approach (*univariate analyses*). Since diet is a complex exposure, it calls for multiple approaches to examine the relationship with disease risk.

4.6 An integrated approach for assessing and analysing dietary intake

Considerable advances in concepts of dietary assessment have occurred over time, aiming to prevent or minimise the effects of measurement error in usual dietary intake estimates. This is particularly, but not exclusively, the case for large population-based studies. These approaches are based on the integration and combination of different dietary (self-report) assessment methods and biomarkers, with the ultimate purpose of optimising their strengths while balancing their weaknesses (see Section 4.2). Furthermore, integrated approaches for assessing and analysing dietary intake require the matching of food consumption data to related food composition tables.

Combining different dietary intake assessment methods

In nutritional epidemiology, the use of self-reported dietary questionnaires (e.g. FFQs) on their own has been challenged. New approaches increasingly favour the use of repeated short-term and open-ended dietary assessment methods, such as quantitative 24-hour

Table 4.3 Characteristics of methods of deriving dietary patterns.

Method	Aim	Common principles and method-specific strengths and weaknesses
Hypothesis-oriented (a priori) methods	Evaluating adherence to dietary guidelines, specific diets or guidelines for prevention of a chronic disease	Theoretically defined according to a priori knowledge for a healthy diet; main example: diet quality indices or scores. **Strengths:** Monitoring of overall adherence to dietary guidelines; evaluation of overall effects of dietary interventions, especially where simultaneous changes in the diet can be expected; subgroups in a population at risk of poor dietary quality are more easily identified; diet quality can be assessed even if only limited dietary information is available or obtainable; evaluation of whether current guidelines for a healthy diet have a protective effect against diseases and to estimate the magnitude of overall effect. **Weaknesses:** Overall diet is not necessarily captured since scores usually focus on specific aspects of the diet; correlations between dietary variables are at best not fully considered.
Exploratory (a posteriori) methods	Explaining as much variation in intake of a dietary variable as possible	(1) Dietary variables (e.g., foods, nutrients) are combined into fewer factors based on their linear relationship; main example principal component analysis (PCA). (2) Individuals with similar diets are aggregated into non-overlapping subgroups (clusters); main example cluster analysis. (3) Combination of PCA and factor analysis; main example treelet transform. **Strengths:** Interactive effects of foods eaten in combination on bioavailability and circulating levels of nutrients are more easily captured; alleviates problems of model over-fitting (multicollinearity between individual dietary variables in a single model), of loss of statistical power in detecting diet–disease association, and of confounding of a single dietary variable by dietary patterns. **Weaknesses:** Not necessarily related to health outcomes; lack of reproducibility of patterns over time and/or between different researchers due to many arbitrary and impacting decisions during the process of deriving patterns; outcomes cannot be linked to a single dietary variable.
Hybrid methods	Explaining as much variation in a response variable as possible	Patterns depend on a priori knowledge in selecting a response variable (e.g. biomarker of disease) and the correlation structure of dietary variables; main example reduced rank regression (RRR). **Strengths:** Consideration of a priori knowledge of biological pathways; these methods should be thus more predictive of disease risk. **Weaknesses:** Requires response information (e.g. biomarker), which may not be available in many studies; potential confounding of biomarker by dietary pattern.

dietary recalls or food records. This new design, initially proposed in European and US food surveillance studies, introduced several innovative statistical methods to estimate individual intakes and population means and distributions more effectively when a limited number of repeated dietary measurements (24-hour dietary recalls or food records) are used. The new statistical models assume that usual intake is equal to the probability of consumption on a given day times the average amount consumed on a consumption day.

Among those developed in connection with 24-hour dietary recalls are the National Cancer Institute Method (NCI), the Multiple Source Method (MSM) and the Statistical Program to Assess Dietary Exposure (SPADE). All these methods combine quantitative data from repeated 24-hour dietary recalls (at least two) with additional covariate information. For example, non-quantitative FFQs or food propensity questionnaires (FPQs), querying only the frequency of consumption, are employed for identifying habitual users of less frequently consumed foods, hence providing important covariate information aiming to reduce within-person variability (i.e. random errors).

Thus, in contrast to linear regression calibration approaches – which regress 24-hour dietary recall data collected from a representative subsample of the study population on FFQ derived data and apply the derived calibration coefficients to correct for population mean differences and for deattenuation of the relative risk estimates (see Section 4.4) – these newer, combined approaches were designed to use short-term dietary assessment methods for measurement of individual intake in the whole study population.

However, the use of repeated interviewer-administered 24-hour dietary recalls on a large scale is costly and implies high logistical demands. So far, the combined approaches have therefore been applied more frequently in monitoring surveys that often include smaller study populations (several thousands) as compared to epidemiological studies (tens or hundreds of thousands). Although the methodological value of the combined approaches still requires further exploration – for example in terms of precise estimation of the probability of consumption – they seem to be promising approaches for deriving individual usual intake and population mean and distribution. The advent of new technologies fosters both the application

of web-based self-reported 24-hour dietary recalls (particularly as the substitute for or complement to traditional FFQs in large study settings), as well as web-based infrastructures to facilitate the conduct and maintenance of traditional interviewer-administered 24-hour dietary recalls.

All self-reported dietary assessment methods are prone to error and none of them alone appears to be suitable for assessing individual usual food intake. The inclusion of recovery or concentration biomarker information (e.g. nutritional biomarkers and increasingly food or other related metabolites) in the estimation of individual usual dietary intake therefore warrants further investigation (see Section 4.4).

In conclusion, the promising direction towards integrated approaches benefiting from advanced technologies to enhance the assessment of usual dietary intake should include, in an optimal study design, short-term repeated dietary assessment methods (i.e. repeated 24-hour dietary recall or food records) for measuring individual dietary intake and population mean and distribution; a complementary food propensity questionnaire (or FFQ) for estimating infrequently consumed foods; biomarkers of diet or its metabolites as independent measurements; and new statistical modelling for integrating the dietary assessment methods and related measurements (Figure 4.8).

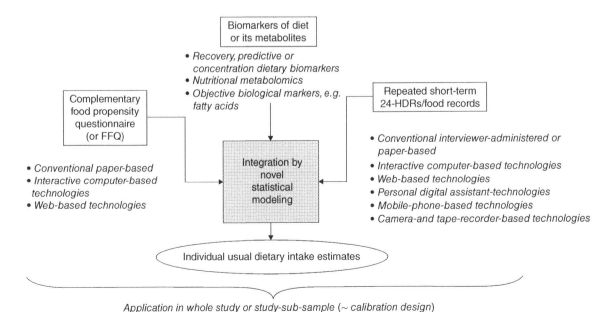

Figure 4.8 Towards an integrated approach to measure diet in international epidemiological studies. From Illner, A.K., Freisling, H., Boeing, H. *et al.* (2012) Review and evaluation of innovative technologies for measuring diet in nutritional epidemiology. *International Journal of Epidemiology*, **41** (4), 1187–1203, by permission of Oxford University Press.

Food composition tables and food matching

Dietary intake is usually assessed at the food intake level, but also at nutrient or other food component levels (e.g. chemicals, additives, contaminants), depending on the research interest. It is therefore necessary to convert collected food consumption data into nutrient intake, through matching to related food composition tables (or databases if in electronic format). In this food-matching process, the best match is sought between food consumption data (e.g. individual food items, ingredients or recipes) and equivalent/similar items in the food composition databases or other occurrence databases. Expert knowledge is required for this process and the related work should not be underestimated. The importance of internationally harmonised food composition databases should also be emphasised, especially in studies aiming at pooling data for analyses at nutrient or food component levels.

These and other requirements and activities related to food composition are detailed in Chapter 5.

References and further reading

Amft, O. and Troster, G. (2008) Recognition of dietary activity events using on-body sensors. *Artificial Intelligence in Medicine*, **42**, 2, 121–136.

Arab, L., Wesseling-Perry, K., Jardack, P. *et al.* (2010) Eight self-administered 24-hour dietary recalls using the Internet are feasible in African Americans and Whites: The energetics study. *Journal of the American Dietetic Association*, **110**, 6, 857–864.

Baranowski, T., Baranowski, J.C., Watson, K.B. *et al.* (2010) Children's accuracy of portion size estimation using digital food images: Effects of interface design and size of image on computer screen. *Public Health Nutrition*, **15**, 1–8.

Beasley, J.M., Davis, A. and Riley, W.T. (2009) Evaluation of a web-based, pictorial diet history questionnaire. *Public Health Nutrition*, **12**, 5, 651–659.

Beasley, J., Riley, W.T. and Jean-Mary, J. (2005) Accuracy of a PDA-based dietary assessment program. *Nutrition*, **21**, 672–677.

Bingham, S.A., Luben, R. and Welch, A. (2003) Are imprecise methods obscuring a relation between fat and breast cancer? *Lancet*, **362**, 212–214.

Boeckner, L.S., Pullen, C.H., Walker, S.N. *et al.* (2002) Use and reliability of the World Wide Web version of the Block Health Habits and History Questionnaire with older rural women. *Journal of Nutrition Education and Behavior*, **34**, Suppl 1, S20–S24.

Dodd, K.W., Guenther, P.M., Freedman, L.S. *et al.* (2006) Statistical methods for estimating usual intake of nutrients and foods: A review of the theory. *Journal of the American Dietetic Association*, **106** (10), 1640–1650.

Fowles, E.R. and Gentry, B. (2008) The feasibility of personal digital assistants (PDAs) to collect dietary intake data in low-income pregnant women. *Journal of Nutrition Education and Behavior*, **40**, 374–377.

Freisling, H., Knaze, V. and Slimani, K. (2013) A systematic review of peer-reviewed studies on diet quality indexes applied in old age: A multitude of predictors of diet quality. In V.R. Preedy, L.-A. Hunter and V.B. Patel (eds), *Diet Quality: An Evidence-Based Approach, Volume 2, Nutrition and Health*, Springer, New York.

Fukuo, W., Yoshiuchi, K., Ohashi, K. *et al.* (2009) Development of a hand-held personal digital assistant-based food diary with food photographs for Japanese subjects. *Journal of the American Dietetic Association*, **109**, 1232–1236.

Gibney, B.J., Margetts, B.M. and Arab, L. (2004) *Public Health Nutrition*. Blackwell, Oxford.

Heath, A.L., Roe, M.A., Oyston, S.L. and Fairweather-Tait, S.J. (2005) Meal-based intake assessment tool: Relative validity when determining dietary intake of Fe and Zn and selected absorption modifiers in UK men. *British Journal of Nutrition*, **93**, 3, 403–416.

Higgins, J.A., LaSalle, A.L., Zhaoxing, P. *et al.* (2009) Validation of photographic food records in children: Are pictures really worth a thousand words? *European Journal of Clinical Nutrition*, **63**, 1025–1033.

Hu, F.B. (2002) Dietary pattern analysis: A new direction in nutritional epidemiology. *Current Opinion in Lipidology*, **13** (1), 3–9.

Illner, A.K., Freisling, H., Boeing, H. *et al.* (2012) Review and evaluation of innovative technologies for measuring diet in nutritional epidemiology. *International Journal of Epidemiology*, **41**, 1187–1203.

Jia, W., Chen, H-C., Yue, Y. *et al.* (2014) Accuracy of food portion size estimation from digital pictures acquired by a chest-worn camera. Public Health Nutrition, **17**, 1671–1681.

Kipnis, V., Subar, A.F., Midthune, D. *et al.* (2003) Structure of dietary measurement error: Results of the OPEN biomarker study. *American Journal of Epidemiolpgy*, **158** (1), 14–21.

Kristal, A.R. and Potter, J.D. (2006) Not the time to abandon the food frequency questionnaire: Counterpoint. *Cancer Epidemiology, Biomarkers and Prevention*, **15**, 1759–1760.

Kristal, A.R., Peters, U. and Potter, J.D. (2005) Is it time to abandon the food frequency questionnaire? *Cancer Epidemiology, Biomarkers and Prevention*, **14**, 2826–2828.

Lambert, N., Plumb, J., Looise, B. *et al.* (2005) Using smart card technology to monitor the eating habits of children in a school cafeteria: 1. Developing and validating the methodology. *Journal of Human Nutrition and Dietetics*, **18**, 4, 243–254.

Lassen, A.D., Poulsen, S., Ernst, L. *et al.* (2010) Evaluation of a digital method to assess evening meal intake in a free-living adult population. *Food & Nutrition Research*, **54**.

Lindquist, C.H., Cummings, T. and Goran, M. (2000) Use of taperecorded food records in assessing children's dietary intake. *Obesity Research*, **8**, 2–11.

Margetts, B. and Nelson, M. (1997) *Design Concepts in Nutritional Epidemiology*. Oxford University Press, New York.

Matthys, C., Pynaert, I., De, K.W. and De, H.S. (2007) Validity and reproducibility of an adolescent web-based food frequency questionnaire. *Journal of the American Dietetic Association*, **107**, 4, 605–610.

McClung, H.L., Sigrist, L.D., Smith, T.J. *et al.* (2009) Monitoring energy intake: A hand-held personal digital assistant provides accuracy comparable to written records. *Journal of the American Dietetic Association*, **109**, 1241–1245.

Murtaugh, M.A., Ma, K.N., Greene, T. *et al.* (2010) Validation of a dietary history questionnaire for American Indian and Alaska Native people. *Ethnicity & Disease*, **20**, 4, 429–436.

Newby, P.K. and Tucker, K.L. (2004) Empirically derived eating patterns using factor or cluster analysis: A review. *Nutrition Review*, **62** (5), 177–203.

Ocké, M.C. (2013) Evaluation of methodologies for assessing the overall diet: Dietary quality scores and dietary pattern analysis. *Proceedings of the Nutrition Society*, **72** (2), 191–199.

Popkin, B.M. (2006) Global nutrition dynamics: The world is shifting rapidly toward a diet linked with noncommunicable diseases. *American Journal of Clinical Nutrition*, **84**, 289–298.

Popkin, B.M., Lu, B. and Zhai, F. (2002) Understanding the nutrition transition: Measuring rapid dietary changes in transitional countries. *Public Health Nutrition*, **5** (6A), 947–953.

Rivera, J.A., Barquera, S., González-Cossío, T. *et al.* (2004) Nutrition transition in Mexico and in other Latin American countries. *Nutrition Review*, **62**, S149–S157.

Schatzkin, A., Kipnis, V., Carroll, R.J. *et al.* (2003) A comparison of a food frequency questionnaire with a 24-hour recall for use in an epidemiological cohort study: Results from the biomarker-based Observing Protein and Energy Nutrition (OPEN) study. *International Journal of Epidemiology*, **32**, 1054–1062.

Schatzkin, A., Subar, A.F., Moore, S. *et al.* (2009). Observational epidemiologic studies of nutrition and cancer: The next generation (with better observation). *Cancer Epidemiology, Biomarkers and Prevention*, **18**, 1026–1032.

Schulze, M.B. and Hoffmann, K. (2006) Methodological approaches to study dietary patterns in relation to risk of coronary heart disease and stroke. *British Journal of Nutrition*, **95** (5), 860–869.

Schwerin, H.S., Stanton, J.L., Smith, J.L. *et al.* (1982) Food, eating habits, and health: A further examination of the relationship between food eating patterns and nutritional health. *American Journal of Clinical Nutrition*, **35** (5 Suppl), 1319–1325.

Stumbo, P.J., Weiss, R., Newman, J.W. *et al.* (2010) Web-enabled and improved software tools and data are needed to measure nutrient intakes and physical activity for personalized health research. *Journal of Nutrition*, **140**, 2104–2115.

Subar, A.F., Thompson, F.E., Potischman, N. *et al.* (2007) Formative research of a quick list for an automated self-administered 24-hour dietary recall. *Journal of the American Dietetic Association*, **107**, 6, 1002–1007.

Six, B.L., Schap, T.E., Zhu, F.M. *et al.* (2010) Evidence-based development of a mobile telephone food record. *Journal of the American Dietetic Association*, **110**, 74–79.

Sun, M., Fernstrom, J.D., Jia, W. *et al.* (2010) A wearable electronic system for objective dietary assessment. *Journal of the American Dietetic Association*, **110**, 1, 45–47.

Thompson, F.E. and Subar, A.F. (2013) Dietary assessment methodology. In Coulston, A.M., Boushey, C.J. and Ferruzzi, M.G. (eds), *Nutrition in the Prevention and Treatment of Disease*, 3rd edn. Elsevier, Philadelphia, PA.

Touvier, M., Kesse-Guyot, E., Mejean, C. *et al.* (2011) Comparison between an interactive web-based self-administered 24 h dietary record and an interview by a dietitian for large-scale epidemiological studies. *British Journal of Nutrition*, **105**, 7, 1055–1064.

Vereecken, C.A., Covents, M., Matthys, C. and Maes, L. (2005) Young adolescents' nutrition assessment on computer (YANA-C). *European Journal of Clinical Nutrition*, **59**, 5, 658–667.

Waijers, P.M., Feskens, E.J. and Ocké, M.C. (2007) A critical review of predefined diet quality scores. *British Journal of Nutrition*, **97** (2), 219–231.

Weiss, R., Stumbo, P.J. and Divakaran, A. (2010) Automatic food documentation and volume computation using digital imaging and electronic transmission. *Journal of the American Dietetic Association*, **110**, 42–44.

Willett, W.C. (2013) *Nutritional Epidemiology*. Oxford University Press, New York.

Willett, W.C. and Hu, F.B. (2006) Not the time to abandon the food frequency questionnaire: Point. *Cancer Epidemiolody, Biomarkers and Prevention*, **15**, 1757–1758.

Williamson, D.A., Allen, H.R., Martin, P.D. *et al.* (2004) Digital photography: A new method for estimating food intake in cafeteria settings. *Eating and Weight Disorders*, **9**, 1, 24–28.

Wong, S.S., Boushey, C.J., Novotny, R. and Gustafson, D.R. (2008) Evaluation of a computerized food frequency questionnaire to estimate calcium intake of Asian, Hispanic, and non-Hispanic white youth. *Journal of the American Dietetic Association*, **108**, 3, 539–543.

World Cancer Research Fund (2008) *Food, Nutrition and the Prevention of Cancer: A Global Perspective*. WCRF and American Institute for Cancer Research, Washington, DC.

Yon, B.A., Johnson, R.K., Harvey-Berino, J. and Gold, B.C. (2006) The use of a personal digital assistant for dietary self-monitoring does not improve the validity of self-reports of energy intake. *Journal of the American Dietetic Association*, **106**, 1256–1259.

Zoellner, J., Anderson, J. and Gould, S.M. (2005) Comparative validation of a bilingual interactive multimedia dietary assessment tool. *Journal of the American Dietetic Association*, **105**, 8, 1206–1214.

5
Food Composition

Barbara Burlingame and U Ruth Charrondiere

Food and Agriculture Organization of the United Nations

Key messages

- Food composition work is research in its own right, and it is the fundamental underpinning to nearly all other research activities in nutrition.
- Food composition covers nutrients, bioactive non-nutrients, anti-nutrients and chemical contaminants in foods.
- Without robust food composition data, dietary surveys cannot be analysed, nutritional epidemiology cannot derive associations/

causality, nutrition interventions cannot be properly targeted, nutrient requirements cannot be determined and food labels cannot be validated.
- The International Network of Food Data Systems (INFOODS), in operation since 1983 and based at FAO, provides the infrastructure for food composition data standards, harmonisation, advocacy and communication.

5.1 Introduction

Food composition activities include sampling and sample preparation, data generation, data compilation, data dissemination and data use.

Historically, food composition activities were limited to data on a small subset of nutrients, usually classified as proximates, vitamins, minerals, and occasionally fatty acids and amino acids. Increasingly, food composition work deals with data for any component found in food that can be measured chemically, biologically or physiologically: a greater range of conventional nutrients and different forms/activities of those nutrients, bioassay data such as measurements of protein quality or glycaemic index, bioactive non-nutrients, anti-nutrients, pesticide residues, heavy metals, additives and more. A single food composition database, with proper documentation, can accommodate data on all these types of components. However, these data are rarely combined and published in a single database.

5.2 Sectors

Food composition data are useful to many sectors and professions within those sectors. Health, agriculture, environment and trade (including the food industry) are

the most notable sectors. The agriculture sector has had a dominant role over many decades in food composition research and service. The Food and Agriculture Organization of the United Nations (FAO) has a long history of food composition work dating back to its inception in the 1940s and it has been the United Nations (UN) agency host for the International Network of Food Data Systems (INFOODS) since 1998. The UK and USA have even longer histories in food composition work dating back to the late nineteenth century, again in the agriculture sector, with responsible agencies being the Ministry of Agriculture, Fisheries and Food and the United States Department of Agriculture (USDA) respectively.

The other historically dominant sector is health. More than half the participants in food composition conferences, and the researchers publishing food composition papers and books, are health-sector professionals. It is often the health sector that provides a high percentage of the funding for food composition work, and the sector that claims the highest percentage of data users.

Involvement of the environment sector is becoming increasingly important as it relates to the composition of food biodiversity; that is, food described at the taxonomic level below species, and wild, neglected and

Nutrition Research Methodologies, First Edition. Edited by Julie A Lovegrove, Leanne Hodson, Sangita Sharma and Susan A Lanham-New.
© 2015 John Wiley & Sons, Ltd. Published 2015 by John Wiley & Sons, Ltd.
Companion Website: www.wiley.com/go/nutritionsociety

under-utilised species. The environment sector also has a leading role in determining and monitoring chemical contaminants in the food supply.

Last, trade has emerged as a sector with a great interest in food composition. Nutrient information panels on processed foods have become regulatory requirements in many countries, and analytical data on both nutrient and contaminant content are necessary documentation for global food trade. Food retailers, restaurants and other food service providers are using food composition data in response to consumer demand.

More details on the importance of food composition to different sectors are provided later in this chapter in the section on data use.

5.3 The Organizational Elements

The international level

INFOODS was established in 1983 by the United Nations University (UNU), with an organisational framework and international management structure that include a global secretariat and regional data centres. Its mandate is the 'Promotion of international participation and cooperation in the acquisition and dissemination of complete and accurate data on the composition of foods, beverages and their ingredients, in forms appropriate to meet the needs of the various users (government agencies, nutrition scientists and educators, health and agriculture professionals, policy makers and planners, food producers/processors/retailers and consumers)'. In the mid-1990s, FAO joined UNU in partnership for INFOODS. The main activities of INFOODS at the international level include the development of technical food composition standards, guidelines and tools, often through expert consultation processes; the development of technical publications and manuals; assistance to regional data centres and individual countries in developing their food composition activities; capacity development through classroom and online courses; and the biennial International Food Data Conference, which has been held in alternate years since 1993, with each second conference as an official satellite to the IUNS International Congress of Nutrition.

The regional level

There are 17 regional data centres in operation, most with well-established and effective coordination. Important activities include the preparation and updating of regional food composition tables, in both electronic and printed form (e.g. in West Africa, Pacific Islands, ASEANFOODS, LATINFOODS), convening of regular food composition coordination activities and technical task forces involving all the individual countries in the region, and participating in standard-setting consultation convened by the INFOODS Secretariat.

The national level

Most countries have food composition activities of one form or other. A national food composition programme is usually the result of the combination and coordination of activities, within some defined administrative framework, related to food composition data generation, compilation, dissemination and use. A steering committee is a useful structure, functioning well in many countries. This steering, or advisory, committee is ideally composed of individuals directly involved in food composition work: data generators, data compilers and data disseminators. Crucial to the effectiveness of a steering committee is the involvement of data users. The users can be selected from among dietitians, nutritionists, food industry personnel and consumer group representatives.

Often a single organisation holds the overall responsibility for managing a national food composition programme, yet it is rare that a single organisation accomplishes all the activities itself. Regardless of their affiliations, the laboratory-based data generators must interact closely with the data compilers, and the compilers must interact closely with the data users. The data compilers therefore serve the central function of, and usually serve in the role of, data disseminators (that is, they publish the data, electronically and/or as printed tables). In most countries there are other agencies with activities that have direct or indirect relationships with food composition data, but operate in concert with the national programme. In addition to the desirability of a coordinated national approach for accomplishing essential activities, it is productive and important for a national food composition programme to operate in conjunction with its regional data centre, and with ongoing international activities.

5.4 Technical elements

Data generation is the process whereby foods are sampled, prepared for analysis and analysed in the laboratory. Data compilation is the process whereby the data from the laboratory and other sources are examined, manipulated and incorporated into a food composition database. Data dissemination refers to the preparation and publication of books and electronic data products, which are made available to users in the various sectors.

Data use also includes the application of these data to tasks, projects and programmes in the various professional sectors.

Data generation

Sampling

Sampling – that is, the process and procedures for obtaining foods that are representative of those available and consumed – is fundamental to any food composition activity. Preparation of a sampling plan often requires the involvement of all the major contributors to a food composition programme. Data generators must be involved in sample collections, or at least the scheduling of sample collections, so that samples may be immediately and properly prepared for analysis. Data compilers must be involved because information on the sampling plan, and details such as when and where sampling took place, are important parts of a food composition database's metadata. Data users must be involved because they have the best appreciation of the foods that need to be analysed, and often of the location from which the samples should be collected. The services of a statistician are useful for developing a sampling plan, because representativeness is dictated by the number of food units collected – and analysed – to achieve the goal. The goal might be to compare compositional differences between cultivars, or to achieve year-round, nationwide mean values for a food composition database. The overall quality of food composition data is determined largely by the sampling plan.

The collected samples must be properly handled so that they arrive at the laboratory without changes that might affect their composition. The key component, crucial to the correct determination of almost all other food components and most easily affected by improper handling and storage, is water (moisture). Once samples are delivered and documented, they are prepared for analysis. Preparation may involve separation of the edible from the inedible portion (for example, removal of bones from fish, or skins and seeds from pumpkins); kitchen-type preparation (for example, boiling rice); or combining of many samples into fewer samples (for example, combining five brands of similar biscuits into one representative composite sample). After this type of preparation, samples will be stored or immediately analysed. As with sample collection and sample handling, proper documentation of all aspects of sample preparation is essential.

Analyses

Most laboratories undertake a limited range of analyses for food composition purposes. This includes a set of core components and then additional components of interest, for example laboratory research dealing with diet-related health problems. Core nutrients usually include the complete range of proximate components (water, nitrogen for the protein calculation, fat, available carbohydrate, dietary fibre, ash, alcohol where relevant, and an energy value using factors applied to the energy-yielding proximates), some vitamins and some nutrient elements. Additional components of interest often include cholesterol, individual fatty acids and aggregations of fatty acids (for example, total saturated fatty acids), carotenoids (both provitamin A carotenoids and antioxidant carotenoids with no provitamin A activity), other bioactive non-nutrients, heavy metals and some so-called anti-nutrients (for example, phytates). Proper laboratory practices must be strictly adhered to, and laboratory quality assurance and quality control procedures, and details of analytical methodologies, must be properly documented.

Table 5.1 provides an overview of analytical methods commonly used for macronutrients, along with their applications and limitations. Table 5.2 provides an overview of commonly measured food components, their recommended units of measure for most food composition purposes, and INFOODS tagnames, the use of which will minimise misinterpretation of the food component.

Data compilation

Data compilation requires a relational database management system and adherence to international food composition standards where they exist. The database should accommodate numerical data, text and graphics. Ideally, all the raw analytical data, and their attendant documentation, should be captured. The system should then be able to manipulate these data in many different ways. The same data system should provide an exhaustive reference database and any number of abridged user databases to satisfy the broad range of user requirements for food composition data. Many compilers only capture mean values, a practice that will satisfy many users. Other compilers provide more information, and therefore higher-quality databases, by including the number of samples and some expression of their variability (standard deviation [SD] or standard error [SE]). Other compilers are able to capture all the analytical data and prepare user databases with ranges (that is, high and low values), medians and many different statistical expressions of the data, satisfying a broader spectrum of users and ensuring the highest-quality database.

Some compilers publish their databases by listing calculated components – for example, a calculated value for vitamin A in retinol equivalents (RE) without individual values for retinol, provitamin A carotenoids and

Table 5.1 Macronutrient analysis.

Food component	Available method of analysis	Limitation	Application
Water (moisture)	Air oven*	Caramelisation of sugars, degradation of unsaturated fat, loss of volatiles	This method is applicable to all foods at 60°C. At 100°C, it is applicable to all foods except those rich in fat and sugar
	Vacuum oven*	Loss of volatiles	
	Freeze-drying*	Slow. Care must be taken to avoid residual water in samples	Applicable to most foods
	Microwave oven	Charring	Applicable to medium- or high-moisture foods only
	Dean and Stark distillation	Safety of solvents used	Applicable to foods high in volatiles*
	Karl Fisher		Applicable to low-moisture, hygroscopic foods
	Physical methods (NMR, NIR)	High cost and needs calibration for each food group	NMR is applicable to most foods. NIR is only established for cereals and some other foods
	Chromatography (GLC, GSC)	High cost	GLC is applicable to meat and meat products only. GSC is applicable only to some meat products
Total fat	Continuous extraction (single solvent, also called Soxhlet)	Time consuming. Extracts cannot be used for fatty acid studies. Incomplete extraction from many foods (dry analytical samples). Non-comparable value for cereals	Applicable to low-moisture foods and non-cereal foods
	Acid hydrolysis	Some hydrolysis of lipids. Extracts cannot be used for fatty acid studies	Applicable to all foods except dairy and high-sugar products
	Acid hydrolysis and capillary GLC	High cost. This method is NLEA-compliant	Applicable to most foods
	Mixed solvent extraction*	Complete extraction from most foods. Extract often needs clean-up	Applicable to most foods and extract can be used for fatty acid analysis
	Alkaline hydrolysis		Validated for dairy foods only
	NIR	High cost. Requires extensive calibration against other methods	Established only for cereals
Fatty acids	HPLC	High cost	
	GLC*	Moderate to high cost	Applicable to all foods. If used for *trans* fatty acids, capillary techniques are required
	Infrared absorption (for *trans* fatty acids)	High cost. Some interference	Applicable to all foods
Total nitrogen/ protein	Kjeldahl (for total nitrogen)*	Minor interference from inorganic nitrogen. Toxic wastes	Applicable to all foods
	Dumas (for total nitrogen)*	High cost, inclusion of inorganic nitrogen and analytical portion size	Applicable to all foods
	Radiochemical methods (for total nitrogen)	Very high cost of instrumentation	Applicable to most foods
	Formol titration; Biuret; Folin's reagent (for protein)	Specificity	Applicable to dairy products only
	Alkaline distillation (for protein)	Specificity	Applicable to cereals only
	Dye-binding (for protein)	Specificity	Applicable only to specific foods, and some cereals and legumes
	NIR (for protein)	High cost. Number of calibration samples	Applicable to some foods
Amino acids (AA)	GLC, preceded by acid hydrolysis for most AA. Alkaline hydrolysis required for tryptophan. Special hydrolysis conditions required for sulphur AA and acid-sensitive AA.	Moderate to high cost. Choice of derivative is critical. AA need to be derivatized prior to chromatography	Applicable to most foods

Food component	Available method of analysis	Limitation	Application
	HPLC,* preceded by acid hydrolysis for most AA. Alkaline hydrolysis required for tryptophan. Special hydrolysis conditions required for sulphur AA and acid-sensitive AA. AA usually derivatised prior to chromatography	High cost	Applicable to all foods
	Ion-exchange chromatography,* preceded by acid hydrolysis for most AA. Alkaline hydrolysis required for tryptophan. Special hydrolysis conditions required for sulphur AA and acid-sensitive AA.	High cost. Hydrolytic losses of more labile AA and slow release of branched-chain AA	Applicable to all foods
	LC-MS	High cost	Applicable to all foods
	Colorimetry (Tryptophan and sulphur containing AA, lysine)	Not sensitive enough	Applicable to all foods
	Microbiological assays	Tedious, time-consuming, non-reproducibility	Applicable to all foods
Alcohol	Distillation*	Interference with volatiles	Applicable to all foods
	GLC*		Applicable to all foods
	Specific enzyme method*		Applicable to all foods
Sugars, total (mono- and disaccharides)	Density	Accurate for sucrose	Applicable to sugar solutions
	Refractive index	Empirical calibration required	Applicable to sugar solution
	Polarimetry	Close attention to standardised methods is essential	Applicable to single sugars or simple mixtures only
	Reductiometric	Non-reducing sugars, sucrose and invert sugar mixtures	Applicable to reducing sugars
	Colorimetric	Specificity	Applicable to single sugars and simple mixtures
	Specific enzyme method*	Reagents can be expensive	Applicable to glucose and complex mixtures
	GLC	Need for derivatives	Can be applied to complex mixtures
	HPLC*	Moderate to high cost. Choice of columns, detectors are crucial	Can be applied to complex mixtures
Polyols	Specific enzymatic method	Specificity of enzymes	Limited to a few polyols only
	HPLC*	Moderate to high cost. Lack of standardised procedures; choice of column	Can be applied to complex mixtures
	Microbiology	Acyclic polyol only	All foods
Oligosaccharides	Specific enzymatic procedures	Moderate to high cost	Applied for selective hydrolysis and separation
	GLC	Moderate to high cost. Choice of column	Can be applied to complex mixtures
	HPLC	Moderate to high cost	Can be applied to complex mixtures
Starch	Polarimetry	Needs very careful calibration	Applicable only to some cereal foods
	Dilute acid hydrolysis using a general sugar method	Interference from any NSP present	Applicable to highly refined foods that are low in NSP
	Dilute acid hydrolysis and glucose-specific method	Presence of β-glucans	Applicable only to foods low in β-glucans
	Enzymatic hydrolysis and glucose-specific method*	Choice of enzymes and conditions	Applicable to all foods

(Continued)

Table 5.1 (*Continued*)

Food component	Available method of analysis	Limitation	Application
Dietary fibres			
Total dietary fibre	AOAC method for dietary fibres (Prosky *et al.*),* an enzymatic–gravimetric method	Time-consuming	Applicable to all foods
Non-starch polysaccharides (NSP)	Enzymatic hydrolysis and removal of starch. Acid hydrolysis of NSP, GLC, HPLC separation of component monosaccharides. Colorimetric analysis of monosaccharide (Englyst *et al.*)	Moderate to high cost. Resistant starch must be treated before hydrolysis. GLC requires preparation of derivatives. Gives only total values. This method is not robust	Applicable to all foods
Resistant starch	Enzymatic hydrolysis of starch before and after treatment with alkali or DMSO	Choice of enzymes and conditions	Applicable to all foods

Inorganic material analysis: applicable to all foods after defatting and drying, especially for food high in fat and/or water content

Food component	Available method of analysis	Limitations
Total ash	Dry ashing	Not suitable for mineral analysis of volatile minerals because of their partial loss
	Wet ashing	Small sample throughput
Cations		
Na*, K*, Ca, Mg	Flame photometry	Interference
Na, K, Ca*, Mg*, Fe*, Cu*, Zn*, Mn*, Co*, Cr*	Atomic absorption spectrometry (AAS) with electrothermal furnace	Moderate to high cost. Interferences from anions; special suppression techniques
Se*	Hydride-generation AAS	Moderate to high cost
	Fluorimetry	
all cations	Plasma-emission spectrometry (=inductively coupled plasma spectroscopy ICP) ideally coupled with mass spectrometry (MS)*	Very high cost. Matrix effects need to be controlled
K, Mg, Fe, Cu, Zn	Colorimetry	Extracting techniques. Difficult for K and Zn
Ca and Mg	Classical precipitation and titration	Size of analytical sample; skilled techniques
Anions		
Phosphorus	Colorimetry	
	ICP-MS	Very expensive
Chloride	Titrimetric	
	Ion-specific electrode (ISE)	Interference
	ICP-MS	Very expensive
	Automated conductimetry	High cost
Iodine	Microdistillation	Laboratory contamination
	ISE	
	ICP-MS	Very expensive
	Alkaline dry-ashing	
	GLC	High cost
Fluorine	Microdistillation	Time-consuming
	ISE	
	Polarography	
Sulphur	Gravimetric	
	X-ray fluorescence	High cost
	ICP-MS	Very expensive
Nitrite	Colorimetry	
	ISE	
Nitrate	HPLC	High cost

Vitamin analysis: applicable to all foods

Food component	Available method of analysis	Limitations
Retinol	Colorimetry	Obsolete (Carr and Price 1926). Low recoveries of retinoids
	HPLC*	Moderate to high cost
Carotenoids	Open column chromatography	Identification of carotenoids. Lack of resolution of some geometrical isomers (lutein/zeaxanthin) and stereo-isomers (cis/trans)
	HPLC*	Moderate to high cost. Identification of carotenoids
Vitamin D	Bioassay	For low level only; animal facilities required
	Colorimetry	Lack of precision and sensitivity
	GLC	New procedures under development
	HPLC*	High cost. Lipid interference; two stages, preparative followed by analytical separation needed for most foods
	Radio-immunoassay	High cost
Vitamin E	Colorimetry	Interfering compounds
	GLC	Derivation prior to chromatography required
	HPLC*	High cost. Extraction techniques
Vitamin K	Colorimetry	Lack of specificity
	Column chromatography, GLC*	Moderate to high cost for GLC
	HPLC*	High cost. Lipid interference
Vitamin C	Dye titration	Measure ascorbic acid only; pigments interfere; value lower as HPLC but comparable values for fresh fruits and vegetables
	Colorimetry	Measures inactive compounds also
	Fluorometry	Does not separate ascorbic and dehydroascorbic acid
	GLC	Derivitisation prior to chromatography required
	HPLC*	High cost. Clean-up and separate detection of homologues add delays
Thiamin/Riboflavin	Microbiological*	Time
	Fluorometry	
	HPLC*	High cost
Niacin	Microbiological*	Time
	Colorimetry	Hazardous reagent
	HPLC*	High cost
Vitamin B6	Microbiological*	Time; response to different vitamers may not be equal; total values only
	HPLC*	High cost
	Radiometric-microbiological	High cost
Vitamin B12	Microbiological*	
	Radio-isotopic	High cost
Folates	Microbiological*	Response to different vitamers may not be equal; total values only
	HPLC	High cost. Not all vitamers measured properly
	LC-MS	Very high cost, but this method is able to quantify the different isomers of folates
Pantothenic acid	Microbiological*	
	HPLC	High cost
Biotin	Microbiological*	
	Isotope dilution	High cost
	Radiometric-microbiological	High cost
	Radio-immunoassay	High cost
	Protein-binding	High cost
	HPLC	High cost

Analysis of other components

Food component	Available method of analysis	Limitations
Hemagglutinins/Lectins	RBC agglutination	Not all blood samples of one animal species will react in an identical manner owing to the existence of several blood groups. Agglutination dilution test semi-quantitative
	Spectrophotometric methods	
	Radioactive labelling of lectin molecules	Requires specialised handling

(Continued)

Table 5.1 (*Continued*)

Analysis of other components

Food component	Available method of analysis	Limitations
Phytic acid	Anion exchange	Inability to resolve inositol phosphates adequately
	HPLC	High cost
	GLC	Detects derivatised volatile inositol phosphate forms only after separation by ion-exchange chromatography
	Capillary electrophoresis	Not applicable to all foods
	NMR-MS	High costs. Specialised application
Oxalates	Capillary electrophoresis	Not good for low oxalate content < 1.8 mg/100 g. Meant for routine monitoring
	Ion chromatography	High running cost
	GLC	Some forms of oxalate are difficult to methylate; high instrument cost
	Enzymatic	Not applicable to all foods
	Colorimetry (AOAC)	Interference from other acids
	HPLC	High cost
Tannins (grouped into condensed tannins also called proanthocyanidins, hydrolysable and derived tannins)	UV-Spectrometry Vanillin HCL reagent	Parameters like extraction time, temperature, vanillin and HCL concentration need to be strictly controlled
	UV-Spectrometry Folin-Denis reagent	Non-specific as they can react with any phenol present in plant tissue
	UV-Spectrometry Prussian blue reagent	Non-specific as they can react with any phenol present in plant tissue, qualitative test
	HPLC	Modest success for smaller compounds of derived tannins
	Colorimetry	Limited to basic compounds of hydrolysable tannins
Saponins	Spectrophotometric method	Not suitable for determination of medicagenic acid for which titrimetric method for the quantitative determination of this aglycone content has to be employed
	Bioassays	
	HPLC	Identification of individual saponins
Trypsin inhibitor	Colorimetric	Does not differentiate between the different protease inhibitors
	ELISA method using monoclonal antibodies derived from mice	
Flavonoids	HPLC	Sample hydrolysis required for optimum resolution and quantisation of quercetin, kaempferol, myricetin, luteolin and apigenin. Separate extraction without hydrolysis required for analysis of anthocyanidins and flavan-3-ols
	LC-MS	Hydrolysis not required as long as masses of individual flavonoid conjugates differ by more than mass resolution of mass spectrometer
Isoflavones** and coumestrol	HPLC	Complex conjugates, and their numbers may be difficult to resolve with some reversed-phase columns and simple mobile-phase programmes (isocratic)
	LC-MS	Hydrolysis not required as long as masses of individual conjugates differ by more than mass resolution of mass spectrometer
Lignans	HPLC	Isolariciresinol, pinoresinol, secoisolariciresinol and matairesinol
	GLC-MS	Only for matairesinol, secoisolariciresinol and shonanin in foods as trimethylsylyl derivatives

*recommended method.

**Isoflavones are a subclass of flavonoids, but because they have different and unique biological activities than other subclasses of flavonoids, they are analysed and compiled as a separate group.

DMSO, dimethyl sulfoxide; GLC, gas-liquid chromatography; GSC, gas-solid chromatography; GLC-MS, gas-liquid chromatography coupled with mass spectrometry; HPLC, high-performance (formerly high-pressure) liquid chromatography; ICP-MS, inductively coupled plasma mass spectrometry (or plasma emission spectrometry) coupled with mass spectrometry; ISE, ion-specific electrode; LC-MS, liquid chromatography with mass spectrometry; NIR, near infrared reflectance; NMR, nuclear magnetic resonance.

Table 5.2 Commonly measured food components, recommended units and INFOODS tagnames. For more information and additional tagnames see INFOODS (2012b), Klensin et al. (1989) and Charrondiere et al. (2011ab, Module 4b).

Component	INFOODS tagnames	Unit*	Comments	European Food Information Resource (EuroFIR) component identifiers (MI = method indicator)

Edible portion	**EDIBLE:** edible portion coefficient		• It is recommended that values for the edible part (or the inedible part/refuse) are recorded in the user table/database for each food entry (if information is available)
			• These values are needed:
			  ○ for a good food description
			  ○ to transform the weight of foods as purchased to the edible parts of the food
			  ○ to facilitate correct food matching
			• Different terms (e.g. edible portion, inedible portion/refuse) and modes of expression (e.g. % or coefficient) exist
			Examples of how to calculate edible coefficients for cooked foods based on raw foods (for foods where the inedible part is not discarded, e.g. meat and fish with bones) are given in INFOODS, 2012a, p.45.
				EDIBLE

Energy	**ENERC:** energy, total metabolisable; calculated from the energy-producing food components More tagnames exist, but are generally not used in user tables/DB	kJ (kcal)	• Energy values of foods presented in the user table/DB should always be calculated in one's own DB, by applying the 'metabolisable energy' conversion factors from Atwater (1910). Different metabolisable energy conversion factors are listed in *Annex 3* (p. 36). INFOODS recommends using the 'General Atwater factors including for dietary fibre' for use in user tables/DB It is not advisable to calculate kJ energy values from energy values in kcal because this may introduce bias. Energy conversion factors in kJ are neither exactly 4.184 nor 4.2 times higher than energy conversion factors in kcal; it may just give an indication	**ENERC**
Water	**WATER:** water Synonyms: moisture	g	• Values for water are required at all levels of data management including archival, reference and user table/DB. Water is the most important component to check and be published in user tables/DB • Water is required to calculate the nutrient values to per 100 g fresh weight of edible portion (EP) when, in the literature, nutrient values were reported on a dry matter basis (DM) • DM values are not published in user tables/DB, but in the scientific literature nutrient values are often reported per 100 g DM. Values reported in DM can be recalculated to fresh weight, if the DM value or the water value of the fresh food is given. Example: Calculate values from per DM to per 100 g EP: Nutrient value (NV) (g/100 g EP) = NV(g/100 g DM) × (100−water)/100	**WATER**

(Continued)

Table 5.2 (*Continued*)

Component	INFOODS tagnames	Unit*	Comments	European Food Information Resource (EuroFIR) component identifiers (MI = method indicator)
Protein and nitrogen components	**PROT** (formerly PROCNT): protein, total; calculated from total nitrogen **XN**: conversion factor for calculating total protein from total nitrogen **NNP**: non-protein nitrogen **PROCNP**: protein, total; calculated from protein nitrogen **NT**: nitrogen, total	g	• Values for protein are required at all levels of the data system (archival, reference and user DB) • Protein is usually a calculated value derived from total nitrogen value multiplied by nitrogen conversion factors • Nitrogen to protein conversion factors (XN) are given in *Annex 3* (p. 36). Nitrogen, total (NT) should be part of archival, reference and comprehensive user table/DB, but must not necessarily be part of a concise/abridged user table/DB.	- **PROT** + MI - Conversion factors are method parameters - no correspondence for NNP - **PROT** + MI NT

Total fat, fatty acids and lipid components	**FAT**: fat, total. Sum of triglycerides, phospholipids, sterols and related compounds. The analytical method is a mixed solvent extraction.
	Synonym: total lipid
	FATCE: fat, total; derived by analysis using continuous extraction. The Soxhlet method has often been used to analyse for total fat using continuous extraction. This method tends to underestimate the total fat value of a food.
	FAMS: fatty acids, total monounsaturated
	FAPU: fatty acids, total polyunsaturated
	FASAT: fatty acids, total saturated
	FATRN: fatty acids, total *trans*
	FAPUN3: fatty acids, total n-3 polyunsaturated
	FAPUN6: fatty acids, total n-6 polyunsaturated
		g	**Fat**
			• Fat values are required at all levels of the database management (archival, reference and user DB)
			• Fat values are highly method depended
			  ○ FAT is the preferred method
			  ○ FATCE: fat, total, Soxhlet, should be avoided since it leads to incomplete extraction and therefore results in lower values, in particular for foods with high amounts of polar and bound lipids
			• Fat and water values are important to check the food description and the concordance between foods. Fat contents of foods need to be compared when estimating values for fat-soluble components (e.g. fat-soluble vitamins, fatty acids) from other sources. If the difference in fat values between the food in the own DB and in the referenced source is higher than 10% the values for fat soluble components need to be adjusted
			Fatty acids
			• Individual fatty acids should be included in the reference DB. In concise user tables/DB the fatty acids may be grouped in total saturated, total monounsaturated and total polyunsaturated fatty acids
			Fatty acid should be expressed in mg/100 g fresh weight of the edible portion (EP). In the literature fatty acids are often expressed differently, including per g or 100 g fatty acids or fat. See the FAO/INFOODS Guidelines on Conversion among different units, denominators and expressions (FAO/INFOODS, 2012a) for further information
				FAT + MI
				
				FAT + MI
				
				FAMS
				FAPU
				FASAT
				FATRS
				FAPUN3
				FAPUN6

Carbohydrates	CHOAVL: carbohydrates, available. This value includes the free sugars plus dextrins, starch, and glycogen	g	**Carbohydrates** • Values for carbohydrates are required throughout the entire database system (archival, reference and user DB)	CHO + MI
	CHOAVLM: carbohydrates, available; expressed in monosaccharide equivalents. This value includes the free sugars plus dextrin, starch and glycogen		• The main difference in carbohydrates relates to: ○ whether or not fibre is included ○ if it is analysed or calculated by difference ○ if the value is expressed in anhydrous form or monosaccharide equivalents	CHO + MI + unit
	CHOAVLDF: carbohydrates, available; calculated by difference. This value is calculated: 100 − (weight in grams [water + protein + fat + ash + alcohol + dietary fibre] in 100 g of food)		• Generally, available carbohydrates are always preferred to total carbohydrates, because available carbohydrates represent only the carbohydrates available to the human body	CHO + MI
	CHOCDF: carbohydrates, total; calculated by difference. This value is calculated: 100 − (weight in grams [water + protein + fat + ash + alcohol] in 100 g of food)		• The most recommended expression is available carbohydrates by summation (CHOAVL). However, this method demands analytical values; in case analytical data are not available for most foods, it is recommended to use 'carbohydrates, available by difference' (CHOAVLDF; FAO, 2003) **Starch** • Starches including glycogen and polysaccharides should be part of a comprehensive user DB	CHOT + MI
	CHOCSM: carbohydrates, total; calculated by summation. This value is the sum of the sugars, starches, oligosaccharide and dietary fibre		**Oligosaccharides** • Are defined as carbohydrates with 3 to 9 monomeric units • Some oligosaccharides can be included in dietary fibre, if they are resistant to digestion in the intestine • In many foods oligosaccharides are in small amounts and are, therefore, not included in user tables/DB **Sugars total** • In many user tables/DB sugars are defined as mono- and disaccharides Sugars should be part of a concise user table/DB and individual mono-, di- and oligosaccharides as well as polyols should be part of a comprehensive user table/DB	CHOT + MI

(Continued)

Table 5.2 (Continued)

Component	INFOODS tagnames	Unit*	Comments	European Food Information Resource (EuroFIR) component identifiers (MI = method indicator)
Fibre	**FIBTG**: fibre, total dietary; determined gravimetrically by the AOAC total dietary fibre method (Prosky method). Sum of the water-soluble components and the water-insoluble components of dietary fibre **FIBTS**: fibre, total dietary; sum of non-starch polysaccharide components and lignin (Southgate method) **PSACNS/NSP**: non-starch polysaccharide, (Englyst fibre). This includes non-starch polysaccharides but excludes lignin, resistant starch and resistant oligosaccharides **FIBAD**: fibre; determined by acid detergent method. Includes cellulose, lignin and some hemicellulose **FIBADC**: fibre, acid detergent method, Clancy modification **FIBINS**: fibre, water insoluble. Sum of insoluble components from the AOAC total dietary fibre method; includes primarily lignin, cellulose, and most of the hemicelluloses **FIBSOL**: fibre, water soluble **FIBND**: fibre; determined by neutral detergent method. Includes lignin, cellulose, and insoluble hemicellulose **FIBC**: fibre, crude	g	• Dietary fibre values are required at all levels of the database system (archival, reference and user DB) • The values for fibre are method dependent and therefore need to be identified by the method used. Any calculation including fibre (e.g. sum of proximates, or carbohydrates calculated by difference) will be affected by how the fibre content was determined • New methods for dietary fibre have been developed that include all residual starch and resistant oligosaccharides. As these methods are still under development, it is suggested that one waits for finalisation before including those values in the Food Composition Database (FCDB). As Codex definition for dietary fibre may include resistant oligosaccharides, they may have to be included in FCDB in future • INFOODS recommends using total dietary fibre by AOAC Prosky (Greenfield *et al.*, 2002) • Dietary fibre by Prosky (FIBTG) captures most completely the components with dietary fibre functions, followed by FIBTS and PSACNS/NSP It would be best to phase out the use of FIBAD, FIBADC, FIBND and FIBC in favour of one of the other methods for determining total dietary fibre, such as FIBTG. New fibre methods are being developed including non-digestible oligosaccharides for which new tagnames will be needed, once fully approved and used in FCTs	**FIBT + MI** **FIBT + MI** **NSP + MI** **FIBT + MI** **FIBT + MI** **FIBINS + MI** **FIBSOL + MI** **FIBT + MI** **FIBC + MI**
Ash	**ASH**: ash	g	**Ash** • Ash values are used in internal checks on the sum of proximates, in the calculation of available or total carbohydrates, by difference. Therefore, it should be part of the archival and reference DB, but is often not included in a concise user table/DB. Ash values should be reported, if carbohydrates are calculated by difference. If no ash value is available, an ash value needs to be estimated from a similar food • Ash values give an approximation of the total inorganic material **Inorganic constitutes** Sodium, potassium, calcium, magnesium, iron, zinc etc. should be part of a concise user table/DB. Iodine and selenium should be included if they are a public health concern	**ASH**

Vitamin A and pro-vitamins		mcg	

VITA_RAE: vitamin A; calculated by summation of the vitamin A activities of retinol and the active carotenoids.

Total vitamin A activity expressed in mcg retinol activity equivalent (RAE) = mcg retinol + 1/12 mcg β- carotene + 1/24 mcg other provitamin A carotenoids

(or RAE = mcg retinol + 1/12 mcg β- carotene equivalent)

VITA: vitamin A; calculated by summation of the vitamin A activities of retinol and the active carotenoids.

Total vitamin A activity expressed in mcg retinol equivalent (RE) = mcg retinol + 1/6 mcg β-carotene + 1/12 mcg other pro-vitamin A carotenoids

(or RE = mcg retinol + 1/6 mcg β- carotene equivalent)

CARTA: alpha-carotene.
All-trans alpha-carotene only
CARTB: beta-carotene.
All-trans beta-carotene only
CRYPXB: beta-cryptoxanthin
CARTBEQ: beta-carotene equivalents. This value is the sum of the beta-carotene + 1/2 quantity of other carotenoids with vitamin A activity.

β-carotene equivalent = 1 β-carotene + 0.5 α-carotene + 0.5 β-cryptoxanthin

Vitamin A   VITA + MI + unit
- Total Vitamin A (VITA_RAE) or total vitamin A (VITA) are the recommended definitions to be used in user tables/DB
- Vitamin A expressed in international units (IU) is obsolete and should not be used any more; however, if IU are used, it must be explicitly stated
- For conversion from IU to mcg retinol, β-carotene or other provitamin A carotenoids and vitamin A in RE and RAE see FAO/INFOODS Guidelines on Conversion among different units, denominators and expressions (FAO/INFOODS, 2012a)

Retinol   VITA + MI + unit
- In the UK, for retinol 'All-trans retinol equivalent' in mcg is used = mcg all-trans retinol + 0.75 mcg 13-cis retinol + 0.90 mcg retinaldehyde

β-carotene/ β-carotene equivalent
- It would be best to phase out β-carotene equivalents in favour of reporting individual carotenes and vitamin A
- In archival and reference DB, β-carotene equivalent should not be listed alone in the DB, but together with all contributing components
- In the user tables (CARTBEQ) might be better to state, as it is more comprehensive, and in user DB (CARTBEQ) should be accompanied by α-carotene, β-carotene and β-cryptoxanthin   CARTA
- Components that are needed to calculate Vitamin A values: retinol, β-carotene, α-carotene, β-cryptoxanthin, their conversion factors to calculate VITA, VITA_RAE and CARTBEQ (β-carotene equivalent is not needed, if values for the single provitamins are given in the DB)   CARTB
Lutein, lycopene and zeaxanthin do not have vitamin A activity   CRYPXB
                                                                              CARTBEQ

(Continued)

Table 5.2 (Continued)

Component	INFOODS tagnames	Unit*	Comments	European Food Information Resource (EuroFIR) component identifiers (MI = method indicator)
Vitamin D	**VITD**: vitamin D; calculated by summation of ergocalciferol and cholecalciferol. This definition is mostly used **VITDEQ**: vitamin D; Vitamin D3 + D2 + 5 × 25-hydroxycholecalciferol **VITDA**: vitamin D; determined by bioassay. The nutrient values are generally higher than the values determined chemically **ERGCAL**: ergocalciferol (D2); occurs in plant foods **CHOCAL**: holecalciferol (D3); occurs in animal foods **CHOCALOH**: 25-hydroxycholecalciferol	mcg	• VITD is mostly used; some DBs also use VITDEQ (e.g. Danish or British food composition databases) • Vitamin D expressed in IU is not preferred; however, if used IU must be explicitly stated IU divided by 40 should be the value for vitamin D reported in mcg (1 IU vitamin D = 0.025 mcg vitamin D (VITD)/vitamin D3 (CHOCAL). See also FAO/INFOODS Guidelines on Conversion among different units, denominators and expressions (FAO/INFOODS, 2012a)	VITD + MI VITD + MI VITD + MI ERGCAL CHOCAL CHOCALOH
Vitamin E	**VITE**: vitamin E; calculated by summation of the vitamin E activities of the active tocopherols and tocotrienols; expressed as α-tocopherol equivalents = α-tocopherol + 0.4 β-tocopherol + 0.1 γ-tocopherol + 0.01 δ-tocopherol + 0.3 α-tocotrienol + 0.05 α-tocotrienol + 0.01 γ-tocotrienol **(mostly used)** = α-tocopherol + 0.5 β-tocopherol + 0.1 γ-tocopherol + 0.3 α-tocotrienol = α-tocopherol + 0.4 β-tocopherol + 0.1 γ-tocopherol + 0.01 δ-tocopherol **VITEA**: vitamin E; determined by bioassay **TOCPHA**: α-tocopherol	mg	• Generally user tables/DB use VITE. However, some user tables/DB report TOCPHA (e.g. USDA) In archival and reference DB, vitamin E (VITE) should not be listed alone in the DB, but together with all contributing components It should be noted that the latest version of the DRIs published by NAS/IOM state that α-tocopherol is the active form of vitamin E and that the use of α-tocopherol equivalents is discontinued	VITE + MI VITE + MI TOCPHA
Niacin	**NIA**: niacin, preformed **NIAEQ**: niacin equivalents, total. Preformed niacin plus niacin equivalents from tryptophan **NIATRP**: niacin equivalents, from tryptophan. 1/60 × tryptophan	mg	Total niacin equivalent (NIAEQ) = niacin preformed (NIA) + 1/60 tryptophan (TRP)	NIA NIAEQ + MI + unit NIATRP

Nutrient	Description	Unit*	Code
VIT B6	**VITB6C**: vitamin B6, total; calculated by summation. Pyridoxal plus pyridoxamine plus pyridoxine **VITB6A**: vitamin B6, total; determined by analysis	mg	VITB6 + MI VITB6 + MI
Folate	**FOL**: folate, total. Includes both conjugated and free folate (determined by microbiological assay). Folate, total: food folates + fortified folic acid (if any) in processed food **FOLSUM**: folate, sum vitamers. It includes mostly tetrahydrofolate, 5-methyltetrahydrofolate, 5-formyltetrahydrofolate, 10-formylfolic acid, 10-formyldihyrdofolate and folic acid (determined by HPLC) **FOLAC**: folic acid, synthetic folic acid used in fortification **FOLFD**: folate food, naturally occurring food folates (determined by microbiological assay) **FOLDFE**: folate, dietary folate equivalents. = food folate + 1.7 × synthetic folic acid	mcg	FOL + MI FOL + MI FOLAC FOL + MI FOL + MI
	• FOL is the recommended expression and generally yields higher values than FOLSUM • FOLFD is to be used if FOL, FOLAC and/or FOLDFE are also reported. This is to distinguish the folate content in the food from the fortificant amount		
Vitamin C	**VITC**: vitamin C. L-ascorbic acid plus L-dehydro-ascorbic acid. Usually analysed by HPLC **ASCL**: L-ascorbic acid. Titrimetry can only analyse L-ascorbic acid **ASCDL**: L-dehydro-ascorbic acid (=oxidised form of VITC)	mg	VITC ASCL ASCDL
	• VITC generally yields highest values. In fresh food, however, VITC and ASCL should give comparable results, since the oxidised form of VITC, if existing, is very low • In fresh foods the reduced form (ASCL) is the major one present, but the amount of the dehydro-form (ASCDL) increases during cooking and processing		

*Recommended unit.

conversion factor – whereas other compilers provide the analytical data for the individual components, in addition to the calculated components. This latter practice should be encouraged, since conventions for calculating these values based on biological activity change, and many of these individual components, have other functions in addition to their roles as provitamins.

In data compilation, all available food composition data can be included in the database. Complete information for all components in all foods is not necessary. Ideally, a database should have complete information for selected 'core' nutrients, but should also be able to accommodate miscellaneous data for other components in the foods listed.

The early work of INFOODS included the development of standards and guidelines for compiling food composition databases for national and regional use (Rand *et al.* 1991), standards for unambiguously identifying food components (Klensin *et al.* 1989) and standards for ensuring international comparability and interchange of food composition data (Klensin 1992). These standards are being maintained and further developed by INFOODS expert committees and consultative groups (see the INFOODS website, http://www.fao.org/infoods/en/).

Data dissemination

With appropriate data compilation, food composition data can be disseminated in many different forms to satisfy all user requirements. Data disseminated as a set of relational files offers users with very specific needs, or those with customised software, the opportunity to use the data as they wish. Other common dissemination formats include printed abridged and unabridged publications, web-accessible databases, spreadsheet or PDF files, all of which provide different levels of information required by different user groups.

Data use

Food composition data are the basic, most fundamental information resource for most nutrition activities. Some of the specific uses of food composition data, along with examples of their uses, are listed here by sector.

Health

Food composition data are used in *health protection* or food safety activities in most countries in the world. 'Food control' laboratories monitor mostly harmful components of foods. Other health protection activities include food composition activities involving total diet surveys or 'market basket surveys' designed to determine the risk to populations from intakes of selected nutrients,

anti-nutrients and contaminants. The sampling, sample preparation, sample handling, analyses and reporting requirements are virtually identical to the requirements of other food composition activities.

Health promotion activities include campaigns aimed at reducing or increasing the intake of certain nutrients in certain populations. Examples include healthy heart campaigns, typically using energy, fat, fatty acid and cholesterol compositional data, to educate the public about diet-related cardiac morbidity and mortality. In many developing countries, health promotion focuses on micronutrient data, including the necessity for including iodine in salt and provitamin A carotenoids from fruits and vegetables.

Food composition data are central to *clinical care and clinical research* trials. Examples include studies focusing on amino acid digestibility in ileostomy patients, vitamin A intake in breast-fed infants and serum cholesterol levels in vegetarians. Knowledge of the composition of the test and control food(s) and/or diet(s) is fundamental to these studies. Clinical dietitians must know the composition of foods in order to provide meals in a clinical setting. Special diets for patients are often based on individual nutrients in the foods: low-sodium diets for hypertensive patients, diets low in saturated fats for heart disease patients, diets containing proper ratios of protein, fat and carbohydrate for diabetics, high-protein diets for burn patients, diets containing low phenylalanine for phenylketonuric patients and so forth.

Nutritional epidemiology addresses food intakes and relates them to the nutrient content of the diet and the incidence of diseases. Dietary intake studies and food consumption surveys (e.g. food frequency questionnaires, diet histories, 24-hour recalls, food diaries, household budget surveys) derive their most important interpretations from food composition data, whether the issue is diet-related chronic diseases or intakes of individual nutrients.

Many *public health policies* relating to non-communicable disease focus on food composition. Such policies set forth nutrition goals and guidelines and include recommended dietary intakes (RDI). An example of such goals and guidelines is 'Choose a diet low in fat, saturated fat and cholesterol'; an example of an RDI is 'Females between the ages of fourteen and eighteen should get 15 mg of iron daily'. In order for such recommendations to be useful, both health professionals and the public must have access to data on the nutrient composition of foods.

Nutrition interventions may take the form of fortification of the food supply or supplementation of the population. Examples of food fortification include the addition of iodine to salt (most countries), vitamin A to sugar (for example, in Guatemala) and addition of minerals and B vitamins to refined cereal products (USA, UK).

It also includes nutrients in the form of injections, sprinkles and ready-to-use therapeutic formulations. Such interventions should only be made after the nutrients in the food and water supply of a country or community have been studied, and a baseline position has been established and carefully monitored over a period of time.

Food security, and more recently food and nutrition security, is an issue that spans several sectors. Knowledge of the nutrient content of the foods in a country's food supply, and those consumed by a household, is a precondition for assessing national and household food and nutrition security.

Consumers' awareness of nutrition is very high and consumers are demanding more and better food composition data, whether it be from food labels or other sources. The internet offers many sites where consumers can enter their food consumption details, for example food source, portion size, frequency of consumption, and receive analyses of their nutrient intakes compared to nutrient requirements and/or nutrient reference values. Often the food composition data supplied is that of the USDA Standard Reference, which does not have worldwide applicability.

Agriculture
The intensive livestock industries require accurate nutrient composition data on the feeds used. These data are generally far more extensive than those required for human foods, and include many micronutrients and individual amino acids. 'Performance' in these animals usually refers to weight at time of slaughter; muscle tissue to fat tissue ratios; and, in the case of milk-producing animals, an accurate profile of the proximate composition (protein, fat, lactose, water and ash).

National and global food and nutrition security is generally considered an agriculture-sector issue related to food production, rural development, irrigation, fertiliser and pesticide use, crop yields and so on. A common tool used to assess national and global food and nutrition security is the FAO food balance sheets, which examine, at the commodity level, the amount of food available to a country. The amount of food is then converted into individual components and reported as the amount of protein, fat and energy available per person per day from the domestic food supply. Food composition data assigned to the commodity data are the basis for many food and nutrition security assessments, including FAO's yearly report on the number of under-nourished people in the world.

The agriculture sector is responsible for ensuring that food exports meet the regulatory requirements of the intended market. Food composition data are important, as product specifications (for example, the fat content of butter) and as nutrition label panels.

Agriculturalists have long professed that malnutrition is not merely a health problem, but also an agriculture problem. Increased consumption of imported food commodities has brought about changes in food patterns and diets that have contributed to the increase in certain diet-related health problems previously unheard of in certain parts of the world. Agricultural extension workers are combating the incidences of diet-related diseases in some developing Pacific Island countries by using nutrient composition data in family food production, helping families in designing home garden projects to supply nutrients that would otherwise be consumed in insufficient quantities.

Breeding has been carried out to modify certain nutrients in foods. Familiar examples include corn bred for higher lysine and cattle bred for a lower fat content of the carcass.

Environment/biodiversity
In the past, generic food composition data were considered sufficient for most purposes. Now there is more awareness of the need for carrying out food composition studies that take biodiversity into account – that is, at the taxonomic level below species (e.g. variety, cultivar, and breed). Thousandfold differences are not uncommon, for example in different cultivars of fruits. Some important authorities and processes have acknowledged the importance of differentiating not only between species, but also between cultivars and varieties of the same species. With respect to rice varieties, the International Rice Commission has recommended the following:

- The existing biodiversity of rice varieties and their nutritional composition need to be explored before committing to transgenic varieties of rice.
- Nutrient content needs to be among the criteria in cultivar promotion.
- Cultivar-specific nutrient analysis and data dissemination should be systematically undertaken.
- The evaluation of the composition and consumption of rice cultivars should continue for the development of food biodiversity indicators to guide agro-biodiversity conservation and human nutrition.

Other bodies have emphasised the importance of undertaking food composition work at the level of the genetic resource, including FAO, Bioversity International, the Convention on Biological Diversity, the Commission on Genetic Resources for Food and Agriculture, INFOODS and its regional bodies, and more. To facilitate this endeavour, FAO has developed the FAO/INFOODS Food Composition Database for Biodiversity (BioFoodComp) as a global repository of nutrient data on food biodiversity to support the evidence basis on the nutrient content of food biodiversity. This database includes analytical data on nutrients and beneficial bioactive non-nutrients for plant varieties/cultivars and animal breeds as well as for neglected and underutilised species and wild foods. The entire database can be downloaded free of charge from the INFOODS website (http://www.fao.org/infoods/en/) and users are able to easily incorporate these data into national or specialised food composition databases.

Knowledge of the nutrient composition of the native diet of endangered animal species is an important requirement for protecting them. In New Zealand, scientists have undertaken studies to determine the nutrient composition of the original diets of birds in their native habitat, to ensure that the same nutrients in the same quantities and proportions were being supplied in their human-made offshore island sanctuaries and other protected, artificial habitats.

Climate change also influences food composition. Ozone depletion affects both food production and the composition of crops and agricultural products. Like ozone depletion, global warming affects agriculture in terms of production implications. Its other major effect, now and in the future, is the creation of conditions that will permit certain food products to be cultivated where temperature conditions did not permit their cultivation previously. This will alter the food supply, and along with it the nutrient composition of certain foods in certain countries. Food composition data have been used as markers in modelling and predicting environmental change, for example monitoring the changes in fatty acid composition of fish to chart the climatic phenomenon of El Niňo.

Trade

Trade has emerged in recent years as one of the more important and demanding of the sectors involved in food composition activities. Food composition in various forms features in World Trade Organization agreements, the Codex Alimentarius Commission and several of its committees, multilateral and bilateral trade agreements, and national food regulations and standards. More than other sectors, trade has illustrated most poignantly the need for standards and harmonisation in technical food composition activities. Many trade-related court cases have involved food composition data, both in the charges filed and in evidence presented, and many of the food product detentions and rejections at US borders are due to the absence of the Nutrition Facts panel of nutrient content data.

5.5 Limitations

A common limitation in food composition data is the lack of statistical reliability of the resultant values. Ideally, a sampling protocol should be designed for representativeness, with a sufficient number of independent samples collected and analysed, and a sufficient number of analytical replicates for each sample to ensure precision. Too often, mainly for reasons of financial limitations, only a single sample is collected and analysed. Documentation needs to include, at the very least, the number of samples analysed (n) for each value and, presuming n = 3 or more, the variation (e.g. a standard deviation) around the central value. Sometimes the reasons for differences are empirical – they relate to differences in methodology, for example in dietary fibre analyses, or in the form of the nutrient, for example total folate vs folic acid. INFOODS tagnames provide much of the necessary documentation to avoid empirical confusion.

Even when a comprehensive sampling and analytical programme is in place, there can be many reasons why the actual nutrient content of a food is different from the data provided in food composition databases. The reasons can often be understood when proper and complete food descriptors are provided – for example, the dietary fibre content related to the part of a plant such as peas with or without pod; processing related to vitamin B enrichment of flour; vitamin C differences with stages of maturity of mangoes; different fat contents for different grades of beef; or beta-carotene differences among different cultivars of sweet potatoes. Part, process, maturity, grade and scientific name (genus, species, variety) should all be part of a food name in a well-documented food composition database.

Even with appropriate metadata, with details of sampling, sample handling and preparation, analytical method and conditions, there will still be limitations in all food composition databases. This is a feature of the rapidly changing food supply, the heterogeneity of agricultural conditions (e.g. soil composition) and practices (use of agricultural chemicals), climatic conditions, seasonal variations, animal husbandry and food regulations (e.g. fortification policies). However, in spite of these limitations, food composition databases are indispensable tools for nutritionists operating in all sectors.

References and further reading

AOAC International (2012) *Official Methods of Analysis of AOAC International, 19th edn. AOAC International*, Gaithersburg, MD.

Atwater, W.O. (1910) Principles of nutrition and nutritive value of foods. U.S. Department of Agriculture, Washington, DC. NAL Call Number 1 Ag84F no.142.

Burlingame, B. (2004). Fostering quality data in food composition databases: Visions for the future. *Journal of Food Composition and Analysis*, **17** (3–4), 251–258.

Burlingame, B. (2008) Measuring nutrients in foods: The importance of international standards and the needs of diverse user groups. In *International Conference on Metrology of Environmental, Food and Nutritional Measurements*, 9–12 Sept 2008, Budapest, 70–72.

Carr, F. H. and Price, E. A. (1926) Color reactions attributed to vitamin A. *Biochemical Journal*, **20**(3): 497–501.

Charrondiere, U.R., Chevassus-Agnes, S., Marroni, S. and Burlingame, B. (2004) Impact of different macronutrient definitions and energy conversion factors on energy supply estimations. *Journal of Food Composition and Analysis*, **17** (3–4), 339–360.

Charrondiere, U.R., Burlingame, B., Berman, S., Elmadfa, I. (2011a) *Food Composition Study Guide. Questions and exercises, volume* **1**, 2nd edn. FAO, Rome.

Charrondiere, U.R., Burlingame, B., Berman, S., Elmadfa, I. (2011b) *Food Composition Study Guide. Questions and exercises, volume* **2**, 2nd edn. FAO, Rome.

Englyst, H.N. and Cummings, J.H. (1988) Improved method for measurement of dietary fiber as non-starch polysaccharides in plant foods. *Journal of the Association of Official Analytical Chemists*, **71**(4), 808–814.

FAO (2013) *Review of Key Issues on Biodiversity and Nutrition.* Commission on Genetic Resources for Food and Agriculture, CGRFA-14/13/8. http://www.fao.org/docrep/meeting/027/mf917e.pdf (accessed June 2014).

FAO/INFOODS/Bioversity International (2008) *Expert Consultation on Nutrition Indicators for Biodiversity 1. Food Composition.* FAO, Rome.

Greenfield, H. and Southgate, D.A.T. (2002) *Food Composition Data: Production, Management, and Use*, 2nd ed. FAO, Rome.

INFOODS (2012a) FAO/INFOODS Guidelines on Conversion among different units, denominators and expressions, version 1, FAO, Rome.

INFOODS (2012b) http://www.fao.org/infoods/infoods/standards-guidelines/food-component-identifiers-tagnames/en/

INFOODS (2013) http://www.fao.org/infoods/en/.

Kennedy, G. and Burlingame, B. (2003) Analysis of food composition data on rice from a plant genetic resources perspective. *Food Chemistry*, **80**, 589–596.

Klensin, J.C. (1992) *INFOODS: food composition data interchange handbook*. United Nations University Press, Tokyo, Japan.

Klensin, J.C., Feskanich, D., Lin, V. *et al.* (1989) *Identification of Food Components for INFOODS Data Interchange*. United Nations University Press, Tokyo.

Prosky, L., Asp, NG., Furda, I., DeVries, J.W., Schweizer, T.F. and Harland, B.F. (1984) Determination of total dietary fiber in foods and food products and total diets: Interlaboratory study. *Journal – Association of Official Analytical Chemists*, **67**, 1044.

Rand, W.M., Pennington, J.A.T., Murphy, S.P., Klensin, J.C. (1991) *Compiling data for food composition data bases*. United Nations University Press, Tokyo, Japan.

6
Biomarkers of Intake

Gunter G C Kuhnle

University of Reading

Key messages

- Nutritional biomarkers offer an alternative assessment method for dietary intake.
- Nutritional biomarkers can be measured objectively and can be used independently – or in combination with other assessment methods – to estimate intake.
- Recovery biomarkers – that is, urinary nitrogen, sodium and potassium – can be used to determine dietary intake directly, while most other biomarkers only allow ranking of intake.
- Biomarkers require careful planning of specimen collection and analytical method to avoid the introduction of additional bias.

6.1 Introduction: Biochemical markers of intake

Biomarkers – short for biochemical markers – are commonly used as surrogate markers for an event that cannot be observed directly. These events are mainly clinical endpoints, for example disease progression or mortality, or exposure, for example diet.

A nutritional biomarker, or biochemical marker of intake, is an indicator of nutritional status that can be measured in any biological specimen. It is not restricted to a specific compound or groups of compounds, and can be interpreted broadly as a physiological consequence of dietary intake. These markers can be used to assess different aspects of nutrition, for example intake – or status – of micronutrients, specific foods or dietary patterns. In nutritional epidemiology, these biomarkers are commonly used as reference measurements to assess the validity and accuracy of other dietary assessment instruments (Prentice *et al.* 2009; Kuhnle 2012).

An ideal nutritional biomarker should reflect dietary intake – or status – accurately and should be specific, sensitive and applicable to most populations. The biomarker should allow the objective and unbiased assessment of intake, independent of all biases and errors associated with individuals and other dietary assessment

methods. However, such an ideal biomarker does not exist, and all biomarkers available have some limitations. Nevertheless, they provide useful information and are commonly used in nutritional epidemiology and other research areas where dietary assessment is important. The three main applications for biomarkers in nutritional sciences are as a measure of nutritional status; as a surrogate marker of dietary intake; and to validate other dietary assessment instruments. These different applications will be discussed in the next section.

6.2 Types of biomarkers and their application

Biomarkers are commonly divided into categories depending on their relationship with intake (Jenab *et al.* 2009). *Recovery biomarkers*, based on the total excretion of the marker over a defined period of time, have a well-known relationship with intake and this relationship is consistent between individuals, with low inter-individual variability. *Predictive biomarkers*, a category introduced 2005 (Tasevska *et al.* 2011), also have a consistent, well-known relationship with intake, but an incomplete and low recovery. In *concentration biomarkers*, this relationship

Nutrition Research Methodologies, First Edition. Edited by Julie A Lovegrove, Leanne Hodson, Sangita Sharma and Susan A Lanham-New.
© 2015 John Wiley & Sons, Ltd. Published 2015 by John Wiley & Sons, Ltd.
Companion Website: www.wiley.com/go/nutritionsociety

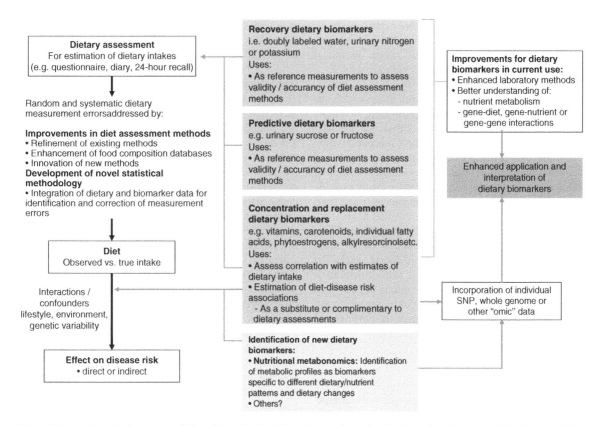

Figure 6.1 Overview of different types of biomarkers of intake, their main properties and application to investigate associations between intake and diseases risk. Jenab *et al.* (2009) Biomarkers in nutritional epidemiology, *Human Genetics*, **125** (5–6), 507. With kind permission from Springer Science and Business Media.

is less well known and more variable, with very high inter-individual variability. A summary of different types of biomarkers is shown in Figure 6.1.

Recovery biomarkers

Recovery biomarkers are the most important category of biomarker available, because they can provide an estimate of absolute intake levels. This type of marker requires a metabolic balance between intake and excretion over a defined period of time and a precise, quantitative knowledge of the physiological relationship. As suggested by the name, recovery markers are based on compounds that can be recovered completely – or almost completely – following consumption, mainly in 24-hour urine samples. For these biomarkers, the inter-individual variability in the excretion of the marker is negligible: for example, the excretion of urinary nitrogen in 24-hour urine is approximately equal to 80% of nitrogen intake in the same time period in any individual in energy and protein balance. A limitation of these biomarkers is that

they are only suitable for individuals who are in a steady state; that is, individuals who do not increase or decrease in body mass as do young or old people or pregnant women. These biomarkers are also sensitive to a number of diseases that affect their excretion, in particular kidney diseases. Currently, only a few recovery biomarkers of dietary intake are available, for example urinary nitrogen, potassium and sodium.

Concentration biomarkers

In contrast to recovery markers, which rely on the total excretion of a specific compound over a defined period of time, concentration biomarkers are only based on the biomarker concentration in the respective specimen. While recovery biomarkers can normally only be measured in 24-hour urine samples, concentration biomarkers can be measured in almost all specimens available. These biomarkers do not have a consistent relationship between intake and excretion, and therefore high inter-individual variability; they also do not have a time dimension. For this reason, concentration biomarkers cannot easily be translated into absolute dietary intake, but are only utilised to compare different levels of intake; additional information is usually required to provide a reference.

Concentration biomarkers are often used to investigate associations between diet and disease risk, as these markers can lead to a better ranking of intake than other assessment instruments that rely on self-reporting. In contrast to dietary data, biomarker concentration determined in blood or urine takes into account bioavailability, metabolism, nutrient–nutrient interaction and excretion, and therefore might provide better information on the bioavailable nutrient than dietary data.

These biomarkers are the most common type of biochemical marker currently available, as they can be measured in a wide range of specimens and do not require the collection of 24-hour urine samples. Many micronutrients can be used as concentration markers of their own intake (see later in this chapter). Other concentration markers include urinary phytoestrogens (isoflavones and lignans) and alkylresorcinols (for wholegrain).

Predictive biomarkers

Predictive biomarkers are the latest category of biomarkers that have been developed. They have an incomplete recovery but a stable and time-dependent correlation with intake. While they allow an estimation of absolute intake, they are not as reliable as recovery markers. Currently, urinary sucrose is the only predictive biomarker available.

Functional markers

Functional markers are an alternative type of biomarker. In contrast to most biomarkers described here, functional markers measure the physiological effect of specific foods as a surrogate marker of intake. A commonly used functional marker is EGRAC (erythrocyte glutathione reductase assay coefficient; Dror, Stern and Komarnitsky 1994) for Vitamin B2 status (see later in this chapter), but other markers are also available.

6.3 Specific biomarkers

Macronutrient and energy intake

There is only one recovery biomarker currently available to assess the intake of the primary three macronutrients, urinary nitrogen for protein intake. While the intake of fat can be determined to some extent by the analysis of fatty acids (see later in this chapter), there is currently no biomarker for the intake of total carbohydrates except for sucrose.

Urinary nitrogen as a biomarker of protein intake

The assessment of protein intake by total urinary nitrogen is based on the assumption that subjects are in nitrogen balance and that there is neither accumulation nor loss due to growth, starvation, diet or injury. The application of urinary nitrogen was described in 1924 by Denis and Borgstrom in a study to investigate the temperature dependence of protein intake in medical students. Since then, this biomarker has been investigated further and it is now commonly used (Bingham 2003).

Several validation studies have been conducted to investigate the association between intake and excretion, and urinary nitrogen is probably one of the best-validated biomarkers available. When taking into account nitrogen losses via faeces and skin, there is an almost complete agreement between long-term intake and urinary nitrogen (as shown by a correlation coefficient of 0.99 for a 28-day diet). The biomarker underestimates intake at higher levels of protein intake and overestimates it at lower levels, but when taking into account the factors described above, urinary nitrogen excretion is on average around 80% of dietary intake, and this ratio can be used for its determination.

Daily individual variations require the collection of urine samples on several days, as an individual is unlikely to be in nitrogen balance on any one day. When using only the sample of a single day, a correlation between intake and biomarker of approximately 0.5 can be expected, with a coefficient of variation of 24%. However, this improves to a correlation coefficient of 0.95 and a coefficient of variation of 5% when using 8 days of urine collection and 18 days of dietary observation.

A key limitation of 24-hour urinary nitrogen is the collection of 24-hour urine samples, which is often not feasible in studies. Urinary nitrogen in partial 24-hour urine collections, and even spot urine samples, has been used, but the results depend on the timing of diet and meal consumption.

The standard method for urinary nitrogen is the Kjeldahl method, developed by the Danish chemist Johan Kjeldahl in 1883. In this method, all nitrogen present in the sample is converted into ammonium sulphate and then analysed; it therefore determines not only protein nitrogen, but all nitrogen present in the sample. The method is very robust and reproducible, and can be automated for the analysis of larger numbers of samples.

An important disadvantage of this method is that it can only provide information on total protein intake, not intake of specific amino acids or the source of proteins (such as plant or animal protein). Additional markers, such as stable isotope ratios, are required to obtain more information on protein sources, although there is still a paucity of validated markers.

Fatty acids as a biomarker of fat intake

While nitrogen intake can be measured with a single biomarker, urinary nitrogen, there is no such biomarker for total fat intake. Individual fatty acids can be measured in a variety of different specimens, and the fatty acid composition can be used to make inferences regarding dietary fat intake.

Fatty acids are mainly present as triacylglycerol, phospholipids and cholesterol esters, and they are found in membranes, adipose tissue and also plasma (as free fatty acids). Their distribution –among both different molecules and tissues – depends largely on the type of fatty acid, and it is mainly the fatty acid profile that is used to make inferences on intake. As fatty acids undergo extensive metabolism, it is important to take this into account when interpreting different biomarkers. While many fatty acids – in particular saturated fatty acids (SFA) – can be synthesised endogenously, this is rare in people consuming more than 25% of their energy as fat and thus storage in adipose tissue tends to reflect dietary consumption. Essential polyunsaturated fatty acids (PUFA), such as members of the $\omega-6$ (linoleic acid) and $\omega-3$ (α-linoleic acid) family, cannot be synthesised *de novo* by humans, and therefore they can also be used as a marker of intake. However, the majority of fatty acids in human tissues are non-essential and can be either endogenously produced or supplied via the diet. The transport of fatty acids into adipose tissue is presumed to be non-selective, and therefore the relative distribution of fatty acids there is often considered to be the strongest biomarker of long-term intake. However, non-selective transport cannot be assumed for all tissues, and this has to be taken into account when interpreting data.

Fatty acids in adipose tissue and blood

Adipose tissue has a half-life of approximately 1–2 years, therefore the fatty acid composition in adipose tissue reflects intake within this period of time (Hodson, Skeaff and Fielding 2008). While this is advantageous when assessing diet, it makes the validation of these biomarkers more complicated, as assessing diet over such a long time frame is difficult. In contrast, the half-life of erythrocytes is approximately 60 days and therefore erythrocyte membrane fatty acids are more suitable to assess medium-term diet. Studies have shown significant correlations between the relative intake of PUFA and PUFA content in adipose tissue, erythrocytes and plasma, in particular n-3 and/or n-6 fatty acids. However, the chain length can affect the association between

intake and concentration, for example the plasma concentration of ALNA (alpha-linoleic acid, C18:3 n-3) does not reflect intake, while EPA (C20:5 n-3) and DHA (C22:6 n-3) do. Strong correlations between intake and biomarker in adipose tissue or blood have also been observed for other types of fatty acids, such as *trans* fatty acids, SFA and monounsaturated fatty acids (MUFA), although the observed correlation coefficients vary widely between less than 0.1 and more than 0.7 (Hodson, Skeaff and Fielding 2008). Concentration of pentadecanoic acid (C15:0) and heptadecanoic acid (C17:0) in adipose tissue correlates well with dairy intake, with correlation coefficients of approximately 0.3.

Fatty acid analysis

The analytical methods for lipids depend to some extend on the specimen used. Thin layer chromatography (TLC) or silica cartridges are commonly used to separate different lipid fractions; alternatively, samples are extracted using a chloroform:methanol mixture (1:1) and purified by solid-phase extraction (SPE). Fatty acids are then normally converted into their methyl-ester (FAME, fatty acid methyl ester) by transesterification and analysed using gas chromatography (GC) or high-performance liquid chromatography (HPLC). While mass spectrometric detection facilitates the identification of individual fatty acids, flame-ionisation detectors (FID) are most commonly used and fatty acids are identified by their relative retention time. This is sufficient for most applications; however, it is often difficult to separate *cis*- and *trans*-isomers of fatty acids and to identify compounds with low abundance.

The results of fatty acid analyses are usually given as a fatty acid profile with the relative contribution of each fatty acid, either as mol% (mol fatty acid per mol total fatty acids) or weight%. The former, mol%, are biologically more meaningful, in particular when molecular ratios of fatty acids or long-chain fatty acids are being considered (Hodson, Skeaff and Fielding 2008). Alternatively, the absolute concentration of individual fatty acids can be given, and this data can also be used as a fatty acid profile. However, the absolute concentration cannot be used as a marker of total dietary fat intake.

Recent developments in mass spectrometry have resulted in novel methods for the analysis of fatty acids that do not require laborious sample preparation. In *lipidomics*, samples are usually separated by HPLC and identified by their fragmentation spectrum using tandem mass spectrometry (MS). While this method can provide detailed information about lipids present in the sample, there are several disadvantages, for example differential loss of lipids and lipid–lipid interactions that can affect ionisation efficiency. An alternative method is shotgun lipidomics, where samples are analysed without prior separation and lipids are identified using tandem MS. This approach has several advantages, for example no differential loss of compounds during liquid chromatography (LC) separation and – when using nano-electrospray – virtually unlimited analysis time, even with small amounts of sample. However, lipidomics relies extensively on bioinformatics for the identification of lipids and interpretation of results, as the generated data can be very complex (Griffiths and Wang 2009; Han, Yang and Gross 2012).

Urinary sugars

There is currently no biomarker for total carbohydrate intake, partially due to the complex nature of these nutrients and their extensive metabolism. However, a *predictive* biomarker exists for total sugar intake – the sum of urinary sucrose and fructose. This biomarker has been validated in several dietary intervention studies as well as the Observing Protein and Energy Nutrition (OPEN) study. The correlation between mean sugar intake and mean sugar excretion is approximately 0.84, even though the recovery is low (~0.05% of total intake). However, this biomarker is more sensitive to extrinsic sugars than to intrinsic sugars. In 24-hour urine samples, the association between total sugar excretion and dietary intake has been estimated to be:

$$\log M_i = 1.67 + 0.02 \times S + 1.00 \log T_i - 0.071 \times A_i + u_{Mi} + \varepsilon_{Mi}$$

where M: biomarker; S = 0 for men; S = 1 for women; A: age; T: true intake; u: person-specific bias; ε: within-person random error
This association can be used to estimate dietary intake.

While urinary sugars are a *predictive* biomarker when determined in 24-hour urine, they are *concentration* biomarkers when determined in spot urine samples. While urinary creatinine can be used to adjust for difference in urine volume in most applications, this is not possible when investigating associations with body mass or body mass index because of the strong correlation between body mass and creatinine excretion. It has therefore been suggested that the ratio of urinary sucrose and fructose should be used as a biomarker of sugar intake.

Urinary sugars are traditionally determined using enzymatic assays, as these are readily available in most clinical laboratories. Alternatively, urinary sugars can be analysed by chromatographic methods such as GC or HPLC. Chromatographic methods have the advantage that they can be used to determine sugars for which no enzymatic methods have been established. In the absence of high-throughput clinical robots, chromatographic methods can also provide a faster sample analysis (Tasevska *et al.* 2005, 2011; Bingham *et al.* 2007).

Fibre and wholegrain

Fibre is an important constituent of diet, but there is still a paucity of easily accessible biomarkers, in particular because of the varied nature of fibre. Two classes of compounds found in fibre-rich foods have been proposed as potential biomarkers of intake: lignans (Lampe 2003) and alkylresorcinols (Marklund *et al.* 2013). As lignans are also found in a number of other foods such as tea and coffee, alkylresorcinols are currently the main candidate biomarker. Alkylresorcinols are phenolic lipids found in particular in cereals, and they are therefore mainly biomarkers of cereal or wholegrain. Validation studies with different assessment instruments, as well as human intervention studies, have shown a significant correlation between wholegrain and the alkylresorcinol metabolite 3-(3,5-dihydroxyphenyl)-1-propanoic acid (DHPPA) and 3,5-dihydroxybenzoic acid (DHBA). In 24-hour urine, alkylresorcinol metabolites correlate well with the intake of both wholegrain (r = 0.3–0.5) and total cereal fibre (r = 0.5–0.6). Alternative biomarkers of fibre intake are stool weight, which correlates well with fibre intake (r = 0.8), and faecal hemicellulose, which also shows a good correlation (r = 0.5). However, these biomarkers require the collection of stool samples and this is not always possible in nutrition studies.

Micronutrient intake

Many micronutrients can be used as their own biomarker of intake, and micronutrient status is often assessed in a number of different specimens. However, for many micronutrients no proper validation studies have been conducted, and there is insufficient information regarding the association between intake and biomarker concentration. Most micronutrients can only act as *concentration* biomarkers – with the exception of potassium and to some extent sodium – as their concentration is affected by a number of different factors.

Vitamin A

Retinol is the bioactive form of vitamin A and can be measured in serum and plasma. Its main dietary sources are retinyl esters, provitamin A carotenoids and vitamin A, the latter mainly from animal sources. Retinol can be measured in blood (serum and plasma), but the concentration has only limited value as it is tightly controlled by the liver. Retinol concentrations are therefore only useful markers of vitamin A status when the liver stores are either saturated or depleted; intervention studies with high intake of retinyl esters in healthy individuals showed only modest changes in plasma concentrations. However, retinol concentrations can be used to detect vitamin A deficiencies and hyporetinolaemia (retinol concentration < 0.7 μmol/L).

Vitamin A – and other carotenoids – are usually analysed using HPLC with ultraviolet (UV), fluorescence or mass spectrometric detection. Carotenoids are sensitive to light and heat, so it is important to store the samples at low temperatures (below –70 °C) and in the dark.

B vitamins

Thiamine (vitamin B1) can be measured in 24-hour urine samples and correlates well with long term (r = 0.7) and short term (r = 0.6) intake. However, because of high between-subject variability, urinary thiamine cannot be used as a recovery biomarker. Similar correlations between short-term intake and urinary excretion (r = 0.4 – 0.7) were also found for other B vitamins except for vitamin B12. The excretion of vitamin B12 appears to be dependent on total urine volume.

The status of vitamin B2 (riboflavin), an important precursor of FAD (flavin adenine dinucleotide), is often determined using a functional biomarker, the erythrocyte glutathione reductase assay coefficient (EGRAC). In this assay, the activity of erythrocyte glutathione reductase is determined with and without the addition of FAD. In subjects with adequate riboflavin intake, only a slight increase occurs, as sufficient FAD is available. However, the ratio increases with lower intake. Alternative measures for vitamin B2 status are plasma or urinary riboflavin, but while EGRAC reflects long-term intake, these measures are more suitable for short-term intake assessment.

Studies using blood samples showed weaker and nonsignificant associations for many B vitamins. However, there are strong correlations between intake of folic acid and folate in red blood cells (r = 0.5), serum (r = 0.6) and plasma (r = 0.6). Erythrocyte folate is generally preferred, as plasma folate varies greatly depending on metabolism and intake, while erythrocyte folate is a measure of long-term intake. Although vitamin B12 status (measured in plasma) has been used as a surrogate marker of intake, there is a paucity of information on the association with intake. Low total serum vitamin B12 (the sum of B12 bound to transcobalamin II and haptocorrin) can be used as an indicator of deficiency.

The standard clinical screening test for the diagnosis of vitamin B12 deficiency, measurement of plasma or serum vitamin B12, has low diagnostic accuracy, while plasma levels of total homocysteine (tHcy) and methylmalonic acid (MMA) are considered more sensitive markers of vitamin B12 status. Holotranscobalamin (holoTC), the portion of vitamin B12 bound to the transport protein transcobalamin (TC) and the related TC saturation (the fraction of total TC present as holoTC), represent the biologically active fraction of total vitamin B12 and have been proposed as potentially useful indicators of vitamin B12 status.

Vitamin C

Vitamin C concentration in blood and urine can be used as a biomarker of overall vitamin C intake, although there are some limitations of urinary vitamin C concentration and this biomarker is mainly assessed in plasma. Even though plasma vitamin C is a commonly used biomarker and is often considered to be well established, there is only a modest correlation between intake and biomarker (r = ~0.4) with a large variation between populations, although this might also be due to other factors such as genotype and lifestyle factors. As vitamin C is one of the most labile vitamins, sampling, storage and analytical techniques are of great importance. The annual loss of vitamin C in plasma during long storage periods has been estimated to be between 0.3 and 2.4 μmol/L depending on the baseline concentration. The stability of vitamin C can often be improved by the addition of protein-precipitating agents such as metaphosphoric acid, but this might not be always possible.

The pharmacokinetic properties of vitamin C are well known, and there are a number of sources of inter-individual variability: vitamin C is absorbed both by diffusion and active transport, the sodium-ascorbate-Co-transporters (SVCT 1 and 2, transporting the reduced form) and hexose transporters (GLUT1 and 3, transporting dehydroascorbic acid), and genetic polymorphisms are a large source of variation. Other factors such as age and smoking status can also affect vitamin C status, as well as the consumption of certain foods and drugs. Furthermore, the relationship between intake and absorption is linear only for intakes below approximately 100 mg/day and reaches a plateau at intakes above 120 mg/day; at lower plasma vitamin C concentrations, renal excretion is minimised, further affecting biomarker concentration (Jenab et al. 2009).

Vitamin D

Vitamin D can either be absorbed from the diet or synthesised in the skin using UV radiation; the precursor of endogenously formed vitamin D, 7-dehydrocholesterol, is thereby converted into cholecalciferol (vitamin D3). The main sources of dietary vitamin D are fortified foods, in particular margarines, animal products (vitamin D3) and plant-based foods (vitamin D2, from the irradiation of ergosterol). The activated form of vitamin D, 25-hydroxyvitamin D (25(OH)D), is commonly used as a measure of vitamin D status. Due to the combination of endogenous and exogenous sources of vitamin D, the plasma level of 25(OH)D can only provide information on total status but not dietary intake (Jones 2012; see also Figure 6.2 for details).

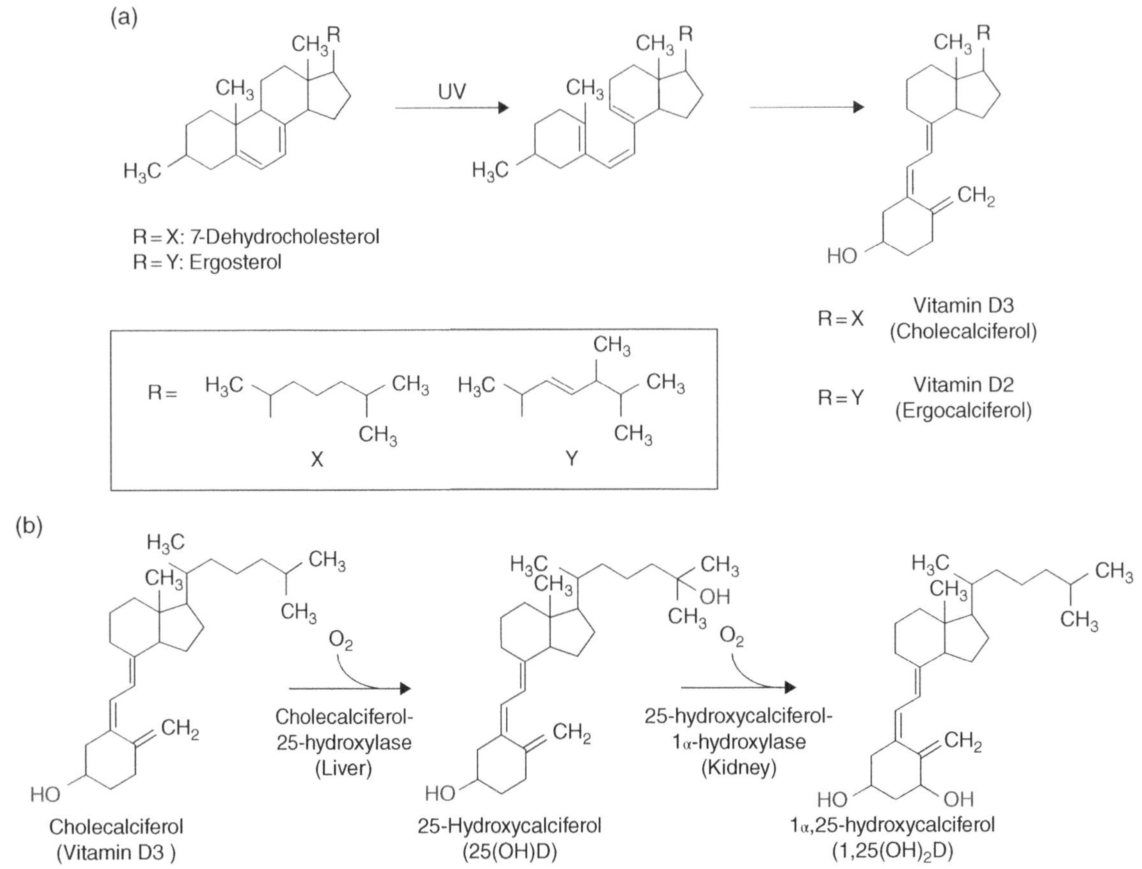

Figure 6.2 Formation and activation of vitamin D. (a) The precursor of vitamin D (7-dehydrocholesterol) is formed non-enzymatically in the skin through photolysis to vitamin D3. The plant sterol ergosterol is activated is also formed by UV irradiation in the plant to form vitamin D2. (b) Vitamins D2 and D3 are active and need to be activated in the liver and kidney to 1α,25-hydroxycalciferol (1,25(OH)$_2$D). 25-hydroxycalciferol (25(OH)D) is the main circulating metabolite and is therefore often used as a biomarker of vitamin D status.

Vitamin E

The main dietary forms of vitamin E are α- and γ-tocopherol. Both can be determined in blood, but there is a strong correlation between them and blood lipids, in particular total cholesterol; it is therefore important to adjust measurements for blood lipids. Using repeated measures, the correlation between lipid-adjusted α-tocopherol and intake adjusted for blood lipids is approximately 0.5, lower than without adjustment (0.6). As a lipid-soluble vitamin, vitamin E can also be measured in erythrocytes (highly correlated with plasma vitamin E) and adipose tissue; however, in adipose tissue γ-tocopherol shows a higher correlation intake (0.4) than α-tocopherol (0.2).

Vitamin K

Vitamin K is a group of lipid-soluble vitamins that are involved in the clotting cascade. Dietary sources (meat, dairy products and green leafy vegetables) and the intestinal flora are the main sources of vitamin K. Significant correlations between the intake of phyllo-quinone – vitamin K from dietary sources – and plasma concentration have been reported, although the strength of the correlation was very variable (0.1–0.5).

Calcium

Blood calcium is under tight homoeostatic control and is therefore not suitable as a biomarker of intake. While urinary calcium depends to some extent on dietary intake, the association is very weak. In observational studies with 7-day diet diaries and 24-hour urine collection, correlation coefficients of less than 0.2 between dietary and urinary calcium were observed.

Chromium

Plasma chromium levels are very low and changes are therefore difficult to detect, even without deficiency.

Urinary chromium appears to be associated with intake, but the relationship is not sufficient to allow urinary chromium to be used as a biomarker of intake. Chromium concentrations in hair are associated with exogenous and endogenous (e.g. hip replacement) exposure, and therefore might be suitable as a biomarker of intake.

Copper

Copper status is usually assessed using plasma copper or ceruloplasmin. These concentrations can indicate deficiency states, but they are not suitable to determine intake at normal levels of intake. Urinary excretion of copper is also very variable and therefore not suitable as a marker of intake. Copper can also be detected in hair and nail samples, but there are currently insufficient data to show an association with intake.

Iodine

The standard method to determine iodine status is the measurement of urinary iodine, as more than 90% of dietary iodine is excreted via the kidneys. Urinary iodine reflects dietary intake within the past days, and concentrations unadjusted for creatinine are often considered to be sufficient for population screening.

Iron

The metabolism of iron is tightly controlled, and intestinal absorption depends on the iron available in the body's stores. Iron status can be determined in several different ways: serum ferritin is the principal iron storage protein and can therefore be used as a marker of stored iron. Increased serum ferritin can be a marker of iron overload, but otherwise there are no significant associations between the intake of iron and its concentration; however, serum ferritin is associated with the intake of haem iron ($r = 0.1$) and red meat ($r = 0.2$). In contrast to the storage protein, serum iron is highly variable, even within a short time (20% within 10 minutes in one study) and therefore is not a suitable marker of intake. Other markers of iron status are erythrocyte protoporphyrin, mean corpuscular volume and haematocrit. Apart from dietary intake, the major determinant of iron status is blood loss – for example from blood donations or menstruation – and this has to be taken into account when interpreting the relationship between iron status and intake.

Magnesium

Magnesium is homoeostatically controlled, but there is a weak correlation with intake ($r = 0.2$). As urinary excretion is one of the methods of homoeostatic control, urinary magnesium is a better marker of intake, and stronger correlations ($r = 0.3$) with intake have been found in 24-hour urine collections.

Manganese

The plasma concentration of manganese reflects dietary intake. However, as it is primarily excreted via bile, urinary manganese is unlikely to be a suitable biomarker of intake. Toenail and hair manganese have been used to measure environmental exposure, and it is possible that – depending on intake and exposure – they can be used as markers of intake as well.

Molybdenum

No direct biomarkers of molybdenum deficiency are currently known, but there are decreased levels of urinary sulphate and uric acid and concomitantly increased levels of sulphite, hypoxanthine and xanthine.

Potassium

Potassium in blood is tightly regulated and therefore is not suitable as a marker of intake; however, urinary potassium excretion – approximately 77% of intake – can be used as a *recovery* marker of potassium intake. As with other biochemical markers, several measurements are required to obtain a reliable estimate of intake.

Selenium

Selenium has an important role in many biochemical pathways and can be found in many selenoproteins. Blood selenium levels are correlated with intake, and erythrocyte selenium is a suitable measure for long-term intake. Other markers of long-term selenium intake are hair and nail samples, which also show a good correlation with intake.

A functional marker of selenium intake is the activity of selenium-dependent glutathione peroxidase, which increases with increasing selenium status. However, this marker is only useful for individuals with low selenium intake, as the activity plateaus with medium and high selenium intake. Furthermore, the activity of the glutathione peroxidase can decrease during storage, while selenium, as an inorganic element, is not prone to degradation.

Sodium

Sodium is a tightly regulated electrolyte, and therefore blood sodium levels provide only very limited information on intake. In contrast, urinary sodium levels are strongly associated with intake and therefore are a good measure of short-term intake, considered to be one of the few *recovery* biomarkers available, with a urinary excretion of 86%. Average urinary output is a better indicator of intake, however, as urinary excretion is directly dependent on recent intake and therefore has very high day-to-day variation; furthermore, sodium excretion follows a long-term (monthly and longer) cycle. Multiple measurements are therefore necessary to obtain reliable estimates of intake (Stamler 1997). As multiple 24-hour urine samples are often difficult to collect, overnight urine samples are sometimes used as a surrogate, and calibration studies have shown a very strong correlation between these samples ($r = 0.8$). Where only casual or spot urines are available, sodium excretion can be standardised using urinary creatinine (see later in this chapter).

Zinc

Dietary zinc can affect plasma levels, but the association is not suitable for making inferences on dietary intake, in particular since zinc levels do not always decrease following deprivation. The concentration of zinc in blood does not only depend on intake, but also on non-dietary factors, and it is subject to tight homoeostatic control. However, despite its poor sensitivity and specificity, plasma zinc is still the most widely used biomarker of zinc status. Zinc in hair is associated with intake, and this might be an alternative biomarker, in particular for long-term exposure.

Other compounds

Many other food components have – or are likely to have – an effect on health and accurate assessment of intake is therefore important. In contrast to many micronutrients, these compounds are rarely under homoeostatic control; concentrations in plasma are very variable and therefore might be a good indicator of intake. However, many of these compounds undergo extensive metabolism, both by the gastrointestinal microbiome and on absorption, and consequently extensive research might be required to identify suitable candidate biomarkers (Figure 6.3). Furthermore, the absorption of many of these compounds is affected by other factors, in particular food composition, and therefore high inter- and intra-individual variability can be observed. For these reasons, all of these biomarkers are *concentration* markers and can only be used accordingly.

Many of these compounds are not only used as a marker for their own consumption, but also as a marker for specific foods, food groups and dietary patterns, and they are therefore discussed in the following section.

Foods, food groups and dietary patterns

Fruit and vegetables

The evidence from observational studies showing beneficial effects of fruit and vegetable intake is often weak, and the World Cancer Research Fund (WCRF) downgraded the likely protective effect of fruit and vegetables in its 2007 report due to accumulating evidence tending towards null, in particular in observational studies. While this effect – or lack thereof – might be real, it con-

tradicts the opinion of many experts and might be due to the attenuation of risk associations because of measurement errors associated with dietary assessment instruments. For this reason, alternative assessment instruments of fruit and vegetable intake are important for future research. The most commonly used biomarkers, carotenoids, vitamin C and polyphenols, are discussed in this section. The limitations of each of these biomarkers – in particular the bias introduced by differences in food composition – make it important to assess results carefully and combine data from several biomarkers.

Carotenoids

Carotenoids are lipid-soluble pigments that are synthesised exclusively by photosynthetic organisms. Structurally, all carotenoids are tetraterpenoids and because of their conjugated double bonds are usually yellow, brown, red or violet. Only about 10% of all known carotenoids can be converted into vitamin A and therefore carotenoid status is distinctly different from vitamin A status; major carotenoids with vitamin A activity are the carotenes and cryptoxanthin. Despite the large number of known carotenoids, food composition tables usually only contain data for a few compounds, primarily β-carotene and lycopene.

The bioavailability of these compounds is largely determined by their lipophilicity, and therefore the fat content in the food matrix can affect absorption; other factors such as colonic metabolism and in particular hormonal factors affect absorption as well. Indeed, intervention studies have found absorption rates of less than 10% to more than 50% of intake, with a modest correlation between intake and blood concentrations (0.2 to over 0.5). This correlation is stronger in normal-weight than in obese individuals, possibly because of differences in the distribution volume. Despite this large variability, blood carotenoid levels are very sensitive to intake as they are not under homoeostatic control. As some carotenoids can be metabolised to retinol, blood carotenoid levels can be influenced by vitamin A status, in particular in individuals with lower status. There is also competition between different carotenoids and β-carotene – given as supplements – which can result in lower blood levels of other carotenoids.

The application of carotenoids as biomarkers of overall fruit and vegetable consumption is impeded by differences in food composition. While carrots and (red) peppers contain large amounts of carotenoids (4–12 mg/100 g), only small amounts are found in foods such as onions or beetroot. Validation studies to investigate the association between carotenoids and fruit and vegetable intake are often conducted using self-reported dietary assessment instruments and might therefore not provide sufficient information. However, these studies show that plasma

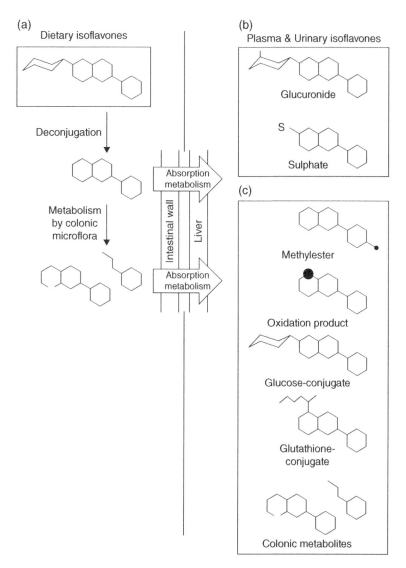

Figure 6.3 The effect of absorption and metabolism on biomarker analysis. Dietary isoflavones (a) are deconjugated and metabolised in the intestinal tract and on absorption. Therefore a variety of different metabolites are circulating. However, most analytical methods only analyse a small number of metabolites (b) and all other metabolites remain undetected (c), resulting in increased variability depending on metabolism and an underestimation. Reprinted from Ward, H.A. and Kuhnle, G.G. (2010) Phytoestrogen consumption and association with breast, prostate and colorectal cancer in EPIC Norfolk, *Archives of Biochemistry and Biophysics*, **501** (1), 170–175, with permission from Elsevier.

concentration is associated with dietary intake; although the correlation coefficients found were modest (0.1–0.4) they were significant, especially for fruit intake.

Flavonoids

Flavonoids are secondary plant metabolites that are ubiquitous in most plant-based foods. They are a diverse group of compounds, comprising monomeric (for example anthocynanidins, isoflavones, flavan-3-ol, flavonols or flavanones) and polymeric (for example proanthocyanidins, theaflavins) compounds. While these compounds are normally present as glycosides in food, they are deconjugated in the intestinal tract and undergo extensive metabolism by the intestinal microbiome and on absorption. Even though flavonoids can be found in most plant-based foods, the actual composition of individual foods is very variable and can be very specific: for example, anthocynanidins are mainly found in berries and isoflavones in legumes. For this reason, flavonoids are not only used as summary markers for total fruit and vegetable intake, but also to identify the intake of specific food groups or even individual foods.

Total excretion of phenolic compounds, measured with a modified Folin–Ciocaltaeu assay, showed a significant relationship with total fruit intake in an observational study, but there is still a paucity of data to validate this biomarker properly. More research has been undertaken to investigate the relationship between diet and biomarker for individual compounds; however, the correlation between intake and biomarker is rather modest. For soy, the main source of dietary isoflavones in the European diet, the correlation coefficient in many studies is below 0.3, and this is similar for other food and biomarker combinations: the correlation between self-reported apple intake and urinary phloretin concentration is between 0.2 and 0.3, and for self-reported citrus fruit intake and the citrus flavonoid hesperetin it is 0.4. A possible explanation for these modest correlations is not only the large variability in food composition and extensive metabolism, but also the very short half-life of these compounds.

Vitamin C

Plasma vitamin C is currently the most commonly used biomarker of fruit and vegetable intake. This is based on the assumption that the main sources of vitamin C in the diet are fruit and vegetables, and its intake is therefore associated with fruit and vegetable intake. As with other biomarkers of food groups, differences in food composition are a major source of variation and are likely to lead to misclassification; in the case of vitamin C, this is exacerbated by the frequent use of vitamin C–containing food supplements. Despite the limitations of vitamin C as a biomarker, it is still the most commonly used biomarker of fruit and vegetable intake.

Meat and fish

Meat intake and fish intake have both been associated with opposing health effects. While fruit and vegetables contain very specific compounds that can be used as candidate biomarkers, this is more difficult with foods of animal origin. Modified amino acids, in particular 1- and 3-methyl-histidine, have been proposed as biomarkers of meat, and they show a significant relationship in dietary intervention studies. As 3-methyl-histidine is also a marker of muscle breakdown, 1-methyl-histidine is more suitable as a biomarker of meat intake.

The ratio of stable carbon ($\delta^{13}C$) and nitrogen ($\delta^{15}N$) isotopes is commonly used in archaeology to assess meat and fish intake, and these biomarkers are becoming more commonly used in the nutritional sciences (Kuhnle et al. 2012). The urinary isotope ratio changes quickly with dietary changes and can therefore be used to assess short-term dietary intake. Conversely, the longer half-life of albumin and in particular red blood cells makes the whole-blood isotope ratio a better marker of medium-term intake. Isotope ratio analyses can also be conducted

on hair and nail samples and they thereby provide long-term information on dietary intake. As this method assesses mainly the protein source, it is not easily possible to distinguish between meat and dairy intake.

6.4 Methodological considerations

Biochemical markers of intake can be analysed in a wide range of specimens. A key advantage of biomarkers is that they can be analysed retrospectively in samples for which no other – or no relevant – dietary information is available. However, careful consideration of collection, storage and analytical methods is necessary to avoid any additional bias.

Specimens

Biochemical markers can be analysed in many different specimens, and each specimen has specific advantages and disadvantages (Table 6.1). While it is not possible for practical reasons to change the type of specimens collected in studies conducted in the past, the choice of specimen in current or future studies is often dictated by the funding available and the feasibility of storage and collection.

There are a number of factors to consider when choosing a specimen:

- The distribution of biomarkers in different specimens depends on a number of factors, e.g. homoeostatic control, active excretion and physico-chemical properties such as lipophilicity. It is therefore important to choose a specimen where the biomarker can be detected.
- Biomarker concentration in blood is often metabolically controlled and is therefore affected by not only dietary intake but also metabolism. The excretion in 24-hour urine samples is often a better indicator of intake, especially for compounds that are readily excreted.
- While 24-hour urine samples are often preferable, they are difficult to collect and many studies rely on spot urine samples. This can increase the variability, in particular for biomarkers with a very short half-life. Furthermore, spot urine samples require an adjustment for urine volume, which can often be achieved by using creatinine.
- Many biomarkers – in particular those with a low lipophilicity – have only a short half-life in the usual specimens such as urine and blood. Hair and nail samples provide an alternative specimen to measure long-term intake (see Figure 6.4 for a comparison of the time frame covered by different dietary assessment methods).

Table 6.1 Summary of main specimens used for biomarker analysis and their advantages and disadvantages.

Specimen	Advantages	Disadvantages
Adipose tissue	Long-term marker of fat intake	Invasive, requires specialist staff for collection
Whole blood, serum and plasma	Most commonly used specimens, infrastructure for collection is often available; reflect directly bioavailability of biomarker; can also be used for genotyping and to determine clinical markers	Invasive, require specialist staff for collection; need to be stored at very low temperature (often liquid nitrogen) to ensure long-term stability; homoeostatic control can affect many candidate biomarkers; timing of sample collection can affect outcome (especially with biomarkers with short half-life); only limited volume available
Hair	Long-term marker of intake, non-invasive collection	Only limited number of biomarkers available; can be affected by hair treatment or lack of hair
Nails	Long-term marker of intake, non-invasive collection	Only limited number of biomarkers available
24-hour urine	Non-invasive collection, does not require specialist staff; large volume available for multiple analyses; stable at −20 °C; no homoeostatic control of most candidate biomarkers	Large volume often requires aliquotation; collection is often considered tedious by volunteers; difficult to assess completeness
Spot urine	Non-invasive collection, does not require specialist stuff; commonly used specimen; stable at −20 °C	Requires adjustment for total urine volume (e.g. using creatinine); biomarkers with short half-life might not be found in all specimens; timing of sample collection can affect outcome (especially with biomarkers with short half-life)

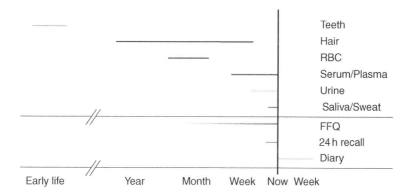

Figure 6.4 Time frame of biomarkers detected in different specimens and different dietary assessment methods (not to scale). Reprinted from Kuhnle, G. (2012) Nutritional biomarkers for objective dietary assessment, *Journal of the Science of Food and Agriculture*, **92** (6), 1145–1149.

Blood

Capillary blood samples can easily be collected in most study settings, as they do not require venepuncture. These samples are ideally suited to rapid analyses such as blood glucose or blood haemoglobin. Capillary blood is usually stored as dried blood spot on filter paper developed for blood spot storage. Dried blood spot can be stored in the dark at room temperature, and many analytes remain stable under these conditions for a long time, for example vitamin D (as 25OHD) or retinol.

Venous blood samples are more commonly collected in nutrition studies, and facilities for their collection and processing can be found in most laboratories. Venous blood samples can then be processed into a number of different specimens, in particular serum, plasma, buffy coat and red blood cells. When collecting blood samples,

it is important to specify the type of tube and in particular the type of anticoagulant used, if any. Whether fasting blood samples are required depends on the nature of the analysis and they are often not necessary. Blood samples should be processed quickly and then stored under appropriate conditions, usually at −80 °C or in liquid nitrogen. To avoid frequent freeze–thaw cycles, these samples should be stored in multiple aliquots.

Blood samples are not suitable for all biochemical markers, in particular not for those under tight homoeostatic control, as their concentration is not affected much by intake. For biomarkers that are rapidly eliminated by the kidneys, urine samples are preferable as they can provide information over a long period of time. However, blood samples are ideal for biomarkers with a long half-life, in particular fatty acids or lipophilic compounds, which can be found in erythrocytes. Recent research has also shown that some hydrophilic biomarkers such as flavonoids can be found in erythrocytes, but more research is required to investigate this. As erythrocytes have a lifetime of 120 days, biomarkers detected in erythrocytes can provide dietary information for approximately 60 days.

Urine

Urine samples are also commonly used for biomarker analysis. While the availability of blood samples is often limited by the volume that can be collected, such a restriction rarely applies to urine samples. In contrast to blood samples, the concentration of biomarkers in urine samples is not controlled homoeostatically and, indeed, compounds underlying homoeostatic control are excreted via the kidneys and their presence in urine is often related to intake. Urine samples are suitable for all hydrophilic – and to some extent also lipophilic – biomarkers that are excreted by the kidneys. Urine samples are mainly useful for markers of short-term intake, as urinary excretion is often more directly related to dietary intake, in particular when the body is in equilibrium.

For the analysis of nutritional biomarkers, 24-hour urine is generally preferable as the total excretion in 24 hours can be measured. There are different protocols for the collection of 24-hour samples, some including the first morning urine, some excluding morning urine samples altogether. While 24-hour urine is less invasive than venous blood samples, volunteers often find the collection of urine samples tedious and prefer venepuncture. To ensure the completeness of 24-hour urine sample collection, p-amino-benzoic acid (PABA) tablets are often given. PABA is excreted readily and can be recovered from urine. A quick photometric test can be used to measure recovery, and often a recovery of less than 85% is used to identify incomplete collections (Bingham and Cummings 1983). However, PABA might not be suitable in elderly participants, as the recovery is lower, and it is not suitable in participants with certain allergies. It is also not known whether PABA affects the metabolism of biomarkers or the stability of urine samples.

Spot urine samples can easily be collected and are therefore preferable – from a volunteer's point of view – when compared with 24-hour urine samples. Biomarker concentration in spot urine samples depends on urine volume; to be able to compare concentration between individuals, concentrations are often normalised using urinary creatinine. This normalisation is based on the assumption that creatinine excretion is constant and therefore any difference in concentration is only based on total urinary volume. However, creatinine excretion is not constant and depends on a number of factors, in particular body mass. Normalising urinary concentrations

with creatinine can therefore introduce additional bias, in particular when investigating associations with body mass or obesity, or related factors.

Faeces

Faeces are not commonly used as specimens for nutritional biomarker analysis. The main biochemical markers of intake analysed in faeces are markers of fibre intake, although other markers can be detected in faecal samples as well, in particular compounds excreted via the bile. The collection of faecal samples can be facilitated with specially designed collection devices such as the Fecotainer® to minimise the contact with the sample for the study participant.

Tissue

Tissue samples are more often used for the analysis of markers of exposure than for markers of intake. However, some biochemical markers of intake, such as carotenoids or fatty acids, can also be measured in adipose tissue. Tissue samples can often provide information on long-term dietary intake – with an average half-life of 1–2 years, fatty acids in adipose tissue can provide information about average dietary intake within this period.

Hair

Hair samples are more commonly used to detect exposure to drugs than for dietary intake, but with a growth rate of approximately 1 cm/month, hair can provide detailed information on long-term dietary exposure. As the composition of hair does not change after formation, a longitudinal analysis of hair can be used to identify dietary changes, such as those between seasons. Biomarker concentration in hair depends not only on dietary intake but also on other factors, in particular colour and thickness. For hair analysis, careful cleaning is necessary to avoid any contamination from environmental compounds or cosmetic products. Hair samples can be stored at room temperature in the dark, but care must be taken to ensure that information on the direction of growth is maintained.

Nails

Like hair, nail samples can be used to obtain information on long-term exposure. Unlike hair samples, nails have to be collected regularly to obtain this information.

Sample collection and storage

The stage of collection and storage of samples is often the first to introduce bias and increase the measurement error. It is therefore important that sample collection and storage should follow a standardised protocol to minimise measurement error. The following aspects need to be addressed:

- The sample-collection procedure should be standardised. For urine samples, this should specify what type of urine (morning, mid-stream etc.) should be collected; for blood samples, this should specify whether capillary or venous blood should be collected and what type of anticoagulant – if any – should be used. Furthermore, it is important to specify whether fasting or non-fasting samples are collected; a record of the collection time and the time of the previous meal can help to explain additional variability.
- Preservatives, such as boric acid or iodoacetamide, might be useful, but they can affect analytical techniques. While the techniques intended for use might not be affected by preservatives, it is possible that other techniques are, and it is prudent to keep unmodified samples in case they are required for future research.
- Samples should be processed without any delay and the process (e.g. separation of plasma) should follow standardised procedures.
- The storage condition – both before processing and for long-term storage – should prevent any degradation of the sample, including degradation by light. For example, vitamin C deteriorates rapidly in the absence of preservatives such as metaphosphoric acid. While some samples – such as hair – can be stored at room temperature, other samples require storage in liquid nitrogen. Long-term stability tests should be conducted to establish the best type of storage.
- Samples should always be stored in aliquots to prevent unnecessary freeze–thaw cycles. The size of each aliquot should be sufficient to conduct one or several analyses.
- Samples should be stored in containers that are easily retrievable while requiring as little space as possible. For the European Prospective Investigation into Cancer (EPIC) study, plastic straws were used to store more than 6 million plasma, serum, red cell and buffy coat samples in liquid nitrogen; these straws allow the storage of large numbers of samples in a small place. Recent developments in automated storage systems allow the storage of specimens in vials identified by barcode or RFID tags, as well as the automated retrieval of samples.

Sample stability

Sample stability is an important aspect to consider, in particular when analysing specimens from prospective studies. These samples are often stored for long periods of time and – depending on the number of aliquots available – undergo several freeze–thaw cycles. Furthermore, it is often not feasible to analyse the entire cohort for specific biomarkers and therefore not all samples will have had the same number of freeze–thaw cycles. For this reason, it is important to investigate the stability of candidate biomarkers in the specimens used. While it is often not possible to test the stability directly over a long period of time, alternative methods are available such as accelerated ageing (using higher temperatures and humidity).

Analytical methods

The analytical method used for biomarker analysis depends on a number of different factors, for example the availability of equipment and expertise, and the required sensitivity. However, the choice of analytical method can have a significant effect on the outcome, not only because of differences in the sensitivity of different methods, and thus in the level of quantification, but also because of differences in variability and specificity.

Sensitivity and selectivity

The sensitivity of analytical methods can have a significant influence on the interpretation of biomarker data, in particular when biomarkers are present at low concentrations. A high lower limit of quantification (LLOQ) will reduce the variability and therefore the observed relationship between biomarker and intake. Furthermore, a low sensitivity often increases the noise – in particular at low concentrations – and thereby introduces additional measurement error. Even though sensitive methods normally require more elaborate sample preparation and are often more expensive, more sensitive methods are usually preferable.

While a higher sensitivity is usually desirable, this is not always the case for selectivity. Some compounds used as biomarkers are extensively metabolised, and it might be necessary to determine the sum of all metabolites; with very selective methods, this requires the identification of each analyte and the development of an appropriate method. The Kjeldahl method for total urinary nitrogen is an example of a non-selective (or only element-specific) method that provides more useful information than the analysis of each individual nitrogen-containing compound. For other biomarkers very selective methods are crucial, as isomers or even enantiomers have to be separated. This degree of selectivity often requires either the use of enzymatic methods or of specialised equipment such as chiral or affinity chromatography.

Throughput

The throughput of analytical methods is of particular concern when analysing large numbers of samples from clinical trials or observational studies. High-throughout methods are usually highly automated and therefore require standardised protocols. While the set-up and maintenance of high-throughput equipment are expensive, results are usually very consistent and of high quality, as there are fewer sources of variation.

Comparability, validation and quality control

Good laboratory practice requires a thorough validation of any analytical method, and a cross-validation when combining data from different laboratories or different methods. Details on method validation can be found elsewhere, for example in the US Food and Drug Administration's *Guidance for Industry*.

Cross-validation is very important for multi-centre studies or when results are also used for diagnostic purposes. It is often sufficient to analyse the same samples in different laboratories or with different methods and compare the results, but for more complex studies this should be done regularly and with blinded samples. An important factor to consider – in particular when comparing different methods – is difference in sensitivity and selectivity. While results might be in agreement across the common range of both methods, the introduction of an artificial cut-off point – that is, the LLOQ of the less-sensitive method – might have an adverse effect on the results.

In addition to the usual quality control samples in analytical batches, it is common practice to place up to 10% blinded QC samples randomly within the normal samples. This will provide additional information about the quality of the analytical method (in particular intra-batch variability) and about the analysis.

6.5 Biomarker development

The development of new nutritional biomarkers is important not only for nutritional research, but also for clinical practice, for instance to monitor compliance with dietary prescriptions. This development can be broadly divided into two parts: biomarker discovery and biomarker validation.

Biomarker discovery is often divided broadly into *hypothesis-driven* and *discovery-driven* approaches (Figure 6.5 shows a work flow for both). In the *hypothesis-driven* approach, candidate biomarkers are selected based on information available about the respective foods. This requires detailed knowledge of the composition of foods or food groups, as well as the *in vivo* metabolism of these compounds, as only the most common metabolites are chosen as candidate biomarkers. Conversely, the *discovery-driven* method does not require any a priori knowledge of potential candidate biomarkers; it uses multivariate techniques to identify candidate biomarkers

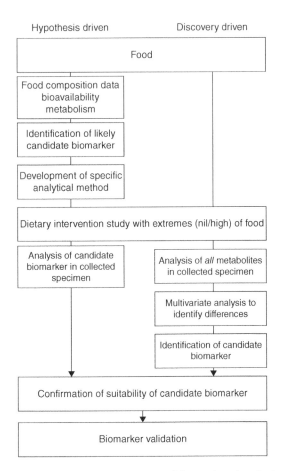

Figure 6.5 Biomarker discovery normally follows either a hypothesis- or a discovery-driven strategy. Both strategies require carefully controlled dietary intervention studies, but use different approaches for the identification of candidate biomarkers. Reprinted from Kuhnle, G. (2012) Nutritional biomarkers for objective dietary assessment, *Journal of the Science of Food and Agriculture*, **92** (6), 1145–1149.

by comparing metabolites in specimens following intervention diets high and low in respective foods (an example of this is the discovery of proline betaine as a biomarker of citrus fruits; Heinzmann *et al*. 2010). As multivariate techniques are very sensitive, it is important to ensure that the only difference between intervention groups is diet and not other factors. Standardised protocols must therefore be followed.

6.6 Biomarker validation

The validation of biomarkers prior to use is important in order to be able to interpret results properly. However, despite this necessity, many biomarkers are used without or with insufficient validation. Of particular concern is that many biomarkers are only validated against self-reported intake, a method that is known to be biased. The validation of a biomarker should address the issues discussed in this section.

Relationship with intake

A relationship with intake is the most important requirement for a biochemical marker of intake, and any validation process must establish this relationship. It does not necessarily have to be direct and a specific metabolic response to intake might also be suitable as a biomarker. Blood concentrations are often controlled by homoeostatic mechanisms, therefore the sensitivity of a biomarker to intake can only be established in some specimens, not all.

The relationship with intake can be established either experimentally with intervention studies or using prior knowledge of the metabolism. A combination of both is generally preferable, as for many candidate biomarkers only limited knowledge of their metabolism is available and intervention studies are often too small to allow generalisation. The relationship with intake of the *predictive* biomarker of sugar intake, urinary sucrose, has been established using a combination of prior knowledge – that is, the sucrose is absorbed intact from the intestinal tract and excreted unmetabolised – and intervention studies where a dose–response effect was established. These dose–response studies were extended to participants with characteristics important for future research – that is, obese participants – to ensure that this relationship was not dependent on body mass.

In addition to a direct dose–response relationship, it is important to estimate the time frame covered by individual biomarkers. Biomarkers that are very sensitive to intake and change almost immediately with consumption might be beneficial to investigate short-term dietary changes, but, in particular in nutritional epidemiology, chronic nutrient exposure is of more interest. It is therefore important to establish the relationship between biomarker, intake and time. It might thus be necessary to establish pharmacokinetic parameters such as the half-life and investigate different specimens such as 24-hour urine samples, red blood cells (RBC), adipose tissue or hair. A biomarker with a high sensitivity to recent intake might still be useful if the assessment is repeated frequently, but this has to be established in validation studies.

The relationship between biomarker and intake is often not linear, but follows a more complicated function. It is therefore of great importance to investigate this relationship, in particular whether the biomarker shows a floor or ceiling effect. For example, plasma vitamin C concentration does not increase proportionally with very high vitamin C intake.

Long-term repeatability of a biochemical marker of intake is usually a good indicator that the marker can be used as an estimate of long-term intake. For this reason, it is important to investigate the intra-person variability of nutritional biomarkers over a longer period of time.

Free-living individuals

Biomarker validation studies are usually always conducted in participants with a controlled diet designed to contain different amounts of the respective foods. While it is important to investigate this relationship, the tightly controlled nature of these diets makes it difficult to compare results to free-living individuals. However, in nutritional epidemiology it is the diet of free-living individuals that is most important, and biomarkers should therefore be validated in a similar population. One method for addressing these difficulties is to conduct dietary intervention studies where participants live under controlled conditions but receive their habitual diet. This allows a detailed analysis of their dietary intake while still obtaining the same dietary variability as in a free-living population.

Validation without intervention studies

While detailed validation studies are desirable, it is often not feasible to conduct them and biomarkers have to be validated using specimen and dietary data from existing studies. A high variation of a biomarker in a cross-sectional study is often a good indicator of a relationship with intake, although other factors can explain this association as well. The quality of a biomarker is often assessed using either the intra-class correlation between self-reported and biomarker data or Cohen's kappa statistic. However, these results only show the agreement between different analytical methods, not the association with true intake. Thus, a biomarker might agree well with self-reported intake and be considered a good biomarker of intake while the association with true intake is unexamined and poor.

6.7 Interpretation of results

Limitations and other considerations

Biochemical markers of intake are often considered an *objective* and more reliable dietary assessment method. However, while biomarkers are less subject to bias introduced by self-reporting, they still can introduce bias and measurement error and careful consideration when interpreting the results is important. Unless detailed data from dietary intervention studies are available, a relationship between biomarker and intake is often only assumed based on self-reported data.

A nutritional biomarker is in most cases essentially a marker of bioavailability (except for markers detected in faeces), as only compounds that enter the body can be detected as biochemical markers. This can be advantageous when the bioactivity of specific nutrients is of interest, as the biomarker is often a better measure of exposure than dietary information. However, this is disadvantageous when dietary intake is the primary interest, for example when investigating food choice or the effect of dietary patterns. Biomarker bioavailability can be affected by a number of different factors, for example dietary composition, health, gastrointestinal microbiome or genetic factors. Biochemical markers are therefore ideally suited to investigate associations with specific compounds – or to some extent to specific foods – but are less well suited to investigating dietary patterns or the wider context of associations between diet and health.

Biomarker concentrations are also affected by other factors such as physiological status, disease state and malnourishment. The application of most biomarkers makes the assumption that the body is in homoeostasis, but this is not the case in a number of people, for example pregnant women, people with (long-term) illness or those still growing; malnourishment can also have an impact on the metabolism and thus biomarkers. It is therefore important to take these aspects into account when using biomarkers in human studies.

A further aspect to consider is the metabolism of compounds used as biomarkers. Most analytical methods are developed for individual compounds, and therefore interindividual differences in metabolism can affect the outcome. This might be less of a problem when bioactive metabolites are used as biochemical markers, but in many cases the individual bioactivity of metabolites is not known. As the metabolism can be influenced not only by genetic factors but also by background diet, this is an additional source of variation that must be taken into consideration.

Correlation between intake and biomarker

The association between dietary intake and biomarker is often given as a correlation coefficient. However, a statistically significant correlation does not imply that the correlation is biologically relevant, and a lack of significance does not imply the opposite. A strong and significant correlation is often due to a high variability of biomarker and intake. Therefore, nutrients with a high variability of intake are likely to show a stronger correlation than nutrients that are ubiquitous in most foods and where the variability is therefore much lower. It is thus important to conduct controlled dietary intervention studies with a

wide range of intake to validate candidate biomarkers properly and establish a correlation.

Biomarkers to improve measurement

Biochemical markers of intake are often used to validate other dietary assessment methods, in particular food frequency questionnaires (FFQs) and to a lesser extent diaries. This approach has the advantage that the two assessment instruments used, self-reporting and biomarkers, are less likely to have correlated errors.

For validation of an assessment intake, a true reference value is normally required. However, in nutritional epidemiology, such a value is usually not available unless dietary intake has been observed directly. Validation in this context is therefore the evaluation of the measurement error, which can then be applied to values obtained from the instrument. The relationship between two measurements is usually determined by calibration. In nutritional epidemiology, this is the relationship between a measurement – that is, self-reported data or a biomarker – and the habitual intake; however, the latter cannot be observed directly. For this reason, calibration in this context can often be assumed to be the estimation of a correction factor that can be applied to a dietary measurement to determine the habitual diet. *Recovery biomarkers* are most suited to method validation and calibration, as they allow a direct estimation of intake and therefore permit the determination of a correction factor, but *concentration biomarkers* have also been used for measurement error correction. Urinary nitrogen – as a recovery marker of total protein intake – has been used in the OPEN study as a reference instrument to investigate the measurement error structure of self-reported dietary assessment instruments, FFQs and 24-hour recall.

The measurement error introduced by the inaccuracies of dietary assessment methods affects the observed association between diet and disease, the so-called regression dilution bias. Information obtained using nutritional biomarkers can be used to correct observed associations for this bias. A commonly employed method is *regression calibration*, where the true value of the intake is predicted using a measurement – such as biomarkers – and relevant confounders (Freedman *et al.* 2010). More information about the statistical methods used for measurement error correction can be found in the references and further reading.

Biomarkers to monitor compliance

Biochemical markers of intake can also be used to monitor compliance in dietary intervention studies. The choice of biomarker depends largely on the type of intervention and the length of the study: for specific intervention foods – such as cruciferous vegetables – a single biomarker such as glucosinolates (or their *in vivo* metabolites) might be suitable, whereas for more complex dietary interventions a battery of biomarkers might be more appropriate (for example vitamin C, carotenoids and polyphenols for a diet with increased fruit and vegetable intake). In short-term studies, it is often sufficient to conduct spot checks and collect samples at random time points to ensure compliance. In these instances, the nature of the biomarker, long or short term, is less important. For longer-term and chronic studies, however, a closer monitoring of compliance is often desirable. This can be achieved either by the regular collection of samples at intervals determined by the physiological half-life of the compound, or the collection of specimens that provide long-term dietary information.

6.8 Outlook

Nutritional biomarkers of intake are an important tool in nutrition research, in particular in nutritional epidemiology. They are an established method to improve dietary assessment methods, but there is still a paucity of properly validated biomarkers, in particular for specific foods or food groups. Future research will therefore focus on the development of more complex markers of intake, employing methods similar to those used in metabonomics.

Another important field of biomarker research is the development of biomarkers of long-term intake. While multiple sampling can provide information about long-term intake and repeatability, this is often not feasible in large observational studies and it is not possible to conduct retrospectively.

References and further reading

Bingham, S.A. (2003) Urine nitrogen as a biomarker for the validation of dietary protein intake. *Journal of Nutrition*, **133** (Suppl. 3), 921S–924S.

Bingham, S.A. and Cummings, J. (1983) The use of 4-aminobenzoic acid as a marker to validate the completeness of 24 h urine collections in man. *Clinical Science*, **64**, 629–635.

Bingham, S.A., Luben, R., Welch, A. *et al.* (2007) Epidemiologic assessment of sugars consumption using biomarkers: Comparisons of obese and nonobese individuals in the European Prospective Investigation of Cancer Norfolk. *Cancer Epidemiology, Biomarkers and Prevention*, **16**, 1651–1654.

Dror, Y., Stern, F. and Komarnitsky, M. (1994) Optimal and stable conditions for the determination of erythrocyte glutathione reductase activation coefficient to evaluate riboflavin status. *International Journal for Vitamin and Nutrition Research*, **64**, 257–262.

Freedman, L.S., Tasevska, N., Kipnis, V. *et al.* (2010) Gains in statistical power from using a dietary biomarker in combination with self-reported intake to strengthen the analysis of a diet–disease association: An example from CAREDS. *American Journal of Epidemiology*, **172** (7), 836–842.

Freedman, L.S., Midthune, D., Carroll, R.J. *et al.* (2011) Using regression calibration equations that combine self-reported intake and biomarker measures to obtain unbiased estimates and more powerful tests of dietary associations. *American Journal of Epidemiology*, **174** (11), 1238–1245.

Griffiths, W.J. and Wang, Y. (2009) Mass spectrometry: From proteomics to metabolomics and lipidomics. *Chemical Society Reviews*, **38**, 1882–1896.

Han, X., Yang, K. and Gross, R.W. (2012) Multi-dimensional mass spectrometry-based shotgun lipidomics and novel strategies for lipidomic analyses. *Mass Spectrometry Reviews*, **31**, 134–178.

Heinzmann, S.S., Brown, I.J., Chan, Q. *et al.* (2010) Metabolic profiling strategy for discovery of nutritional biomarkers: Proline betaine as a marker of citrus consumption. *American Journal of Clinical Nutrition*, **92**, 436–443.

Hodson, L., Skeaff, C.M. and Fielding, B.A. (2008) Fatty acid composition of adipose tissue and blood in humans and its use as a biomarker of dietary intake. *Progress in Lipid Research*, **47**, 348–380.

Jenab, M., Slimani, N., Bictash, M. *et al.* (2009) Biomarkers in nutritional epidemiology: Applications, needs and new horizons. *Human Genetics*, **125** (5–6), 507–525.

Jones, G. (2012) Metabolism and biomarkers of vitamin D. *Scandinavian Journal of Clinical and Laboratory Investigation*, **243**, 7–13.

Kjeldahl, J. (1883) Neue Methode zur Bestimmung des Stickstoffs in organischen Körpern. *Zeitschrift für Analytische Chemie*, **22**, 366–382.

Kuhnle, G.G.C. (2012) Nutritional biomarkers for objective dietary assessment. *Journal of the Science of Food and Agriculture*, **92**, 1145–1149.

Kuhnle, G.G.C., Joosen, A.M.C.P., Kneale, C.J. and O'Connell, T.C. (2012) Carbon and nitrogen isotopic ratios of urine and faeces as novel nutritional biomarkers of meat and fish intake. *European Journal of Nutrition*, **52** (1), 389–395.

Lampe, J. (2003) Isoflavonoid and lignan phytoestrogens as dietary biomarkers. *Journal of Nutrition*, **133** (Suppl. 3), 956S–964S.

Marklund, M., Landberg, R., Andersson, A. *et al.* (2013) Alkylresorcinol metabolites in urine correlate with the intake of whole grains and cereal fibre in free-living Swedish adults. *British Journal of Nutrition*, **109**, 129–136.

Ocke, M.C. and Kaaks, R.J. (1997) Biochemical markers as additional measurements in dietary validity studies: Application of the method of triads with examples from the European Prospective Investigation into Cancer and Nutrition. *American Journal of Clinical Nutrition*, **65** (Suppl. 4), 1240S–1245S.

Potischman, N. (2003) Biologic and methodologic issues for nutritional biomarkers. *Journal of Nutrition*, **133** (Suppl. 3), 875S–880S.

Potischman, N. and Freudenheim, J.L. (2003) Biomarkers of nutritional exposure and nutritional status: An overview. *Journal of Nutrition*, **133** (Suppl. 3), 873S–874S.

Prentice, R.L., Huany, Y., Tinker, L.F. *et al.* (2009) Statistical aspects of the use of biomarkers in nutritional epidemiology research. *Statistics in Biosciences*, **1**, 112–123.

Stamler, J. (1997) The INTERSALT study: Background, methods, findings, and implications. *American Journal of Clinical Nutrition*, **65**, 626S–642S.

Tasevska, N., Runswick, S.A., McTaggart, A. and Bingham, S.A. (2005) Urinary sucrose and fructose as biomarkers for sugar consumption. *Cancer Epidemiology, Biomarkers and Prevention*, **14**, 1287–1294.

Tasevska, N., Midthune, D., Potischman, N. *et al.* (2011) Use of the predictive sugars biomarker to evaluate self-reported total sugars intake in the Observing Protein and Energy Nutrition (OPEN) study. *Cancer Epidemiology, Biomarkers and Prevention*, **20**, 490–500.

Willett, W. (2012) *Nutritional Epidemiology*. Oxford University Press, Oxford.

7
Methods of Data Analysis

Graham Horgan

Biomathematics and Statistics Scotland, Rowett Institute of Nutrition and Health,
University of Aberdeen

Key messages

- The aim of nutritional data interpretation is to understand the variation in the data, to describe this variation and investigate its association with other information.
- The standard error quantifies the uncertainty in a summary statistic due its being based on a sample.
- Regression modelling is a technique for investigating the factors explaining variation in an outcome variable.

- In multiple regressions with more than one explanatory variable, the marginal effect of each variable is estimated, with the effects of other variables accounted for.
- Logistic regression models a binary yes/no outcome.
- Principal component analysis can help to reduce the dimensionality when many variables are recorded.

7.1 Introduction

This chapter considers the analysis of nutritional data. This includes summarising such data, producing estimates of effects and differences and testing them. It also includes techniques such as principal component analysis that are exploratory, looking for patterns in data. This essentially is statistics, which may be defined as the study of variation. Any collection of nutritional data will certainly show variation. Intake data will vary between subjects (different people eat different things and different amounts) and within subjects (between days, or between baseline and endpoint in an experiment, for example). Food composition will also vary among samples of food items. Our task is to summarise this variability and draw conclusions in its presence. Some of it we will be able to explain. Dietary intakes vary because of a person's age, gender and weight, for example, and perhaps because of dietary interventions in which they are participating. We try to quantify these effects and test whether we can be sure they are present. Other variations we will be unable to explain. A person will not eat the same things every day. Some of this we can account for (day of the week, activity level and so on, if we have recorded this information), but some of it always remains unaccounted for. Such variation is termed random.

Many varied things in people's day-to-day life (work patterns, social life, the weather) will determine what they eat on different occasions, but since these are unrecorded in our data, we cannot use them to account for the dietary variation.

This chapter covers a number of topics in the handling and interpretation of nutritional data. All of them are deserving of a whole chapter, indeed a whole book, in themselves, so we will of necessity have to be brief. Much of what is presented therefore raises issues or questions, rather than offering a detailed discussion of their treatment.

7.2 The basics of statistics

Statistics is a scientific discipline. Here we aim to cover the main topics briefly and put them in the context of nutritional data. There are many excellent textbooks that give a good introduction to statistics and those aimed at scientific disciplines allied with nutrition are probably the most useful. We would mention Campbell (1989) and Bland (2000), although there are many others. As may be expected, they vary in style, level of detail and extent of mathematical treatment, and each scientist will need to find one that suits him or her individually.

Nutrition Research Methodologies, First Edition. Edited by Julie A Lovegrove, Leanne Hodson, Sangita Sharma and Susan A Lanham-New.
© 2015 John Wiley & Sons, Ltd. Published 2015 by John Wiley & Sons, Ltd.
Companion Website: www.wiley.com/go/nutritionsociety

Types of variables

Data variables can be of different types and as this affects how they are handled, it is worth keeping in mind for each variable which type it is. A continuous variable, also known sometimes as a variate or a vector or an interval variable, denotes a quantity of some sort. Larger numbers will denote more of something, and we can speak about differences between values. For values obtained from physical measurements, these variables will usually have units (cm, gram, hour, kg/week and so on). Often a zero value of the variable is possible, and ratios may sensibly be calculated (in which case the term 'ratio variable' can be used). The unit scale is usually arbitrary: it is not important whether height is recorded in metres or centimetres, or energy intake in kJ or kcal. A change of scale by multiplying by a constant will not affect a statistical analysis, other than those parts that should scale accordingly. On other occasions variables may be defined that represent quantities that cannot be accessed directly, such as appetite or a psychometric score. These will usually not have units and their values are determined by recording something else (a visual analogue scale, answers in a questionnaire). For most purposes, there are treated in the same way as physical measurements.

The other common type of variable is categorical (sometimes termed factor or group), meaning that it records to which of two or more groups an observation belongs. If there are only two groups, the variable is termed binary (e.g. gender, or any yes/no outcome). In a trial where a treatment is offered at different doses, we sometimes regard these as categorical or sometimes as a continuous variable.

Finally, an intermediate type of variable is ordinal. In this case the categories follow a natural order. Volunteers may record how much they like a food as 'not at all', 'only a little', 'somewhat', 'a lot'. There is a natural ordering here, for which we may wish to account in presenting and analysing the data. Opinions are often recorded as the extent of agreement with a statement, and a similar scale results.

Biological and measurement variability

Observed values are subject to variation, which may either be biological in origin or due to the measurement technique being used. Biological variation is what is generally of interest, whereas measurement variation is typically a nuisance. Measurement variation, sometimes termed technical variation, is the variation that would be observed if several measurements are made on each biological sample, or on an individual person if it is something that is believed to be constant in that individual, at least over the time scale of the measurements. Technical variability can be quite small (e.g. an individual's height) or substantial, possibly even greater than the biological variation (as in some methods of determining protein expression, for example). If measurement variation is large, and time and costs permit, there may be benefits in doing several repeat measurements on each sample. However, it is important to remember that these are not true replicates, and in any analysis it is the mean of the repeat measurements that should be used. Furthermore, it is almost never a good idea to take repeated technical measurements if it is at the expense of true biological replication.

Populations and sampling

Throughout this chapter it is important to keep in mind that there is some population to which we want the information generated by our research to apply. This may be as wide as humanity in general, or it may be some subset, such as those within a certain age range, or with some specific characteristics (such as obesity). Whatever it may be, we cannot collect data on all of humanity or of the subset. We study a sample. If that sample is representative of a wider population, then we can claim that our conclusions are valid for that population. This representativeness may partly be based on the sample having been selected at random. However, it is often the case in nutritional research that those studied are volunteers or patients, from some geographical region, and their representativeness of any population in particular is an assumption that we need to make, but about which the data cannot inform us. The validity of this generalisation of the results should be discussed when the results are presented.

Distributions, transformations and outliers

The distribution is a fundamental concept in statistics. It specifies all the details of how some quantity varies. Figure 7.1 shows the observed distribution of body mass index (BMI) in a sample of about 200 adults. It allows us to see the relative proportions of individuals in each range of 2 BMI units (kg/m^2). If the sample is representative of some population, we can estimate the probability that an individual in that population will have a BMI in any specified range. The histogram allows us to observe characteristics of the distribution such as skewness (asymmetry), multimodality (more than one peak) and outliers. The most commonly used measure of variability is the standard deviation, defines as the square root of the mean squared deviation of observations about the mean $\bar{x}$:

$$SD = \sqrt{\frac{1}{n-1}\sum\left(x-\bar{x}\right)^2}$$

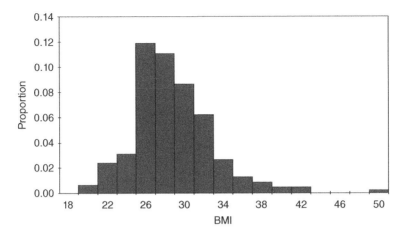

Figure 7.1 Histogram of BMI.

The divisor of n-1, termed the degrees of freedom, is used because the deviations are not independent but are constrained to sum to zero.

For many purposes in data analysis, it is convenient if random variation has a roughly normal (also termed Gaussian) distribution, one that is symmetrical and bell shaped. Note that it is the distribution of the random unexplained variation that needs to be normal, not necessarily the original values, although the shape of the distribution is usually similar for both. The calculations done in statistical testing, for example, tend to assume this normality. If data depart substantially from this, it may be more reliable to work with a transformed version. There are many possibilities here, but the log transform is by far the most widely used. It tends to make positively skewed distributions more symmetrical, and can be thought of as transforming multiplicative effects and differences into additive ones. If some data values are zero, add a small constant to all values (the smallest non-zero value, for example) before taking logs. If some values are negative, this usually is because they are differences, in which case take logs before calculating differences.

A histogram will also alert you to outliers, observations far from the rest of the distribution. These should be checked in case they are errors, or in some way unrepresentative of what you intend to study. However, they cannot be removed without good justification. For example, in Figure 7.1 we might want to check that the BMI observation about 50 is correct. If it had been 5 or 500 we would have been sure that it must have been wrong, and we would either correct it if we could, or omit it if we could not. There are no standard tests to help identify outliers. Scientists must use their own judgement and knowledge of how the data were collected.

Quantiles

Sometimes it can be convenient to handle continuous variables by chopping the range of values into intervals to define an ordered categorical variable. The main reason for doing this is convenience. It can be easier to discuss the differences between these categories than to talk about the effects of gradual changes in the continuous variable. In some cases, statistical analysis using the categories is more easily able to account for effects such as non-linearity, which require more care on the continuous scale. Non-linearity occurs when a response does not change at a constant rate as an explanatory variable changes.

The definition of the intervals can be done in various ways. Dividing age into decade intervals (20–30, 31–40 etc.) seems natural and easy to remember. BMI is traditionally divided into intervals of < 18, 18–25, 25.1–30 and > 30 as a choice of readily remembered round numbers, and these are used by the World Health Organization. The > 30 range is sometimes further subdivided. Dietary intakes are sometimes split according to whether they meet specified recommendations or not. Splitting the range of values according to the observed distribution is also widely done. This involves choosing dividing points so that the same proportion of observations falls into each interval. The usual choices are three intervals (tertiles) or four (quartiles) or five (quintiles) and occasionally ten (deciles). The advantage of defining categories in this way is that it is objective and frees scientists from the need to choose values themselves. It also ensures an equal number of observations in each category, which is optimal for statistical power.

There is a disadvantage to turning a continuous variable into categories, and that is the loss of information that it implies. The usual BMI categories, for example, imply

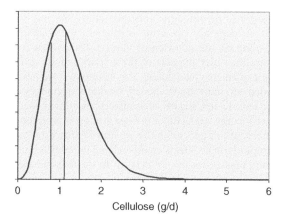

Figure 7.2 Example of representing a continuous variable (dietary cellulose) as quartiles. The lowest and particularly the highest contain values with considerable variability.

no difference between two individuals with BMIs of 25.5 and 29.5, while the latter is in a different category from someone with a BMI of 30.5. There is also an information loss if the analysis does not account for the ordering of the categories, which very often it does not. In terms of variance information discarded, defining tertiles discards about 21% of the variability, quartiles discards about 14% and quintiles about 10%. This loss of information is illustrated in Figure 7.2. More quantiles result in less loss of information, but more result details have to be presented, and fewer observations per quantile increase the uncertainty about each result. Four quantiles (i.e. quartiles) seem to be the most common choice.

Standard error and confidence interval

For anything we want the research to tell us – which is typically the mean of a variable, the effect of a treatment, the difference between two population subgroups or the risk of some adverse outcome – we suppose that there is some true value for this quantity. Then there is the value that we estimate in our study.

The classic statistical view is that this estimated quantity is subject to variability. If we repeated the whole study, changing nothing but sampling a different but equally representative set of subjects, we would obtain results that were somewhat different. The amount by which an estimated quantity is subject to variability in this way is termed its standard error. We do not need to repeat the study in order to obtain it, as it can be calculated from the information in a single study.

The value of a standard error (SE) is that it tells us the reliability of the (single) estimate that we have obtained of some quantity. If the SE is low, then we know that any repeated study would produce a similar estimate, so it

must be close to the true value (assuming of course that there is no bias).

A standard error can be obtained for any quantity that is calculated from a sample. The most often quoted are the standard error of the mean (SEM = $SD / \sqrt{n}$) or that of the difference in two means (SED = $SD\sqrt{\dfrac{1}{n_1} + \dfrac{1}{n_2}}$), but it can also be calculated for a proportion or regression coefficient or anything else calculated from a sample. A common way of presenting the same information is to quote a confidence interval. This is based on the fact that the variability in estimates has a normal distribution, and this distribution encompasses 95% of observations within about 2 standard deviations. So if we quote an interval of plus or minus 2 × SE about an estimate, it will include the true value 95% of the time. In fact, allowing for the SD being estimated rather than known exactly, the correct multiplier is not exactly 2 and depends on the sample size. However, it will not be greatly different from 2, and will be between 1.96 and 2.2 as long as the sample size is at least 10.

Standard errors and confidence intervals may also be calculated for proportions, such as the proportion of individuals who meet a dietary recommendation. If the proportion in the sample of size n is p, then the SE is $\sqrt{p(1-p)/n}$, and the confidence interval is calculated as for the mean.

Tests and p-values

Very often the central question in a nutritional investigation is whether or not there is an effect (of one variable on another) or a difference (between two intervention groups) or an association (between two variables). This question is assumed to have an answer 'yes' or 'no'. This is the usual view, although some experts would argue (Nester 1996) that there is always an effect or difference of some sort, even though it may be small. Perhaps we can say that if a difference is small enough that our study cannot even tell whether it is positive or negative, we will regard it as effectively zero.

The p-value is based on considering what might be observed if there was no difference or effect or association. Suppose we are comparing an intervention and a control group in a situation where the intervention really has no effect. Ideally, the mean of the outcome of interest would be the same in both groups. In practice, because of random variation, the difference in means will not be exactly zero. Let us call this difference D. The p-value asks the question: 'How likely are we to observe a value of D as large as this in the absence of any intervention effect?' The answer is a probability, the p-value. If this is small, we have observed something that is unlikely in the absence of an effect, and so we conclude that there is an effect. Indicating significance using * for p < 0.05, ** for p < 0.01 and *** for p < 0.001 is common.

How small does a p-value need to be in order to draw this conclusion? There is no answer to this, and the p-value is a continuous scale of evidence for or against the existence of the effect. There is a convention that 5% is the value below which the evidence is enough. In practice, the p-value calculated should be presented, and the discussion should then proceed to weighing the strength or weakness of the evidence against the consequences of deciding whether or not there is an intervention effect.

One final subtlety of the p-value is related to the phrasing in the question: 'a value of D as large as...'. Conventionally, this is taken to include both positive and negative differences of the specified magnitude, and the test is termed 'two-sided'. Rarely, we may declare that we are only interested if differences are in one particular direction and a one-sided test results, with half the p-value of the corresponding two-sided version. For example, we could claim that we are only interested in a dietary supplement if it reduces cholesterol, and would declare that it had no effect if evidence pointed to a significant increase. In reality, any such outcome would be noteworthy. Two-sided tests are always recommended.

A t-test is the most basic statistical test and is most often used to compare two groups, but it can also compare a single sample against some specified constant. An example is comparing the mean intake against some dietary reference value, a recommended level of intake that many governments and nutritional organisations promote. For example, this might be an Estimated Average Requirement (EAR), published by the Institute of Medicine of the US National Academy of Sciences, expected to satisfy the needs of 50% of the people in that age group and used to assess the contributions of food items to nutritional needs. Also published are Recommended Dietary Allowances (RDA), the daily dietary intake level of a nutrient considered sufficient to meet the requirements of 97.5% of healthy individuals in a group, and this is usually about 20% higher than the EAR.

7.3 Regression modelling

Regression modelling is the most commonly used technique for linking one variable to others. Other techniques such as analysis of variance (see Section 7.4) are also built around regression-type models. In regression we select one specific variable that we regard as

the response or outcome, and then study the way in which it depends on other explanatory variables. Depending on the question of interest, things that we measure may play the role of the response or the role of the explanatory variable(s). For example, if we have recorded an individual's dietary intake of retinol, we might seek to investigate what affects that intake: age, gender, income level, choice of food groups, experimental interventions and so on. Or we may be interested in how retinol intake affects health-related outcomes such as blood pressure or even mortality. In the former case, retinol is the outcome; in the latter, it is blood pressure or whatever. The outcome variable may be of any of the types listed above, as may the explanatory variables. Here we will only consider the simpler cases where the outcome is continuous or binary and the explanatory variables are continuous or categorical or a mixture of these.

For a continuous outcome, consider the simplest model where there is one explanatory variable (let us call it X) and the outcome or response variable (call it Y). We then suppose that

$$Y = A + B X + \varepsilon$$

where A and B are constants that we estimate from the data, and ε denotes random variation, whose variability we also estimate. We assume its mean to be zero. The model is linear in that the effect of changing X is independent of the value of X: an increase of one unit in X is associated with a mean increase of B in Y, regardless of what X is. The constant A is the mean value of Y if X is zero, although as often as not this does not have any practical meaning.

Regression can be carried out in almost any statistical software, and will produce various results in the output. These will include:

- Estimates of the values of A and B.
- Standard errors of these estimates.
- P-values to test whether the values differ significantly from zero.
- Estimate of the variance of ε, the random variation.
- R^2 – this may be interpreted as the proportion of the variance of Y that can be explained by the variability in X.

Figure 7.3 shows a plot of bodyfat and triceps skinfold thickness in 20 women (see Neter *et al.* 1996). We expect these to be related and can see that they are. A plot such as this allows us to judge whether or not a linear model is appropriate. There are ways to test this formally, but that is not discussed here (see Chaterjee and Hadi 2012, §4.7). Examining a plot should always be the first step.

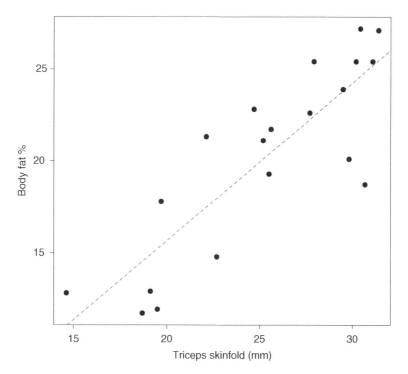

Figure 7.3 Plot of body fat % against triceps skinfold.

A linear model seems a reasonable choice to fit here. However, it is not completely clear which variable should be the explanatory and which the response. If the purpose is to predict body fat (which we want to measure, although this is not easy) from skinfold thickness (which is easy) then body fat should be the response, if the subjects are representative of those for whom we plan to use the prediction. Figure 7.3 shows the output

from fitting a linear regression using the open-source R statistical programming language (R Core Team 2012).

Thus, A is estimated to be -1.5% and B to be 0.86%/mm, and they have standard errors of 3.32% and 0.13%/mm respectively. The t-value is the ratio of the estimate to its standard error and provides the basis for the p-value that tests the parameter. B is significantly different from zero, which was hardly in doubt in this case as it was

```
> summary(lm(Fat~Triceps))
Call:
lm(formula = Fat ~ Triceps)
 Residuals:
    Min       1Q   Median      3Q      Max
-6.1195   -2.1904  0.6735   1.9383   3.8523
Coefficients:
             Estimate   Std.  Error t value Pr(>|t|)
(Intercept)  -1.4961         3.3192  -0.451    0.658
Triceps       0.8572         0.1288   6.656 3.02e-06 ***
---
Signif. codes:  0   '***' 0.001  '**' 0.01 '*' 0.05 '.' 0.1 ' ' 1
Residual standard error: 2.82 on 18 degrees of freedom
Multiple R squared: 0.7111,     Adjusted R-squared: 0.695
F-statistic:  44.3 on 1 and 18 DF,  p-value: 3.024e-06
```

clear from the plot that there was an association. The random variation is estimated to have a standard deviation of 2.82%, indicating the uncertainty if the model is used for prediction. We can say that 71% of the variation in fat percentage can be explained or predicted by triceps skinfold, and a version of this adjusted for what is explained by chance patterns in the random variation is 69.5%. The final p-value quoted is the same as in the test for the effect of triceps, as it is the only explanatory variable.

If it seems odd that the constant A has no direct meaningful interpretation, it may be helpful to note that the model can be rewritten in terms of the mean values of X and Y, which we will write as Xmean and Ymean. The linear model is then

$$(Y - Y\text{mean}) = B(X - X\text{mean}) + \varepsilon$$

so that B relates deviations of Y from its mean to deviations of X from its mean. They are scaled by a constant B, and there is additional random variation.

Multiple regression

Very often we have more than one explanatory variable. We can examine how each of them separately is related to the outcome variable, using the single linear regression described previously. We can also consider fitting a single model that describes how the response is related to the whole set of explanatory variables. The generalisation looks fairly straightforward, although much greater care is needed in interpreting the estimates. The issue of deciding which variables should be included in the model and which omitted may also be important. The complexities arise because the explanatory variables are usually correlated with each other. While there are many possibilities for modelling the effect of several explanatory variables on an outcome, the first model usually examined is the multiple linear regression model.

For this, the single linear regression model is extended to more variables by adding additional linear terms. For example, if we suppose that we have not one explanatory variable X but three, which we label X, U and V, then the model for outcome variable Y becomes

$$Y = A + BX + CU + DV + \varepsilon$$

where we now have two additional parameters, C and D, to estimate. C may be interpreted as the mean change in Y per unit change in U, with this change being the same regardless of the value of U, or of X or V. It is also important to remember that these parameters estimate the marginal effect of changing one of the variables, with the other held constant, even though correlation

Table 7.1 Multiple regression with three variables.

```
Call
lm(formula = Fat ~ Triceps + Thigh + Mid-arm)
Residuals
Min        1Q        Median    3Q        Max
-3.7263    -1.6111   0.3923    1.4656    4.1277
Coefficients
              Estimate Std     t-value Pr(>|t|)
                       error
(Intercept)  117.085   99.782   1.173   0.258
Triceps        4.334    3.016   1.437   0.170
Thigh         -2.857    2.582  -1.106   0.285
Mid-arm       -2.186    1.595  -1.370   0.190
Residual standard error: 2.48 on 16 degrees
of freedom (Df)
Multiple R-squared:  0.8014
Adjusted R-squared:  0.7641
F statistic:  21.52 on 3 and 16 Df
p-value:  7.343e-06
```

among the predictor variables means that changes in one tend to be accompanied by changes in the other. What the model shows is the marginal effect of changes in each variable.

Fitting multiple regression models is not difficult and any statistical software will have the facility for doing this. As an example, we can look again at the triceps and body fat data used earlier. In addition to triceps skinfold, the mid-arm and thigh circumference were also recorded. These are likely to be associated with body fat and may provide information that can improve the prediction compared with using triceps alone. A multiple regression with all three variables gives the results in Table 7.1.

The F statistic quoted shows that the regression model explains more variation in body fat than can be explained as a chance finding. The t-value (ratio of estimate to its standard error) and associated p-value indicate the significance of each variable. Perhaps surprisingly, none of the variables has a value significantly different from zero. This is because given the other two, each variable adds nothing more to the prediction.

Further exploration of the different possible choices of variables can help in the selection of a suitable model. If two measurements are enough, then we may prefer not to take the trouble of recording all three. In a model with just mid-arm and triceps, both are significant (see Table 7.2).

Some caution is needed as this is a small dataset; it is possible that a larger study might find that the other measurements (and other potential measurements) do have something to add. Here we are able fairly readily to examine all eight possible combinations of variables, null included. However, the number of possible models

Table 7.2 Multiple regression with two variables.

	Estimate	Std error	t-value	Pr(>|t|)
(Intercept)	6.7916	4.4883	1.513	0.1486
Triceps	1.0006	0.1282	7.803	5.12e-07***
Mid-arm	-0.4314	0.1766	-2.443	0.0258*

doubles for each additional variable, and this rapidly becomes unmanageable.

Good statistical software will have tools for navigating among all these models. For up to 16 or so variables (at the time of writing) it is possible for all models to be checked and a summary produced so that the best by some criterion can be chosen. For more than this, some sort of stepwise procedure is usually recommended. This starts with either an empty model (no explanatory variables) or a full model (all variables included) and then sequentially adds or removes variables according to a protocol until the procedure terminates. Such algorithms have the advantage of providing an objective means of choosing a model, but the disadvantage of being over-optimistic about how good the final model selected really is (see for example Rencher and Pun 1980).

Sometimes the variables included in a regression model are not all of primary interest in themselves, but may be included as they explain some of the variation in the outcome. For example, if we are studying the effect of dietary variables on blood pressure, we would usually include information such as age and BMI in the model as well. This is not to investigate their effect, which has been examined many times before, but to adjust for them. Since diet patterns differ between age groups, this means that the effects of dietary variables in the model are clearer because their effect is estimated within age groups. The effect of this adjustment can be assessed by comparing the model with one in which age is not included.

Calibration

Regression is often used for calibration of measurement methods. Indeed, the example we used earlier is likely to have arisen in this way, if the measurements were obtained in order to validate the use of skinfold measurements to estimate body fat, rather than to study the physiology of fat distribution. Assuming that calibration was the intention, then the regression provides a prediction of body fat from the other measurements. Another version of calibration sometimes used for laboratory measurements is to take samples made with known values of (for example) concentration of a compound, and then to measure some indicator of the concentration

from these samples. In this case the regression should be of the indicator as outcome and the concentration as explanatory, and the resulting regression function inverted for routine use.

Measurement error in explanatory variables

Measurement error is often present, so the variables we are studying in the regression are not the true values of the quantities in which we are interested, but vary somewhat about these. When we use these measured values in a regression, what we obtain will be a model linking the measurements, rather than the true but unobserved quantities. There are ways of accounting for this, particularly if the amount of measurement variation is known, but they are beyond the scope of this chapter. Any regression textbook will cover them and whole books (e.g. Fuller 1987) have been devoted to the topic. It is an issue that is often ignored in nutritional studies (unlike some other areas of science). One effect is that associations between variables will often appear weaker than they really are, due to the extra random variation arising from the measurement process.

7.4 Analysis of variance

Analysis of variance, often shortened to ANOVA, is, along with regression, one of the standard ways of analysing and interpreting nutritional (or any other scientific) data. Looked at closely, it is similar to regression in that it models the variation in an outcome, and it is a linear model in terms of what affects the outcome. It often appears different, however, in that the emphasis is generally on the categorical factors rather than continuous measurements, and these factors often represent the interventions in an experiment. The principal result of ANOVA is an analysis of variance table. This shows how the total variability in the outcome can be broken down into the amount of variation that can be explained by various sources. Tests of whether these sources explain a significant amount of variation (more than is likely to be due to chance) are part of the table. Tables of means and standard errors are usually produced as well.

There are columns in the ANOVA table for Df (degrees of freedom, the amount of information about the source of variation), the sum of squares (of deviations about the mean), mean square (sum of squares divided by Df) and an F value (the ratio of the mean square for that row to the mean square for the residual term). Finally, a p-value helps to assess whether a term really is producing any variation, or if it can plausibly be explained by the random variation.

As an example of ANOVA, we look at some data on systolic blood pressure (SBP) measured in volunteers who were assigned to one of three diets: a control low-fibre diet, a diet enriched with wholegrains, or one enriched with wholegrains and oats. See Tighe *et al.* (2010) for more details. Table 7.3 shows an ANOVA table of SBP change after 12 weeks, a table of means and the standard errors.

The ANOVA table has a row for each source of variation. There is a row for gender (differences between males and females, averaged across diets), one for diet (differences between diets, averaged over males and females) and an interaction term. The interaction term is based on the extent to which the differences in the outcome due to one factor (diet) vary according to another factor (gender). The residual term is the remaining variation once these factors have been accounted for, and is considered random.

We see that there appears to be a diet effect, since the p-value of 0.00463 is considerably less than 0.05. There is no evidence for gender differences (p-value about 0.18) or interaction between gender and diet (p-value about 0.31). So although a wholegrain diet appears to produce a bigger drop in SBP relative to control in males than in females, this can reasonably be explained from the random variation within each diet and gender combination.

The standard errors that follow the table of means are based on a pooled estimate of within-group variation (from the residual mean square $\sqrt{61.6} = 7.8\,\text{mmHg}$)

and vary a little due to different numbers of volunteers in each group. We can calculate standard errors of difference (SED) in this situation from the square root of the sum of the squares of the two SE values. (In more complex designs, this may need to be calculated in a different way, but will usually be produced by the software being used.)

In the ANOVA in Table 7.3, we have accounted for variation in the baseline SBP at week 4 by subtracting it from the endpoint SBP at week 16. A more flexible way to do this is to perform an ANOVA of the endpoint SBP and include the baseline value as a *covariate* in the analysis. This approach, which involves fitting a regression model to the association between baseline and endpoint values, adapts to however strong or weak this association is, whereas subtracting the baseline assumes a strong association. The second approach results in the ANOVA table shown in Table 7.4. The variation in endpoint values that can be explained by the variation present at baseline appears as an extra term (SBP_4).

We can see that for these data the effect of diet is more clearly significant, and a difference between genders now appears. The very highly significant variation explained by the baseline is as expected.

ANOVA can be a great deal more complex than in the examples shown here, if the design of the experiment is more complex. For example, a cross-over design is one in which each volunteer experiences all treatments, changing

Table 7.3 Analysis of variance in SBP change after 12 weeks.

```
ANOVA table
```

	Df	Sum Sq	Mean Sq	F value	Pr(>F)	
Gender	1	112	111.6	1.811	0.17987	
Diet	2	681	340.3	5.523	0.00463	**
Gender:Diet	2	144	72.2	1.172	0.31199	
Residuals	199	12262	61.6			

```
Table of means (units are change in mmHg)
```

Gender	Control	Wholegrain	W+Oats
Male	0.00	−5.18	−4.22
Female	−2.79	−4.52	−7.15

```
Standard errors
```

Gender	Control	Wholegrain	W+Oats
Male	1.35	1.24	1.27
Female	1.21	1.29	1.33

Table 7.4 ANOVA table including baseline value as covariate.

	Df	Sum Sq	Mean Sq	F value	Pr(>F)	
SBP_4	1	23920	23920	456.396	<2e-16	***
Gender	1	329	329	6.272	0.013071	*
Diet	2	899	449	8.576	0.000268	***
Gender:Diet	2	189	94	1.802	0.167674	
Residuals	198	10377	52			

between them in different time periods. For an ANOVA of such an experiment, we would have different treatments at different time periods in each volunteer, as well as differences between groups of volunteers (male and female, for example). In such a design there are two levels of random variation (between and within volunteer), with different factors being assessed at each level. The ANOVA must be constructed based on this structure, although once this is done the interpretation follows the same lines as in the earlier example.

7.5 Adjusting for energy intake and other lifestyle factors

When examining data on intakes of nutrients, some of the variability in their values will be due to overall dietary intake. A 100 kg person will eat more overall than a 60 kg person, so it is likely that they will eat more of most nutrients because of this: more vitamins, minerals, phytochemicals and so on. This is of course not a deterministic association, since diet composition varies, but greater food intake is associated with greater intake of all nutrients. However, for some purposes we may wish to have a measure of relative intake.

In most studies of nutrients and disease, the primary dietary exposure of interest is adjusted for energy instead of using the absolute dietary intake. Because of the high inter-correlation of dietary intake with energy, energy adjustments in dietary investigations reduce the variation in dietary intake resulting from differences in body size, metabolic efficiency and physical activity.

Figure 7.4 shows a plot of reported intake of calcium against total energy intake in a sample of 50 people. The positive correlation is clear, but there is a large amount of variation not accounted for. Individual A has an intake greater than would be expected given their overall intake, while B has a lower than expected intake. If we want to look at factors affecting intake, or the association that intake may have with health outcomes, we might wish to look at this relative intake rather than overall intake.

It may be enough to obtain relative intakes simply by dividing the nutrient intake by the total energy intake, to obtain a nutrient density. However, sometimes this does not reflect the association between nutrients and energy. Looking at Figure 7.4, we see that a doubling of the total energy intake does not on average lead to a doubling of calcium intake. Dividing by total intake would leave an adjusted value that tended to be lower at a higher intake. Instead, we carry out a linear regression.

It is usual to suppose that the association between nutrient and energy intake is linear. It is worthwhile to check this by examining a scatter plot. In the case of Figure 7.4, it appears that a linear association is reasonable. If the association is non-linear, then a non-linear curve rather than a straight line should be fitted to the data. This can be done either by non-linear curve fitting, or possibly by transformation of one or both variables. In either case, the basic idea of obtaining residuals is the same, but more care is needed with the mathematics.

The residuals that are obtained from the regression will be a mixture of positive and negative numbers, with a mean of exactly zero. As such they may look a little odd: we do not expect nutrient intakes to be negative. We can deal with this by adding a constant value to all of them. The usual choice is the overall mean value for the nutrient before adjustment. The values obtained from this can be interpreted as the nutrient intake that

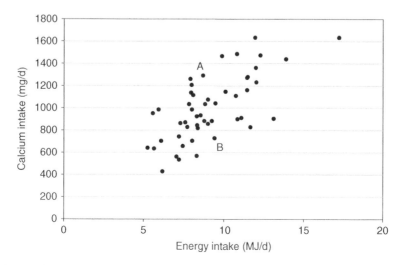

Figure 7.4 Plot of calcium intake against total energy intake.

individual would have had if their overall energy intake had been average (if such a hypothetical statement can be accepted). Since the same constant is added to all residuals, it will have no effect on the use of the adjusted values in statistical modelling. Another way of visualising the adjustment is to think of it as like sliding an observation parallel to the regression line until it reaches the position of mean intake.

Adjusting for energy intake is the most common type of adjustment, but we can in the same way adjust for any other variable we wish. Adjusting for total body weight may be of interest, but anything we have recorded, such as resting metabolic rate or fat-free mass, is also possible. The adjustment is done in exactly the same way. It is also possible to adjust for more than one variable at the same time. We carry out multiple linear regression with more than one explanatory variable and obtain the residuals in the same way.

7.6 Morbidity/mortality data

Morbidity and mortality can be regarded as outcomes in an experiment or observational study that have the characteristic of being binary: for each individual they occur or they do not. For mortality, a more long-term view is that death will occur eventually for all of us and the outcome is not whether or not but when it occurs. A complication in that view is that for many individuals we do not know when it occurs by the time the study is concluded, only that it has not occurred yet. Such observations are termed 'censored' and this type of data is referred to as 'survival data'.

The most widely used regression model for binary outcomes is logistic regression, a special case of the wider class of models known as generalised linear models. (The standard reference is McCullough and Nelder 1989, where the treatment is fairly mathematical.) The outcome is binary and we refer to alternatives as 'no' and 'yes'. The probability P of a yes outcome depends on a predictor variable, X, via the formula:

$$P = \frac{\exp(A + BX)}{1 + \exp(A + BX)}$$

It is a transformed version of the linear function $A + B X$ and with a little manipulation we have:

$$\frac{P}{1 - P} = \exp(A + BX)$$

The term $P/(1 - P)$ is termed the 'odds' (this is also used as an everyday term). If X increases by one unit, the linear expression will increase by B and the exp term on the right-hand side will be multiplied by $\exp(B)$, this being a property of the exp function. Thus the ratio of the odds associated with this increased value of X, to the odds associated with the original value, is $\exp(B)$. It is natural to express the effect in terms of odds ratios, rather than on the original scale of probabilities.

The model is similarly constructed for a categorical explanatory variable. If X specifies two categories (male and female, for example), we can consider them coded as 0 and 1. In that case, $\exp(B)$ is the odds ratio associated with being in the category labelled 1 relative to the category labelled 0. If X specifies three or more categories then, as in linear regression, one is a reference category and the model specifies the odds ratios associated with being in each of the other categories, relative to that of being in the reference category. These categories may be quantiles of some continuous variable. More often than not, this is the way in which continuous variables are handled in logistic regression.

To illustrate the results produced by logistic regression, we investigate the association between dietary fibre intake and incidence of coronary heart disease, here recorded as incidence = no or yes. The data are described in more detail in Clayton and Hills (1993). We first show (Table 7.5) a logistic regression fit treating fibre as a continuous variable, so estimating the effect associated with a unit increase (g/day) in fibre.

Thus the odds ratio for a unit increase in fibre intake is $\exp(-1.12) = 0.326$. To get a confidence interval for this, we take a confidence interval for the value of $B = -1.12$ using 1.96 times the SE to get $(-1.87, -0.37)$ and apply the $\exp()$ function to give $(0.154, 0.688)$. The z-value is the ratio of the estimate to its standard error. Alternatively, we can divide the range of fibre intakes into quartiles and fit this as a categorical variable to give the values in Table 7.6.

Here the upper three quartiles are compared with the lowest quartile, and odds ratios may be calculated as before.

Survival data

As already explained, survival data analysis is concerned with how long individuals survive after the start of a study. The observed outcome is the time of death (or possibly some other event) if it occurs, or otherwise the time at which the individual is lost to further observation (which is often but not always at the conclusion of the study). This type of data is widely collected in medical research, where the individuals observed have some medical condition and are usually termed patients rather than subjects. It is not as common for such data to be collected in nutritional studies, and so we will not cover any of the details of these models here.

Table 7.5 Logistic regression fit of the association between dietary fibre intake and incidence of coronary heart disease.

```
glm(formula = chd ~ fibre, family = binomial)
```

Deviance residuals

Min	1Q	Median	3Q	Max
-0.8880	-0.5900	-0.4949	-0.3619	2.3823

Coefficients

	Estimate	Std error	z-value	Pr(>|z|)	
(Intercept)	-0.04852	0.60364	-0.08	0.93594	
fibre	-1.12160	0.38150	-2.94	0.00328	**

```
---
Null deviance: 263.76 on 332 degrees of freedom
Residual deviance: 253.53 on 331 degrees of freedom
4 observations deleted due to missingness
```

```
Signif. codes: 0 '***' 0.001 '**' 0.01 '*' 0.05 '.' 0.1 ' ' 1
Dispersion parameter for binomial family taken to be 1
```

Table 7.6 Logistic regression fit of the association between quartiles of dietary fibre intake and incidence of coronary heart disease.

```
glm(formula = chd ~ f4, family = binomial)
```

Deviance residuals

Min	1Q	Median	3Q	Max
-0.7210	-0.5837	-0.4502	-0.3525	2.3704

Coefficients

	Estimate	Std error	z-value	Pr(>|z|)	
(Intercept)	-1.2144	0.2613	-4.648	3.34e-06	***
f4(1.36,1.67]	-1.0236	0.4545	-2.252	0.02432	*
f4(1.67,1.94]	-0.4691	0.3993	-1.175	0.24011	
f4(1.94,5.35]	-1.5328	0.5302	-2.891	0.00384	**

```
---
Null deviance: 263.47 on 331 degrees of freedom
Residual deviance: 251.77 on 328 degrees of freedom
5 observations deleted due to missingness
```

```
Signif. codes: 0 '***' 0.001 '**' 0.01 '*' 0.05 '.' 0.1 ' ' 1
Dispersion parameter for binomial family taken to be 1
```

In survival analysis, the primary object of interest is the survival function. This is the probability that an individual will survive for a specified amount of time (after he or she enters the study). After data is collected, this function may be estimated up to some time point, since we know for any amount of time what proportion of individuals survived for at least that amount of time. Related to this is the hazard function, which for a specified time is the rate (per unit of time) at which deaths occur among those who have survived to that time. In a survival study, we are interested in what factors affect the survival and hazard functions. As for continuous and binary data, there are many ways in which this may be modelled. One of the common choices is the proportional hazards model, which assumes that variables and factors affect the hazard function through being proportional to the exponential of a linear function of the explanatory variables. The same proportionality applies at all times – that is, for some value of the explanatory variable, the hazard is always increased or reduced by the same proportion. This, of course, is an assumption that will need to be checked.

Many other models are possible and there are many textbooks on survival data analysis, mostly with a medical viewpoint (e.g. Collett 2003).

7.7 Principal component analysis and other multivariate methods

The methods described in this section differ from all those covered earlier in that we are no longer developing a model for an outcome or response variable. We have a number of measurement variables, possibly a very large number, and are interested in exploring the patterns in their variability. The assessment of dietary patterns represents an alternative to the more usual approach, which focuses on single foods and nutrients, and allows evaluation of the effects of combinations of many foods simultaneously. We do not regard one of them as a response, but consider all on an equal basis. We are also not aiming to test hypotheses or validate models, so no p-values are produced. There are many multivariate methods, depending on the structure of the data and the patterns of interest. We will explain the basics of only one of these here, principal component analysis (PCA). The ideas on which it is based form the foundation of many other multivariate methods.

PCA can be viewed in a number of ways, but the usual one is as a way of reducing the dimensionality of a data set with many variables, which are usually correlated with each other. The idea is that although we may have recorded, say, 30 variables, there are not really 30 dimensions of important interesting variability in the data. We suspect that the variation of interest can be captured in fewer dimensions, and PCA aims to find these.

To see how this might be done, consider Figure 7.5, which shows a scatterplot of intakes of butter and cheese in different European countries in 2008. Clearly, these intakes are highly correlated. A line is shown fitted to the scatterplot. If we record where an observation is along this line, we will have captured most of the variability in two variables (butter and cheese intakes) in a single

variable (position along the line). This is the first principal component. Formally, it is the linear combination of the variables that maximises the variability. It does not, of course, capture *all* of the variability. There is some variation perpendicular to the first component line. This perpendicular displacement is the second principal component. Formally, it is the linear combination perpendicular (and hence statistically uncorrelated) to the first that maximises variability. And with two original variables, this is as far as we can go. Calculating these first two components can be seen as rotating the axes of the plot so that as much as possible of the variation is along the first axis. The maximum number of components is the number of original variables (or the number of observations minus one, if that is fewer). If we use all of these, we have not achieved a dimensionality reduction. The hope is that the first few will contain all the variation of interest and the rest can be ignored. Reducing two variables to one, as we have done here, does not achieve much. However, reducing 30 variables to 4, for example, would make discussing the patterns of variation much more tractable.

One point to note is that the line in Figure 7.5 is *not* the regression line. The first principal component is symmetrical with respect to the two variables, whereas linear regression is not: it treats one variable as explanatory and the other as the response. The resulting fitted lines are different.

Standardising the variables as part of PCA is a common choice. This means scaling them all to have the same variance (standard deviation), so that those that are numerically more variable do not contribute more to the calculation of components. It is the usual choice when the variables being examined have different units. We do not, for example, want it to matter whether height is recorded in metres or centimetres. If the variables do in fact all have the same units, then not standardising should be considered, if those variables with greater variability are more important because of this. Standardising or not is often expressed as basing the PCA on the correlation or covariance matrix respectively; which the default is varies in different statistical software packages.

PCA is often used with food intake data to look for patterns in the amounts of different foods reported as consumed by different individuals. The example in Table 7.7 was done with food item data from the UK NDNS data set, arranged into 23 food types. The first four components were extracted from a scaled version of the data, and the resulting components were defined from the linear combination weightings (termed loadings).

These loadings indicate how each food item contributes to the calculation of the component value (termed the score). The task here is to interpret these loadings. For example, we see that the first one has the highest

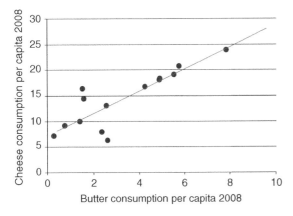

Figure 7.5 Butter and cheese consumption in EU countries. Source: Eurostat.

Table 7.7 Principal component loadings for different foods.

	PC1	PC2	PC3	PC4
Bacon	−0.063	0.291	−0.088	0.015
Beef	−0.089	0.081	0.375	−0.138
Beer	−0.220	0.338	0.099	−0.163
Biscuits	0.085	0.115	0.249	0.567
Butter	−0.049	0.015	−0.021	−0.236
Cheese	0.053	0.195	0.232	0.283
Chocolate	−0.040	0.247	0.030	0.377
Chicken	0.040	0.295	−0.514	0.102
Eggs	0.054	0.178	−0.563	0.107
Fruit	0.436	0.132	0.023	−0.008
FruitJuice	0.095	0.210	0.136	−0.179
Bf Cereals	0.213	−0.173	0.153	−0.030
Low Fat Spread	0.046	−0.087	0.126	0.178
Fish	0.306	0.149	0.041	−0.202
Salad	0.368	0.201	0.070	−0.024
Milk	0.202	0.051	−0.042	0.069
Low Cal Drinks	−0.110	0.206	0.050	0.249
Soft Drinks	−0.246	0.347	0.089	−0.055
Spirits	−0.153	0.358	0.095	−0.171
Tea Coffee	0.370	−0.021	−0.084	0.094
Vegetables	0.266	−0.030	−0.063	−0.169
Wine	0.129	0.294	0.038	−0.300
Yogurt	0.292	0.146	0.210	−0.019

positive weight for fruit and salad, and is also high for vegetables, fish, tea and coffee, while it is negative for soft drinks and beer. We might then interpret this as assessing an aspect of how healthy a diet is. An individual will get a high score (calculated value of the component) if they eat more than average of those items with positive weights and less than average of those with negative weights. Other components are interpreted in the same way. We could then proceed to investigate how component scores are linked to individual characteristics such as age, gender, income level and so on.

Factor analysis

Factor analysis is closely related to PCA. It has its origins in, and is mainly used with, sociological and psychological research. In these and related branches of science, many of the quantities of interest (personality attributes, for example) cannot be observed directly, but must be studied by recording measurable data (questionnaire answers, for example) that are influenced by these quantities. Factor analysis can then be seen as a way to access and estimate these unmeasurable quantities.

Other multivariate methods

There are many other methods that can be used for exploring multivariate data, depending on the structure of the data and the questions of interest. *Canonical covariate* analysis forms components like PCA, but with the intention of maximising separation between groups, such as different treatment groups. Related to this is *discriminant analysis*, where the interest is in using the measurements to assign or classify future observations of an unknown group to whichever group is most likely, and to assess how well this will work. It is used when searching for biomarkers of disease status or dietary intake. *Partial least squares* looks at relating one set of variables, or possibly a single variable, to another set of variables. For example, we might want to relate an outcome such as vitamin status to a large set of gene or protein expression values. *Cluster analysis*, of which there are many variations, attempts to arrange the observations into a number of groups or clusters. It could be used with dietary intake data if it is thought that the individuals sampled are of distinct but unknown types. Last, *multidimensional scaling* takes information on the similarities or differences between a number of items – subjectively scored similarities between different foods, for example – and attempts to represent this in terms of a set of components where more similar items have more similar component scores.

7.8 Bayesian statistics

This chapter has presented statistics from the 'classical' viewpoint, the one most often used in nutritional research. There is another, termed 'Bayesian statistics', because of its foundation on Bayes' theorem (Bayes and Price 1763). Its use in many areas of science has increased in recent years, partly due to the greater availability of the computing power that makes its implementation easier.

The traditional view in statistical data analysis is that the truths of nature are fixed, whereas the data we collect is variable. Conclusions are based on studying the likelihood of observing the data as a function of different possibilities for the truth. The Bayesian viewpoint largely turns this around. Once collected, the data are fixed, and it is the truth of nature that is uncertain. The best way to discuss this uncertainty is to express it using probability. So we base our conclusions on probabilities regarding the unknown truth, given the data. This differs from the classical approach, which calculates probabilities regarding the data, given the truth.

The Bayesian viewpoint can thus be seen as closer to what we really want to know. For example, we want to know how likely it is that an effect is of a certain magnitude given the data, not how likely the data are given statements about the effect. Conclusions based on this Bayesian viewpoint therefore enjoy greater properties of mathematical and logical consistency. It is natural, then, to ask why Bayesian statistics has not replaced the traditional approach. One reason is the natural inertia that scientists – like everyone else – have about the way they do things. Another is that the computational requirements are greater and software and algorithms to implement Bayesian statistics are more demanding to use. Yet another is that the Bayesian method requires us to specify some prior statement quantifying our uncertainty regarding the quantities of interest before we study the data. This can seem subjective and appears to allow the conclusions to be influenced by our prior beliefs rather than the data alone. Nevertheless, it is usually possible to make this prior specification quite vague and uninformative, and in any case the sensitivity of our conclusions to it can be examined. Those who promote Bayesian methodology believe that its advantages outweigh these disadvantages.

Readers wishing to know more can find examples in the wider medical and health-related literature. A good introduction is Spiegelhalter, Abrams and Miles (2004). It may be that the Bayesian approach to presenting evidence will become more widely used in nutritional research, as has occurred in other areas of biological science.

Acknowledgements

I would like to acknowledge the support of the Scottish Government's Rural and Environment Science and Analytical Services Division (RESAS).

References and further reading

Bayes, T. and Price, R. (1763) An essay towards solving a problem in the doctrine of chance. By the late Rev. Mr. Bayes, communicated by Mr. Price, in a letter to John Canton, M.A. and F.R.S. *Philosophical Transactions of the Royal Society of London*, **53**, 370–418.

Bland, J.M. (2000) *An Introduction to Medical Statistics*. Oxford Medical Publications, Oxford.

Campbell, R.C. (1989) *Statistics for Biologists*. Cambridge University Press, Cambridge.

Chatterjee, S. and Hadi, A.S. (2012) *Regression Analysis by Example*. John Wiley & Sons, Inc., New York.

Clayton, D. and Hills, M. (1993) *Statistical Models in Epidemiology*, Oxford University Press, Oxford.

Collett, D. (2003) *Modelling Survival Data in Medical Research*, 2nd edn. Chapman & Hall, London.

Ferreira de Moraes, A.C., Adami, F. and Falcão, M.C. (2012) Understanding the correlates of adolescents' dietary intake patterns: A multivariate analysis. *Appetite*, **58** (3), 1057–1062.

Fuller, W.A. (1987) *Measurement Error Models*. John Wiley & Sons, Inc., New York.

McCullough, P. and Nelder, J.A. (1989) *Generalized Linear Models*, 2nd edn. Chapman & Hall, London.

Nester, M.R. (1996) An applied statistician's creed. *Journal of the Royal Statistical Society. Series C (Applied Statistics)*, **45** (4), 401–410.

Neter, J., Kutner, M.H., Nachtsheim, C.J. and Wasserman, W. (1996) *Applied Linear Statistical Models*. McGraw-Hill, New York.

Panagiotakos, D.B., Pitsavos, C., Skoumas, Y. and Stefanadis, C. (2007) The association between food patterns and the metabolic syndrome using principal components analysis: The ATTICA study. *Journal of the American Dietetic Association*, **107** (6), 979–987.

R Core Team (2012) *R: A Language and Environment for Statistical Computing*. R Foundation for Statistical Computing, Vienna. http://www.R-project.org/ (accessed June 2014).

Rencher, A.C. and Pun, F.C. (1980) Inflation of R^2 in best subset regression. *Technometrics*, **22**, 49–54.

Spiegelhalter, D.J., Abrams, K.R. and Myles, J.P. (2004) *Bayesian Approaches to Clinical Trials and Health-Care Evaluation*. John Wiley & Sons, Inc., New York.

Tighe, P., Duthie, G.G., Vaughan, N.J. *et al.* (2010) Effect of increased consumption of whole-grain foods on blood pressure and other cardiovascular risk markers in healthy middle-aged persons: A randomized controlled trial. *American Journal of Clinical Nutrition*, **92** (4), 733–740.

8
Considerations for Including Different Population Groups in Nutrition Research

Maria J Maynard

Leeds Beckett University

Key messages

- There is no internationally agreed definition, terminology or method of assessing ethnicity. When including different ethnic groups in research studies, definitions should be explicit.
- Further development of portion size and food composition data for minority ethnic groups in the UK and elsewhere is required.
- Cultural influences such as maintenance of traditions, religious dietary laws and acculturation are of major importance in the food habits of ethnic minorities. Such influences should be considered in the context of structural social processes such as socio-economic status, income and education.
- Research in developing countries requires consideration of a number of logistical, cultural, ethical and methodological challenges ranging from travel to remote areas, to adaptation and translation of study materials and gaining trust.
- Migration studies (studies in both home and destination countries of migrants) can tell us a great deal about the role of context and the relative importance of genetic, social and environmental factors that influence the patterning of health and diet among migrant groups.
- Assessing dietary patterns among children and the elderly poses many of the same challenges, with cognitive difficulties influencing

the ability to report intakes. Overall, it appears that valid studies capturing habitual diet are not precluded among older people. A number of computer-based methods have been developed for use with children and adolescents. In addition to their acceptability, their validity requires further exploration, particularly among diverse groups.
- Validation studies indicate that understanding the potential for systematic under-reporting of energy intake is necessary among different ethnic groups, in low- as well as high-income countries, and at all stages of the life course. Limited evidence suggests that factors associated with systematic bias in Caucasian European populations, for example overweight and obesity, appear also to be important in these diverse groups.
- There is debate around the sensitivity and specificity of measures of body size and body composition among different ethnic groups and at different stages of the life course. Suggestions have been made for alternative, associated cut-points/predictor equations for body fat estimation from anthropometric and other indices (e.g. BMI, bio-impedance) to accommodate these differences, but none has been universally adopted.

8.1 Introduction

In developing initiatives to improve health and address health inequity, additional consideration may have to be given to ensuring that diverse populations are included. For some population groups, particularly ethnic minorities, there has been limited research on what is acceptable in terms of diet and nutrition assessment tools and intervention materials. This chapter explores the factors that need to be taken into account when including different ethnic groups, conducting studies in developing countries and working across regions or countries in migration studies. In addition, it describes considerations when including individuals at different stages of the life course – during pregnancy, in childhood and at older ages. Indicators of the quality of reporting in dietary assessment methods are crucial across all population groups, and there is a particular issue with dietary energy misreporting across some groups. Issues around body size and body composition measures across groups are also addressed in this chapter.

Nutrition Research Methodologies, First Edition. Edited by Julie A Lovegrove, Leanne Hodson, Sangita Sharma and Susan A Lanham-New.
© 2015 John Wiley & Sons, Ltd. Published 2015 by John Wiley & Sons, Ltd.
Companion Website: www.wiley.com/go/nutritionsociety

8.2 Ethnicity in research methods

Defining ethnicity

The term ethnicity comes from the Greek word 'ethnos', which means 'nation' or 'people', and refers to a shared identity through common cultural traditions (typically language, religion and diet), nationality, geography, ancestry and history. 'Ethnic minority' refers to a numerical minority, but also to those in a position of disadvantaged power relations (Platt 2011). Ethnicity is therefore a fluid, social construct that may vary according to context. For example, migrants' and indigenous minorities' offspring may be deemed to be of their parents' ethnic group(s), but may themselves also perceive their identity as relating to the majority community while remaining distinctive, for example 'British Asian' or 'Asian American'. Ethnicity is often used interchangeably with the term race, which has its origins in the concept of biological categorisation of groups. Due to difficulties with the use of race, the term race/ethnicity is also frequently seen. Researchers therefore need to be clear on the specific definition and the intended meaning in the use of these terms in their work.

Measuring ethnicity

Ethnic groupings are imprecise and fluid, so any definitions used must be made explicit at the outset of a research project and will vary according to the requirements of the research. There is no universal consensus on assigning ethnic groups. In the UK, consistent groups are commonly created by permitting people to assert their own identity, in addition to using parental and grandparental place of birth. The contrasts in approaches to measuring ethnicity between the UK and the USA are shown in Table 8.1.

Ethnicity classifications provide a way of highlighting important differences and inequalities between groups. Some ethnic groups are at a higher risk than the majority population of nutrition-related chronic diseases such as obesity, cancer, type 2 diabetes and cardiovascular conditions. These ethnic differences are a key feature of health inequalities in developed countries and have been well documented among migrant and indigenous minority groups in the UK, USA and Australia (Nazroo 2010). Many populations are dynamically enriched by a range of ethnic groups and such minority groups should be key targets when tackling inequalities in health.

Table 8.1 UK and US ethnicity/race census questions and response categories.

UK census 2011 ethnicity question and response categories	US census ethnicity/race question and response categories
What is your ethnic group or background?	**1. Are you of Hispanic, Latino, or Spanish origin?**
Choose one option that best describes your ethnic group or background	No not of Hispanic, Latino, or Spanish origin
White	Yes, Mexican, Mexican Am., Chicano
English/Welsh/Scottish/Northern Irish/British	Yes, Puerto Rican
Irish	Yes, Cuban
Gypsy or Irish Traveller	Yes, another Hispanic, Latino, or Spanish origin – *print origin, for*
Any other White background, please describe	*example Argentinean, Colombian, Dominican, Nicaraguan,*
Mixed/Multiple ethnic groups	*Salvadoran, Spaniard, and so on*
White and Black Caribbean	
White and Black African	**2. What is your race? Mark one or more boxes**
White and Asian	White
Any other Mixed/Multiple ethnic background, please describe	Black, African Am., or Negro
Asian/Asian British	American Indian or Alaska Native – *print name or enrolled*
Indian	*or principal tribe*
Pakistani	Asian Indian
Bangladeshi	Chinese
Chinese	Filipino
Any other Asian background, please describe	Japanese
Black/African/Caribbean/Black British	Korean
African	Vietnamese
Caribbean	Other Asian – *Print race for example Hmong, Laotian,*
Any other Black/African/Caribbean background,	*Thai, Pakistani, Cambodian, and so on*
please describe	Native Hawaiian
Other ethnic group	Guamanian or Chamorro
Arab	Samoan
Any other ethnic group, please describe	Other Pacific Islander – *print race, for example, Fijian, Tongan,*
	and so on

The main problems associated with using ethnicity as a research variable include errors of measurement and the degree of heterogeneity of groups. Senior and Bhopal (1994) suggest a number of ways in which the value of ethnicity as a research variable can be improved. Recommendations include recognising the limitations of classification methods; giving at least equal weight to consideration of socio-economic differences as to ethnic differences; not generalising the results of research on ethnicity and health over time, generations or populations with different histories of migration; and following descriptive research with detailed examination of environmental, lifestyle, cultural and genetic influences.

Measuring socio-economic status among minority groups presents its own challenges. Occupational socio-economic status alone may not be an adequate measure among minority ethnic groups, as some groups are more likely to be in manual occupations than the general population; in some cases this is despite being well educated and having previous professional jobs in their home countries (this is known as downward mobility). Multicomponent proxy measures may be more appropriate: in addition to occupation and education measures, these can include access to standard-of-living items. To ensure consistency, multicomponent and traditional measures can be compared in the same study and with national data on, for example, socio-economic status.

Conducting ethnicity and health research

Agreeing core principles for the conduct of ethnicity and health research has been a challenge to date, with a number of disciplines represented in this field. A Delphi exercise was undertaken among a range of academics and practitioners to explore the possibility of deriving common principles for ethnicity and health research (Mir *et al.* 2013). A Delphi exercise involves the creative exploration of ideas in a structured process of collecting information from an expert panel, usually with a series of questionnaires and opinion feedback, with the aim of attempting to reach consensus (Adler and Ziglio 1996). The ten key principles devised by this group for framing, undertaking and using ethnicity and health research (known as the Leeds Consensus Principles) are shown in Table 8.2. The group acknowledged that study design and data-collection decisions are likely to be shaped by disciplinary norms and practical constraints. However, there was widespread consensus on the need to avoid the replication of patterns of social exclusion, stereotyping and stigmatisation, and that research efforts should contribute to better healthcare experiences and better health outcomes.

Study design

Nutrition-related research among minority ethnic groups can include the whole range of study designs: quantitative (cohort, intervention and so on) and qualitative

Table 8.2 The Leeds Consensus Principles for research on ethnicity and health. Mir, G., Salway, S., Kai, J. *et al.* (2013) Principles for research on ethnicity and health: The Leeds Consensus Statement. *European Journal of Public Health*, **23** (3), 504–510.

Importance and purpose

1. Ethnicity is often associated with disadvantage and ill-health. Researchers consequently have both a professional and ethical responsibility to incorporate evidence on ethnicity into their work and recommendations.
2. The purpose of research on ethnicity and health should be for the well-being and betterment of populations being studied and equity should be the guiding ethical principle. Researchers must be alert to the dangers of discriminatory thinking and behaviour and guard against actual and potential harm resulting from their research.

Framing and focus

3. It is important to be explicit about the assumptions and theories that underlie research on ethnicity and health.
4. There is a need for research to, where appropriate, examine diversity within ethnic groups and avoid homogenization. For example, age, gender, religion, education, socio-economic position, geography or time of migration may all impact on the generation of ethnic health inequalities. Investigation of ethnic health inequalities should pay due regard to the ways in which ethnicity intersects with other forms of difference in order to understand how and why it may be relevant.
5. There is a need to improve the participation of minority ethnic communities in all stages of the research process. Appropriate participation should be defined by these communities, then promoted by researchers and statutory agencies and resourced by funding bodies.

Data collection and analysis

6. The use of ethnic categories and labels should be meaningful in relation to the particular experiences and outcomes being explored.
7. Census categories are often useful for exposing disadvantage, but additional measures may be needed to explore the processes through which disadvantage is created.
8. Analysis of health inequalities should pay attention to the social context in which ethnic differences in health outcomes are measured and health behaviours occur.

Future priorities

9. There is a need to focus on intervention studies that help identify effective ways of reducing inequalities.
10. More research is needed on appropriate models for involving minority ethnic communities throughout the research process. For example, models for community capacity building, empowerment, representativeness and continuity of engagement.

(interviews, focus groups). However, a number of design issues need to be considered and addressed. Commonly there are limited sampling frames for minority ethnic groups and therefore convenience, pragmatic and quota sampling is common (Chaturvedi and McKeigue 1994). Alternative methods for identifying target groups include name-recognition software for surname analysis, which is useful for those groups (mainly South Asian) whose names are most distinctive. Surname analysis cannot disaggregate populations according to place of origin, however, and as exogamy (marriage outside one's own group) increases, additional methods will need to be developed. Frequently used sampling frames include general practitioner lists in the UK, which now feature ethnic monitoring, electoral registers (to determine areas of high ethnic density) and samples of occupational groups, as well as mailshots with registered mail envelopes, followed by door-knocking or screening to confirm the ethnicity of household members. The latter screening method was used to good effect to boost ethnic minority samples in the Health Survey for England 2004 (http://www.hscic.gov.uk/pubs/hse04ethnic), which included diet and nutrition related health indicators.

Additional activities are often needed to gain support for studies, particularly in terms of community acceptance and trust. Community participation or community assets approaches refer to improving the understanding of community needs and assets among partners, service providers, local policymakers, other influential community members and the broader community. These approaches are particularly useful for engaging hard-to-reach groups in order to establish trusting relationships between researchers and communities. As the ethos of the community assets approach is one of mutual benefit, improving community health and enhancing community involvement should also be goals in addition to achieving the academic research objectives. The overarching aim in this approach is therefore equitable community participation with the highest level of community involvement that is feasible or practical. Non-traditional venues for targeted community research and interventions to engage minorities, such as places of worship and barber shops, have been used extensively in the USA, but require further exploration in the UK and elsewhere (Maynard et al. 2009). Frameworks for engaging communities (including minority communities) such as Ownership, Control, Access and Possession (OCAP) in Canada, Community Based Participatory Research (CBPR) in the USA and the UK's People-Centred Public Health principles could usefully be applied to the nutrition research context (Schnarch 2004; Minkler and Wallerstein 2010; South et al. 2013).

8.3 Ethnic minority diets

Cultural influences

Culture – the behaviours, traditions, beliefs and values of a particular group – has a major influence on the diet choices, food preparation, food preferences and eating habits of different ethnic groups. Traditional foods can play an important part in the diet as they contribute to the maintenance of cultural customs, social networks in destination countries and links with home countries. Among many ethnic groups it is also traditional for families to eat together.

Religion is a key cultural influence on food-related habits for a number of ethnic groups. Religious dietary laws proscribe the consumption of non-*halal* foods (known as *haram*) among Muslims (mainly Pakistanis and Bangladeshis, but also other South Asian and African groups). Other related practices include washing the hands and the mouth before and after meals and before prayers, and using the right hand for eating, the left for washing the body. Among Hindus (mostly Indians), the cow is sacred so beef is not consumed. Strict Hindus are vegetarian due to their belief in reincarnation; some avoid additional foods such as onions, garlic, eggs and coconut, often on specific days. The religious laws of Sikhism, originating from the Punjab region of India, advocate refraining from alcohol and ritually slaughtered meat. Vegetarian meals (*langar*) served free of charge at Sikh *gurdwaras* (temples) can be an important component of the diet of this group. Seventh-Day Adventism is one of the largest Christian denominations among Africans, Caribbeans and African Americans. Many Adventists are ovo-lacto vegetarians and non-vegetarians avoid pork and fish without fins or scales. Some avoid tea, coffee and other caffeinated drinks and most avoid alcohol.

Acculturation describes the multidimensional and dynamic process by which a minority adopts the behavioural patterns of the majority group (Satia 2010). A number of studies have shown the consequences of dietary acculturation to be detrimental. Examples include the increased intake of saturated fat and energy-dense convenience foods among Black Caribbeans in the UK, potentially increasing disease risk (Sharma et al. 1999), and similarly the increase in 'Western' eating habits and decrease in traditional food practices among the Inuit of the Canadian Arctic, consistent with a rise in diet-related disease (Hopping et al. 2010). Nevertheless, it is important to bear in mind that the influences are not all negative or one-way: mutual exchange of food habits means that while minorities are influenced by the food culture of the majority, they contribute to the availability of an ever-increasing range of new food items in shops and restaurants. There are varying degrees of acculturation between ethnic groups, and within-group variation such as in different generations should be considered, with minority children more likely to engage in majority food cultures than their parents (Khokhar *et al.* 2013).

While considering 'culture' as an explanation of differences in health outcomes or behaviours between groups, structural social processes such as socio-economic status, income and education should also be borne in mind.

Dietary intake assessment

The above cultural and other influences have a number of practical implications for assessing dietary intake among minority groups (Vyas *et al.* 2003; Ngo *et al.* 2009; Sharma 2011). Concomitantly, weaknesses in food and nutrient assessment in ethnic groups most commonly include limitations in recipe information, portion sizes and food composition data. Improvements in these areas are needed in order to carry out accurate dietary assessments and the requirement for standardised dietary assessment tools needs to be balanced with specific cultural tailoring. The acceptability and appropriateness of techniques and instruments as well as their validity are under-researched in nutrition-related studies among some minority groups. Translating study materials (see Section 8.4) may be a necessary part of the cultural tailoring of methods for those who do not speak the language of the host country. It may also be important as a mark of respect for some groups, particularly among elders. Clear descriptions of methodologies and their adaptation are required in research dissemination materials (papers, reports and so on) to enable replication and wider implementation.

Lists of the most commonly reported foods, portion sizes and food preparation methods need to be field tested for the development of retrospective methods such as food frequency questionnaires (FFQs). Confirming recipes and cooking practices with the target populations is essential, as public sources (cookery books, the internet) may differ significantly from day-to-day practices at home. A number of foods will have the same name across cultures, but have different compositions and nutrient intakes, indicating the importance of using the correct terminology for both foods and portion size. Account needs to be taken of the increasing availability of culturally specific convenience and fast foods; additional prompts may be needed in assessment methods for these and for high-energy snack foods such as patties, fried dumplings and pakoras, as well as sugary drinks.

It should not be assumed that data on 'average' food portion size for the majority population are applicable to minority populations, either for commonly consumed or ethnic-specific foods. There is no consistent evidence on the most appropriate method of portion size assessment among ethnic minority groups. However, use of visual aids such as food photographs or food models is considered important to avoid assumptions based on majority population data. For prospective methods employing estimated portions, differences between groups in common household measures will need to be documented.

Food composition databases designed for the majority population usually lack foods and dishes commonly consumed by minority ethnic groups. Cross-country collaborative efforts such as the European Food Information Resource Network (EuroFIR) have increased the scope, reliability and validity of minority ethnic food composition data in national databases in France, Israel, Spain, Denmark, Italy, the Netherlands, Belgium and the UK. The UK arm of EuroFIR, focusing on South Asian diets, has demonstrated that key sources of nutrients (based on chemical analysis of foods), portion sizes and eating practices differ significantly among children and adults in South Asian ethnic groups compared to Caucasian British (Khokhar *et al.* 2013). Among Black Caribbeans in the UK, varying portion sizes have been identified compared to the Caucasian population for local 'British' foods such as potatoes, and average portion size data have been established for local and ethnic-specific foods and composite dishes (Sharma *et al.* 2002). Ethnic differences in trends in the portion size of energy-dense foods have been identified in the USA, with the greatest increases among African American and Hispanic groups. There is, however, much scope for further development of portion size and food composition data for a number of ethnic groups. The diets of the growing UK Black African populations represent a distinct gap in the literature in Britain. The largest of these groups are from Nigeria and Ghana, with long-established communities in the UK, other European countries, the USA and Canada, but relevant dietary data are sparse. Research has been conducted updating UK food tables with the nutritional composition of commonly consumed Ghanaian dishes in London and Accra, Ghana, including folate content determined by microbiological assay (Owusu *et al.* 2010). The sodium content of Nigerian, Ghanaian and Caribbean takeaway meals has also been analysed. Studies of East Asian minorities have largely been carried out in the USA, with few studies in Europe, and there are a limited number of large-scale studies among migrant Eastern Europeans. Extensive development of food composition databases has been carried out for minority groups in Bangladesh, American Indian and Alaskan Native populations in the USA, for diverse ethnic groups in Hawaii and for indigenous people in Canada (see for example Kolonel *et al.* 2000; Hopping *et al.* 2010; Illner *et al.* 2012).

8.4 Research in developing (low- and middle-income) countries

Countries are categorised by the World Bank according to gross national income (GNI) into low-, middle- and high-income countries, and this is useful in research terms for classifying nations. In some instances the terms low- and middle-income countries (LMICs) have tended to replace the term developing countries, and are employed in this chapter, but they are often also used interchangeably.

In the past there has been a logical emphasis on malnutrition (under-nutrition) and micronutrient deficiency in nutritional research in low-income countries. However, the 'nutrition transition' in a number of poorer countries has changed the landscape of nutrition-related research. The term denotes a shift towards energy-dense foods and low energy expenditure, contributed to by the globalisation of food production and distribution and internal migration from rural to urban centres (Satia 2010). Such changes in dietary patterns and food availability have been deemed causal factors in the rise of nutrition-related disease, particularly obesity, in LMICs (Popkin, Adair and Ng 2012).

Nutrition-related research conducted in low-income countries requires a number of logistical, cultural, ethical and methodological issues to be taken into consideration. Logistical issues include time required for travel to remote rural areas and problems related to low income (water, food and fuel scarcity). Research in hard-to-reach areas can be worth pursuing if such logistics can be overcome. Residents may be highly willing to participate if the motivations and purpose of the research are clear, and in communities where needs have been previously neglected projects can make a significant contribution to health inequalities (Cameron and van Staveren 1988). Ethical concerns can range from gaining trust, ensuring informed consent (especially where there is cross-cultural working between an external research team and the study population) and managing expectations of the benefits of the study. Written materials or methods requiring written records may have to be avoided in areas of limited literacy and where there may be difficulties in accommodating a variety of dialects.

Awareness of local customs is required, including religious and tribal customs, particularly those related to food practices and food taboos; food composition databases may need to be further developed. Employing local professionals, such as interpreters and other members of the community, is often invaluable in obtaining rigour in the research process, and where possible should

be combined with activities that may make a lasting contribution to the health and empowerment of communities. Researchers do need to be aware, however, that there may also be potential drawbacks to research being conducted by those with an 'insider identity', including respondent concerns about confidentiality. The focus of this section is on low-income countries; however, similar issues may be faced in research among peoples in remote areas of high-income countries, such as Inuit and Aboriginal populations in Canada and Australia. The time and costs involved in travelling long distances, challenges to participant recruitment such as geographical isolation and identifiable populations leading to confidentiality issues are all potential difficulties in the research process.

Translation of study materials/data

The aim of rigorous translation is to achieve 'content equivalence' – that is, for the content and meaning to be the same in both languages. However, a number of translation methods exist and there is no accepted 'gold standard'. Long-standing methods include back-translation, the bilingual technique, the committee approach and the pre-test procedure (Cha, Kim and Erlen 2007). Back-translation is a resource-intensive iterative process involving blind translation by one translator, then retranslation from the target to the original language by a second translator. The original and the retranslated version are then compared and if an error is found, a further translator retranslates, continuing until no errors are found. The bilingual technique involves administering both the original and the translated tool to bilingual members of the target population and comparing their responses. The key limitation of this method is that the bilingual participants may differ from the monolingual participants in socio-economic status, degree of acculturation and so on. The committee process involves a group of bilingual experts (usually three or more) who translate from the original to the target language, the benefit being that a committee member's mistake may easily be picked up by other members. However, it requires the availability of a number of bilingual individuals, with similar limitations to the bilingual method in terms of the lack of representativeness of the target group. Focus group and 'think aloud' techniques extending the committee method have also been tested (Daniel, Miller and Wilbur 2011). The pre-test procedure involves a pilot study of participants from the target population in which potential issues and problems are identified, such as by probing participants on their view of the meaning of individual items.

8.5 Multi-centre migration studies

Nutrition-related diseases, including cardiovascular disease and some cancers, vary across and within countries. Among migrant populations the patterns of health and disease are transferred to the new host country, potentially explained, at least in part, by the shared genetic background. The 'healthy migrant effect', a form of selection bias whereby the healthiest individuals are able to migrate, is posited as the reason why migrants initially have better health profiles compared to those of host populations. Increasing length of residence, however, is generally associated with the health patterns of migrants moving towards that of the host population. For health outcomes such as type 2 diabetes, prevalence rates begin to exceed those of the host population and, for some groups, of people in their country of origin (Tillin *et al.* 2013). This phenomenon indicates the significance of environmental factors, rather than, or at least interacting with, genetic factors. Putative factors include dietary patterns and dietary acculturation (see Section 8.3), potentially interacting with determinants of fetal origin. Comparison studies of health and its influences among migrant groups in both home and destination countries allow for the exploration of the relative importance of genetic, social and environmental factors and the interaction between these entities.

Findings from a multicentre study of hypertension and diabetes in four populations (rural and urban Cameroon, Jamaica and the UK) of adults of African origin demonstrate the complexity of context, and the intersectionality between social, environmental and cultural factors, in relation to diet and adiposity across sites. A gradient in overweight and obesity was seen among women, with the lowest prevalence of excess weight among rural Africans in Cameroon and the highest rates among African Caribbeans in the UK. The gradient was less prominent among men, with Jamaican men having lower rates of overweight and obesity than those in urban Cameroon. Energy intake and percentage energy from fat were greatest in rural Cameroon, despite the lowest rates of overweight, probably due to greater energy expenditure. Overweight was positively associated with education levels in Cameroon and in Jamaica, which is common in countries undergoing the nutrition transition. Lower rates of obesity with increased education, as seen in the general UK population, were not evident among the UK Black Caribbeans in this study, indicating that the social mechanisms influencing overweight and obesity in high-income countries may not operate in the same way across all ethnic groups (Jackson *et al.* 2007). An inverse association between energy intake and obesity in the UK sample may be influenced by energy under-reporting (see Section 8.7).

Differences in methodology, population groups and age categories can make it difficult to compare data across regions and countries. Therefore there is a requirement for standardised methods that are cost-effective and have the lowest possible respondent burden. Methods and analysis databases need to be able to capture geographical and cultural dietary diversities.

8.6 Stages of the life course

Conducting nutrition research among the young and the old is key in identifying where in the life course the aetiology of diet-related disorders occurs, and the appropriate points for effective intervention. The challenges of dietary assessment, which may include reliance on memory, the concept of time, literacy, mathematical ability, knowledge of food groups, food identification and portion estimation, are even more of an issue when conducting research with young people and older members of the population. While the core methods for the measurement of diet in these age groups have been in place for some decades (see Chapter 4), a number of methods based on new technology have emerged in recent years. Key developments to aid research among children and in old age are described in this section.

Due to the particular physiological changes during pregnancy and the additional ethical and safety concerns regarding the unborn fetus, pregnant women are sometimes excluded from research studies. However, nutritional research focused on pregnancy offers the opportunity to influence the health of both mother and child. Renewed interest in nutrition during pregnancy has been generated by the hypothesis that adult disease has its origins in early life and thus by the opportunity for long-term influence of the health of a number of generations. As with all studies, a clear health-and-safety protocol needs to be in place in research with pregnant women regarding research tools, substances, venues, travel and so on to ensure that there is no harm to the woman or her unborn child. No specific regulations are directed to research involving lactating women. It is notable that breast milk itself can provide nutrient indices that may reflect nutrient status and in some cases intakes. Some dietary components such as vitamin A can be a more sensitive indicator of intake in breast milk than plasma levels.

Childhood and adolescence

Valid and reliable methods for assessing diet in childhood are essential for revealing the impact of diet on health, addressing issues such as childhood obesity, and to identify dietary change as the result of interventions. A number of the methods used with adults (24-hour recalls, estimated diaries, diet histories and so on) have been used with children, therefore working with children does not necessarily mean different methods. However, some methods may be more appropriate than others in particular contexts and in different age groups. It is generally considered that children under 7 years cannot report on their dietary intake with sufficient accuracy. For this age group it is common to use surrogate reports. Research suggests that combining child and parent reports may give better information than either alone. Also useful with children are observation methods, which have most commonly been used to validate diary intakes, but are resource intensive and therefore not suitable as a sole method for assessing intake in large-scale studies. The demographic and other socioeconomic data required to interpret the findings will need to be obtained from parents, carers and school records. For young people under the age of 16–18 years, it is necessary to obtain consent from parents. In addition, at the time of data collection it is usual to obtain written assent from each child.

In terms of research settings, schools provide a 'captive' audience for research projects and are a key location, particularly for nutrition-related interventions. Enhancement of the school curriculum by the appropriate integration of research projects into core topics, for example science lessons and those that deal specifically with health such as personal, social and health education (PSHE), increase the acceptability of the research and provide additional benefit and motivation for schools to take part. As much school-based research will be planned as group or whole-class activities, care must be taken that children do not feel under an obligation to take part, for example by being aware of body language indicating a passive opt-out even if there has been no verbal refusal.

Dietary assessment among children

Portion size assessment

Estimated portion size rather than a weighed portion is preferable in nutrition research with children to reduce the burden on the subject. Visual estimation of portion size requires a high level of cognitive skills and among children, as with adults, can therefore result in error associated with under- and overestimation. Techniques used to aid portion size estimation among children include drawings, food models and digital images such as food photographs. Food photographs developed for adults have been shown to be unsuitable for use with children, however (Frobisher and Maxwell 2003; Foster *et al.* 2006). Three age-specific portion size assessment

tools – food photographs, food models and the interactive portion size assessment system (IPSAS, described in the next section) – have been compared, testing perception, conceptualisation and memory (Foster *et al.* 2008). Food photographs and IPSAS performed well among children aged 4–16 years.

Novel methods of assessing intake

The benefits of computer-based methods include standardisation, significantly reduced administrative and data-processing costs, facilitation of large-scale data collection and increased acceptability of methods among young people. Table 8.3 shows a number of recently developed computerised methods for assessing dietary intake among children. Methods have been developed in the UK, elsewhere in Europe and in the USA, based on 24-hour recalls, estimated records and a food frequency questionnaire. Two of the methods reviewed combine reporting of dietary and physical activity habits. Most are self-complete methods and as such are suitable for children aged over 10 years for the reasons outlined earlier. At younger ages reporting is completed by parents or carers (e.g. portion size assessment using IPSAS for children aged 1.5–11 years) or reporting is kept simple (e.g. the Synchronised Nutrition and Activity Program, which does not incorporate portion size assessment and has been developed for children as young as 7 years).

The acceptability of these methods among child participants appears to be high, most likely due to the general popularity of communication and gaming technology and familiarity with the computer interface, as well as the opportunity for reporting habits in private in self-complete methods. Few of the studies have tested the suitability of these methods for use among ethnic minority children, and the suitability to other social groups, such as the less well-off, needs to be explored further. In particular, in settings where computer ownership is closely related to socio-economic status, web-based studies may not be representative of all social groups. Most of the studies reported on the relative validity of the tools, but often using methods with a similar error structure to the test method. Additional validation research incorporating independent measures such as biomarkers of intake is necessary to ensure that innovative dietary assessment technologies are beneficial in terms of increased accuracy as well as appeal.

Older ages

Populations around the world are rapidly ageing and have increasing life expectancy. The global population aged 65 years and over, estimated to be 524 million in 2010, is projected to be 1.5 billion by 2050 (World Health

Table 8.3 Computerised methods of assessing intake in children.

Method (reference); country	Acronym	Target age group (years)	Key features	Validation method (sample size) and results
Researcher administered				
Interactive Portion Size Assessment System (Foster *et al.* 2014b); UK	IPSAS	1.5–16	• Portion size assessment only • Researcher administered during an interview for a food diary or 24-hour recall (with parents at age 1.5–4 years; with parents and children at age 4–16 years) • Displays digital images of foods to estimate the amount served and amount left over • Needs to be used with a parent for children aged 10 years or younger	• 4-day weighed records kept by parents and researcher, in-school/nursery observations (n = 262) • Food weights were overestimated using IPSAS by 1–3% among adults and 2–5% among children • Energy intake was overestimated by 1% among children aged 4–11 years and was otherwise underestimated by 3–5% among parents and children • Limits of agreement from Bland–Altman plots ranged from −33% to +72%. Precision was greater among parents at ages <11 years but greater for children at age 11+ years
Self-completed				
Self-Completed Analysis and Recall of Nutrition (Foster *et al.* 2014a); UK	SCRAN24	11–16	• Based on multi-pass 24-hour recall • 25–30 min completion time to recall 1 day's intake • Free-text search for foods • Food composition code and weight of selected items automatically allocated and stored. • Portion size assessment based on IPSAS (see above) • Prompts if no food recorded in a 3-hour time frame or <3 drinks throughout the day • Additional prompts and probes for commonly forgotten and associated foods • Designed to allow development for web-based delivery • Received well by children • Not recommended for use with children aged <11 years • Small-scale validation study – more extensive validation required	• Parent recorded 1-day weighed food diary (n = 38) • Low intrusion rate of foods (6%) • 26% of foods omitted, mostly drinks, confectionery and spreads • 20% underestimation of energy intake

(Continued)

Table 8.3 (Continued)

Method (reference); country	Acronym	Target age group (years)	Key features	Validation method (sample size) and results
Self-completed (web-based)				
Web-based Dietary Assessment Software for Children (Biltoft-Jensen et al. 2014); Denmark	WebDASC	8–11	• Based on 7-day record • Interactive features (animation, cartoons and computer games) maintain motivation • Category browse and free-text search to locate foods • Meal-based approach – shows pictures of foods commonly eaten at a given meal • Includes foods commonly consumed by ethnic minorities in Denmark • Portion size estimation based on a range of digital images or pictures of small packaged items • Reminder email sent to parents if a diet record is not completed	• Well accepted by children in preliminary testing but needs to be validated
Young Adolescents' Nutrition Assessment on Computer (Vereecken et al. 2005); Belgium-Flanders	YANA-C	11–14	• Based on 24-hour recall • Meal-based approach embedded in questions about usual daily activities (e.g. getting up in the morning) • Portion amount typed into a text box or modification of a standard portion size (linked to food photographs) using 'more' or 'less' buttons • Additional prompt and probes for condiments, spreads, drinks etc.	• 1-day food record (n=145) and standard 24-hour recall (n=103) • Food intrusions ranged from 0–18%, omissions from 0–28%. Kappa statistic ranged from 0.38–0.92 (mean 0.73 food record, 0.70 recall) • For energy and nutrients YANA-C overestimated intakes compared to food records, mean kappa 0.44; very little significant difference in intakes compared to recall, mean kappa 0.50
Food Intake Recording Software System, version 4 (Baranowski et al. 2014); USA	FIRSSt4	> 10	• Based on multi-pass 24-hour recall • Animated avatar to guide and maintain motivation • Digital images aid portion size estimation • Optional modules query location of meals, whether meals were eaten alone or with others, television and computer use during meals, and supplement intake • Simplified wording (e.g. 'bubbly water' instead of 'carbonated water'); phonetic spell-check • Acceptability assessed among White, Hispanic and Black American children. Hispanic children were more likely to report problems with using the tool compared to other groups • Available to researchers via US National Cancer Institute as ASA-kids 24 http://riskfactor.cancer.gov/tools/instruments/asa24/respondent/childrens.html#adapting	• Original version validated against school meal observation and 24-hour diet records (n=138) (Baranowski et al. 2002) • 24% intrusion, 30% omission compared to observation; 17% intrusion, 24% omission compared to recall

Study	Tool	Age	Description	Validation/Findings
Synchronised Nutrition and Activity Program (Moore *et al.* 2008); UK	SNAP™	7–15	• Based on diet and physical activity 24-hour recalls • Completion time 15–40 min (dependent on reading ability and internet connection speed) • Segmented-day format structured around daily activities and the school day to enhance recall • Location of eating occasion queried to aid recall • Pictures provided visual memory prompts • Intake assessed by count – no assessment of portion size • Small pilot study – more extensive validation required • Positive feedback from participants in anonymous questionnaires	• Researcher-administered multi-pass 24-hour recall (n = 121) • SNAP underestimated mean counts but mean difference between methods was < 1 count for most food except for confectionery and cakes, total energy-dense foods and total carbohydrate-rich foods • Between method agreement within +1 count ranged from 0.40–0.99
Web-Survey of Physical Activity and Nutrition (Storey and McCargar 2012); Canada	Web-SPAN	11–15	• Based on 24-hour recall • Digital images for portion size estimation • Additional cues, virtual meal plate and meal summary features to aid recall	• 3-day estimated diet records (n = 370) • Weak correlations for energy and nutrients (r = 0.24–0.40) but mean differences were small • Tended to overestimate compared to validation method • Authors state social desirability may have reduced the accuracy of reporting in the validation method
Healthy Lifestyle in Europe by Nutrition in Adolescence food frequency questionnaire (Vereecken *et al.* 2010); Belgium	HELENA FFQ	13–17	• Based on Netherlands EPIC FFQ and FFQ from local studies • 137 items/food groups on 21 screens • Response categories: units per day/week/during the last 30 days • Digital images to aid portion size estimation of amorphous foods	• 24-hour recall measured by YANA-C (see above) (n = 48) • Spearman's correlations between methods were > 51 for all dietary components except fibre (r = 0.23), % energy from fat (r = 0.30) and vitamin C (r = 0.40) • HELENA overestimated a number of food groups resulting in overestimation of energy, fibre, iron and vitamin C; % energy from fat was underestimated

Organization and US National Institute of Aging 2011). High-income countries have the oldest population profiles, but the most rapidly ageing populations and the majority of older people are found in low- and middle-income countries. Research on the influence of diet, nutrition and the food environment on health in old age, using validated methods, will therefore become increasingly important, but presents a number of challenges. Nonetheless, the elderly, generally defined as those aged 65 years and over, should be considered a heterogeneous group, including, for example, people in their 60s who are fit, healthy, active and living independently (and who may not consider themselves 'elderly') as well as centenarians who rely on full-time care. Old age on its own should therefore not be used as a criterion for individuals' ability to consent, although care must be taken to ensure that the burden on the respondents is balanced by the potential benefits to the target group of taking part. General considerations include ensuring that study information, consent forms, questionnaires and so on are in large enough print for the visually impaired. In the particular situation of the institutionalised elderly, additional time and care should be taken to ensure voluntary and informed consent and there needs to be awareness of where additional efforts may have to be made in the research process, such as in ensuring privacy. The underrepresentation of ethnic minority groups in research among older people is as marked as at other ages and so diversity should be improved in this area of nutrition research to ensure equity of research benefits.

The usual limitations to dietary and nutritional assessment, present at any age, need to be considered, but there are also particular issues associated with the ageing process. General issues that may influence eating habits and/or the ability to report intake include an increase in health problems, disabilities or impairment such as loss of hearing and sight or poor dentition, and methods need to be adapted accordingly. Of major importance in old age is the potential for age-related cognitive decline to contribute to bias in the results of diet studies. Some mental capabilities are well maintained into old age; however, from early adulthood onwards some capabilities begin to decline, such as short-term memory, executive function (the set of cognitive abilities that control and regulate other abilities and behaviours), processing speeds and reasoning. This decline could potentially have an impact on a range of studies: for example, impaired short-term memory may lead to a tendency to report previous food habits rather than current food habits. In addition, the increasing interest in the role of nutrition in cognitive decline per se means that accurate measures of diet are required so that associations between diet and cognitive decline are not biased. Studies that have examined the role of cognitive ability in choice of measure and the quality of dietary assessment measures have shown conflicting results. Studies validating an FFQ with 24-hour recalls in the elderly aged 68–99 years (Morris et al. 2003) and 4-day weighed records (McNeill, Winter and Jia 2009) showed no influence of cognitive function on validity, whereas cognitive ability was inversely associated with potential errors in reporting total energy intake in a large study of 70–79-year-olds (Pope et al. 2007).

Consumption habits among the elderly may be very different from those in other age groups. Surveys among older people have shown them to have regular eating routines (which may aid in dietary assessment), although this may vary according to other factors such as age (the just retired and the very elderly may have different habits), living alone and socio-economic status. Compared to younger adults, older people are also currently more likely to eat at home and cook meals from basic ingredients. Although this picture may represent many older people's lifestyles in high-income countries, it is important not to have a stereotypical view of the habits of the elderly. For example, Maynard and Blane (2009) report that freedom of choice associated with life transitions such as the death of a spouse can influence eating habits. For subsequent generations of people at all stages of old age there may be significant changes in cooking and eating habits, including more fast food or convenience meals and eating out more frequently, making it more difficult than for earlier generations to report intake in detail. Supplement taking increases significantly with age, which can further hamper accurate characterisation of intakes.

Choice of methods

The factors already discussed need to be taken into account in the choice of dietary assessment methods. The 24-hour recall is popular for use with the elderly, as it is with other age groups, because it does not rely on participants' literacy and ability to write if interviewer administered. It does, however, rely on short-term memory, and has therefore been speculated to be a poor choice of method for use with older people, although this has not been explored in detail. The diet history method may be particularly useful as the level of respondent burden is low. Skilled interview techniques such as patient and effective probing are particularly important due to potential issues such as poor memory or hearing impairment. Social isolation is common in old age and so the opportunity to talk that the interview provides may mean that additional time needs to be factored into study designs that incorporate interview methods. The FFQ is another potentially useful tool among the elderly since it does not rely on short-term memory and may be less challenging than the recall of specific foods, as in the 24-hour recall. Adaptations to questionnaires and associated processes have been made, such as combining frequency and amount responses, using age-specific portion size data and picture-sort techniques to represent frequency of use (whereby coloured picture cards are sorted into trays). For the institutionalised elderly, observation techniques are useful (Thompson and Subar 2008).

Data quality issues have been assessed in a cohort study of people in early old age, where those omitting answers on an FFQ were more likely to be female and aged over 70 years, but were not more likely to be overweight (Maynard and Blane 2009). Telephone follow-up of those with missing items was a successful way of reducing missing data on regularly consumed foods. As with other groups, FFQs for those in early old age need to be comprehensive enough to capture a varied diet while not deterring completion through being too onerous. Researchers have examined the particular challenge of dietary assessment in the 'oldest old' (that is, people aged 85 years or more), the largest increase in the ageing population being predicted to be among this group. Considerable overestimation associated with the FFQ compared to multi-pass 24-hour recalls has been reported in a study of over 85-year-olds in Newcastle, UK (Adamson *et al.* 2009). The 24-hour recall also had a higher acceptability rating than the FFQ. However, the recall was highly resource intensive with regard to interviewer time, training, quality assurance and data processing, a significant factor for consideration, particularly in large-scale studies.

The use of new technology has not been as well explored with older populations as with young people, although many of the challenges of dietary assessment are similar. Information and communication technology use among older people is on the rise and age should therefore not necessarily be seen as a barrier to the use of new technology in research. One UK example is the Novel Assessment of Nutrition in Ageing (NANA) project, which aims to improve self-report dietary assessment among the elderly, integrated with physical and mental health and cognitive function measures, using touch-screen technology (Astell *et al.* 2012).

Nutrition screening tools are a useful alternative to dietary assessment by self-report, especially if the research question involves identifying those at risk of malnutrition. A range of validated tools for use among adults have been identified and rated (Phillips *et al.* 2010). Of these, the Mini Nutritional Assessment–Short Form (MNA-SF), the Malnutrition Universal Screening Tool (MUST) and the Seniors in the Community: Risk Evaluation for Eating and Nutrition-II (Screen II) received a 'good' rating. MNA-SF is based on six items (BMI, weight loss, food intake decline in past three months, mobility, psychological distress or disease, neuropsychological problems); iPhone/iPad apps and self-complete versions are available. MUST is a three-item tool incorporating BMI, weight loss and acute illness or disease leading to reduced dietary intake, and is available in a number of European languages. SCREEN II includes 14 items encompassing frequency of consumption of selected foods and fluids, weight loss, factors affecting food intake such as physical problems (swallowing, chewing), food access and food preparation, but does not incorporate a measure of adiposity such as BMI.

Existing studies of nutritional assessment among the elderly include a range of research in terms of aims, study designs and participants, therefore it is difficult to draw general conclusions regarding the most appropriate methods. Overall, it appears that valid studies capturing habitual diet are not precluded among older populations; however, the main concern is the use of methods that depend on good short-term memory.

8.7 Dietary energy misreporting in different population groups

The misreporting, particularly under-reporting, of energy intake can significantly reduce the accuracy of dietary intake measures, with the resulting bias leading to lack of detection of diet–disease associations or, in the case of systematic bias, spurious associations. The studies reviewed in this section indicate that energy misreporting is also an issue across the population groups addressed in this chapter. Plausibility cut-offs based on predicted energy requirements should be incorporated into dietary studies among different ethnic groups, in low-income as well as high-income countries and across the life course, particularly at the extremes of childhood and old age, in order to quantify misreporting.

Among ethnic minority groups

The factors associated with under- and over-reporting in ethnic minority groups are not well elucidated. Possible assumptions relating to a greater acceptance of larger body size, applied to migrant groups in destination countries, are poorly supported empirically but may nevertheless have seen a cultural shift to the 'Western' norm of valuing thinness. There may therefore be the same association of under-reporting with larger body size as in the majority population, compounded by a greater prevalence of overweight and obesity among some ethnic groups. In the study described earlier comparing populations in rural and urban Cameroon, Jamaica and Black Caribbeans in the UK (Jackson *et al.* 2007), the UK group had the highest prevalence of overweight and obesity, and also by far the highest rates of under-reporting. Further research in this area is required, but this study indicates the plausibility of acculturation leading to a status view of thinness and associated effects on dietary assessment among ethnic minority groups in high-income countries (Jackson *et al.* 2007). It is also imperative to explore how these ideals are shifting in home countries in parallel with globalisation and the nutrition transition.

In LMICs

Under-reporting of dietary intake in studies conducted in developing countries has been reviewed by Scagliusi, Ferriolli and Lancha (2006). Methodological heterogeneity aside, it appears that levels of under-reporting varied within and between studies, but were lower than those in 'Western' countries; key limitations were the lack of independent comparison and of analysis by socio-economic factors. Few studies in LMICs have been conducted on under-reporting using independent biomarkers such as doubly labelled water (DLW). One such study among women in Brazil showed that, as in higher-income countries, systematic under-reporting was associated with high BMI, and also with social desirability, body dissatisfaction and low income (Scagliusi *et al.* 2009). Qualitative methods have also been used in Brazil to explore factors associated with under-reporting by women. Focus group participants reported changing food habits and negative feelings towards their true diet during recording, high respondent burden associated with the food diary method, and difficulty with portion size assessment, particularly among the overweight participants. Issues associated with dietary assessment may therefore be similar in some LMICs to those in high-income countries. Funding constraints in exploring ways of addressing dietary reporting errors in high-income countries are greatly compounded in LMICs and so this area is not likely to be addressed without a commitment to policy, funding and collaboration with colleagues in wealthier nations.

Across the life course

The prevalence of under-reporting of energy intake in pregnancy has been examined in a small number of studies in the UK and Ireland, USA and Indonesia (Winkvist, Persson and Hartini 2002; Derbyshire *et al.* 2009; Nowicki *et al.* 2011; McGowan and McAuliffe 2012). Sample size ranged from n = 72 to n = 998. Most were conducted among the majority population of the country, except the US study that included 'White', 'Black' and 'Other' ethnic groups. The range of dietary assessment

methods used included 3-day diaries, FFQs, 4–7-day weighed intake and repeat 24-hour recalls. All studies used energy intake/basal metabolic rate (EI/BMR) equations to estimate under-reporting; over-reporting was examined in one study. Under-reporting of energy intake ranged from around 20% to 45%. Where measured, the factors associated with under-reporting commonly included overweight and obesity, as well as low educational attainment. Additional factors included being married and high levels of physical activity. In the US study the proportion of high-energy reporters was also assessed, being on average 13% and predicted by underweight, African-American ethnicity, low educational attainment and depressive symptom score. Particularly in early pregnancy, nausea can lead to lack of appetite and decreased intake, leading to a genuinely low intake for that period, confirmed by lack of weight increase.

A review of the available literature shows that children and adolescents tended to under-report energy, particularly in food records, and this appears to be more common than among adults (Forrestal 2011). A number of potential predictors have been examined, with the most consistent findings being age (inverse association) and adiposity (positive association). Gender and social desirability, important predictors for adults, were not consistent factors among children and adolescents. Over-reporting also tended to be more common than it is among adults.

Among the elderly, studies validating dietary assessment methods against DLW and biomarkers are very limited. Some of the existing studies appear to indicate that, as with younger adults, the overweight elderly appear to have a tendency towards greater energy under-reporting than normal-weight elderly, although other studies have shown no association with increased BMI (Thompson and Subar 2008). Education may also be inversely associated with under-reporting, as with younger adults.

8.8 Body size and composition measures

Measuring body size and body composition helps in the understanding of nutrition and growth status in relation to diseases, particularly obesity, and their treatment (see Chapter 11). Resource-intensive direct or criterion methods such as isotope dilution or dual-energy X-ray absorptiometry (DXA) are not usually available for routine surveillance or large-scale research projects. DXA is also not used during pregnancy due to the perceived radiation hazard. More commonly, relatively simple, indirect measures such as anthropometry, skinfold thickness and bioimpedance analysis (BIA) provide estimates of body composition based on their relationship with directly measured components. The appropriateness of indirect body composition measures among different ethnic groups and across the life course are discussed in this section.

Anthropometry

Ethnic groups

It is widely recognised that for a given BMI, South Asian populations have more body fat and a greater risk of central obesity compared to Caucasian Europeans. By contrast, Black African origin groups have lower fat mass and greater lean body mass compared to Caucasians, at the same BMI level. Such ethnic-dependent relationships between BMI and percentage body fat may also be influenced by differences in leg length and body frame, and are evident in both adults and children. BMI cutpoints, based on the association between BMI and mortality and with risk factors for disease in Caucasian European populations, may therefore be error prone for different ethnic groups. For non-Caucasian populations, particularly South Asian groups, different cut-points have been suggested and debated, but as yet there is no consensus on the routine use of these alternatives.

Similar issues beset the use of skinfold thickness to predict percentage body fat in different ethnic groups, since their accuracy depends on the assumption that the representativeness and patterning of subcutaneous fat do not vary by ethnicity. Studies in the USA show differences in the distribution of fat between Black Americans and Caucasians, with less subcutaneous fat on the extremities and more subcutaneous fat on the trunk apparent for Black Americans. These findings suggest that the prediction equations may not be valid across ethnic groups (Deurenberg and Deurenberg-Yap 2003).

Pregnancy

Much of the interest in maternal weight gain and changes in body composition is as the correlate of perinatal outcomes such as birthweight, gestational diabetes and gestational hypertension. The use of skinfold thickness measures during pregnancy has been widely reported. These are low-cost, portable measures and have been validated against more direct measures such as magnetic resonance imaging. The key limitation is the change in skinfold thickness during pregnancy that does not reflect the amount of subcutaneous fat, leading to a tendency to over-estimate percentage body fat. The validity of predictor equations typically developed in non-pregnant populations is also not well established.

Children

Growth monitoring is a key clinical tool in child health, including in the detection and monitoring of overweight and obesity. BMI is the most frequently used index for assessing whether children are overweight or obese, as well as underweight or of healthy weight. High BMI for age has been consistently shown to be associated with high specificity (low false positives) but low to moderate sensitivity (moderate to high false negatives) among children. High specificity is a major advantage for clinical use, but low sensitivity is problematic for public health applications. A systematic review and critical appraisal of co-morbidities of paediatric obesity concluded that high BMI for age is clinically and biologically meaningful and constitutes 'a state of increased risk of morbidity' (Reilly 2006).

In identifying BMI thresholds for overweight and obesity for children, age and sex need to be taken into account, and are usually derived from a reference population known as a child growth reference. Growth reference charts illustrate how BMI varies and provide gender-specific average BMI and the distribution of measurements above and below this value (see for example http://www.rcpch.ac.uk/growthcharts). Individual children can be compared to the reference population and the degree of variation from the 'norm' can be calculated.

BMI thresholds for overweight and obesity are usually defined in terms of a specific z-score, or a centile on a growth reference chart. A z-score or standard deviation (SD) score indicates how many units (of the SD) a child's BMI is above or below the average for their age and sex group, using the equation z-score = (measurement − mean)/SD. For example, a z-score of 1.5 indicates that a child is 1.5 SD above the average value; −1.5 means that they are 1.5 SD below. There is, however, no universally accepted system for the classification of childhood obesity, although a number of child growth references are available and many countries have their own population-specific thresholds. Such thresholds are generally expressed in whole number of SDs or centiles; a key exception is the International Obesity Task Force (IOTF) thresholds, which are derived to line up with the adult BMI thresholds for overweight and obesity (25 and 30 kg/m² or greater), and these are recommended for research projects. To address the weaknesses of BMI, it has been suggested that waist circumference or waist–hip ratio should be added to studies, in combination with BMI (Must and Anderson 2006). Evidence has also shown waist–height ratio to be a valid height-adjusted measure of central adiposity in children.

Elderly

The natural processes of ageing include a decrease in lean tissue and thus an increase in the ratio of fat to lean muscle; as such, the relationship between BMI and body fat becomes increasingly discrepant with age.

Additionally, problems such as shrinkage and kyphosis (curvature) of the spinal vertebrae can make measurement of stature difficult. Alternative measures to standing height commonly used among the elderly include knee height, ulna length and demispan. However, the associated prediction formulas were once again developed in younger adults. Self-reported height and weight have been employed where direct measurement was not feasible. In a study comparing self-reported and measured height and weight among a cohort of elderly men and women, overweight individuals tended to under-report and the short and underweight tended to over-report their height and weight. Underestimates of the associations between disease and height and weight may occur if self-reported measures are used (Gunnell *et al.* 2000). The correlation between skinfold thickness and total body fat at older ages is also generally lower than in younger adults. Prediction equations are therefore likely to underestimate body fat, with particularly large error rates associated with measuring obese individuals.

Bioimpedance analysis (BIA) across population groups

The validity of bioimpedance measures of body water compartments may be influenced by relative limb length, as leg length is known to vary by ethnic group (Rush, Freitas and Plank 2009). The degree of total impedance in subjects with relatively long limbs is high compared to the amount of total body water, therefore predicted body fat percentages using BIA are likely to be overestimated if the formula used was developed in a population with relatively shorter limbs.

Valid estimates of fat-free mass have been demonstrated using BIA among children, with equations for the estimates derived in 5–11-year-olds (Clasey *et al.* 2011), and have been deemed appropriate for use with diverse ethnic groups. BIA measures are also safe to use in pregnancy and validate well against isotope dilution techniques. BIA indices can identify women at risk of gestational hypertension and inadequate fetal growth, and have been shown to be directly related to birthweight. Suitable regression equations to calculate total body water (TBW), and a predictor formula to calculate extra-cellular water (ECW), have been developed for use with pregnant women (Segal *et al.* 1991; Lukaski *et al.* 1994); as with all other groups, intra-cellular water is calculated as the difference between ECW and TBW.

8.9 Conclusions

A number of considerations for incorporating different population groups in nutrition-related research have been summarised in this chapter. When including different ethnic groups in research studies, definitions of ethnicity need to be explicit. Of the range of factors that influence the diets of ethnic groups, cultural mores such as religion and other traditional beliefs are key and need to be taken into account in the design, conduct and interpretation of research studies. However, before applying 'culture' as an explanatory model of differences in health outcomes or behaviours between groups, it is also crucial to simultaneously consider structural social processes such as socio-economic status, income and education. To this end, carefully conducted migration studies can tell us a great deal about the role of context and the relative importance of genetic, social and environmental factors that influence patterning of health among migrant groups.

Across the life course, studies at all ages are crucial in determining when diet–disease associations emerge and the opportune timing of interventions, but they also present a number of challenges. Assessing dietary patterns among children and the elderly poses many of the same issues: the very young and the very old may have difficulties with cognition (memory, conceptualisation, perception), all of which have an impact on their ability to report intakes.

Novel methods of dietary assessment show promise in terms of acceptability, particularly among the young; however, further validation of dietary and body composition measures across age, ethnic and social groups are key areas for future research. Overall, avoiding stereotypical views and acknowledging diversity within and between groups is paramount for the meaningful inclusion of different populations in research.

References and further reading

Adamson, A., Collerton, J., Davies, K. *et al.* (2009) Nutrition in advanced age: Dietary assessment in the Newcastle 85+ study. *European Journal of Clinical Nutrition*, **63**, S6–S18.

Adler, M. and Ziglio, E. (1996) *Gazing into the Oracle: The Delphi Method and Its Application to Social Policy and Public Health*. Jessica Kingsley, London.

Astell, A., Adlam, T., Hwang, F. *et al.* (2012).Validating NANA: Novel assessment of nutrition and ageing. *Gerontechnology*, **11** (2), 243.

Baranowski, T., Islam, N., Douglass, D. *et al.* (2014) Food Intake Recording Software System, version 4 (FIRSSt4): A self-completed 24-h dietary recall for children. *Journal of Human Nutrition and Dietetics*, **27** (Suppl. 1), 66–71 (epub 2012).

Biltoft-Jensen, A., Trolle, E., Christensen, T. *et al.* (2014) WebDASC: A web-based dietary assessment software for 8–11-year-old Danish children. *Journal of Human Nutrition and Dietetics*, **27**, 43–53 (epub 2012).

Cameron, M. and van Staveren, W. (1988) *Manual on Methodology for Food Consumption Studies*. Oxford University Press, Oxford.

Cha, E.S., Kim, K.H. and Erlen, J.A. (2007) Translation of scales in cross-cultural research: Issues and techniques. *Journal of Advanced Nursing*, **58** (4), 386–395.

Chaturvedi, N. and McKeigue, P.M. (1994) Methods for epidemiological surveys of ethnic minority groups. *Journal of Epidemiology and Community Health*, **48** (2), 107–111.

Clasey, J.L., Bradley, K.D., Bradley, J.W. et al. (2011) A new BIA equation estimating the body composition of young children. *Obesity*, **19** (9), 1813–1817.

Daniel, M., Miller, A. and Wilbur, J. (2011) Multiple instrument translation for use with South Asian Indian immigrants. *Research in Nursing and Health*, **34** (5), 419–432.

Derbyshire, E., Davies, G., Costarelli, V. and Dettmar, P. (2009) Habitual micronutrient intake during and after pregnancy in Caucasian Londoners. *Maternal and Child Nutrition*, **5** (1), 1–9.

Deurenberg, P. and Deurenberg-Yap, M. (2003) Validity of body composition methods across ethnic population groups. *Acta Diabetologica*, **40** (1), s246–s249.

Forrestal, S.G. (2011) Energy intake misreporting among children and adolescents: A literature review. *Maternal and Child Nutrition*, **7** (2), 112–127.

Foster, E., Matthews, J.N., Nelson, M. et al. (2006) Accuracy of estimates of food portion size using food photographs: The importance of using age-appropriate tools. *Public Health Nutrition*, **9** (4), 509–514.

Foster, E., Matthews, J., Lloyd, J. et al. (2008) Children's estimates of food portion size: The development and evaluation of three portion size assessment tools for use with children. *British Journal of Nutrition*, **99** (1), 175–184.

Foster, E., Hawkins, A., Delve, J. and Adamson, A. (2014a) Reducing the cost of dietary assessment: Self-Completed Recall and Analysis of Nutrition for use with children (SCRAN24). *Journal of Human Nutrition and Dietetics*, **27** (suppl. 1), 26–35 (epub 2013).

Foster, E., Hawkins, A., Simpson, E. and Adamson, A. (2014b) Developing an interactive portion size assessment system (IPSAS) for use with children. *Journal of Human Nutrition and Dietetics*, **27** (suppl. 1), 18–25 (epub 2013).

Frobisher, C. and Maxwell, S. (2003) The estimation of food portion sizes: A comparison between using descriptions of portion sizes and a photographic food atlas by children and adults. *Journal of Human Nutrition and Dietetics*, **16** (3), 181–188.

Gunnell, D., Berney, L., Holland, P. et al. (2000) How accurately are height, weight and leg length reported by the elderly, and how closely are they related to measurements recorded in childhood? *International Journal of Epidemiology*, **29** (3), 456–464.

Hopping, B., Mead, E., Erber, E. et al. (2010) Dietary adequacy of Inuit in the Canadian Arctic. *Journal of Human Nutrition and Dietetics*, **23** (s1), 27–34.

Illner, A., Freisling, H., Boeing, H. et al. (2012) Review and evaluation of innovative technologies for measuring diet in nutritional epidemiology. *International Journal of Epidemiology*, **41** (4), 1187–1203.

Jackson, M., Walker, S., Cruickshank, J.K. et al. (2007) Diet and overweight and obesity in populations of African origin: Cameroon, Jamaica and the UK. *Public Health Nutrition*, **10** (2), 122–130.

Khokhar, S., Ashkanani, F., Garduño-Diaz, S. and Husain, W. (2013) Application of ethnic food composition data for understanding the diet and nutrition of South Asians in the UK. *Food Chemistry*, **140** (3), 436–442.

Kolonel, L.N., Henderson, B.E., Hankin, J.H. et al. (2000) A multiethnic cohort in Hawaii and Los Angeles: Baseline characteristics. *American Journal of Epidemiology*, **151** (4), 346–357.

Lukaski, H.C., Siders, W.A., Nielsen, E.J. and Hall, C.B. (1994) Total body water in pregnancy: Assessment by using bioelectrical impedance. *American Journal of Clinical Nutrition*, **59** (3), 578–585.

Maynard, M. and Blane, D. (2009) Dietary assessment in early old age: Experience from the Boyd Orr cohort. *European Journal of Clinical Nutrition*, **63**, S58–S63.

Maynard, M.J., Baker, G., Rawlins, E. et al. (2009) Developing obesity prevention interventions among minority ethnic children in schools and places of worship: The DEAL (DiEt and Active Living) study. *BMC Public Health*, **9** (1), 480.

McGowan, C. and McAuliffe, F. (2012) Maternal nutrient intakes and levels of energy underreporting during early pregnancy. *European Journal of Clinical Nutrition*, **66** (8), 906–913.

McNeill, G., Winter, J. and Jia, X. (2009) Diet and cognitive function in later life: A challenge for nutrition epidemiology. *European Journal of Clinical Nutrition*, **63**, S33–S37.

Minkler, M. and Wallerstein, N. (2010) Community-based Participatory Research for Health: From Process to Outcomes. John Wiley & Sons, Inc., San Francisco, CA.

Mir, G., Salway, S., Kai, J. et al. (2013) Principles for research on ethnicity and health: The Leeds Consensus Statement. *European Journal of Public Health*, **23** (3), 504–510.

Moore, H.J., Ells, L.J., McLure, S.A. et al. (2008) The development and evaluation of a novel computer program to assess previous-day dietary and physical activity behaviours in school children: The Synchronised Nutrition and Activity Program™ (SNAP™). *British Journal of Nutrition*, **99** (6), 1266–1274.

Morris, M.C., Tangney, C.C., Bienias, J.L. et al. (2003) Validity and reproducibility of a food frequency questionnaire by cognition in an older biracial sample. *American Journal of Epidemiology*, **158** (12), 1213–1217.

Must, A. and Anderson, S. (2006) Body mass index in children and adolescents: Considerations for population-based applications. *International Journal of Obesity*, **30** (4), 590–594.

Nazroo, J. (2010) Health and health care. In Bloch, A. and Solomon, J. (eds), *Race and Ethnicity in the 21st Century*. Palgrave Macmillan, Basingstoke.

Ngo, J., Gurinovic, M., Frost-Andersen, L. and Serra-Majem, L. (2009) How dietary intake methodology is adapted for use in European immigrant population groups: A review. *British Journal of Nutrition*, **101** (Suppl. 2), S86–S94.

Nowicki, E., Siega-Riz, A.-M., Herring, A. et al. (2011) Predictors of measurement error in energy intake during pregnancy. *American Journal of Epidemiology*, **173** (5), 560–568.

Owusu, M., Thomas, J., Wiredu, E. and Pufulete, M. (2010) Folate status of Ghanaian populations in London and Accra. *British Journal of Nutrition*, **103** (3), 437–444.

Phillips, M.B., Foley, A.L., Barnard, R. et al. (2010) Nutritional screening in community-dwelling older adults: A systematic literature review. *Asia Pacific Journal of Clinical Nutrition*, **19** (3), 440–449.

Platt, L. (2011) *Understanding Inequalities: Stratification and Difference*. Polity Press, Cambridge.

Pope, S., Kritchevsky, S., Morris, M. et al. (2007) Cognitive ability is associated with suspected reporting errors on food frequency questionnaires. *Journal of Nutrition, Health and Aging*, **11** (1), 55–58.

Popkin, B.M., Adair, L.S. and Ng, S.W. (2012) Global nutrition transition and the pandemic of obesity in developing countries. *Nutrition Reviews*, **70** (1), 3–21.

Reilly, J. (2006) Diagnostic accuracy of the BMI for age in paediatrics. *International Journal of Obesity*, **30** (4), 595–597.

Rush, E.C., Freitas, I. and Plank, L.D. (2009) Body size, body composition and fat distribution: Comparative analysis of European, Maori, Pacific Island and Asian Indian adults. *British Journal of Nutrition*, **102** (4), 632–641.

Satia, J.A. (2010) Dietary acculturation and the nutrition transition: An overview. *Applied Physiology, Nutrition, and Metabolism*, **35** (2), 219–223.

Scagliusi, F.B., Ferriolli, E. and Lancha, A.H. (2006) Underreporting of energy intake in developing nations. *Nutrition Reviews*, **64** (7), 319–330.

Scagliusi, F., Ferriolli, E., Pfrimer, K. et al. (2009) Characteristics of women who frequently under report their energy intake: A doubly labelled water study. *European Journal of Clinical Nutrition*, **63** (10), 1192–1199.

Schnarch, B. (2004) Ownership, control, access, and possession (OCAP) or self-determination applied to research. *Journal of Aboriginal Health*, **1** (1), 80–95.

Segal, K.R., Burastero, S., Chun, A. *et al.* (1991) Estimation of extracellular and total body water by multiple-frequency bioelectrical-impedance measurement. *American Journal of Clinical Nutrition*, **54** (1), 26–29.

Senior, P.A. and Bhopal, R. (1994) Ethnicity as a variable in epidemiological research. *British Medical Journal*, **309** (6950), 327.

Sharma, S. (2011) Development and use of FFQ among adults in diverse settings across the globe. *Proceedings of the Nutrition Society*, **70** (2), 232–251.

Sharma, S., Cade, J., Riste, L. and Cruickshank, J.K. (1999) Nutrient intake trends among African-Caribbeans in Britain: A migrant population and its second generation. *Public Health Nutrition*, **2** (4), 469–476.

Sharma, S., Cade, J., Landman, J. and Cruickshank, J.K. (2002) Assessing the diet of the British African-Caribbean population: Frequency of consumption of foods and food portion sizes. *International Journal of Food Sciences and Nutrition*, **53** (5), 439–444.

South, J., White, J. and Gamsu, M. (2013) *People-Centred Public Health*. Policy Press, Bristol.

Storey, K. and McCargar, L. (2012) Reliability and validity of Web-SPAN, a web-based method for assessing weight status, diet and physical activity in youth. *Journal of Human Nutrition and Dietetics*, **25** (1), 59–68.

Thompson, F.E. and Subar, A.F. (2008) Dietary assessment methodology. In Coulston, A., Boushey, C. and Ferruzzi, M. (eds), *Nutrition in the Prevention and Treatment of Disease*. Academic Press, San Diego, CA.

Tillin, T., Hughes, A.D., Godsland, I.F. *et al.* (2013) Insulin resistance and truncal obesity as important determinants of the greater incidence of diabetes in Indian Asians and African Caribbeans compared with Europeans. The Southall And Brent REvisited (SABRE) cohort. *Diabetes Care*, **36** (2), 383–393.

Vereecken, C., Covents, M., Matthys, C. and Maes, L. (2005) Young adolescents' nutrition assessment on computer (YANA-C). *European Journal of Clinical Nutrition*, **59** (5), 658–667.

Vereecken, C., De Bourdeaudhuij, I. and Maes, L. (2010) The HELENA online food frequency questionnaire: Reproducibility and comparison with four 24-h recalls in Belgian–Flemish adolescents. *European Journal of Clinical Nutrition*, **64** (5), 541–548.

Vyas, A., Greenhalgh, A., Cade, J. *et al.* (2003) Nutrient intakes of an adult Pakistani, European and African-Caribbean community in inner city Britain. *Journal of Human Nutrition and Dietetics*, **16** (5), 327–337.

Winkvist, A., Persson, V. and Hartini, T. (2002) Underreporting of energy intake is less common among pregnant women in Indonesia. *Public Health Nutrition*, **5** (4), 523–530.

World Health Organization and US National Institute of Aging (2011) *Global Health and Aging*. WHO, Geneva.

9
Use of Biobanks in Nutrition Research

Kurt Zatloukal,[1] Pieter van't Veer,[2] Christian Viertler,[1] Marc-Jeroen Bogaardt[3] and Peter Hollman[2]

[1]Institute of Pathology, Medical University of Graz
[2]Division of Human Nutrition, Wageningen University
[3]DLO Foundation, Agricultural Economics Research Institute, Wageningen University and Research Centre

Key messages

- Biobanks provide access to quality-defined biological samples and associated health-related information as well as data generated by analysis of biological samples. These resources are critical for biological and medical research and for the advancement of human health.
- Biological specimen and associated health information complemented with dietary assessment of food and nutrient intake offer unique opportunities for the objective assessment of internal exposure, thereby allowing nutrition to be related to health outcomes.

- Biological samples are needed to identify markers of the early biological effects of nutrition. They are crucial in understanding the causal pathways underlying the impact of nutrition on health and disease.
- The standardisation and international harmonisation of biological specimen and data collection, as well as the design and governance of biobanks, are prerequisites for international collaboration. Eventually, the scientific value of biobanks established in different countries can be exploited via meta-databases that describe the stored specimens in the biobanks as well as dedicated databases with the analytical results of selected specimens.

9.1 Introduction

Biobanks for medical research are collections of essentially any type of human biological sample, such as blood, tissues (e.g. liver biopsies, visceral and subcutaneous adipose tissue, intestinal biopsies, tumours), urine or saliva, and data on the sample characteristics as well as on the health/disease status of the sample donor (Box 9.1). On the one hand, biobanks have been established in the context of prospective population cohort studies comprising hundreds of thousands of samples and data from a certain population that is followed up on disease incidence and outcome for many years to decades. On the other hand, biobanks emerged from collections established in the context of health care (e.g. collection of serum or tissue samples from patients treated at hospitals; Figure 9.1).

Historically, valuable collections of biological samples from patients have been established by individual scientists to support their research work. However, there are several differences between the personal collection of an individual scientist and modern biobanks. These differences include the implementation of a governance structure for the biobank, defining responsibilities, access conditions and ethical and legal compliance. Furthermore, quality management is essential to guarantee proper sample quality. In general, individual scientists are not in a position to provide such a professional environment for their collections, and this led to the establishment of institutional biobanks or biobanks as common research infrastructures for whole universities or companies (Asslaber and Zatloukal 2007; Harris et al. 2012). Personalised medicine with its smaller and smaller disease subentities created a demand for increased collaboration among biobanks nationally and across borders, because single biobanks could not provide sufficient numbers of samples for a given disease subentity to achieve statistical significance in studies of single biobanks. Furthermore, increasing interest in

Nutrition Research Methodologies, First Edition. Edited by Julie A Lovegrove, Leanne Hodson, Sangita Sharma and Susan A Lanham-New.
© 2015 John Wiley & Sons, Ltd. Published 2015 by John Wiley & Sons, Ltd.
Companion Website: www.wiley.com/go/nutritionsociety

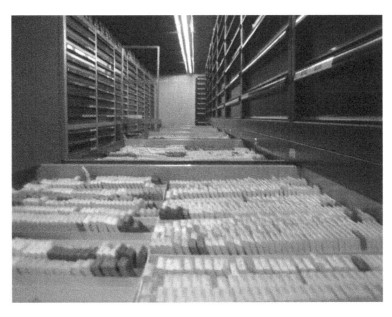

Figure 9.1 Biobank containing a large collection of human formalin-fixed paraffin-embedded tissues representing a broad spectrum of human diseases that were established in the context of health care (BioBank Graz).

Box 9.1 OECD biobank definition

A collection of biological material and the associated data and information stored in an organised system, for a population or a large subset of a population.

Box 9.2 Standardisation and harmonisation

To improve the international interoperability of biobanks, standards and harmonised procedures are required.

Ethical and scientific quality standards are needed for designing, conducting, recording and reporting of research. Standards are developed by national, regional (CEN) or international (ISO) organisations.

Principles for conducting research with humans are often translated into a guideline. Guidelines define the state of the art, but it is not mandatory to follow a guideline.

Harmonised procedures are those that are aligned. This can be achieved by implementing standards and following guidelines.

Several institutions and organisations, such as the Organisation for Economic Co-operation and Development (OECD; 2007, 2009), the World Health Organization's International Agency for Research on Cancer (WHO/IARC; Caboux, Plymoth and Hainaut, 2007), the International Society for Biological and Environmental Repositories (ISBER; 2012) and the National Cancer Institute (NCI; 2007), have produced guidelines related to the various aspects of biobanking in order to establish a common basis for biobanks to facilitate collaboration.

understanding the impact of the genetic make-up of populations with different ethnic origins, as well as the increasing importance of environmental and lifestyle factors, made international collaboration mandatory. This development has gone hand in hand with the requirement for international quality standards and harmonised procedures to improve the interoperability of biobanks (Box 9.2).

In Europe, in the roadmap of the European Strategy Forum for Research Infrastructures (ESFRI) member states have prioritised a pan-European research infrastructure for Biobanking and Biomolecular Resources (BBMRI; Yuille *et al.* 2008). BBMRI was established by the European member states and the European Commission under the recently created legal entity the European Research Infrastructure Consortium (ERIC) in 2013. BBMRI-ERIC is the only ESFRI research infrastructure for biobanking for the whole of Europe that will provide access to quality-defined human biological samples and associated information following internationally harmonised standards and procedures. BBMRI-ERIC offers a common framework and a single access

point to foster high-level scientific collaboration that requires access to various types of human biological samples, ranging from blood or deoxyribonucleic acid (DNA) samples from large cohort studies, tissues from cancer biobanks, serum, plasma or urine collections to samples containing pathogens or microbiomes. Furthermore, the scope of BBMRI-ERIC comprises biological resources, such as cell lines, gene clone collections, protein libraries or antibodies. All samples are linked to comprehensive information on the health or disease condition of the sample donor and related to sample quality. A minimal data set that has to be linked to each sample has been defined (Brochhausen *et al.* 2013). The data management infrastructure of BBMRI-ERIC is designed to handle not only data related to sample origin, but also the massive data generated by sample analyses using modern -omics technologies. A specific challenge in this context is also to meet ethical and legal requirements, particularly to guarantee the privacy of sample donors. It is noteworthy that BBMRI-ERIC is a research infrastructure owned by the European member states and should be in operation for several decades, thereby providing sustainable access to a key resource for the advancement of human health, medicine and related industries.

Biobanks provide a broad spectrum of solutions that are also relevant for nutrition research. For example, several EU or nationally funded research programmes have put major effort into developing proper data-management concepts, including solutions for data protection and privacy. Furthermore, useful expertise has been developed in the effective consideration of different ethical and legal systems in multinational study designs (reports are available at www.bbmri-eric.eu). Several biobanks have linked their sample-associated data with health, disease and death registries, which has resulted in a marked enrichment of biobanks. This is of particular importance in establishing the relationship between molecular alterations identified in samples and health or disease outcomes. Expertise in sample management is mandatory for each biobank. Proper collection, processing, aliquotting, stabilisation and storage of samples are prerequisites to ensure that analytical data are reliable and reflect the status of biological processes within the body (Figure 9.2). The rapid advancement of analytical technologies requires a continuous co-development of quality standards for biological samples in order to deliver the full analytical capacities, because even the most advanced technologies cannot produce better results than the quality of the samples analysed.

Furthermore, biobanking has extended its scope from blood and tissue to a variety of other sample types, such as urine and saliva as well as the intestinal microbiome, allowing a comprehensive investigation of individuals' biological response to environmental and lifestyle factors. Each of these sample types requires specifically optimised standard operating procedures for handling and specific quality controls, resulting in a comprehensive body of knowledge that has to be established in the context of the operation of biobanks. This knowledge has often been generated in parallel in various biobanks, resulting in unnecessary duplication of effort or, even worse, in different procedures that are not compatible between biobanks and thus impede collaboration. Therefore, a major emphasis is currently being placed on overcoming the fragmentation of the biobanking landscape by improving interoperability and coordinating developments (Harris *et al.* 2012).

9.2 Biomarkers in nutrition research

A substantial amount of evidence on diet–health relationships is based on population cohort studies assessing dietary intake and subsequent health outcomes. However, these observational studies are hampered by unavoidable errors in dietary assessment methods. Randomised controlled trials circumvent this problem, but their duration is usually limited and risk factors or intermediate endpoints are used instead of 'hard' clinical endpoints. As indicators of dietary intake, biomarkers can fulfil a role in the validation of dietary assessment or as a proxy for dietary intake. As effect markers they are relevant as intermediate or proxy endpoints for the disease outcome. Thus, biomarkers can be seen as signals of subsequent biological events between the consumption of foods, the impact on metabolism and health, and the eventual occurrence of disease (Box 9.3). In this way, they are crucial in substantiating the biological and pathophysiological models of nutrition-related diseases.

In the context of environmental protection, Hulka *et al.* (1990) provide a framework for biomarkers that distinguishes biomarkers of internal dose, of the biologically effective dose, early response, and altered structure and function, with all the relationships between these being modified by inherited or acquired susceptibility. In nutrition research the framework translates to familiar concepts, for instance for vitamin B12 we distinguish biochemical indicators of short-term intake (B12 concentration in plasma) or long-term intake (B12 concentrations in erythrocytes), biomarkers of nutrient status (liver stores quantified by B12 concentration), early indicators of altered metabolic responses or deficiency (methylmalonic acid, MMA) and clinical alterations (megaloblastic anaemia) causing tiredness and weakness. Susceptibility is increased when there is insufficient hydrochloric acid to separate B12 from food proteins, or because of intrinsic factor insufficiency prohibiting the absorption of the intrinsic factor–B12 complex (pernicious anaemia), or impaired absorption resulting from coeliac disease or Crohn's disease.

Biomarkers can be used for numerous objectives and in various research settings. For the validation of dietary assessment, there is a distinction between recovery markers and concentration markers. Examples of recovery markers are urinary nitrogen excretion for validation of protein intake assessment, and urinary sodium and

(a)

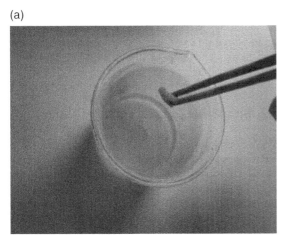

(b)

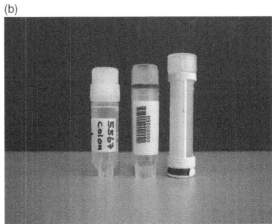

(c)

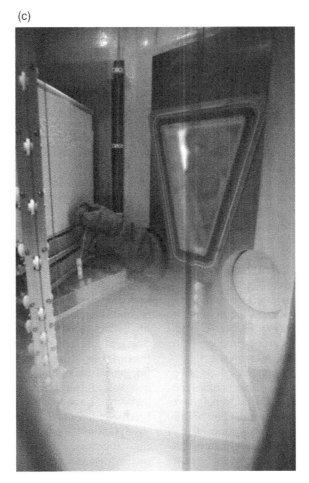

Figure 9.2 Biobanking of cryopreserved tissues. (a) Snap freezing of a tissue sample in metylbutane pre-cooled by liquid nitrogen. (b) Different types of storage containers and labelling (handwritten, barcode, radiofrequency identification). (c) Liquid nitrogen storage system with cooled retrieval unit to prevent temperature shifts of samples (BioBank Graz).

potassium; the doubly labelled water technique can be used for validation of energy expenditure. Recovery markers are based on the principle of nutrient balance and are expressed in amount per day. They are measured in urine; in the ideal situation, 24-hour urine should be collected. If this is not available spot urine can be used, but should be corrected for creatinine excretion. If the objective is to validate assessment methods for nutrition surveillance, the estimated intake is compared to excretion and the conclusion is on the average amount (or percentage) of over- or underreporting. If the objective is to estimate the strength of association between dietary intake and health outcomes in, for example, a cohort study, the degree of attenuation of the observed association can be estimated by regression of the recovery marker on the assessed intake (calibration factor).

Concentration biomarkers are relevant to validation studies, epidemiological research and intervention studies. Examples of concentration markers are B12 or folate levels in plasma or erythrocytes, vitamins A and E, 25-hydroxy vitamin D and carotenoids in plasma, fatty acid patterns in serum triglycerides, cholesteryl esters, erythrocytes or even fat tissue (Hunter 1998). The choice of the type of biological material used for the determination of the biomarker is critical, as plasma or serum mostly reflects short-term intake, whereas blood fractions such as erythrocytes or cholesteryl esters, or fat tissue, may reflect medium- to long-term exposure. In validation studies a direct comparison with calculated nutrient intake is not possible as daily intakes and concentrations are fundamentally different. However, concentration markers can provide an indication of whether the dietary assessment suffices to rank people according to their reported intake. In epidemiological studies, biomarkers can be used as proxies for exposure to nutrients or as indicators of food groups (carotenoids, fish fatty acids).

Further development of biomarkers as predictors of nutrient and food intake could be of interest to complement dietary assessment in epidemiological studies. In intervention trials, concentration or recovery markers can be used as objective indicators of compliance on top of other methods (e.g. pill counts, indicator nutrients or compounds from prescribed foods). As an example, metabolites of the compound used in the intervention may be followed in plasma or urine. In the past few years high-throughput technologies have developed tremendously, which has enabled the measurement of vast amounts of metabolites, transcripts and proteins in intervention studies (Hedrick *et al.* 2012; Rubio-Aliaga, Kochhar and Silva-Solezzi 2012; Wild, Scalbert and Herceg 2013). This multitude of data is promising for the identification of new biomarkers of exposure and (early) effect. However, a new so-called nutrigenomics approach is needed in which transcriptomics, metabolomics, proteomics and epigenomics have to be integrated. Ultimately, there is an urgent need to link these innovative markers to established markers and to evaluate their predictive potential, as indicators of either exposure or disease risk.

A key issue in the practical application of biomarkers in nutrition research is the choice of the biological specimen for biomarker determination. In research practice, the type of biological specimen needed has direct implications for the feasibility of sample collection, including ethical issues (e.g. invasiveness). In nutrition research, only more easily accessible biospecimens such as blood, urine or faeces can generally be obtained. For very specific questions, fat tissue or muscle tissue can be sampled, which requires very invasive procedures. However, it has to be realised that the health effects may take place in tissues not accessible for sampling (e.g. the vessel wall, glandular breast tissue, liver etc.). For the interpretation of biomarkers it is therefore important to realise that biomarkers measured in plasma or urine may only weakly reflect the biological processes in the target tissue. In order to use biomarkers for the underpinning of biological pathways, their predictive validity for the target tissue must be evaluated in terms of their external determinants, biological variation, and random and systematic errors.

9.3 Biobanking for nutrition research

Collection of specimens

Protocols for the collection of specimens should be well described and accessible in the databank. Special considerations for specimen-collection procedures will depend on the type of biological sample (International Society for Biological and Environmental Repositories 2012). For blood sampling, the primary decision made in the biobank determines whether anticoagulated (plasma/buffy coat/erythrocytes) whole blood or coagulated (serum/clot) is available. The blood clot may be used as a source of DNA for genotyping and other DNA-related studies. The buffy coat from blood collected with anticoagulant may be used to isolate ribonucleic acid (RNA) for gene-expression studies. In addition, various anticoagulants can be chosen, which may have consequences for the analysis of the biomarker of interest. As blood sampling may occur at locations remote from storage, special precautions should have been taken during temporary storage and transport. For urine, spot samples or 24-hour collection samples may be available. This has major consequences for the predictive value of the urinary biomarker to be determined. Ideally, 24-hour samples should be accompanied by data on the completeness of the urinary collection, for example a recovery marker like para-amino benzoic acid (PABA).

Sample pre-analytics

It is becoming increasingly important in biomedical research to extend analysis from single molecules to signatures of nucleic acids, proteins and metabolites in a variety of human biological samples. However, the profiles of these molecules can change during collection, preservation, transport and storage, leading to unreliable results because the analytical assay will not determine the *in vivo* situation, but rather reflects an artificial profile generated during sample processing. Therefore, standardisation of the entire pre-analytical process from sample collection to analysis is needed (Box 9.4).

The pre-analytical phase of biological samples, archived in biobanks and used for research and diagnostics, is increasingly the focus of international initiatives, as it has been recognised that pre-analytical variables could have a major impact on the validity of analytical results. One of the recent major activities in this field is SPIDIA (Standardisation and improvement of generic pre-analytical tools and procedures for in-vitro diagnostics, www.spidia.eu), a large-scale European collaborative project involving industry and academia within the Seventh EU Framework Programme to investigate the impact of such critical pre-analytical variables of biological samples on molecular analyses. SPIDIA has developed comprehensive scientific evidence for new standards for pre-analytical sample processing for molecular diagnostics.

The requirements for quality control and standardisation of the pre-analytical workflow and subsequent implications for standard operating procedures in biobanks depend on the sample type and analytical platform used. For instance, metabolic profiles can be seen as the final response of the human body to environmental changes, particularly nutrition, since they are the end products of cellular regulatory processes. However, their value in biomedical and nutrition research, biomarker discovery programmes and future clinical applications depends on the extent to which the metabolome measured actually reflects the original *in vivo* metabolic state. The metabolome may be sensitive to a number of variables of the pre-analytical phase that influence enzymatic activity, chemical reactions or apoptotic processes before

---

Box 9.4 Sample pre-analytics

The pre-analytical processing of biological samples to be used in research and diagnostics could have a major impact on the analytical results. The pre-analytical processing of biological samples comprises three different phases:

- The pre-acquisition phase, before the primary sample is being collected, is influenced by patient-related factors such as genotype, lifestyle, nutritional state of individuals from whom specimens are being collected (e.g. fasting or postprandial samples), medications and underlying diseases. It may also involve medical treatment, anaesthesia, different surgical procedures and intraoperative ischemia (in case of tissues), blood loss and transfusions. Most of these variables cannot be standardised because they are related to individual patient conditions and specific treatments. Nevertheless, all of these parameters may have an impact on subsequent analytical results for research and diagnostics, thus it is important that scientists are aware of these variables.
- The acquisition phase starts when biobank personnel receive the specimen and is influenced by for instance different transport conditions (e.g. temperature) and times or processing procedures in the lab.
- The post-acquisition phase covers registration and annotation of the sample in the biobank database, different storage conditions and time, as well as quality assurance and control of archived samples, and isolation procedures of analytes for subsequent examination.

In contrast to the pre-acquisition phase, the acquisition and post-acquisition phases of the whole pre-analytical workflow are more accessible to standardisation by the use of evidence-based best practice protocols.

---

and during collection, transport, sample handling and storage. Therefore, the impact of pre-analytical effects must be evaluated, monitored and, if possible, minimised. It was recently shown how ischaemia during and after surgery led to alterations of the metabolic profile of human liver tissue samples during the pre-analytical phase (Cacciatore *et al.* 2013). Such studies have implications for biobanking in nutrition research and biomarker development, and researchers should be aware of the impact of pre-analytics in the context of the biological samples, analytes and analytical platforms with which they are working.

To summarise, emerging developments in analytical techniques together with a better understanding of preanalytical effects, standardisation and optimisation of workflows offer new possibilities for nutrition research, but also lead to new requirements for biobanking in this field, for instance for the collection of samples and clinical data, pre-analytical sample treatment, storage conditions and quality control. There are ongoing activities at the European Committee for Standardization (CEN), based on the results of projects like SPIDIA, to develop new technical specifications for ISO standards regarding standardisation of the pre-analytical workflow, best handling procedures and quality assurance in molecular analyses of different sample types and analytes.

Sample storage

A variety of storage systems are available for specimen collection (e.g. for storage in liquid nitrogen, in the gas phase of liquid nitrogen, at –80 °C, –20 °C, 4 °C or at room temperature; from manual systems to fully automated systems; Figure 9.1). Selection of the most suitable equipment should be based first of all on the optimal conditions that guarantee stability of the specimens and the biomarkers of interest. However, many other factors should be taken into consideration: the anticipated length of storage, the intended use of the specimens, the total amount (depending on detection limit) and number of specimens to be stored, sample entry and retrieval, and quality issues (International Society for Biological and Environmental Repositories 2012). Important quality aspects are continuous monitoring of the storage temperature and measures taken to prevent accidental rises in that temperature. These measures should be appropriate, because the stored specimens potentially represent significant scientific and economic value. Another aspect that is becoming increasingly important is the energy efficiency of storage systems, since ultra-low-temperature freezing systems consume more energy. Therefore, techniques for the preservation of biomolecules that allow sample storage at room temperature are currently being explored, which may complement or even replace ultra-low-temperature storage.

Governance of biobanks

Biobanks are considered as a key resource for the advancement of human health. They are typically established by using public funding and rely on donation of samples. Consequently, biobanks represent a common good, which is kept in the public non-for-profit domain. The governance of biobanks should guarantee that this valuable resource is properly maintained and that access is available in a fair and transparent manner. This requires defined processes and rules as well as clear responsibilities. The OECD best-practice guidelines for biological resource centres (OECD 2007) define key personnel (director, data protection officer, quality manager), their qualifications and responsibilities in operating a biobank. Furthermore, a biobank requires appropriate infrastructure and equipment that guarantees proper preservation of samples and data. All

procedures need to be specified in standard operating procedures and biobanks should be accredited or at least certified. The whole governance system should properly address the scientific and technical needs of biobanks and their user communities and also guarantee ethical and legal compliance (Box 9.5). In this context it is important that biobank governance provides solutions for protecting samples and data from destruction or unauthorised access, guarantees sample and data integrity and quality, provides fair and open access to samples and data for excellent research projects, and ensures sustainable funding. Furthermore, the involvement of stakeholders (e.g. sample donors, medical doctors who contribute to sample and data collection, user communities from academia and industry) as well as public engagement is becoming increasingly important.

Emerging research infrastructures for nutrition and health research

Biobanks often emerge from single studies with specific research questions and different protocols and practices for sample collection, treatment and storage. In nutrition research, the collection, processing and storage of dietary intake data are also highly study specific. Methods range from single/multiple-day records or 24-hour recalls to nutrient-tailored or general food frequency questionnaires (FFQs); web-based or mobile devices are also being introduced. The diversity in protocols, lab methods and data handling limits comparability between studies and increases the need for standardisation. Even if laboratory analysis and food composition are eventually conducted by standardised methods or in a central laboratory, there remains a need to compare results between studies at, for instance, the single-country, European or global levels. In the area of dietary assessment, two major drivers are shaping the field: the standardisation of food composition databases (FCDBs); and validation and calibration of dietary assessment, as for example in the EPIC multicentre cohort. These are connected via nutritionally relevant and chemically well-characterised food components: FCDBs enable the conversion of food intake data from different foods to chemically well-characterised nutrients; calibration enables the comparison of nutrient intake data obtained with different dietary assessment instruments.

Harmonisation of food composition data in Europe was initiated by the European Food Information Resource Network project (2005–10; EuroFIR). This was a Network of Excellence (NoE) comprising 48 partners from academia, research organisations and small and medium-sized enterprises in 27 countries, funded by the EC Sixth Framework Programme. It developed, for the first time in Europe, a single online platform with up-to-date food

Box 9.5 Ethical and legal requirements for biobanks in Europe (key documents)

Relevant EU legislation

- The Charter of Fundamental Rights of the EU
- Directive 95/46/EC of 24 October 1995 on the protection of individuals with regard to processing of personal data and the movement of such data
- Directive 2001/20/EC of 4 April 2001 on clinical good practice
- Directive 2001/20/EC of the European Parliament and of the Council of 4 April 2001 on the approximation of the laws, regulations and administrative provisions of the member states relating to the implementation of good clinical practice in the conduct of clinical trials on medicinal products for human use
- Directive 2004/33/EC with regard to information to be provided to prospective donors, information required from donors, eligibility of donors; storage, transport and distribution conditions for blood and blood components; quality and safety requirements for blood and blood components
- Directive 98/44/EC of the European Parliament and of the Council of 6 July 1998 on the legal protection of biotechnological inventions
- Directive 2000/54/EC of the European Parliament and of the Council of 18 September 2000 on the protection of workers from the risks related to exposure to biological agents at work (7th individual directive within the meaning of Article 16(1) of Directive 89/391/EC)

- Directive 2004/23/EC of the European Parliament and of the Council on Setting standards of quality and safety for the donation, procurement, testing, processing, preservation, storage and distribution of human tissues and cells, code number 2002/0128 (COD), Strasbourg, 31 March 2004
- Directive 2002/98/EC setting standards of quality and safety for the collection, testing, processing, storage and distribution of human blood and blood components

International conventions, declarations and guidelines

- Helsinki Declaration in its latest version
- Convention of the Council of Europe on Human Rights and Biomedicine signed in Oviedo on 4 April 1997, and the Additional Protocol on the Prohibition of Cloning Human Beings signed in Paris on 12 January 1998
- Recommendation Rec(2006)4 of the Committee of Ministers to member states on research on biological material of human origin
- UN Convention on the Rights of the Child
- Universal Declaration on the human genome and human rights adopted by UNESCO
- OECD Best Practice Guidelines for Biological Resource Centres (OECD 2007)
- OECD Guidelines on Human Biobanks and Genetic Research Databases (OECD 2009)

---

composition data across the continent. Most partners continued in the subsequent longer-term non-profit international association EuroFIR AISBL, based in Brussels. The main aim of this institution is to support and promote the development, management, publication and application of food composition data through international cooperation and harmonisation. In 2010, the EC's Seventh Framework Programme funded EuroFIR Nexus to develop this initiative further in order to harmonise research into relationships between food, diet and health in Europe. Its main aim is to improve the application of validated food data and tools for pan-European nutrition studies, and to promote the use of standards and best practice.

The European Prospective Investigation into Cancer (EPIC) was designed to investigate the relationships between diet, nutritional status, lifestyle and environmental factors and the incidence of cancer and other chronic diseases. As the largest European study on diet and health to date, it has recruited over 500 000 people from 23 centres in 10 European countries: Denmark, France, Germany, Greece, Italy, the Netherlands, Norway, Spain, Sweden and the UK. Enrolment of the general population cohort was initiated in 1992 and lasted until 1999; it is planned to continue for another decade. At baseline, detailed information on diet and lifestyle was obtained by questionnaires, anthropometric measurements and blood samples, stored in liquid nitrogen. To allow for the widely diverse dietary habits, country-specific FFQs were developed and validation studies were conducted within countries; to calibrate the FFQs, almost 35 000 subjects completed a 24-hour recall using the dedicated EPIC-Soft program.

Together, these two developments have paved the way for European-wide nutritional epidemiology, and simultaneously EPIC-Soft has provided the basis for the emerging pan-European Nutrition Surveillance programme, now being carried forward by the EFSA-coordinated EU-Menu project. At the same time, the pan-European BBMRI, discussed earlier in this chapter, has been constructing an infrastructure that provides access to quality-defined biological samples and associated health-related data (including data on nutrition and physical activity). BBMRI was designed using funding from the EC'S Seventh Framework Programme involving 275 institutions from 33 countries and was established in 2013 under the European Research Infrastructure Consortium (ERIC) legal framework. BBMRI-ERIC is well embedded in European ethical, legal and societal frameworks and is emerging as the leading biobanking initiative with the potential to contribute to a further alignment of data platforms for food, nutrition and health research in Europe.

9.4 From samples to knowledge

Biobanks can be seen as (often literally) frozen bits of biological information, just as databases with information on dietary intake, physical activity, determinants and health effects represent fixed bits of information. All these pieces of information can provide information about the causal process leading from dietary exposure to disease. Basic training in research thus focuses on the proper design, conduct and analysis of separate studies to provide the primary source of information on (causal) relationships. Exploitation of study data requires the formulation of specific hypotheses based on knowledge of nutrition, human biology and pathogenesis, in conjunction with proper study design, for instance specification of explanatory variables, confounders, modifiers and health outcomes. Of course, the strength of any causal claim depends on the reliability of the study design, data gathering and laboratory methods.

Biobanks carry the promise of a wealth of biomarkers that open up the black box between food intake and health outcomes. Different studies do so at different stages in the biomarker framework and at different levels of aggregation, for example the cellular, individual and population levels. At the population level, epidemiologists can analyse separate studies and combine measures of association between a priori defined exposures and (intermediary) health outcomes from similarly designed studies using meta-analysis. At the individual level, clinical studies provide data on disease pathophysiology, either organ specific (e.g. cancer, coronary heart disease) or systemic (e.g. metabolic syndrome). At the cellular level, multivariate nutrigenomics data are analysed and interpreted using the available information on gene sets that are related through their role in biochemical pathways.

Exploitation of the information held in biobanks follows similar strategies to any other study. Research based on biobanks requires background data on their design, conduct and analysis. Laboratory issues of standardisation and calibration have their counterparts in dietary assessment. Specimen retrieval from biobanks shares many characteristics with the retrieval of original data from questionnaires or other data sources. Data analysis of individual studies will focus on a priori hypothesised associations in the grid of the biomarker framework and levels of aggregation. Meta-analysis and evidence appraisal can be used to analyse and evaluate results from similar studies, while the future looks to analyses of the original individual patient data, rather than aggregate meta-analysed data. Nowadays, reviewers take account of evidence appraisal and ensure that the full body of evidence is built using the wisdom of expert committees that integrate different types of evidence from all types of studies, eventually leading to conclusions on the causal role of foods and nutrients in disease aetiology. In future, the causal grid of the biomarker framework and aggregation levels might provide a framework for integrating different types of evidence. This could possibly start with meta-analysed associations, but – as data sharing and exchange are expanding – it could evolve into quantitative analysis of original study data, guided by nutritional mechanisms embedded in pathophysiological models considering the complexity of biological systems.

At the level of the research community, the emerging availability of biobanks requires multidisciplinary and transnational collaborative networks with complementary expertise and skills in the grid of the biomarker framework and aggregation levels. At the level of individual studies, this outlook stresses the importance of meta-data in study design, conduct and methods, as well as data sharing and exchange. This implies that future researchers could build their careers on conducting state-of-the-art individual studies, and then develop either technical and (data) analytical innovations in their part of the grid, or specific skills to integrate the different parts of the grid.

9.5 Future outlook

Biobanking and nutrition research communities have developed valuable complementary expertise and skills. The future integration of these two fields by, on the one hand, the increasing complementing of existing biobanks with quality-defined data on nutrition and, on the other, the enrichment of nutrition data surveys with biological samples and standardised data on health outcomes as provided by biobanks will generate enormous new opportunities to address key problems related to ageing societies and how nutrition could contribute to healthy ageing. It is expected that disease prevention by nutrition will have to consider the specific requirements of individuals as determined by their individual genetic make-up and concrete lifestyle factors. Therefore, biobanks for nutrition research will face very similar challenges to biobanks for personalised medicine.

Acknowledgements

The authors are part of the Determinants of Diet and Physical Activity Knowledge Hub (DEDIPAC KH), funded under the Joint Programming Initiative 'A Healthy Diet for a Healthy Life', a research and innovation initiative of EU member states and associated countries. Part of the work described in this chapter is based on the EuroDISH project 'Studying the need for food and health research infrastructures in Europe'. This project is supported by the European Commission under the Food, Agriculture and Fisheries, and Biotechnology theme of the Seventh Framework Programme for Research and Technological Development (Grant Agreement no. 311788). The overall objective is to provide advanced and feasible recommendations to the European Strategy Forum on Research Infrastructures (ESFRI) and future European funding programmes, as well as other stakeholders for food and health research infrastructure development, and it is dual led, with Stichting Dienst Landbouwkundig Onderzoek as project coordinator and Wageningen University as scientific coordinator. Both are part of Wageningen UR (University and Research Centre). There is more information at http://www.eurodish.eu. Part of the work described in this chapter is based on the European FP7 project SPIDIA (Standardisation and improvement of generic pre-analytical tools and procedures for in-vitro diagnostics; grant agreement n° 222916; www.spidia.eu), in conjunction with the Christian Doppler Laboratory for Biospecimen Research and Biobanking Technology.

References and further reading

Asslaber, M. and Zatloukal, K. (2007) Biobanks: Transnational, European and global networks. *Briefings in Functional Genomics and Proteomics*, **6**, 3, 193–201.

Brochhausen, M., Fransson, M.N., Kanaskar, N.V. *et al.* (2013) Developing a semantically rich ontology for the biobank-administration domain. *Journal of Biomedical Semantics*, **4**, 1, 23.

Caboux, E., Plymoth, A. and Hainaut, P. (eds) (2007) *Common Minimum Technical Standards and Protocols for Biological Resource Centres Dedicated to Cancer Research. Work Group Report 2.* International Agency for Research on Cancer, Lyon.

Cacciatore, S., Hu, X., Viertler, C. *et al.* (2013) Effects of intra- and post-operative ischemia on the metabolic profile of clinical liver tissue specimens monitored by NMR. *Journal of Proteome Research*, **12**, 12, 5723–9.

Harris, J.R., Burton, P., Knoppers, B.M. *et al.* (2012) Toward a roadmap in global biobanking for health. *European Journal of Human Genetics*, **20**, 11, 1105–11.

Hedrick, V.E., Dietrich, A.M., Estabrooks, P.A. *et al.* (2012) Dietary biomarkers: Advances, linitations and future directions. *Nutrition Journal*, **11**, 109.

Hulka, B.S., Wilcosky, T.C. and Griffith, J.D. (eds) (1990) *Biological Markers in Epidemiology.* Oxford University Press, New York.

Hunter, D. (1998) Biochemical markers of dietary intake. In W. Willett (ed.) *Nutritional Epidemiology*, 2nd edn, Oxford University Press, Oxford.

International Society for Biological and Environmental Repositories (2012) 2012 Best practices for repositories: Collection, storage, retrieval, and distribution of biological materials for research. *Biopreservation and Biobanking*, **10**, 2, 79-161.

National Cancer Institute (2007) *Best Practices for Biospecimen Resources.* National Cancer Institute, Washington, DC. http://biospecimens. cancer.gov/global/pdfs/NCI_Best_Practices_060507.pdf (accessed June 2014).

OECD (2007) *OECD Best Practice Guidelines for Biological Resource Centres.* Organisation for Economic Co-operation and Development, Paris. www.cect.org/docs/38777417.pdf (accessed June 2014).

OECD (2009) *Guidelines for Human Biobanks and Genetic Research Databases (HBGRDs).* Organisation for Economic Co-operation and Development, Paris. www.oecd.org/sti/biotechnology/hbgrd (accessed June 2014).

Rubio-Aliaga, I., Kochhar, S. and Silva-Solezzi, I. (2012) Biomarkers of nutrient bioactivity and efficacy. *Journal of Clinical Gastroenterology*, **46**, 545–554.

Vineis, P. (1997) Sources of variation in biomarkers. *IARC Scientific Publication Series*, **142**, 59–71.

Wild, C.P., Scalbert, A. and Herceg, Z. (2013) Measuring the exposome: A powerful basis for evaluating environmental exposures and cancer risk. *Environmental and Molecular Mutagenesis*, **54**, 480–99.

Yuille, M., van Ommen, G.J., Bréchot, C. *et al.* (2008) Biobanking for Europe. *Briefings in Bioinformatics*, **9**, 1, 14–24.

10
Methods Investigating Food-Related Behaviour

Moira Dean,[1] Monique M Raats[2] and Liisa Lähteenmäki[3]

[1] *Queen's University Belfast*
[2] *University of Surrey*
[3] *Aarhus University*

Key messages

- Diet and thus food-related behaviour contributes to health. It is therefore important to understand how people view health in relation to eating and how their health interpretations shape food-related strategies and behaviours.
- Different methods of data collection can be used to investigate food-choice behaviour, including qualitative, quantitative or mixed-method approaches.
- Qualitative and quantitative designs should not be viewed as polar opposites but as different ends of a continuum, with mixed methods in the middle as it incorporates elements of both qualitative and quantitative approaches.
- Qualitative approaches employ emerging methods with open-ended questions and may contain interview data, observation data, document data and audio-visual data that undergo text and image analysis with themes and pattern interpretation.

- Quantitative approaches aim to test objective theories by examining the relationships among variables using pre-determined, instrument-based questions that contain performance data, attitude data, observational data and census data. These are statistically analysed and interpreted.
- Mixed-methods approaches use both pre-determined and emerging methods, with open and closed questions to gather multiple forms of data drawing from all possibilities. Statistical and text analysis are conducted with across-database interpretation.
- Food-choice and eating behaviour differ from many other behaviours in that they contain a number of many small decisions that although separately they may have very little relevance, cumulatively add up to behaviours that have a big influence on health outcome.

10.1 Introduction

In nutrition, the main aim is to measure what and how much people eat and to translate this into information on energy and nutrient intake, which can be used to assess the nutritional quality of the diet. To understand the determinants of food choices and amount eaten, we need to find answers to why people choose what they choose, where they eat, with whom and when. These food-related behaviours are complicated actions governed by a mix of cultural conventions, social interactions, individual perceptions and psychological influences. Food and nutrient systems can be conceptualised as interlinked

systems of producer, consumer and nutrition. Further food choices are inter-related and foods are not selected in isolation. For example, when a food is added to a diet it may replace another; omitting or adding a food that is usually eaten in combination with another food may also result in omitting or adding that other food as well. Thus, when dealing with food-related consumer behaviour, there is a need to address not only eating behaviour but purchasing and preparation as well (Figure 10.1).

As food choices and other diet-related behaviours are determined by cultural, social, individual and food-related factors, there are different models to explain these behaviours depending on the viewpoint taken. The choice

Nutrition Research Methodologies, First Edition. Edited by Julie A Lovegrove, Leanne Hodson, Sangita Sharma and Susan A Lanham-New.
© 2015 John Wiley & Sons, Ltd. Published 2015 by John Wiley & Sons, Ltd.
Companion Website: www.wiley.com/go/nutritionsociety

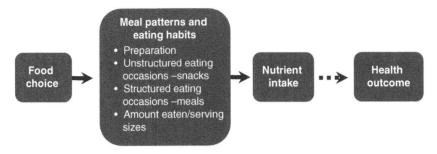

Figure 10.1 The relationship between food and health.

Table 10.1 Levels of influence on food-choice behaviour: the Social Ecological Framework.

Level of influences	Examples of influences
Intrapersonal level	An individual's knowledge, skills, attitudes, values, preferences, emotions, values, behaviour
Interpersonal level	An individual's social networks, social supports, families, peers and neighbours
Community level	Community resources, neighbourhood organisations, social and health services
Organisational level	Businesses, public agencies, churches, service organisations
Public policy level	Legislation, policies, taxes, regulatory agencies, health system, social care system, political/geographical environment

of approach is dependent on the research questions in which we are interested, but typically all these approaches use methods that have a basis in social sciences. The methods help us understand why people choose what they eat; that is, the reasons for the behaviours over and above the intake methods typically used in nutrition. These methods should be able to elicit the types of explanations given for food choice at the individual, societal and/or cultural levels (Table 10.1). In all cases the reasons for food-choice behaviour are usually elicited at the individual level and the impact of societal and cultural reflections on the individual are subsequently discussed.

The methods introduced here should support nutrition studies by providing tools to measure the reasons behind food choices and intake more effectively. Due to limited space, the methods are described as types of approaches. The aim is to cover the general principles in applying the specific methodologies and to demonstrate what information different methods can give us about the factors influencing behaviour, but active application of the chosen method will require further reading and more in-depth exploration.

When interventions are used to change an individual's food-related behaviours, the instruments and scales used in this research should be able to measure the changes in behaviour. Therefore, measurements employed to measure behaviour not only have to be good enough to measure food-choice behaviours, but also sensitive enough to pick up behaviour change as well.

10.2 Types of data in food-choice behaviour

There are three main types of research approaches: qualitative, quantitative and mixed methods. Criteria for selecting a research design for a study will depend on the research problem, the personal experience of the researcher and the researcher's audience. Here qualitative and quantitative designs should not be viewed as polar opposites, but as different ends of a continuum with mixed methods in the middle, as it incorporates elements of both qualitative and quantitative approaches. These approaches differ in:

- the basic philosophical assumptions the researchers bring to the research;
- the types of research strategies used (e.g. qualitative case studies or quantitative experiments); and
- the specific methods employed in conducting these strategies (e.g. collecting data quantitatively on instruments versus collecting data qualitatively through observing a setting).

Qualitative approaches employ emerging methods with open-ended questions and may contain interview data, observation data, document data and audio-visual data that undergo text and image analysis with themes and pattern interpretation. In contrast, *quantitative approaches* aim to test objective theories by examining the relationships among variables using pre-determined, instrument-based questions that contain performance data, attitude data, observational data and census data. These are statistically analysed and interpreted. A *mixed-methods* approach uses both pre-determined and emerging methods with open and closed questions to gather multiple forms of data, drawing from all possibilities. Statistical and text analysis are conducted with across-database interpretation.

In a study design the researcher not only selects a qualitative, quantitative or mixed-methods approach, but also has to decide on a specific strategy of inquiry within each of the approaches.

10.3 Qualitative approaches

When to choose a qualitative approach

Qualitative research explores and understands the meaning that individuals or groups ascribe to a social or human problem. The process of research involves emerging questions, procedures and data collected in the participant's setting. Data are analysed inductively, building from particular to general themes, and the researcher interprets the meaning of the data. Researchers support an inductive style, focusing on individual meaning and the importance of interpreting the complexity of a situation. Qualitative research is thus well placed to answer complex questions about food-related behaviour, as it can investigate how and why individuals act in certain ways. Qualitative approaches are typically applied in studying how consumers relate to novel types of foods, such as functional foods, or to gain a better understanding of cultural practices around food provisioning. Qualitative strategies include:

- *Ethnography*, where the researcher studies an intact cultural group in a natural setting over a prolonged period of time by collecting, primarily, observational and interview data.
- *Grounded theory*, where the researcher derives a general, abstract theory of a process, action or interaction grounded in the views of the participants. This involves using multiple stages of data collection and the refinement and inter-relationship of categories of information.
- *Case studies*, where a programme, event, activity, process or one or more individuals are investigated in depth. Case studies are bounded by time or activity and researchers collect detailed information using a variety of data-collection procedures over a sustained period of time.
- *Phenomenological research*, where the researcher identifies the essence of human experience about a phenomenon described by the participants, by studying a small number of subjects through extensive and prolonged engagement, to develop patterns and relationships of meaning.
- *Narrative research*, where the researcher studies the lives of individuals by asking one or more people to provide stories about their lives. These stories are then re-told and re-storied by the researcher onto a narrative chronology.

Sampling and recruitment in qualitative research

Qualitative research uses some type of *purposive sampling* to recruit a relatively small number of participants (Table 10.2). These people are deliberately selected to address the research aim, as they are considered to be a rich source of data in relation to that aim. They could be selected on personal characteristics such as gender, socio-economic status, nutritional status, health status or their experience of a specific event (e.g. regular shoppers), their behaviour (e.g. organic shoppers) or their attitudes and beliefs (for or against genetic modification). While there are different types of purposive sampling, *theoretical sampling* is commonly used, originating from grounded theory where sampling continues until no new data or properties relating to the construct(s) of interest emerge, a point known as theoretical saturation. *Convenience sampling* (where a group is easily accessible, but not biased) and *snowball sampling* (asking recruits to suggest new participants from among their friends and acquaintances) are also employed in qualitative research; these may be the only practical options when working with vulnerable and hard-to-reach populations.

The adequacy of sample size is determined by the breadth of the phenomenon under study: the broader the phenomenon, the larger the number. Rough indicators of what might be adequate could be obtained from similar published studies in high-quality journals. It has been shown that theoretical saturation could be achieved with six interviews.

Data collection and analysis of qualitative methods

Individual interviews

Interviews are a commonly used technique for data collection in qualitative research and can be described as a 'construction site of knowledge where two individuals discuss a theme of mutual interest'. Interviews can be categorised into four types: the informal, conversational interview; the guided interview or topic approach; the standard open-ended interview; and the co-constructed dialogue interview. The four types vary in the degree to

Table 10.2 Sampling methods used in food-choice research.

Sampling approach	Sample selection strategy
Probability sampling methods where random selection is used to ensure that all members of the group of interest have an equal chance of being selected to participate in the study	
Simple random sampling	Every member of the population being studied has an equal chance of being selected. All of the population needs to be available.
Systematic selection (interval sampling)	Used when a stream of representative people are available, e.g. shoppers in a particular store.
Stratified sampling (proportional and disproportional)	The population is divided into non-overlapping groups ('strata') and samples are taken from within these groups.
Clustered sampling	Used when the population of interest is large and widely geographically dispersed. Clusters within the population are randomly selected, e.g. cities.
Purposive (non-probability) sampling, i.e. sampling with a purpose in mind, usually an interest in particular groups	
Convenience sampling	Participants will be those to whom the researcher has relatively 'easy' access, e.g. students.
Snowball sampling	Participants meeting the study requirements will recommend others with the same characteristics, e.g. members of a club. This method is used when trying to access difficult-to-reach populations.
Quota sampling	Participants are non-randomly selected according to a pre-defined fixed quota. Proportional quota sampling aims to match the proportions of a particular characteristic found in the population as a whole; in no-proportion quota sampling one is less restrictive about matching the population-level figures.
Typical case sampling	Participants are selected to be typical, normal or average for a particular phenomenon.
Theoretical sampling	Participants are selected on the basis of the results of the data collected to date. The goal is develop a deeper understanding of the topic and to develop theory.

which they are structured, with one end of the continuum being unstructured, in-depth interviews where the researcher introduces a topic and then gives the interviewee the freedom to talk, with only occasional prompts and probes. This type of interview allows participants' experiences, meanings, values and priorities to emerge with minimal interference on the part of the researcher, but it may be less useful for answering specific research questions. At the other end of the continuum, structured interviews comprising pre-defined questions are administered in a pre-set order.

Semi-structured interviews seek to obtain descriptions of the life of the interviewee with respect to interpreting the meaning of the phenomenon being described. They consist of a sequence of themes to be covered, as well as some suggested questions, with an understanding that changes to the sequence and form of questions are possible in order to follow up the specific answers given and the stories told by the participants.

Preparation for the interview stage usually involves a script called an *interview guide*, which structures the course of the interview more or less tightly. In a semi-structured interview the guide will include an outline of topics to be covered with suggested questions. Depending on the particular study, the sequence of the questions will be pre-determined and binding, or it can depend on

the judgement and tact of the interviewer, who can follow up the interviewee's answers and any new directions that open up.

The interview questions must be brief and simple. Different types of questions may be used. To allow for an easy start and to build rapport, introductory questions such as 'Can you tell me about…?' or 'Could you describe in detail…?' can be used, followed by questions to which the participants' answers are extended through a curious, persistent and critical attitude on the part of the interviewer. This can be done through direct questioning of what has just been said or by a mere nod or 'mm'. The interviewer can use probing questions such as 'Could you say something more about…?' or 'Can you give a more detailed description?' to pursue the answers without stating what dimensions are to be taken into account. The interviewer may also follow up with more operationalising questions, such as 'What did you actually do?' or 'How did you react?' The interviewer can introduce topics directly, preferably in the later part of the interview. Furthermore, interpretive questions can take the form of rephrasing the question or clarification.

Depending on the participants, some interviews need more careful consideration. For example, when interviewing people from a different culture, specific factors such as asking questions as a means of obtaining information, replying directly, referring to taboo matters, making eye contact when speaking or sending a man to interview a woman and vice versa need to be thought through in detail. Difficulties in recognising disparities in language use, gestures and cultural norms may also arise within the researcher's own culture when interviewing across gender, generation, social class or religion. Although differences between subcultures may not be as pronounced as those between different cultures, if the researcher makes the implicit assumption that everyone belongs to a common culture, intercultural variations may be harder to detect.

When interviewing children, it is important to use age-appropriate questions and to be aware of several difficulties of interviews with adults that may be aggravated, such as the interviewer asking long and complex questions or posing more than one question at a time. In some instances, it may help to interview children while they are carrying out some other task such as drawing, reading a story, or watching TV or a video. See Box 10.1 for an example of a study using interviews.

Group discussions

A commonly used form of group discussion is a focus group, which is defined as a carefully planned discussion designed to obtain perceptions on a defined area of interest in a permissive, non-threatening environment. The focus group presents a natural environment in which participants are influencing and influenced by others – just as they are in real life. The researcher serves several functions in the focus group: moderating, listening, observing and eventually analysing using an inductive process.

The topics of discussion in a focus group are carefully pre-determined and sequenced based on analysis of the situation. This analysis includes an in-depth study of the event, experience or topic in order to describe the context, ingredients and components of the experience. The questions are placed in an understandable and logical order.

Focus groups produce qualitative data that provide insights into participants' attitudes, perceptions and opinions. These results are solicited through open-ended questions, to which respondents are able to choose the manner in which they respond, and from observations of those respondents in a group discussion. The discussions are audio-taped and transcribed. Careful and systematic analysis of the discussions provides clues and insights into how a product, service or opportunity is perceived. The researcher derives understanding based on the discussion as opposed to testing or confirming a preconceived hypothesis or theory. See Box 10.2 for an overview of the strengths and weaknesses of group discussions and Box 10.3 for an example of a study using group discussions.

Laddering

Laddering refers to an in-depth, one-to-one interviewing technique used to develop understanding of how consumers translate attributes of products into meaningful associations, following means–end theory. Salient attributes of product choices are often elicited by asking why one product is chosen over another, followed by asking why these attributes are important in the choice.

Box 10.1 Example of a study using interviews

In a study by Blake et al., (2008) examining how people construct their evening meals, 32 adults were interviewed on nine different occasions, with the first seven interviews asking about their use of food during the previous 24 hours (24-hour recall) and then two weeks later an in-depth in-person interview about how they experienced different eating occasions and contexts. The interview was semi-structured and interviewees identified the eating situations that were most common to them, explaining how these eating occasions were constructed. Based on the individual interviews, a constant comparative method was used to construct different scripts for meals. These were named to describe the content, for instance 'Provider script' or 'Egalitarian script'. Around two months after the in-depth interview, a final interview was carried out to discuss and review the preliminary results with the interviewees, also giving participants the possibility of clarifying their answers. The research used a grounded theory approach and schema theory as a framework.

Box 10.2 Strengths and weaknesses of group discussions (Kelley et al., 2003)

Strengths

- It is a socially oriented research procedure that captures the dynamic interaction between individuals in a group.
- The format allows the moderator to probe and offers the flexibility to explore unanticipated issues.
- There is high face validity.
- They are relatively low cost to run.
- They can provide results quickly.
- The can increase the sample size of qualitative studies.

Weaknesses

- Researchers have less control than in an interview, as participants interact and influence each other.
- Data may be more difficult to analyse, as comments must be analysed and interpreted in context.
- A trained moderator is needed in order to achieve good results.
- Groups can vary significantly, so a reasonable number are needed to balance the idiosyncrasies of individual sessions.
- Groups may be difficult to assemble.
- The discussion needs to be conducted in a conversation-friendly environment, so participants may have to be paid for their travel/time/inconvenience etc.

Box 10.3 Example of a study using group discussions

Flavonoids in fruit and vegetables are compounds that are perceived as beneficial for health. How consumers perceive the idea of enhancing the flavonoid content was studied by Lampila *et al.*, (2009) using focus group discussions in three countries: Finland, the Netherlands and France. Focus groups were selected as a method because consumers are not likely to be familiar with flavonoids as a concept or with their benefits; in focus groups this information can be provided. Focus groups also give information on how consumers discuss these novel components. In total, 6 focus group discussions were carried out in each country, with 130 participants in total.

When consumers were informed about the benefits of flavonoids, their attitudes towards them were positive. This positive attitude was based on the idea that flavonoids are naturally present in fruit and vegetables and that their health benefits are linked to common diseases. Although generally positive, participants discussed the need to enhance the flavonoid content (why to make healthy fruit even healthier?), whether there are risks involved in eating fruit with enhanced flavonoid content, and what kind of breeding and production methods are required to increase the flavonoid content. These factors may interact with the perceived naturalness of fruit and vegetables with enhanced flavonoid content.

There were very few cultural differences in the way flavonoids were discussed in the three countries. The focus group discussions were carried out using an interview guide and by an experienced moderator. Discussions were transcribed and coded into themes with the help of a computer program. The reliability of the coding was checked by an independent second researcher. The results were presented using quotations from the discussions to illustrate the themes.

The second 'why' question elicits what consequences the attributes have for the person; further 'why' questions about the importance of consequences lead to values. With the laddering technique we can find out what product-related attributes signify to a person. Its advantage over other qualitative approaches is that the meanings in the means–ends chain are personally relevant. Therefore, laddering can provide results that are more closely related to preference and choice behaviour.

As described above, laddering uses a tailored interview format employing a series of directed probes, typified by the 'Why is that important to you?' question, with the aim of determining connections between attributes (A), their consequences (C) and values (V). These association networks, or ladders, represent combinations of elements that distinguish between the products in a given product class. The higher-order knowledge structures represented by the A-C-V ladders provide a perspective on how the product information is processed from what could be called a motivational perspective, in that the underlying reasons for an attribute or a consequence being important can be uncovered. If product-related attributes are linked to values via consequences, they are likely to be more central in making decisions over alternatives than those attributes that are not linked to values or even consequences: it is not about what the product is, but what the product can do for you. Laddering interviews have been used extensively in the food domain, although sometimes the level of elicitation has not reached the value level.

The analysis of laddering data involves coding the attributes, consequences and values by a standard content analysis procedure. The summary table constructed represents the number of connections between the elements. From this the dominant connections can be selected and graphically represented in a tree diagram, called a hierarchical value map. Interpretation of this type of qualitative, in-depth information permits an understanding of a consumer's underlying motivations with respect to a given product class. Each unique pathway

Box 10.4 Attributes, consequences and values generated in a laddering study by Ares *et al.*, (2008) on understanding consumers' perceptions of conventional and functional yogurts

- **Attributes:** contains fibre, contains antioxidants, is a regular product, is low in calories, is low in fat
- **Consequences:** lack of need, weight control, improves body functions, prevention of diseases, like, dislike, has no added value
- **Values:** looking good, live longer, better quality of life, well-being, pleasure, healthy life

Box 10.5 Example of laddering study on consumers' orientation to the health and hedonic characteristics of foods

Laddering was used by Roininen *et al.*, (2000) to identify how consumers perceive the health and hedonic aspects of foods. In this study, 47 participants sorted 32 foods into 4 categories: pleasure giving and healthy; pleasure giving but not healthy; not pleasure giving but healthy; and not pleasure giving and not healthy. Within each category, attributes were elicited by asking respondents to describe the most important attributes of foods in that category. Good taste, naturalness and a number of more specific health-related attributes were mentioned, such as obtaining beneficial compounds, the importance of nutrients, reduced fat content and general health effects of foods. Although the vocabulary used for health is wider than that for pleasure, which is mainly described by good taste, it is hedonic characteristics that are of importance and these are linked to pleasure, which in turn is linked to health effects. Physical well-being is an instrumental value linked to most health-related attributes and their consequences, but risk and preventing disease as consequences do not link to values, suggesting that they have lower relevance in consumers' minds

from attribute to value represents an opportunity to understand the values driving food-choice decisions. See Box 10.4 for an example of attributes, consequences and values generated in a laddering study and Box 10.5 for a further example of this kind of research.

Behavioural observations

As opposed to self-reported behaviour, observational techniques allow behaviour to be observed directly. The data obtained is very rich because it includes non-verbal and physical behaviour. Measures of what, when, where and how much is being selected, purchased, prepared, cooked, shared or eaten can be collected by observers by photographing or filming behaviour. Data can be collected in unobtrusive naturalistic or controlled settings, such as observation labs where participants shop, cook or eat in a controlled environment that uses cameras and/or sensors to record behaviour. See Box 10.6 for the strengths and weaknesses of behavioural observations and Box 10.7 for an example of a mixed-methods study that included behavioural observation.

Observational techniques include the 'accompanied shop technique' (Box 10.8), which was originally developed in the consumer sciences as a way of modelling decision-making, where it is generally known as 'shopping with consumers'. An investigation into why price differences failed to predict women's clothing purchases demonstrated the method's ability to elicit the less tangible factors influencing decisions and to reveal how they interact with more obvious influences. Another study a year later showed shoppers' ability and willingness to articulate their choices as they make them.

These early studies also illustrate the flexibility of the basic accompanied shop concept, demonstrating the ways in which it can be customised to address research questions related to food choices. For example, because the researchers in the first clothing study were specifically interested in the factors that moderated the effect of price on dress purchases, they allocated participants specific amounts of money and instructed them to shop within certain product categories. On the other hand, the researcher in the later study avoided imposing any external constraints on shopping behaviour in order to preserve the validity of the exercise, though he also interacted

---

Box 10.6 Strengths and weaknesses of behavioural observations

Strengths

- They provide direct information about the behaviour of individuals and groups.
- They permit the evaluator to enter into and understand the situation/context.
- They provide good opportunities for identifying unanticipated outcomes.

Weaknesses

- They are expensive and time-consuming.
- They require well-qualified, highly trained observers, who may need to be content experts.
- They may affect participants' behaviour.
- The selective perception of the observer may distort the data.
- The investigator has little control over the situation.
- The behaviour or set of behaviours observed may be atypical.

Box 10.7 Example of a mixed-methods study that included behavioural observation

Focused observations were used by Moore et al., (2010) to examine the social, physical and temporal characteristics of primary school dining halls and their implications for children's eating behaviours. The observations were guided by a semi-structured schedule that prompted the observer to consider each of nine aspects of a social scene (space, object, act, activity, event, time, actor, goal, feeling) in isolation (e.g. describe all objects, all places) and in interaction with each other (e.g. how the space is organised by the objects). Notes were written on the observation schedule during the observation. After each session, the notes were expanded into detailed field notes that followed the structure of the observation schedule. In order to capture the temporal aspects of the scene, the notes were time stamped.

On the first observation day in each school, a plan of the empty dining hall was drawn before lunch began. Children who opted out of the study were discreetly identified by staff so that the observations/field notes excluded them. Semi-structured interviews with catering staff and school meal supervisors provided data on what was not observable (e.g. goals and feelings). These interviews sought clarification or expansion on field-note entries. Semi-structured interviews were held with head teachers to establish the organisational context surrounding school meals. School administrative staff made available data relating to meals served (free and paid for).

Box 10.8 Example of an accompanied shopping study

An accompanied shopping method was used by Hollywood et al., (2013) to study the perceptions regarding, and identify the barriers to, conducting a healthful shop. A study with 50 grocery shoppers consisted of three elements: a short pre-shop interview (5–10 minutes before the shop began) and the accompanied shop (15–90 minutes), followed by a post-shop telephone interview (20–45 minutes). Participants were asked to 'think aloud' as they shopped. They were informed that they were being observed as they engaged in their normal shopping activity and were not prompted about the concept of health prior to the shop.

The post-shop interview explored each participant's perceptions of their shop in terms of its healthfulness, their shopping intentions and the shopping experience. It was conducted within a two-week period, to explore participants' lifestyles in relation to their shopping and eating behaviour, and was used to identify perceived barriers to conducting a healthful shop. The results indicated that participants used three criteria to identify a healthful shop: inclusion of healthful foods; avoidance or restriction of particular foods; and achieving a balance between healthful and unhealthful foods. Those participants who took a balanced approach employed a more holistic approach to their diet, while those who avoided or included specific foods might be setting criteria to purchase only certain types of food. Two barriers to healthful shopping identified by participants were lack of self-efficacy in choosing, preparing and cooking healthful foods; and conflicting needs when satisfying self and others.

frequently with his shoppers, exerting a degree of influence that arguably brought that same validity into question.

The need to avoid interfering with the shopping process while still capturing relevant data is a difficulty inherent in the accompanied shop technique that researchers have addressed in many different ways, with varying degrees of success. More hands-off solutions to this problem have included equipping shop assistants with microphones and interviewing shoppers immediately on leaving a supermarket, although neither of these approaches allows immediate access to consumer reasoning around purchasing decisions. Outside the realm of consumer research, more recent studies conducted in public health and food science contexts also indicate the potential of this technique in exploring reasoning around the food purchases of allergic shoppers. For example, think-aloud protocols were found to be highly effective in discovering with which aspects of food labels shoppers engage.

The widespread use of think-aloud protocols in various forms can arguably be traced back to work on 'productive thinking', via attempts to restore verbal data to its rightful place in scientific research. The latter emphasise the crucial distinction between explanations of actions still held in short-term memory and retrospective accounts of past decisions. In many cases, thinking aloud tends to be used as one component of a broader methodology and thus often escapes being assessed as a technique in its own right. The extent to which thinking aloud is assumed to provide insight into actual reasoning processes is likewise rarely addressed beyond what can be implied from the ways in which different researchers have chosen to use it. A key aspect of the variability in how thinking aloud is applied is whether or not it is followed by an interview. Think-aloud exercises and interviews after the fact, 'think afters', have been said to generate very different kinds of data and are best used in conjunction with each other.

The role of the qualitative interviewer

In the qualitative approach the researcher is the instrument. In studies related to food and nutrition, the target of qualitative studies is not overly sensitive, but the points made here still need to be considered.

In both sustained and intensive long-term ethnographies, and in relatively brief but personal in-depth interview studies, researchers enter the lives of the participants, bringing with them a range of strategic, ethical and personal issues that need to be carefully thought through at the design stage. The researchers must think about the degree of *participantness* – the degree of actual participation in participants' daily life, which can vary from full participation, where the researcher goes about ordinary life in a role or set of roles constructed in the setting, to being a complete observer who does not engage in social interaction in the world being studied. All possible complementary mixes of these roles along the continuum are available to the researcher, although some direct and immediate participation in the research environment is important to build rapport.

Researchers also have to consider the level of *revealedness* – the extent to which the participants know about the details of the study, from full disclosure at one end to complete secrecy at the other. While some researchers advocate full disclosure, claiming that participants are seldom deceived or reassured for long by false or partial explanations, revealing the exact purpose may cue people to behave in ways that might undermine the research's qualitative purposes and principles. Many researchers follow the advice to be truthful but vague.

Another dimension is the researcher's *role intensiveness* and *extensiveness* – the amount of time spent in the setting and the duration of the study. Various positions on both dimensions demand certain role considerations. Spending time early to develop trust with participants may make data collection easier and quicker. On the other hand, when researchers are minimally intrusive and present for a short time, they will need to practise and find ways to build bridges and form trusting relationships quickly, as this happens in the first few minutes of an interview and is crucial for gathering good data.

The success of a qualitative study depends primarily on researchers' interpersonal skills. They need to build trust, maintain good relationships and respect norms of reciprocity, sensitively considering ethical issues. This entails an awareness of the politics of organisations, as well as sensitivity to human interactions. Researchers should not use qualitative methods if they cannot converse easily with others, be active, patient and thoughtful listeners or have an empathetic understanding of and profound respect for the perspectives of others. Researchers can undermine the quality of their data if they feel compelled to fill in silences, offer their own opinions or show off how much they know. Finally, researchers' respect and caring for participants can, if unguarded, make them lose their ability to separate themselves from any personal entanglement. Therefore, an exit strategy has to be planned and should be in place.

Qualitative data analysis

Qualitative data analysis can be seen as searching for patterns in the data and for ideas that help explain why those patterns are there in the first place. The approach taken will depend on many factors, including the epistemological position; the research question; the time available; funders' priorities; and what researchers want to get out of the data.

Data analysis strategies can be viewed on a continuum: at one end the researcher takes an objective stance and stipulates the categories in advance; at the other end are emersion strategies in which categories are not pre-fixed and which rely heavily on the researcher's intuitive and interpretive capabilities.

In qualitative studies, data collection and analysis go hand in hand to build a coherent interpretation. The researcher is guided by the initial concepts and a developing understanding that shifts and is modified as the data are collected and analysed. The overall strategy is usually closer to the interpretive/subjective end of the spectrum than the technical/objective end. The researcher should use the preliminary research questions and the related literature as guidelines for data analysis.

Analysis may involve some or all of the following stages, not necessarily in the same order:

- Transcription of tape-recorded material
- Familiarisation with the data through review, reading listening etc.
- Organisation and indexing of data for easy retrieval and identification
- Anonymising sensitive data
- Coding
- Identification of themes
- Re-coding
- Development of provisional categories
- Exploration of relationships between categories
- Refinement of themes and categories
- Development of theory and incorporation of pre-existing knowledge
- Testing of theory against data
- Report writing, including excerpts from original data if appropriate (e.g. quotes from interviews)

Although most qualitative research in nutrition and dietetics to date has been of the descriptive kind, it has been argued that qualitative research in this area should go beyond description and should present a convincing explanation of the original research question. A good example of where this has been achieved is shown in Box 10.9.

Assessing the quality of qualitative studies

The trustworthiness of qualitative data can be demonstrated by four quality criteria: transferability, dependability, conformability and credibility (Lincoln and Gaba, 1985).

Transferability refers to evidence supporting the generalisability of findings to other contexts, such as across different participants, groups, situations and so forth.

> ### Box 10.9 Example of qualitative research going beyond description and presenting a convincing explanation of the original research question
>
> Much of the research in the behaviour change literature focuses on short-term changes. The mechanisms behind sustained changes in behaviour were explored in a study by Ogden and Hills (2008) that used qualitative interviews with participants with 'success stories', including 24 who had lost weight through changes in either diet and exercise and had maintained this change for at least three years. The study found that most participants described their sustained behaviour change as being triggered by a significant life crisis relating to their health, relationships or salient milestones. Sustained behaviour change was dependent on three sustaining conditions being in place: namely, the function of the unhealthy behaviour was disrupted; the individual perceived that their choice over carrying out the unhealthy behaviour had been reduced and they adhered to a behavioural model of their problem; this initial change was then translated into sustained change. These conditions also functioned as a means of enabling a process of re-invention through a shift in identity towards a new healthier self. The authors concluded that the way in which life crisis, sustaining conditions and the process of re-invention interact determines whether or not the individual utilises the opportunity as a means to establish a new, healthier equilibrium. The life crisis offers the chance of an 'epiphany' or a time to 'see the light', and the sustaining conditions influence whether or not this opportunity translates into a shift in both behaviour and self-identity.

Transferability is enhanced by detailed descriptions that enable judgements about a fit with other contexts, comparisons across cases or other units of analysis (classrooms, schools) that yield similar findings. At the theoretical level, transferability can be achieved by evidence of theoretical transference, where the same ideas are shown to apply more widely in other fields.

Dependability is demonstrated by showing evidence that similar findings would be obtained by other researchers by showing audit trails, rich documentation and so on, as well as inter-coder/inter-observer agreement.

Conformability is shown by the researcher's self-reflections and by intentionally seeking potentially contradictory evidence predicted by alternatives, as well as through triangulation.

The *credibility* of the study can be assessed through the quality of the data, their analysis and the resultant conclusions. Qualitative analysis includes three streams of activity to evaluate credibility: data reduction (simplifying complex data by extracting re-occurring themes via coding); data display (e.g. matrices, charts, graphs, stories); and drawing conclusions and verifying them as a means of testing the validity of findings.

Some strategies that promote the trustworthiness of a study are:

- Triangulation, or multiple sources of data as evidence
- Member checks, bringing together those who provided the data to evaluate the conclusions

- Saturation, continuing data collection to the point at which more data add little to regularities that have already surfaced
- Peer review or consultation with experts
- Audit trail, the detailed record of data collection and the rationale for important decisions
- Thick descriptions, rich details of the context of the study
- Plausible alternatives, a rationale for ruling out alternative explanations and accounting for discrepant cases

10.4 Quantitative research methods

When to choose a quantitative approach

Quantitative research is a means of testing objective theories by examining the relationships among variables. These variables can typically be measured on instruments, so that the numbered data can be analysed using statistical procedures. Researchers make assumptions when testing theories deductively, building in protection against bias, controlling for alternative explanations and being able to generalise and replicate findings. Quantitative strategies include experimental and survey research.

Experimental research seeks to determine whether a specific intervention or treatment influences an outcome. The impact is assessed by providing the intervention or treatment to one group and withholding it from another, then determining how both groups scored on an outcome. Experiments include true experiments, with the random assignment of subjects to an intervention or treatment condition, and quasi-experiments, which use non-randomised and single-subject designs. See Table 10.3 for the strengths and weaknesses of experimental research.

Survey research provides a numerical description of the trends, attitudes or opinions of a population by studying a sample of that population. It includes cross-sectional and longitudinal studies using questionnaires or structured interviews for data collection, with the intent of generalising from a sample to a population. See Table 10.3 for the strengths and weaknesses of survey research.

Data collection and analysis of quantitative methods

Experimental studies

An experimental design is used to test the impact of an intervention or treatment on an outcome, controlling for all other factors that might influence that outcome. Conducting experiments allows researchers to judge whether an intervention or treatment, for example exposure to information, changes an outcome variable (e.g. perception, liking, understanding, intention to buy). In a food-choice experiment we are interested in whether the availability of health claims or the type of claims (i.e. the 'independent variable', the variable that is being manipulated) has an effect on behaviour or some other variable (i.e. the 'dependent variable', the response variable). In other words, researchers manipulate an independent variable in an experiment to observe the effect on a dependent variable such as behaviour, attitude or some other variable that is a target response.

A control group is the group of people with whom the people receiving the intervention or treatment, for example nutritional labelling, are compared; that is, it serves as a reference. The control group is similar to the experimental group except that it does not receive the experimental treatment. Experimental control allows researchers to draw conclusions about whether the

Table 10.3 Strengths and weaknesses of quantitative strategies.

Type of research	Strengths	Weaknesses
Experimental	• Often carried out in a place that can be carefully controlled. It is thus easier to estimate the true effect of the variable of interest on the outcome of interest.	• The 'external validity', i.e. the extent to which study findings can be extended beyond the data collected, can be compromised due to frequent use of non-random samples and the artificial nature of the experimental context.
Survey	• Produces data based on real-world observations (empirical data). • Breadth of coverage of many people or events means that it is more likely than some other approaches to obtain data based on a representative sample, and can therefore be generalisable to a population. • Can produce a large amount of data in a short time at a fairly low cost.	• Too much focus on the range of coverage, to the exclusion of an adequate account of the implications of those data for relevant issues, problems or theories; can have an impact on the significance of the data. • Data likely to lack detail or depth on the topic under investigation. • Difficult to achieve a high response rate, particularly when carried out by post, but also when the survey is carried out face to face or over the telephone.

independent variable caused the observed changes in the dependent variable, for instance 'Does nutrition labelling have an effect on understanding or behaviour?'

In an experiment, participants are randomly assigned to the different intervention or treatment groups or groups are balanced according to their characteristics, such as gender or psychological eating styles. This randomisation or balancing cancels out factors other than the independent and dependent variables being studied, thus making it possible to determine whether there is a cause-and-effect relationship between the dependent and independent variables.

There are two fundamental experimental designs that underpin all other, more complex designs. They differ according to the way in which they deal with the control of subject variation and include between-subject (see Box 10.10) and within-subject designs (see Box 10.11). When different people are used in the different experimental conditions, this is known as a between-subject or unrelated design, because the comparison is between the groups of subjects whose scores are unrelated. In between-subject designs the researcher compares two or more groups. When the same subjects are used in all the experimental conditions, this is known as within-subject or related design, because the comparison is within the same group of subjects, the scores from each subject being related. In this design participants are their own control group. For example, in a repeated-measures design participants are assigned to different treatments at different times during the experiments. Between- and within-subject designs can also be mixed.

A factorial design is a variation on the between-subject design that involves using two or more treatment variables to examine their independent and simultaneous effects on an outcome (Box 10.12). This will allow exploration of the effects of each treatment and the combination of treatments. For example, a 2 by 2 design can investigated the effect on intention to buy organic food of providing information (low vs regular fat content information) and type of information (front-of-package claim vs nutrition table) – the main effects – as well as the differences between whether fat information has a different impact on choices if the low-fat information is provided by a claim or a nutrition table – the interaction.

Cross-sectional surveys

Survey research designs allow for the quantitative or numerical description of variables and enable the researcher to make claims about a population, for example what percentage of the population claims to buy wholegrain food, understands what wholegrain is or

---

Box 10.10 Example of an experimental study with a between-subject design

Using self-refilling soup bowls, Wansink *et al.*, (2005) conducted a study with 54 participants examined whether visual portion size cues influenced intake volume without altering either estimated intake or satiation. A between-subject design was employed with two visibility levels – accurate visual cue of a food portion (normal bowl) vs biased visual cue (self-refilling bowl). The soup apparatus was housed in a modified restaurant-style table in which two of four bowls slowly and imperceptibly refilled as their contents were consumed. Intake volume, intake estimation, consumption monitoring and satiety were measured. Those participants unknowingly eating from self-refilling bowls ate more soup than those eating from normal soup bowls. However, despite consuming 73% more, the 'self-refilling' participants did not believe that they had consumed more, nor did they perceive themselves as more satiated than those eating from normal bowls.

Box 10.11 Example of a study with a within-subject design

Blass *et al.*, (2006) used a within-subject design to examine whether the amount of two familiar, palatable, high-density foods (pizza and macaroni and cheese) eaten was increased during a 30-minute meal consumed when watching TV. While watching a TV show of their choice, a group (n = 10) ate pizza and another (n = 10) macaroni and cheese. Television viewing increased the caloric intake of pizza and even more of macaroni and cheese. Eating patterns also differed between conditions: although the length of time to eat a slice of pizza remained stable between viewing conditions, the amount of time before starting another slice was shorter during television viewing. The rate and duration of eating macaroni and cheese were increased during television viewing.

Box 10.12 Example of a study with a factorial design

Provencher *et al.*, (2008) investigated the effects of food-related beliefs about the healthiness of foods, restrained eating and weight salience on actual food intake during an ad libitum snack used a 2 (healthy vs unhealthy) by 2 (restrained vs unrestrained eaters) by 2 (weight salient vs not salient) factorial design. The study participants were 99 female undergraduate students who were invited to taste and rate oatmeal raisin biscuits. Dietary restraint and weight salience were not found to influence the intake of biscuits, but participants ate about 35% more when the biscuit was regarded as healthy than when it was seen as unhealthy. Participants' ratings of the biscuit's 'healthiness', 'capacity to affect weight' and 'appropriateness in a healthy menu' indicated the 'healthy' manipulation to be effective. The 'weight salience' manipulation appeared to influence participants' perceptions about food differently. The restrained eaters evaluated both healthy and unhealthy snack foods more negatively when they received weight feedback before eating, whereas the unrestrained eaters made more positive food evaluations in the feedback-before-eating condition. Despite the fact that the restrained eaters were less convinced that the biscuit was good for them, as was the case when weight was made salient, they nevertheless ended up eating the same amount of food as unrestrained eaters in both the healthy and unhealthy conditions. Being 'restrained' did not prevent them from eating more of the 'healthy' biscuit.

actually uses health claims. From the sample results the researcher generalises or makes claims about the population. The survey design should address the purpose of the survey and how the data will be collected. Possible ways of collecting data include self-administered questionnaires (i.e. completed by respondents themselves), which can be completed on paper or via a computer (online survey-delivery systems can be used; see Wright (2005) for links to 20 of the more prominent packages and services, along with their web addresses), and interviews, which can be done face to face or by telephone. See Table 10.4 for an overview of the advantages and disadvantages of the various survey methods.

It is important to have a full description of the survey instrument used to collect the data. There needs to be clarity about whether it was designed specifically for the study or was a modified instrument, or an intact instrument developed by someone else. See Tables 10.5 and 10.6 for an overview of the types of questions that can be included in surveys.

Socio-demographic and psychological variables

Socio-demographic variables
The most common socio-demographic variables used in quantitative studies are gender, age, education, ethnicity, marital status, employment status, social class, actual socio-economic status and perceived socio-economic status. These variables serve to identify people and check for representativeness, but are also closely related to most outcome variables of interest in food-related behaviours. Thus, studies have to describe the outcome measure in relation to these variables or control for them when making predictions.

Psycho-social and other intervening variables
The Social Ecological Framework (Table 10.1) offers a means for understanding the levels through which people's behaviour can be influenced and the following levels can be distinguished: intrapersonal, interpersonal, community, organisational and public policy.

Psychological factors such as mood (depression, anger, anxiety), emotional eating, distorted body image, low self-esteem, poor self-efficacy dietary restraint, stress, susceptibility to external cues to eat, locus of control and stages of change are some of those that affect individuals' food-choice behaviours. These factors are typically measured by validated scales that consist of a number of verbal statements, which respondents rate along a given response scale. The articles describing the scale also explain how to construct it from single ratings when analysing the results. Some of these measures are stable over time and can be regarded as personal tendencies that can be used to segment respondents according to their responses to the scale. See Table 10.7 for examples of scales that have been used in food-choice research and Box 10.13 for an example of a study in which mood was assessed.

Table 10.4 Strengths and weaknesses of specific survey methods.

Survey type	Strengths	Weaknesses
Mail	• Easy and cost-efficient • No interviewer, respondents may be more willing to share information	• Response rates are typically low • Not appropriate for low-literacy audiences • No interviewer, respondents cannot be probed
Phone	• Large-scale accessibility in many countries • Rapid data collection, particularly with the integration of computer-assisted telephone interviewing (CATI) systems • Quality control • Anonymity • Flexibility	• Lack of visual materials • Call screening is common • Limited open-ended questions or time constraints due to more restricted survey length • Wariness • Inattentiveness
Online	• Low costs • Automation and real-time access • Less time needed • Convenience for respondents • Design flexibility, surveys can be programmed even if they are very complex • No interviewer, respondents may be more willing to share information	• Limited sampling and respondent availability • Possible cooperation problems • No interviewer, respondents cannot be probed
Face to face	• Good response rates • Longer interviews more likely to be tolerated • Attitude can be observed	• Expensive • Time-consuming • May produce a non-representative sample

Table 10.5 Types of open or partially open-ended survey questions.

Question type	Uses	Strengths	Weaknesses	Example
Open-ended questions (essay or short-answer questions)	• Explore respondents' views in depth • Identify relevant issues • Obtain a full range of responses	• Identify issues most relevant to respondents • Generate new ideas about topic • Clarify respondents' positions • Provide detail and depth	• Data analysis and summary can be complex • Data entry can be time-consuming if not collected directly from the participant • Dependent on participants' willingness and ability to articulate a response • Higher respondent burden • May generate incomplete or irrelevant data	Are you aware of any major health problems or diseases that are related to a low intake of fruit and vegetables? If yes, what diseases or health problems do you think are related to a low intake of fruit and vegetables?
Partially open-ended questions (multiple-choice questions with 'other' option)	• Ask many questions in a short time period • Assess learning or attitudes when issues are clear and identifiable • Discover relevant issues	• Enable respondents to create their own response if choices do not represent their preferred response • Fast and easy to complete • Generate new ideas about topic	• Data analysis and summary can be complex • Miss detail and depth • Prior knowledge of the topic is needed in order to develop appropriate questions and responses	Which of these best describes the other adult(s) in your household? The response options included: (1) Partner; (2) Child aged 17 or over; (3) Other adult relative; (4) Other adult (not a relative); (5) Other

Table 10.6 Different types of closed survey questions.

Question type	Uses	Strengths	Weaknesses	Example
Closed-ended questions (multiple-choice or yes/no questions)	• Many questions can be asked in a short time period • Measure knowledge or ability • Where issues are clear, learning or attitudes can be assessed	• Data analysis and summary are less complex • Easy and quick to complete • Easy to implement automated data entry	• Lack detail and depth • Preferred responses may be missing • Require moderate knowledge of the topic to write appropriate questions and responses • Response options are limited	Respondents were given a brief description of the ingredient list and nutrition label and asked whether they pay attention to each type of information. The possible answers were yes and no.
Scaled questions	• Determine the degree of an opinion, response or position	• Easy and quick to complete • Easy to implement automated data entry • More precise than dichotomous measures, e.g. yes/no; true/false	• Require moderate knowledge of the topic to write appropriate questions	When you were making food choices, how important were each of the following in determining which product you chose? The list included calories, saturated fat, trans fat, unsaturated fat, sodium. Each was asked on a 7-point importance scale.
Ranking questions	• Choose among various options • Determine the relative importance to respondents of various options	• Easy to implement automated data entry • Enable respondents to specify the relative importance of choices	• Limit number of response options • May omit a respondent's preferred answer • More difficult to answer	Purchase preference measured by having each study participant rank four brands shown (each with a different nutritional label) in the order that they would buy them if given the opportunity.

Box 10.13 Example of a study in which mood was assessed

A study conducted by McConnon *et al.*, (2013) consisting of an initial eight-week rapid weight-loss phase (800–1000 kcal/day), followed by a six-month weight-maintenance intervention with five different diets varying in protein and glycaemic index (GI) content, included measures of a range of outcomes relating to the experience of the diets in terms of acceptability, experience and mood. It employed an end-of-day questionnaire that included questions assessing the acceptability and tolerability of the weight-control programme and participants' mood, confidence in their ability to lose weight and motivation to lose weight at specific time points during the study to measure the experience of the dietary programme. Participants were asked to rate their responses on a visual analogue scale from 0 to 100 (extremes weighted at each end given in parentheses below) in relation to the following:

- How satisfying/convenient/easy to stick to/motivating/enjoyable you found the weight-loss programme (not at all/very).
- How would you rate your general mood today (very good/very bad)?
- Please rate specific aspects of your mood today on the following four scales: energy (tired/energetic), anxiety (tense/relaxed), happiness (sad/happy) and clear-headedness (dazed/clear headed).

Table 10.7 Examples of scales that have been used in food-choice research.

Psychological factors	Instrument of measurement example
Dutch Eating Behaviour Questionnaire	A validated eating behaviour scale to assess restrained, emotional and external eating behaviour
Eating self-efficacy questionnaire	Factor analysis of the 25-item scale yielded two reliable factors, one concerned with eating when experiencing negative affect and the other with eating during socially acceptable circumstances
Emotional Appetite Questionnaire	Comprises ratings of tendency to eat in response to both positive and negative emotions and situations
Food Choice Questionnaire	Measures food selection determinants
Food Neophobia Scale	Measures a person's distrust towards and avoidance of novel foods, dishes or cuisines
Impact of Weight on Quality of Life-Lite	Measures weight-specific perceived quality of life on five dimensions of daily life (physical functioning, self-esteem, sexual life, public distress and work) and also provides a summary score
Meals	Eight items measuring aspects of meal situations have been associated with better long-term weight-maintenance success
Preoccupying Cognitions	Items have been used to measure preoccupying cognitions related to weight loss and have been shown to be associated with impairments of cognitive functioning in dieters
Profile of Mood State (POMS)	Measure of affective mood state fluctuation
Regulatory Focus Questionnaire	Assesses individuals' subjective history of their health promotion and prevention success
Three Factor Eating Questionnaire	The standard instrument includes 51 Items and results in three scales: restraint, disinhibition, hunger

In addition to these variables, knowledge (understand of what a healthy diet is, awareness of the correlation between diet and disease, nutritional knowledge); beliefs (e.g. about appropriate foodstuffs, relevance of dietary advice to self); role obligations (who does food purchase, preparation, cooking etc.); and other behaviours that have an impact on eating (such as smoking, alcohol consumption, exercise) are often seen as interacting with food-choice behaviours.

Recruitment of the sample

The population from which the study sample is to be drawn must be clearly defined. Clever selection of populations with characteristics that are different from the general population in one or more aspects of lifestyle (e.g. vegetarians, organic consumers) or who have a unique history (e.g. allergy sufferers) may help to achieve the study aims by controlling for or determining exposures that are thought to influence the outcome measures.

How you select your sample will depend on the type of measurement you want to make, the nature of the population being studied, the complexity of the design and the resources available. For most sampling strategies a sampling frame is needed, which is a list of all the members of the population from which a sample can be drawn. A truly representative sample for a survey would be very expensive, hence the sample has to be restricted depending on access, which in turn has implications for the generalisability of the data (Table 10.2).

Classic sampling strategies include *simple random samples*, where each person in the sampling frame has an equal chance of being selected to be in the study. Alternatively *stratified random sampling* can be used, where the initial sample is divided into different subgroups, perhaps using census information (e.g. people who live in high-, medium- and low-income areas). Once this has been done, simple random samples may be drawn from within these strata in proportion to the known sizes of each group in the population. *Cluster sampling* procedures select a small number of cluster units from which samples are then drawn. For example, to study school children's attitude towards wholegrains, schools can be selected as clustering units. These can be selected at random and pupils within these schools sampled. Alternatively, *quota sampling* attempts to create a representative sample by specifying particular types of individuals that need to be included in the study to represent the population. For example, if only 28% of males do the family food shopping, then the sample should contain 28% males and 72% females who do regular food shopping.

When aiming not to estimate population parameters but to develop theory, it may be appropriate to sample groups of people who are most likely to provide theoretical insights. This approach should be used in qualitative studies (Glaser and Strauss, 1967) and where statistical inference is not required. When studying hard-to-reach groups or vulnerable populations, *snowball sampling* may be appropriate. Here a small number of known members of the target population are asked to introduce other members to help with the research.

Reliability and validity

Reliability, also known as reproducibility, refers to a method's ability to produce the same answer when used on different occasions under similar circumstances. To assess reliability, the measurement is repeated on the same subjects after an appropriate length of time. The time interval will depend on the assessment tool; however, it must be long enough for the subjects not to remember their answers and short enough to minimise real change. A more practical method for estimating the reliability of a test is to examine its internal consistency. This is based on the principle that each part of the test should be consistent with all other parts.

Validity refers to the ability of a method to measure what it claims to measure. There are a number of types of validity, including face validity (are the test items relevant here?), content validity (is the content of the test relevant to the characteristics being measured?), construct validity (does the instrument behave as predicted by theory?) and predictive validity (the extent to which the new measure correlates well with future values of the criterion variable). Criterion validity is how well the measure compares to a better measure of the same variable and is the type of validity that is most commonly referred to. The aim is to compare your test method with the truth; however, as the truth can often not be measured, the test method is compared to a gold standard method that is a more accurate (but not perfect) reference method (see Box 10.14 for an example). Criterion

---

Box 10.14 An example of validating a new measure, 'satisfaction with food-related life'

A measure of satisfaction with food-related life was developed by Grunert *et al.*, (2007) and tested in three studies in eight European countries. The scale was tested for reliability, temporal stability and construct validity. Five items were retained from an original pool of seven items since they exhibited good reliability as measured by Cronbach's alpha, good temporal stability, convergent validity with two related measures, and construct validity as indicated by relationships with other indicators of quality of life, including the Satisfaction With Life and SF-8 scales.

---

validity includes both predictive validity and concurrent validity (the extent to which the new measure correlates well with current values of the criterion variable).

How to analyse – some examples from studies

Data from experimental and survey studies are analysed using statistical tests. The choice of methods for statistical analyses is an important point that has to be addressed when designing the study. The researcher should know at the outset what statistical tests would be used to describe the data and to test for associations between variables. This would be informed by the hypothesis and by consideration of the tables and figures that will be used to convey information about the results. Early clarification of the analysis will help to define the characteristics of the variables to be measured (e.g. continuous or discrete) and help to avoid problems of mismatch between the types of data needed for particular analysis. Statistical software programs offer a range of analysis techniques, but it is important that the researcher is familiar with the chosen application and its interpretation.

10.5 Mixed-methods research

Mixed-methods research combines both qualitative and quantitative forms in its assumptions and approach. It does not simply consist of using both qualitative and quantitative data; it involves the use of both approaches in tandem, so that the overall strength of the study is greater than either individual approach. The three general strategies used are described in this section.

When using *sequential mixed methods*, the researcher seeks to elaborate or expand on the findings of one method with another method. For example, the study could begin with a qualitative focus group for exploratory purposes and follow this up with a survey method with a large sample, so that the researcher can generalise the results to the population. Alternatively, the study could begin with a quantitative method where a theory is tested, followed by a qualitative method involving detailed exploration with a few cases or individuals.

In *concurrent mixed methods*, the researcher merges both qualitative and quantitative data to provide a comprehensive analysis of the research problem. Here the researcher collects both forms of the data at the same time and integrates the information in the interpretation of the overall results. The researcher can also embed a smaller form of data collection within a larger data collection to analyse different types of questions (e.g. qualitative for studying the process and quantitative for the outcomes).

Transformative mixed-methods procedures are those in which the researcher uses a theoretical lens as a perspective within a design that contains both qualitative and quantitative data. The lens selects topics of interest, methods for data collection and outcomes or changes anticipated by the study. Here data collection may involve a sequential or concurrent approach.

10.6 Perspectives on the future

In the context of nutrition, food choices are often considered from the perspective of health rather than the other functions that food fulfils, including gastronomic (people eat for the pleasure of food), communication, status, power, safety and security, or magic and religion-related behaviour. Different theoretical models cite various determinants underpinning food-related behaviour. These models do not provide sufficient insight into how much influence the health motivation has on food choice or preference.

To date researchers have used a variety of models of behaviour change from a range of theories. Different models of behaviour change from a range of behavioural science theories contain similar elements and most of these models have been developed within domains other than food, so their direct applicability in explaining food choice or eating behaviour has been limited. It has been suggested that food choice and eating behaviour differ from many other behaviours in that they involve a number of many small decisions that although separately they have very little relevance, cumulatively they add up to behaviours that have a big influence on health outcome. Forcing the complexity of food-related behaviour into models that are developed in other fields of behavioural science may result in artificial actions that have no relevance in the food domain, or alternatively omit important factors.

It has been proposed by Jensen *et al.*, (2012) that in the food context, focusing on understanding the mechanisms of behaviour change is more useful than using single theories (see Table 10.8). Being able to draw on a broad range of theories linked to a particular mechanism offers better insights as to why, for example, information provision is not sufficient to increase awareness. The

Table 10.8 Behaviour change mechanisms facilitating or mitigating change and the major theories/models in which they are used.

Mechanisms affecting belief formation	Mechanisms of intention formation	Adopting and maintaining behaviour	Habit
Behaviour change mechanisms facilitating/mitigating change			
• Cognitive mechanisms: heuristics, loss aversion, framing, hyperbolic discounting, cognitive dissonance and optimistic bias	• Decisional balance • Pros and cons/cost–benefit • Attitudes • Social influences • Model learning, descriptive norms • Subjective norms, injunctive norms • Control mechanisms • (Action) self-efficacy • Perceived behavioural control	• Self-efficacy • Coping self-efficacy • Recovery self-efficacy • Mechanisms of intention formation • Planning and goal setting • Implementation intentions • Action planning • Coping planning	• Accumulated experience with behaviour • Strength of habit • Change in context factors affecting habit
Major theories/models where the behaviour change mechanism is used			
• Behavioural economics • Social psychology	• Health belief model, protection motivation theory • Rational model of man • Social cognitive theory • Theory of planned behaviour • Theory of reasoned action • Trans-theoretical model of change	• Health action process approach	• Theory of interpersonal behaviour

reasons for this can be a result of many cognitive psychological processes, including attention bias (i.e. only paying attention to messages that are considered to be personally relevant), optimistic bias (i.e. people considering themselves to be at lower risk than the average person), hyperbolic discounting (i.e. concentrating on the short-term rewards such as taste as opposed to long-term benefits such as health), as well as others that may be used to disregard the information. A mechanistic approach helps explain why some of the traditional forms of intervention such as providing information may not have been successful in changing food-related behaviour.

References and further reading

Ares, G., Giménez, A. and Gámbaro, A. (2008) Understanding consumers' perception of conventional and functional yogurts using word association and hard laddering. *Food Quality and Preference*, **19**, 636–643.

Blake, C.E., Bisogni, C.A., Sobal, J. *et al.* (2008) How adults construct evening meals: Scripts for food choice. *Appetite*, **51**, 654–662.

Blass, E.M., Anderson, D.R., Kirkorian, H.L. *et al.* (2008) On the road to obesity: Television viewing increases intake of high-density foods. *Physiology & Behavior*, **88**, 597–604.

Crabtree, B. and Miller, W. (1999) A template approach to text analysis: Developing and using codebooks. In B. Crabtree and W. Miller (eds), *Doing Qualitative Research*, Sage, Newbury Park, CA.

Creswell, J.W. (2007) *Qualitative Inquiry and Research Design: Choosing among Five Approaches*, 2nd edn. Sage, Thousand Oaks, CA.

De Vaus, D. (2001) *Research Design in Social Research*. Sage, Thousand Oaks, CA.

Draper, A. and Swift, J.A. (2011) Qualitative research in nutrition and dietetics: Data collection issues. *Journal of Human Nutrition and Dietetics*, **24**, 3–12.

Fade, S. (2004) Using interpretative phenomenological analysis for public health nutrition and dietetic research: A practical guide. *Proceedings of the Nutrition Society*, **63**, 647–653.

Fade, S.A. and Swift, J.A. (2011) Qualitative research in nutrition and dietetics: Data analysis issues, *Journal of Human Nutrition and Dietetics*, **24**, 106–114.

Fereday, J. and Cochrane-Muir, E. (2006) Demonstrating rigor using thematic analysis: A hybrid approach of inductive and deductive coding and theme development. *International Journal of Qualitative Methods*, **5**, 80–92.

Furst, T., Connors, M., Bisogni, C. *et al.* (1996) Food choice: A conceptual model of the process. *Appetite*, **26**, 247–265.

Glaser, B. (1992) *Basics of Grounded Theory Analysis*. Sociology Press, Mill Valley, CA.

Glaser, B.G. and Strauss, A.L. (1967) *The Discovery of Grounded Theory*. Aldine, New York.

Grunert, K.G., Dean, M.S., Raats, M.M. *et al.* (2007) A measure of satisfaction with food-related life. *Appetite*, **49**, 486–493.

Hollywood L.E., Cuskelly G.J., O'Brien M., *et al.* (2013) Healthful grocery shopping. Perceptions and barriers. *Appetite*, **70**, 119–126.

Jensen, B.B., Lähteenmäki, L., Grunert, K.G. *et al.* (2012) Changing micronutrient intake through (voluntary) behaviour change: The case of folate, *Appetite*, **58**, 1014–1022.

Kelley, K., Clark, B., Brown, V. and Sitzia, J. (2003) Good practice in the conduct and reporting of survey research. *International Journal of Quality in Health Care*, **15**, 261–266.

Krueger, R.A. (1994) *Focus Groups: A Practical Guide for Applied Research*. Sage, Thousand Oaks, CA.

Krueger, R.A. and Casey, M.A. (2000) *Focus Groups: A Practical Guide for Applied Research*, 3rd edn. Sage, Thousand Oaks, CA.

McConnon, A., Shepherd, R., Raats, M.M. *et al.* (2013) Experience and acceptability of diets of varying protein content and glycemic index in an obese cohort: Results from the Diogenes trial. *European Journal of Clinical Nutrition*, **67**, 990–995.

Miles, M.B. and Huberman, A.M. (1994) *Qualitative Data Analysis: An Expanded Sourcebook*. Sage, Thousand Oaks, CA.

Lampila, P., Lieshout, M. van, Gremmen, B. *et al.* (2009) Consumer attitudes towards enhanced flavonoid content in fruit. *Food Research International*, **42**, 122–129.

Moore, S.N., Murphy, S., Tapper, K. *et al.* (2010) The social, physical and temporal characteristics of primary school dining halls and their implications for children's eating behaviours. *Health Education*, **110**, 399–411.

Lincoln, Y.S. and Guba, E.G. (1985) *Naturalistic Inquiry*. Sale, Newbury Park, CA.

Ogden, J. and Hills, L. (2008) Understanding sustained behavior change: the role of life crises and the process of reinvention. *Health*, **12**, 419–437.

Patton, M.Q. (2002) *Qualitative Research and Evaluation Methods*, 3rd edn. Sage, Thousand Oaks, CA.

Provencher, V., Polivy, J. and Herman, C.P. (2009) Perceived healthiness of food. If it's healthy, you can eat more! *Appetite*, **52**, 340–344.

Roininen, K., Lähteenmäki, L. and Tuorila, H. (2000) An application of means-end chain approach to consumers' orientation to health and hedonic characteristics of foods. *Ecology of Food and Nutrition*, **39**, 61–81.

Rabiee, F. (2004) Focus-group interview and data analysis. *Proceedings of the Nutrition Society*, **63**, 655–660.

Swift, J.A. and Tischler, V. (2010) Qualitative research in nutrition and dietetics: Getting started. *Journal of Human Nutrition and Dietetics*, **23**, 559–566.

Wansink, B., Painter, J.E. and North, J. (2005) Bottomless bowls: why visual cues of portion size may influence intake. *Obesity Research*, **13**, 93–100.

Wright, K.B. (2005) Researching internet-based populations: Advantages and disadvantages of online survey research, online questionnaire authoring software packages, and web survey services. *Journal of Computer-Mediated Communication*, **10**, 3, article 11. http://jcmc.indiana.edu/vol10/issue3/wright.html (accessed June 2014).

11

Methods for Assessing Nutritional Status and Body Composition

Peter Murgatroyd,[1] Les Bluck[2] and Laura Watson[1]

[1] NIHR/Wellcome Trust Clinical Research Facility
[2] MRC Human Nutrition Research

Key messages

- Body composition assessment aims to quantify the fat, lean, water and bone mass in a body or in regions of a body.
- Measurement techniques may be optimal for measures of change in body composition, rather than absolute masses.
- Some measurements rely on calibration against a criterion method.

- Some methods lack the quality to be useful for individual assessment but work well in population studies.
- Some methods enable the flux of nutrients to and from tissues or organs to be observed and quantified.
- Some approaches help in discrimination between normal or disordered composition.

11.1 Body composition

This chapter aims to explore a range of techniques for the assessment of body composition. The concept of body composition in terms of compartments such as fat and lean will be developed. The chapter will then cover the basic anthropometric measurements, height, mass and body volume, on which many of the subsequent methodologies depend. The first compartmental measure discussed will be total body water, which may be subdivided into its intra- and extra-cellular components. Dual energy x-ray absorptiometry is a precise method for fat, lean and bone quantification, and offers both whole-body and regional analyses. The bone measurement contributes, with height, mass and volume, to multicomponent models that describe the compartmental masses. Magnetic resonance, a very versatile technique, and computed tomography will then be discussed. Next we will look at some lower-technology measurements that may contribute to an understanding of nutritional status and to lower-precision representation of body composition. These

will include muscle mass and strength, anthropometric approaches, ultrasound and bio-electrical impedance analysis. The merits and shortcomings of these approaches will be discussed, with consideration given to those that may be valuable for measurement in individuals and those that may be more appropriate in larger cohort research. Finally, consideration will be given to placing an individual's measurement in the context of reference data.

11.2 Introduction to body composition compartments

The term *body composition* may be used to describe the body from a chemical perspective, in terms of elements, molecules and compounds, from a tissue and organ perspective, or in terms of compartments defined by their physical characteristics and functions. While there is some overlap between these descriptive approaches, the most widely applied methodologies discriminate between fat, lean, bone mineral and fluid spaces.

Nutrition Research Methodologies, First Edition. Edited by Julie A Lovegrove, Leanne Hodson, Sangita Sharma and Susan A Lanham-New.
© 2015 John Wiley & Sons, Ltd. Published 2015 by John Wiley & Sons, Ltd.
Companion Website: www.wiley.com/go/nutritionsociety

From a nutritional perspective these compartments arguably hold most interest. Fat, for example, is the primary energy store and may be found in excess, as in obesity, or may be depleted, as in anorexia or malnutrition. Bone mass may be compromised by deficiencies in calcium or vitamin D. In a broader context, body composition measurements can be characteristic of clinical disorders and contribute to the description of phenotypes. The balance between fat and lean compartments may be atypical, as in some thyroid hormone disorders. Fat storage may be compromised, as in disorders such as severe insulin resistance and in lipodystrophy. A notable, nutritionally important omission from the list of primary compartments is glycogen, which may be stored in liver and muscle. Its diffuse distribution makes it challenging to quantify in mass terms, although its flux can be estimated, as we shall see.

Some measurement methodologies do not separate all the compartments, but may combine lean with water as lean body mass (LBM), or combine all but fat into a single compartment, referred to as fat-free mass (FFM). These combinations reduce the number of discrete compartments to three or two respectively.

Though measurements of total body composition may be valuable, insight into regional distribution may be more so, in some instances in the context of a specific tissue or organ such as liver or skeletal muscle. Water, for example, may be partitioned into intra- and extra-cellular spaces; fat may be subcompartmented into depots such as subcutaneous, intra-muscular, intra-myocellular, visceral and hepatic and its distribution between legs, arms, trunk and so on may also be explored. Many of these subcompartments again have clinical relevance and atypical or ectopic distribution may be characteristic of a range of disorders, as for example in the fatty liver diseases.

11.3 A word about accuracy, precision and limits of agreement

A feature of body composition measurement is the difficulty of determining the absolute accuracy of methods. The characteristics of tissue compartments such as fat and lean used in their measurement are heavily dependent on properties determined by cadaver analysis, and reported cadaver analyses are understandably rather few in number. In practice, a four-component model describing fat or lean mass in terms of body mass, body volume, total body water and bone mass is most usually taken as the criterion against which to assess the absolute accuracy of other methodologies (see Section 11.11). The limits of agreement between this and other methods are often investigated by the Bland–Altman approach, in which neither of the pair of methods being compared is assumed to be superior.

Fortunately, in a nutritional or clinical context absolute accuracy is not always crucial to measurement. The predominant requirements are most commonly either to detect *changes* within an individual or group, or to identify *differences* between groups or between health and disease. Detection of changes and differences is much more dependent on the precision of methods (which may be deduced from analysis of repeated measures) than on their accuracy. In the subsequent methodological descriptions in this chapter the discussion of quality will therefore focus on precision.

It may be worth mentioning here that one methodology stands out when it comes to validating approaches to quantifying changes in total body fat mass. The work of Susan Jebb and colleagues has shown that dietary manipulation over a 12-day period within a whole-body calorimeter can induce changes in composition large enough to be measurable by the better methods discussed here, it can measure these changes with high accuracy, and it can do so with a precision that is at least five times better than comparator methods. In this way the properties of underwater weighing, deuterium dilution, three-component models and skinfold measurement for detecting changes have been explored. It is perhaps regrettable that this approach has not been revisited since the introduction of dual-energy x-ray absorptiometry, air displacement plethysmography, magnetic resonance and impedance methodologies.

11.4 Stature

Measurement of stature (height) forms part of anthropometric assessment and is a parameter in some body composition measurements. The measurement is best performed with a purpose-designed stadiometer, which should be checked regularly for accuracy against an independent standard. The subject should be lightly clad and should stand in bare feet with heels, back and head against the stadiometer, and eyes horizontal. Two measures should be taken, with repositioning of the subject, to confirm the reliability of the measurements, and a third taken if the first two differ by 2 cm or more. Consistency in measurements repeated on different occasions is best achieved by standardising the time of day for all repeat measures. When the difference between repeats is greater than 2 cm, there should be concern about measurement error or poor technique.

11.5 Body mass

Measurement of total body mass underpins most body composition measurement techniques. Technically, mass represents the quantity of matter, and is expressed in kilograms (kg). Most weighing scales measure *weight* through the action of gravity on mass, but are calibrated in kg mass units. Guidance notes for specifying clinical weighing scales recommend scale intervals as broad as 100 g for adults, even where mass measurement is critical to treatment, hence it is rare to find clinic scales that are better than this. For body composition investigations, particularly where changes in composition are of interest, better mass resolution may be beneficial. Masses of 300 kg may be resolved to 10 g or less by an industrial platform scale. Some scales are able to show an average reading taken over a few seconds, thus suppressing the effect of movement on the displayed reading. This is a valuable feature that may repay the additional investment through higher measurement quality. Further improvements in measurement quality can be achieved by weighing the subject in an overnight-fasted, voided state and wearing night clothes or a gown. Later these clothes may be independently weighed and the subject's naked mass derived.

11.6 Body volume

Underwater weighing (UWW)

Measurement of body volume has traditionally been performed by water displacement, an approach that dates from the time of Archimedes, who demonstrated that the apparent loss of weight (mass is unchanged) of an immersed body is equal to the weight of the water displaced. As 1 kg of water occupies close to 1 litre, it follows that, for a *totally* immersed body, the apparent loss of weight equates to its volume. In practice a person usually has positive buoyancy, so the subject must wear supplementary diving weights of known immersed weight w_s to ensure total immersion.

The weight of water w_d displaced by the subject can then be expressed as:

$$w_d = w_a - w_w + w_s$$

where w_a is the subject's weight in air and w_w the weight when immersed.

The volume V is found as w_d/ρ_w, where ρ_w is the density of water at the experimental temperature (typically 0.9957 at a comfortable water temperature of 30 °C). Thus:

$$V = \frac{w_a - w_w + w_s}{\rho_w}$$

This is the gross body volume, which includes the volumes of supplementary weights, air in the lungs and gas in the gut. The latter is usually assumed to be 100 ml, and can be minimised if the subject is fully voided prior

to the measurement. Lung volume is ideally measured at the time the immersed weight is recorded. The residual lung volume may be measured by helium dilution. To do this, a spirometer is prepared by filling to a volume (typically 5 litres) with oxygen and adding a further volume (typically 1 litre) of helium to give a total volume V_s. The resulting mixture is sampled by a helium analyser and its concentration of helium h_o is recorded. During immersion, the subject breathes through a mouthpiece and tube of volume V_t. At the time of weight recording, the subject fully expires and the tube is coupled to the spirometer, from which the subject breathes the helium–oxygen mixture until a new steady concentration of helium h_i is recorded. Carbon dioxide produced by the subject is absorbed and oxygen is replaced as it is consumed, so the initial volume of the spirometer is restored at the end of each expiration. The subject's residual lung volume V_r may then be expressed as:

$$V_r = \left(\frac{h_o}{h_i} - 1\right)V_s - V_t$$

The precision of repeated body volume estimates is typically 0.15 l.

An underwater weighing system may take a number of forms. Some systems adopt vertical immersion, lowering the subject into a tank on a chair suspended from a cable incorporating a tension measurement instrument. Others put the immersion process in the control of the subject, by asking them to lean forwards or backwards into the water while sitting on an immersed platform suspended from load cells. Whatever the design, there will be subjects for whom immersion is not easy or well tolerated and so alternative approaches to volume measurement have been developed. It is also worth noting that in the interests of hygiene it may be advisable to change the water and clean the tank between subjects.

Air displacement plethysmography (ADP)

Air displacement offers one alternative to water displacement for body volume estimation. The BOD POD® is a commercial implementation of this (Cosmed, Rome, Italy). The adult version is described in this section and a smaller version, the PEA POD, is available for neonatal measurements.

The BOD POD consists of two chambers, a large front measurement chamber accessible to the subject and a smaller reference chamber of fixed volume, separated from the measurement chamber by an electronically driven diaphragm – see Figure 11.1. The diaphragm oscillates, causing small, equal-amplitude fluctuations in the volumes of the chambers. These induce pressure

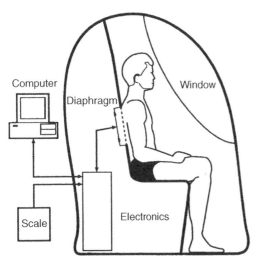

General arrangement of chambers, subject, and diaphragm.

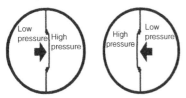

Moving diaphragm produces complementary
pressure changes in the chambers.

Figure 11.1 Schematic diagram of the BOD POD. By courtesy of
COSMED and reproduced with permission.

oscillations such that the ratio of the front to rear pressure
amplitudes is inversely proportional to the ratio of the
respective chamber volumes. The instrument is
calibrated with a standard cylinder of 100 l volume, so
that the change in pressure ratio resulting from this can
be compared to that induced by a subject, thus enabling
the subject's volume to be expressed in terms of the
standard.

This simple theoretical principle becomes more
complex in practice. Throughout most of the system
the pressure and volume changes occur adiabatically –
that is, without the exchange of heat. However, the
system software must correct for surface area effects
where the pressure–volume relationship is isothermal
rather than adiabatic, around the subject's body and
the chamber walls. The isothermal region around the
subject is minimised by reducing clothing to a minimum (e.g. swimwear) and compressing the hair in a
bathing cap.

Lung volume is not directly measured during the body
volume measurement procedure. The body volume
measurement may be expected to take account of lung
volume, but in practice this is isothermal space and

so needs separate consideration, either through prior
independent measurement or alternatively by assignment
of a value estimated from height and body mass. As lung
volume is an isothermal space there is some tolerance of
errors in its estimation; only 40% of an error in lung
volume estimation propagates to the body volume
measurement.

BOD POD measurement is generally better tolerated
and quicker than underwater weighing and is suitable for
subjects up to 225 kg body mass. The measurement
procedure incorporates a body mass measurement so
that body fat and lean content may be calculated by a
two-component model such as that described by Siri,
described later in this chapter. The precision of repeated
measures of body volume by ADP is similar to UWW, in
the order of 0.15 l.

Photonic scanning

Photonic scanning is a recent novel approach to the
estimation of body volume. A three-dimensional image
of the body is generated from reflections of multiple
sources of light in the near infra-red region. Body volume
is computed from the image. Lung volume must also be
measured or estimated and deducted from the superficial
volume. In contrast to ADP, there is no attenuation of
errors in the lung volume estimate. Validation against
UWW and ADP suggests that the average bias in
estimation of body volume by photonic scanning is
small, but that its precision is only half as good: 0.3 l
compared to 0.15 l for ADP.

11.7 Total body water by deuterium dilution

The mass of water within the body may be estimated by
measuring the dilution of a known mass of a tracer into
the body water pool. The most commonly used tracer is
water itself, labelled by enrichment in deuterium (^{2}H), a
stable isotope of hydrogen (^{1}H) with a neutron in its
nucleus. The ratio of deuterium to hydrogen in water
may be determined by mass spectrometry or Fourier
transform infra-red spectrometry (FTIR).

Prior to dosing with labelled water, a sample of body
fluid is taken for baseline ratio analysis, as deuterium is
naturally present in water at an atomic concentration of
about 150 parts per million (ppm) of hydrogen. Body
water may be sampled as urine, blood or saliva – the latter is particularly convenient to collect. The tracer dose is
usually given as a drink containing a known amount of
deuterated water. The dose is typically prescribed as
0.1 g/kg body mass for mass spectrometric analysis or
0.4 g/kg for FTIR. Further samples of body fluid are

taken for ^2H:^1H ratio analysis, usually at 3, 4 and 5 hours post dose. The aim of sample timing is to identify the highest ^2H concentration in body water following absorption of the dose, before the concentration falls again due to dilution by further water, be it produced by metabolism or ingested. An adjustment is made to account for the 4% higher distribution space of ^2H relative to total body water. This is due to exchange of ^2H with non-aqueous hydrogen.

While this section has focused on deuterium dilution, ^{18}O labelled water may also be used as the tracer. The procedure is very similar to that for ^2H dilution, though the dilution space adjustment may be smaller. The cost of ^{18}O labelled water may be higher than for deuterated, but analytical costs may be lower. The precision achievable in total body water estimate is in the region of 0.7% of TBW, or roughly 0.4% of body mass.

11.8 Intra-cellular water by ^{40}K counting

Total body water is distributed between the fluids inside and outside cells. Intra-cellular fluid is characterised by its potassium content. The body contains typically 3500 mmol of potassium with around 98% in cells, where it has a concentration close to 150 mmol/l. Potassium has a naturally occurring radioactive isotope ^{40}K with 0.012% abundance. Its half-life is exceptionally long (1.2×10^9 years), but the 1.46 MeV gamma radiation from its decay may be measured in a whole-body counter. From its decay rate and the intra-cellular potassium concentration, intra-cellular fluid volume may be deduced. The precision of total body potassium (TBK) estimates has been estimated as 1.5–2.3%. As intra-cellular volume reflects cell mass, lean mass may be inferred from TBK and fat mass derived by difference from body mass. Whole-body counters are uncommon and so this methodology may not be generally applicable.

11.9 Extra-cellular water by sodium bromide dilution

Extra-cellular fluid is more easily quantified by a tracer-dilution approach. Sodium bromide is usually the tracer of choice, as bromide ions remain predominantly in the extra-cellular space. Two samples of extra-cellular fluid (plasma) are required, one prior to bromide administration and a second 3 hours after administration of 5 g of 4 mol/l sodium bromide

solution as a drink. Sodium bromide concentrations are analysed in each and the extra-cellular water in g is calculated as:

$$ECW = D \times \left(\frac{C_{dose}}{C_{p2} - C_{p1}} \right) \times 0.9 \times 0.95$$

where D is the dose in g, C is concentration in mmol/l; p1 indicates pre-dose and p2 post-dose sample. The constant 0.9 is a correction for intra-cellular bromide and 0.95 is the Gibbs–Donnan equilibrium factor. Correction may also be made for bromide lost to urine between dosing and sampling. Estimation of extra-cellular water space by bromide dilution has an estimated precision of around 3%.

Bromide is eliminated slowly, so sodium bromide may not be the ideal tracer when measurements must be repeated within a day or two. Inulin has been explored as an alternative tracer to overcome this, but it must be administered by injection or infusion.

11.10 Fat, lean and bone mass by dual-energy x-ray absorptiometry

Principle of measurement

Dual-energy x-ray absorptiometry (DXA) was initially developed to measure bone density, for example in the femoral head or lumbar spine, but is equally effective for the measurement of fat and lean mass and its distribution in the whole body. The principle of DXA measurement, in somewhat simplified form, is as follows. An x-ray beam with two energy spectra (analogous to the light of two colours) is passed through the body towards a detector. Between the source and the detector, body tissues absorb some of the x-ray. The attenuation of the x-ray is proportional to the absorption coefficient μ, which is both tissue and energy specific, and to the tissue path length d. In the case of two tissues, for example fat and lean, each having a characteristic absorption coefficient, the absorbance A may be described at each of the energies as:

$$A_1 \propto d_f \mu_{f1} + d_l \mu_{l1}$$
$$A_2 \propto d_f \mu_{f2} + d_l \mu_{l2}$$

where 1 and 2 represent the energies and f and l represent fat and lean. These expressions are solved by the instrument software to disclose the depths of the respective tissues. The instrument scans the whole body or a subregion to build up a two-dimensional image over which the tissue depths are calculated and integrated to give volumes and subsequently reported in mass units (g, kg). As these two expressions only solve for two unknowns, when bone is detected within the x-ray field it becomes one of the analysed tissues, and soft tissue above and below the bone is treated as the second, being assigned absorption coefficients derived from adjacent fat and lean measurements.

Early DXA instruments employed a narrow 'pencil' x-ray beam. This resulted in rather long total body scan times (20–40 minutes for a whole body). More recent instruments have fan-shaped beams that enable whole-body scan times to be reduced to 5–10 minutes. Scan times of hips and spines for bone density analysis are shorter still. Image resolution has also been improved several fold. The benefit of higher resolution and smaller pixel size is improved measurement precision, particularly in the trunk where spaces between ribs may be comparable with the pixel size of low-resolution instruments. Precision derived from the standard deviation (SD) of repeated measures of total body fat and lean mass has been reported as around 900 g in both pencil and narrow fan beam instruments prior to recent resolution enhancements offered by the GE Lunar iDXA. These have seen reported precision improved more than threefold to 250 g in fat mass and 200 g in lean mass, so that precision is now comparable with that of quantitative magnetic resonance methodology and has roughly twice the power of multicomponent models to detect changes in body composition (see later in this chapter). Agreements between whole-body DXA estimates of fat and lean mass and those of the four-component criterion method (Section 11.11) are generally excellent. Examples of DXA whole-body soft tissue images for a male and a female subject are shown in Figure 11.2. The lines in the figure mark the boundaries of standard subregions for which results are reported. Custom regions may also be defined by the investigator.

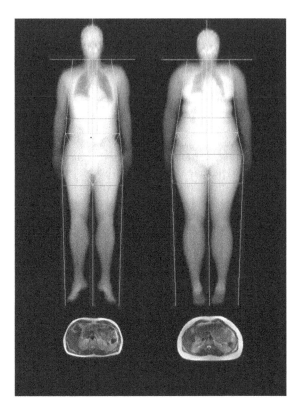

Figure 11.2 Whole-body images of soft tissue made by dual energy x-ray absorptiometry (DXA). On the left is an image of a male subject of 84 kg body weight and on the right a female of body weight 74 kg. Below the DXA images are images of a transverse slice though the abdomen at the level of the fourth lumber vertebra made by magnetic resonance imaging (MRI).

Ionising radiation

DXA involves exposure to ionising radiation. The risks associated with this are related to the effective dose, a measure that is weighted to take account of the sensitivity of different organs and tissues to radiation. The effective dose is expressed in micro Sieverts (µSv) and may be considered in the context of natural background exposure, which typically lies between 4 and 10 µSv/day depending on geographical location. Pencil and earlier narrow fan beam instruments incur a typical effective dose in the range 0.2–0.4 µSv. This may be an order of magnitude greater for whole-body measurements made with wide fan beam and for more recent high-resolution narrow fan beam instruments. Regional scans for bone density are at much higher resolution than those of the

total body and so incur an effective radiation dose that is higher by a factor of 2 to 10 than for the whole body. Even so, the highest doses are comparable to just one day's natural background radiation.

11.11 Multicomponent models of body composition

The masses of the body composition compartments introduced in Section 11.2 may be derived from the measurements described in Sections 11.4–11.10. Underpinning the derivations, which will be explored in this section, are physical characteristics of the body and its tissues that have been deduced from careful analysis of cadavers and animal carcases. These are presented in Table 11.1. Most are the values adopted in the work of Siri, who published derivations of multicomponent models in 1956 and 1961. Other authors suggest slightly different values, particularly for bone mass.

Table 11.1 Characteristics of tissue compartments.

Tissue compartment	Property	Symbol	Value
Fat	Density	ρ_F	0.900 kg l^{-1}
Fat-free body	Density	ρ_{FF}	1.100 kg l^{-1}
Protein (dry lean mass)	Density	ρ_P	1.340 kg l^{-1}
Bone mineral	Density	ρ_M	3.000 kg l^{-1}
Protein + mineral	Density	ρ_{PM}	1.564 kg l^{-1}
Water	Density	ρ_w	0.993 kg l^{-1}
Fat-free body	Hydration by mass		73 %

Body mass and body volume

Body mass (BM) may be compartmented into fat mass (FM) and fat-free mass by a two-component model using body mass and body volume (BV). The densities (mass/volume) of fat ρ_F and fat-free ρ_{FF} compartments differ (see Table 11.1) and so fat mass may be expressed as:

$$FM = \frac{\rho_F}{\rho_{FF} - \rho_F}\left(BV\rho_{FF} - BM\right)$$

or, inserting densities from Table 11.1:

$$FM = 4.95\,BV - 4.50\,BM$$

This expression derives from the work of Siri, published in 1956. Fat-free mass may be deduced by subtracting fat mass from body mass. The model performs well in healthy adults, but underlying it is an assumption that the components of the fat-free body (protein, mineral and water) are in a simple fixed relationship – an assumption to which many exceptions may be conceived. The precision of the fat estimate is primarily limited by the precision of the body volume estimates and is around 0.7 kg when body volume is measured by UWW or ADP. Bias may arise in estimating fat mass changes during longitudinal studies if bone mineral mass does not change at the same rate as other components of the fat-free compartment.

Body mass and total body water

Fat-free mass may be deduced from total body water and the hydration factor for the fat-free body (Table 11.1) as:

$$FFM = \frac{TBW}{0.73}$$

Fat mass is thus:

$$FM = BM - \frac{TBW}{0.73}$$

Note that the hydration factor 0.73 has some associated uncertainty – the literature suggests that it is higher in children, in pregnancy and in patients with oedema or ascites. The precision is limited by that of the TBW methodology and is about 0.5 kg fat. Again, bias may arise during longitudinal studies if bone mineral mass does not change at the same rate as other components of the fat-free compartment.

Body mass, body volume and total body water

When fat mass is estimated from body mass, body volume and total body water combined in a three-component model, the assumed relationship between water, protein and mineral masses in the fat-free body, underlying two-component models, is reduced to one between protein and mineral mass, assigned density ρ_{PM}. Thus the estimation of fat mass is less susceptible to uncertainty in the hydration of lean tissue. The expression for fat mass becomes:

$$FM = \frac{\rho_F}{\rho_{PM} - \rho_F}\left(\rho_{PM}BV - \frac{\rho_{PM} - \rho_W}{\rho_W}TBW - BM\right)$$

or, inserting the densities from Table 11.1:

$$FM = 2.119\,BV - 0.799\,TBW - 1.355\,BM$$

Precision is roughly equally limited by volume and water measurements to 0.5 kg fat.

Body mass, body volume, bone mass and total body water

The remaining compartment combination, between protein and mineral mass, may be resolved if a measure of bone mineral mass M_{Bone} is incorporated into the model. Although this was not possible at the time of Siri's work, it is now quite practical through the development of DXA. The resulting four-component model has become a reference against which the measurements of other methodologies are compared, and in some cases standardised. This is because the model reduces the potential for bias that may arise when assuming protein, water and bone proportions in the lean or fat-free body. This model, based on the values in Table 11.1, describes fat mass as:

$$FM = 2.741\,BV - 0.715\,TBW - 2.045\,BM + 1.132\,M_{Bone}$$

The similarity between the coefficients here and for the three-component expression will be apparent and so the precision of fat mass estimates is similar too. Note that in both the three- and four-component expressions the coefficients of mass quantities are dimensionless, but those for volume have the dimensions of density, mass/volume.

When the aim is to measure changes in fat mass over intervals when bone mass is unlikely to change significantly, it is arguably preferable to derive an expression for the change that assumes constant bone mass. This is because the DXA measurements have some repeated-measures variability (SD in the order of 50 g), which may serve to reduce the precision of the compartmental change estimate a little without contributing any improvement in its accuracy.

11.12 Magnetic resonance

Elements with an odd number of protons, neutrons or both have spin and an associated nuclear magnetic moment. When placed in a magnetic field, the spins of the elemental nuclei align with the field. A pulse of energy at an appropriate radio frequency may displace the spin, and as the original spin state is re-established a signal is emitted at the resonant frequency characteristic of the atom. This frequency is proportional to the magnetic field strength, and may be influenced, through the shielding effect of electrons, by the chemical environment in which the atom is bonded – a phenomenon known as chemical shift. Thus the emitted signal is able to represent both an element and its bonding within a compound. The relaxation of the excited element as it returns to its quiescent state may also be characterised by two time constants, T1 and T2, which can be reflective of the chemical environment of the element. Elements that exhibit magnetic resonance and are of particular interest in a nutritional context include hydrogen, phosphorus and the naturally occurring stable isotope of carbon, ^{13}C (1.1% natural abundance).

Participants who have implanted metallic materials or electronic devices may be excluded from magnetic resonance investigations. The risks of magnetic materials derive in part from the forces exerted on them by the external field. However, all conductors are susceptible to induction of currents by the radio frequency fields. These may result in the generation of considerable heat. Any endogenous metal may have an impact on image or analysis quality through distortion of the magnetic field.

Quantitative magnetic resonance (QMR)

QMR associates protons with their specific chemical environments, such as lipid, on the basis of their relaxation time constants and so is able to determine the quantity of lipid in a sample. QMR instruments are often designed to operate at relatively low magnetic field strengths established by permanent magnets or room-temperature electromagnets. QMR has been applied, at one extreme, to quantify fat in food samples and in unanaesthetised small animals. At the other extreme, it may be used to quantify total body fat mass in humans. QMR does not generate images or analyse subregions within a body or sample. In the human application, QMR has particular merits. It is calibrated against a true lipid tissue substitute (phantom) in the form of rapeseed oil. The measurement is quick (around 5 minutes), comfortable and can accommodate subjects up to 250 kg. Most importantly, the precision of repeated measurements is very high, though there has been discussion about the technique's absolute accuracy. The standard deviation of repeated measures has been reported as 250 g, offering the potential to detect changes of 350 g in fat mass ($\sqrt{2} \times 250$ g). This implies that it has twice the power of multicomponent models to detect changes in body composition.

Magnetic resonance imaging (MRI)

MRI employs the principles described previously to generate high-resolution images. It uses a superconducting electromagnet to generate a high field strength. The spatial information is achieved by introducing additional magnetic fields during a scan so that the signal detected at any time is restricted to a defined region of interest. Image detail may be further enhanced by introducing contrast media, for example to highlight blood vessels. Soft tissue images from MRI can be particularly detailed and yield clear discrimination between adipose tissue and other surrounding tissues and structures. The images are intrinsically greyscale in nature, but image processing may enhance tissue discrimination by the use of colours and may report cross-sectional areas and volumes of tissues and organs.

MRI is an expensive procedure, but is able to offer information on the spatial distribution of tissues within the body that is hard to rival by any other method with the exception of CT (see Section 11.13) and does so without the radiation exposure associated with CT. Images are presented as cross-sectional slices at a defined region of interest. This may be, for example, the abdomen, where a cross-section helps the viewer to visualise and quantify visceral and subcutaneous adipose tissue (Figure 11.2). By acquiring multiple transaxial slice images along the whole body, cross-sectional areas of tissue may be integrated to give regional and total body volumes. Repeated observations allow investigation of depot-specific responses to the passage of time or to weight-modifying interventions.

Magnetic resonance spectroscopy (MRS)

MRS has become one of the most valued tools for *in vivo* investigation of metabolic processes in health and disorders. Its particular value lies in its ability to reveal the relative concentrations of metabolites in localised tissue or organ regions. This methodology can use imaging to identify the location of interest or, when the MR signal is smaller, such as in phosphorus and carbon-13 MRS, a larger volume can be acquired by using a coil, which is placed on the surface of the body to focus MR excitation and signal detection on that location. The detected signal may be displayed as a spectrum showing signal amplitude against chemical shift referenced to a standard, so a range of compounds may be seen through a single test – see Figure 11.3. In this example, the method employs proton (hydrogen) spectroscopy to compare the area under the methylene group spectral peak in lipid to a reference peak from water in a region localised in the liver, thus quantifying hepatic lipid. When the resonance is in phosphorus, metabolites such as phosphocreatine, adenosine triphosphate and inorganic phosphate are visible in the spectrum, and also it permits ATP turnover to be investigated.

The methodology gains further power when natural abundance ^{13}C is measured, as may be seen in the next section on glycogen. ^{13}C may also be administered, at levels well above natural abundance, to label nutrients such as glucose, so the fate of an ingested nutrient may be followed through its storage in and subsequent mobilisation from liver or muscle. Unfortunately, this latter approach carries all the expense of MRI, compounded by the cost of ^{13}C labelled compounds and the specialised ^{13}C coils, but it does open up options for *in vivo* investigation that would be hard to achieve by any other methodology.

Glycogen measurement by natural abundance (^{13}C MRS)

Glycogen is a compartment of nutritional interest in that it represents an energy store whose total capacity equates to roughly one day's total energy requirement and provides a buffer in the regulation of glucose homeostasis. The major glycogen depots are in liver and muscle – typically 100 g and 500 g respectively in adults.

Measurement of glycogen concentration has classically required chemical analysis of biopsy samples. However, MRS methodology has been validated against this and now offers a non-invasive alternative. This approach measures the magnitude (area under curve) of glycogen's ^{13}C spectral signal arising from the 1.1% natural abundance of this isotope of carbon. The method is effective in estimating glycogen fluxes to and from individual muscles or groups and may also be applied to the estimation of hepatic glycogen concentration. Changes in glycogen concentration in response to depletion, for example by exercise, or to dietary intervention may be followed by repeated MRS observations.

11.13 Computed tomography (CT)

CT is an x-ray imaging technique. An x-ray source projects across the diameter of a circular opening towards a detector at the opposite side. The body of the subject under investigation passes through the opening. The source and detector rotate around the opening so that the absorption of x-ray may be determined at all angles. From the absorption data a cross-sectional image slice is constructed. As with MRI (see the previous section), the subject may be moved through the opening so that three-dimensional images may be constructed from multiple slices. The image-processing principles have much in common with those described for MRI.

In most circumstances MRI would be the imaging method of preference over CT due to its freedom from ionising radiation. There are, however, two potential advantages to CT. One is its image acquisition speed, which may lead to clearer images in regions where respiration induces movements. The second is that it may be combined with positron emission tomography (PET), as in recent studies to detect brown adipose tissue. However

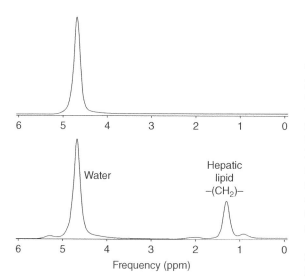

Figure 11.3 Proton magnetic resonance spectroscopy spectra for healthy (upper) and fatty (lower) livers. The water peak is at 4.7 ppm and the methylene peak –(CH$_2$)– of lipid is at 1.3 ppm. The lipid is barely visible in the upper trace – it is typically 1% of the water peak in health. Images by courtesy of Dr Alison Sleigh.

in this, as in most applications of CT to human research, radiation exposure limits the value of the technique by reducing or eliminating the prospect of longitudinal repeat observations.

11.14 Muscle mass

An evaluation of skeletal muscle mass may be made by measuring the rate of loss of creatinine, a metabolite of creatine, in urine. Creatine may be ingested in the diet and may be synthesised in liver and kidneys. It is transported to skeletal muscle where, as creatine phosphate, it contributes to cellular energy supply through the formation of ATP. Roughly 95% of creatine is found in skeletal muscle, where the creatine pool size primarily reflects muscle mass, though with some residual dependence on dietary intake. Regardless of pool size, close to 1.7% of the creatine pool is eliminated as urinary creatinine each day. Thus the rate of creatinine excretion may be used to estimate the creatine pool size and to infer muscle mass. Dietary creatine may contribute to creatinine excretion and so must be taken into account or minimised.

The expression:

$$SM = k \times Cr$$

describes the relationship between skeletal muscle SM mass in kg and creatinine excretion Cr in g per 24 hours. A range of values for the constant k has been proposed, extending from 16–18 kg/g for ad libitum diets where some creatinine derives from the diet to 18.6–20 kg/g on meat-free diets. More recent validations against skeletal muscle mass determined from multiscan computed axial tomography (CT) following a week-long meat-free diet have suggested that the value of k should be 21.8. A slight improvement in the relationship was found by allowing an intercept such that:

$$SM = 18.9 \times Cr + 4.1$$

The protocol averaged creatinine excretion over 3 days to derive the value for Cr in g/24 hours.

An advantage of this methodology is that it incurs a relatively low cost and requires minimal investment in equipment, as it requires only a single creatinine assay, available in most hospital biochemistry laboratories.

11.15 Muscle strength

Under-nutrition may result in protein loss from muscle, with associated loss of function reflected in muscle strength. Assessment of nutritional status may therefore include tests of muscle function, the most common of which is hand-grip strength.

Grip strength is measured using a hand-grip dynamometer, many of which are commercially available. Traditionally the test outcome was displayed by a pointer on an analogue scale, though digital displays now predominate. It is important to adjust the dynamometer to the size of hand prior to testing.

The measurement is usually displayed in kilograms force. Typical grip strength in healthy males is around 40–50 kg and in females 20–30 kg, though it may differ between dominant and non-dominant arms and tends to decline in later years. A literature search will reveal several protocols for hand-grip dynamometry that may differ in the posture, timing and number of test repeats contributing to the assessment. There are many other forms of muscle strength test available. Some, such as the Rotterdam Intrinsic Hand Myometer, enable specific muscle groups within the hand to be tested; others, such as isokinetic dynamometry, enable leg or back muscle strength to be assessed.

11.16 Anthropometric indicators of adiposity and nutritional status

A number of assessments have been developed to relate adiposity and lean mass to anthropometric measurements. These commonly include body mass index, skinfold measurement and waist and hip circumferences. To provide estimates of compartment mass they generally require calibration against a reference method such as has been described in this chapter, and their accuracy and precision are inferior to these.

Body mass index

Body mass index (BMI) derives from the work of the nineteenth-century Belgian mathematician Adolphe Quetelet. It aims to reflect adiposity by expressing body mass in a way that is independent of stature.

BMI is calculated as:

$$BMI = \frac{BM}{H^2}$$

where BM is body mass in kilograms and H is stature in metres.

BMI is widely used for classifying individuals into groups associated with weight-related health risk, as in Table 11.2.

Table 11.2 Classification of weight on the basis of body mass index (BMI).

Group	Underweight	Normal	Overweight	Obese
BMI range	< 18.5	18.5–25	25–30	> 30

Variations in body mass are not solely dependent on adiposity, so BMI-based predictions of body composition compartments such as fat mass are rather poor. When the fat mass of metabolically healthy subjects measured by DXA is regressed on BMI a linear relationship is found, but the standard deviation of residuals is rather high, around 3.2 kg, suggesting that BMI is a poor proxy for fat mass in individuals – see Figures 11.4a and 11.4b. Even so, BMI is often used to assign nutrition research study participants into 'normal' and 'overweight' groups, though there is a real prospect of crossover in the fat masses of groups selected in this way, as may be judged from the figure. A better approach would be to make group assignments on the basis of measured composition.

Waist and hip circumference

Each of waist circumference alone, waist–hip ratio or waist–height ratio offers a predictive association with cardiovascular and metabolic disease through its representation of central or visceral adiposity.

Protocols for the measurement of waist and hip circumferences have been described by the World Health Organization (WHO). Briefly, with the subject standing in a relaxed posture with feet together, the waist circumference is measured at the midpoint between the lower margin of the last palpable rib and the top of the iliac crest. Hip circumference is measured around the widest portion of the buttocks. Measurements should be made at the end of normal expiration. The tape should be parallel to the floor and tension adjusted for a snug fit without compression of body tissues. Measurements are recorded in centimetres. Measurements should be repeated, and a third taken if the first two measurements differ by 2 cm or more. If it is necessary to make measurements over clothing, clothing thickness should be minimised and standardised between visits and pockets should be emptied.

Neck circumference

The risk of developing obstructive sleep apnoea increases with excess weight. Neck circumference is also associated with sleep apnoea and so its measurement may have a place in any study that aims to improve the condition through a weight-loss intervention. Neck

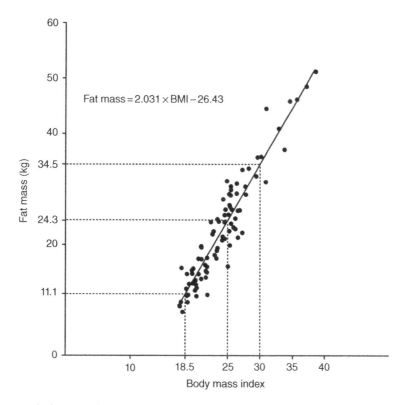

Figure 11.4a Fat mass vs body mass index (BMI) plotted for 89 healthy female subjects. Fat mass data are from dual energy x-ray absorptiometry (DXA).

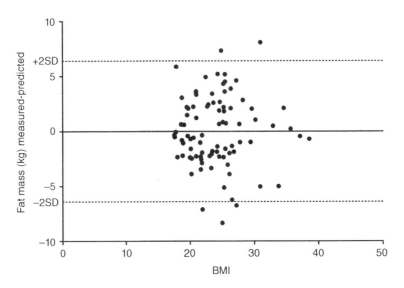

Figure 11.4b Residuals for the regression of fat mass against body mass index for 89 healthy female subjects.

circumference/height has been proposed as an index with independence from body size.

Body mass, height and age

Malnutrition in children presents in a number of ways, depending both on the age at which it occurs and its duration. Several indices based on height, mass and age may help to determine the presence and history of under-nutrition in children. These rely on reference to data from well-nourished populations.

Height is generally less susceptible to under-nutrition than body mass and so short stature (stunting, low height for age) may reflect historical growth failure dating from before birth or due to under-nutrition or repeated infection after birth. Leg length in proportion to stature has been proposed as an indicator of the quality of the growth environment during developmental years. Low mass for height may represent current under-nutrition. Low mass for age may reflect a composite of historical and current under-nutrition.

Growth charts based on the WHO's Child Growth Standards may aid in the interpretation of measurements.

Mid upper-arm circumference

Mid upper-arm circumference is a valuable screen for under-nutrition. It may be used along with weight for height in children to identify current malnutrition, particularly protein-energy malnutrition, in children. It is also valuable for identifying nutritionally compromised adults. The circumference is measured on the triceps

muscle at the midpoint between the shoulder and the elbow, usually on the non-dominant arm.

Skinfold measurements

Skinfold thickness offers an approach to measurement of subcutaneous adiposity. There are many expressions relating fat mass to skinfold thickness, incorporating measurements from sites varying in location and in number from seven (biceps, triceps, sub-scapular, supra-iliac, abdominal, thigh, calf) down to three. Purpose-designed skinfold callipers are used to measure the thickness of a pinch of skin at each site. The callipers use spring tension to grip the skin with a force of $10\,g\,mm^{-2}$. The procedure is as follows.

Take a pinch of skin at the point of interest. The pinch includes a double fold of skin around subcutaneous adipose tissue, but excludes muscle. Grip the skin to the side of the pinch. Allow 2–3 seconds for the skin to compress under the calliper force – the sides of the fold should be parallel between the calliper jaws. Record the reading. Repeat twice, allowing 30 seconds for skin compression to relax between measurements and take the average of three readings. Practice makes perfect!

Where several operators contribute skinfold records to a study, it is important that they rehearse together to achieve minimum inter-observer difference in measurements. It is also good practice that each subject is measured by the same observer when measurements are repeated in longitudinal studies. Even with careful practice, this is a method with limited repeated-measures precision and it can suffer from considerable inter-observer inconsistency.

The principle may be illustrated by the work of Durnin and Womersley, published in 1974, as this included validation against underwater weighing. They measured skinfold thickness in 209 male and 272 female adults, taking a subset of four measurement sites: biceps, triceps, sub-scapular and supra-iliac. Regression expressions relate the log of the sum of skinfolds measured at the four sites to body density (see the two-component volume–mass model in Section 11.11) and show that the relationship is sensitive to both sex and age. They went on to provide a table relating skinfold thickness to fat as a percentage of body mass for males and females across four age bands. The reported standard deviation of difference between repeated measures of the sum of four skinfolds equates to less than 1% of body mass as fat. The variability between %fat estimated from skinfold and from underwater weighing is much greater. Durnin and Womersley conceded a standard deviation of difference between the methods of 3.5% body mass in women, 5% in men. For a 70 kg female this translates to 2.5 kg, for a male 3.5 kg fat.

11.17 Ultrasound

Medical ultrasound uses sound waves with a frequency in the range 2–18 MHz to generate images. The sound waves are transmitted into tissues by a piezoelectric transducer and reflected waves are detected by the same transducer. The incident beam may be focused to produce an arc-shaped wave. Images are constructed from the time and amplitude of the reflected signal. If the target is moving, then Doppler shifts between the frequencies of the incident and reflected signals allow resolution of the motion.

Tissues differ in their impedance to the acoustic waves and the boundaries between tissues of differing impedance generate 'impedance jumps', which enable them to be visualised as changes in brightness in the images. In the abdomen, both subcutaneous tissue and visceral adipose tissue may be visualised and their depths measured. The subcutaneous tissue may be visualised as two compartments, superficial and deep. The measurements of deep subcutaneous and visceral fat are indicators of central obesity and are associated with metabolic and cardiovascular risks.

Subcutaneous fat thickness is defined from the fat/skin barrier to the linea alba. For subcutaneous measurements the probe is positioned on the skin of the epigastrium, with the probe across the body. The scan depth is set to 9 cm. It is important to take pressure off the transducer before freezing the measurements to avoid compressing the skin and the fat together. Visceral fat thickness is measured from the posterior surface of the rectus abdominis muscle to the spine, though some researchers use the anterior wall of the aorta as an end point. The transducer is placed against the skin, parallel to the spine, just above the umbilicus, the scan depth is set to 15 cm and the image is captured at the end of expiration. Figure 11.5 shows some sample images.

The liver is susceptible to fat accumulation and can be assessed by ultrasound to identify steatosis and non-alcoholic fatty liver disease (NAFLD), another potential metabolic consequence of obesity and type II diabetes. A fatty liver is scored visually based on the amount of

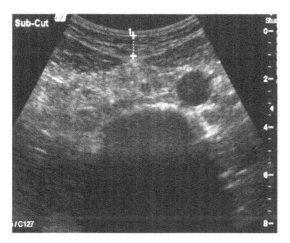 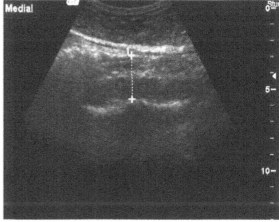

Figure 11.5 Ultrasound images of the abdomen. The left image shows the subcutaneous measurement; the right shows the visceral measurement. The depth or thickness measurements are taken between the points marked + using the scale in cm at the right of each image. Images by courtesy of Dr Emanuella De Lucia Rolfe, MRC Epidemiology Unit, University of Cambridge School of Clinical Medicine.

echogenicity, grade 0 representing normal echogenicity and grade 3 being poor or no visualisation of intra-hepatic vessels. The echogenicity of kidney or spleen is used as a reference.

Ultrasound methodology has been validated against CT and MR imaging, described earlier in the chapter, which provide the criterion reference. It is cost-effective, involves no radiation or risk to the participant and is also portable.

11.18 Bio-electrical impedance methods

The estimation of body composition from bio-electrical impedance analysis (BIA) is a widely available methodology offered by many manufacturers. It offers a low-cost, portable option for composition assessment.

The principle of the method is that the electrical impedance of the body reflects total body water (TBW). An alternating current is passed through the body from electrodes placed at the extremities of arms and legs. The resulting potential difference (voltage) between the electrodes is measured and the impedance R calculated as voltage divided by current. Early instruments used a single frequency, typically 50 kHz, and represented total body water in terms of height^2/R. Developments of the methodology have increased its sophistication, so analysis is now often performed across a range of frequencies (bio-electrical impedance spectroscopy, BIS). The current and voltage differ in phase, and determination of the phase angle enables the impedance to be resolved into in-phase (resistive) and out-of-phase (reactive) components at each frequency. The reactive component is associated with cell membranes that have the properties of capacitors. This offers the prospect of deducing intra- and extra-cellular water spaces.

As already discussed, TBW may be used to estimate lean body mass and, by difference from total body mass, fat mass. A literature search will reveal many publications describing validations of BIA/BIS against other methodologies such as deuterium dilution, and many expressions for estimating fat-free mass and fat mass from BIA and BIS have been developed. These are often specific to gender, age range and/or ethnicity. Many incorporate terms in body mass; some include other anthropometric measurements such as waist circumference.

Repeat measurements should be made on the same day of the week and at the same time of day to optimise consistency. Results may be dependent on the state of hydration, and may be unreliable in pregnancy. The method should not be used in subjects with pacemakers.

Even in carefully conducted, laboratory-based trials, the reported limits of agreement with criterion methods tend to be wide and the quality of composition estimates or their change over time when considered in individuals rather than groups must be considered critically.

11.19 Approaches to assessing individuals

When studying uncommon disorders, it may be challenging to describe the body composition of an individual or small group in the context of a healthy population. Prediction expressions may hold the key. A literature search will reveal a number of body composition prediction expressions for fat or lean masses or their proportions of body weight, based on anthropometric measurements. The relationship between BMI and fat mass (Figure 11.4a) discussed earlier is one such, associating fat mass with BMI by a linear regression. From the data in the figure, the regression equation in females is:

$$FM = 2.031 \times BMI - 26.43$$

Let us see what this reveals about two real-world female patients, one with lipodystrophy, the other with thyrotoxicosis. Their characteristics are given in Table 11.3.

How far do their measured fat masses differ from the prediction? The standard deviation of residuals for the regression is 3.2 kg. A standard deviation score – or Z-score – may be used to describe the difference from expectation, where:

$$Z = \frac{Measured - Predicted}{3.2}$$

For the lipodystrophic subject this indicates a fat mass 7.4 standard deviations below that expected, a Z-score of –7.4, and for the thyrotoxic subject a Z-score of +3.4, on a scale where we would expect to find 95% of people in the range ±2. Thus we can see that both these subjects lie well beyond the range of normality.

Table 11.3 Physical characteristics of two subjects with metabolic disorders.

Disorder	Height (m)	Weight (kg)	BMI (kg m^{-2})	Fat mass (kg)	
				Measured	Predicted
Lipodystrophy	1.60	71.0	27.7	6.1	29.8
Thyrotoxicosis	1.72	73.1	24.85	34.77	24.0

11.20 Summary

This chapter has aimed to provide an introduction to methods applicable to body composition assessment in nutritional research. Table 11.4 summarises the characteristics of the more common of these. The authors would encourage further reading prior to applying any of the methodologies we have described; a starting point for this will be found in References and further reading. Some methodologies are now quite stable, but others, such as photonic scanning, ultrasound and BIA, continue to develop. Our final advice is therefore to look for advances before excluding any methodology on the basis of the performance shortcomings we may have described.

Table 11.4 Summary of characteristics of methods commonly used in body composition assessment.

Method	Components	Outcome	Estimated precision or limits of agreement	Assumes	Benefits	Disadvantages
Body mass and volume by underwater weighing	2	Fat mass, fat-free mass (FFM)	Volume 0.15 l 0.7 kg fat mass	Densities of tissues	Lung volume measured at measurement time	Large, non-commercial apparatus Hygiene
Body mass and volume by air displacement plethysmography	2	Fat mass, FFM	Volume 0.15 l 0.7 kg fat mass	Densities of tissues	Quicker and better tolerated than underwater weighing	Uncertainty in residual volume of lungs and other gas spaces
Total body water (TBW) by isotope dilution	1 TBW and lean 2 Fat mass	TBW, fat mass, FFM	TBW 0.7% 0.5 kg fat mass	Fat mass and FFM assume a hydration factor in fat-free body	Simple in practice	Hydration factor uncertainty
Body mass, volume, TBW	3	TBW, fat mass, FFM	0.5 kg fat mass	Densities of tissues	Overcomes hydration factor uncertainty	
Body mass, volume, TBW, bone mass	4	TBW, fat mass, FFM, bone mass	0.5 kg fat mass	Densities of tissues	Lowest bias potential hence a criterion method	
Dual-energy x-ray absorptiometry	2/3	Fat mass, lean mass, bone mass	0.9 kg fat or lean mass (Lunar iDXA 0.25 kg)	Tissue x-ray absorption coefficients	Fast and well tolerated Whole-body and regional data	Unsuitable in pregnancy Body weight and size limit
Quantitative magnetic resonance		Fat mass	0.25 kg fat mass	Magnetic resonance characteristics of fats	Quick, high precision Well tolerated	Large instrument Expensive
Body mass index		Index of adiposity	Limits of agreement vs criterion method > 3 kg fat	Body mass reflects fat mass	Quick, easy Portable	Limited value in individuals
Skinfolds		Fat mass	Limits of agreement vs criterion method > 2.5 kg fat	Skinfolds reflect total fat mass	Portable	Poor precision Variable between observers
Bioimpedance (BIA)		TBW, fat mass	Limits of agreement vs criterion method > 3 kg fat	Impedance represents total body water	Quick, easy Portable	Poor precision

Acknowledgement

With grateful appreciation of the outstanding work of Dr Les Bluck (1956–2014), formerly of MRC Human Nutrition Research.

References and further reading

Ackland, T.R., Lohman, T.G., Sundgot-Borgen, J. et al. (2012) Current status of body composition assessment in sport: Review and position statement on behalf of the ad hoc research working group on body composition health and performance, under the auspices of the I.O.C. Medical Commission. Sports Medicine, 42, 227–249.

Anon. (2002) Guidance Notes Relating to the Legal Prescription of Medical Weighing Scales. UK Weighing Federation, Northampton.

Anon. (2008) Waist Circumference and Waist–Hip Ratio: Report of a WHO Expert Consultation. World Health Organisation, Geneva.

Anon. (2009) Assessment of Body Composition and Total Energy Expenditure in Humans Using Stable Isotope Techniques. International Atomic Energy Agency, Vienna.

Anon. (2010) Standards for the Weighing of Infants, Children and Young People in the Acute Health Care Setting. Royal College of Nursing, London.

Bland, J.M. and Altman, D.G. (1986) Statistical methods for assessing agreement between two methods of clinical measurement. Lancet, 327, 307–310.

Collins, A.L., Saunders, S., Mccarthy, H.D. et al. (2004) Within- and between-laboratory precision in the measurement of body volume using air displacement plethysmography and its effect on body composition assessment. International Journal of Obesity and Related Metabolic Disorders, 28, 80–90.

Crim, M.C., Calloway, D.H. and Margen, S. (1975) Creatine metabolism in men: Urinary creatine and creatinine excretions with creatine feeding. Journal of Nutrition, 105, 428–438.

De Lorenzo, A., Andreoli, A., Matthie, J. and Withers, P. (1997) Predicting body cell mass with bioimpedance by using theoretical methods: A technological review. Journal of Applied Physiology, 82, 1542–1558.

De Lorenzo, A., Andreoli, A., Serrano, P. et al. (2003) Body cell mass measured by total body potassium in normal-weight and obese men and women. Journal of the American College of Nutrition, 22, 546–549.

De Lucia Rolfe, E., Norris, S.A., Sleigh, A. et al. (2011) Validation of ultrasound estimates of visceral fat in black South African adolescents. Obesity (Silver Spring), 19, 1892–1897.

Dewit, O., Fuller, N.J., Fewtrell, M.S. et al. (2000) Whole body air displacement plethysmography compared with hydrodensitometry for body composition analysis. Archive of Disease in Childhood, 82, 159–164.

Durnin, J.V. and Womersley, J. (1974) Body fat assessed from total body density and its estimation from skinfold thickness: Measurements on 481 men and women aged from 16 to 72 years. British Journal of Nutrition, 32, 77–97.

Ellis, K.J. (2000) Human body composition: In vivo methods. Physiological Reviews, 80, 649–680.

Fuller, N.J., Jebb, S.A., Goldberg, G.R. et al. (1991) Inter-observer variability in the measurement of body composition. European Journal of Clinical Nutrition, 45, 43–49.

Fuller, N.J., Jebb, S.A., Laskey, M.A. et al. (1992) Four-component model for the assessment of body composition in humans: Comparison with alternative methods, and evaluation of the density and hydration of fat-free mass. Clinical Science (London), 82, 687–693.

Fuller, N.J., Sawyer, M.B. and Elia, M. (1994) Comparative evaluation of body composition methods and predictions, and calculation of density and hydration fraction of fat-free mass, in obese women. International Journal of Obesity and Related Metabolic Disorders, 18, 503–512.

Fuller, N.J., Wells, J.C. and Elia, M. (2001) Evaluation of a model for total body protein mass based on dual-energy X-ray absorptiometry: Comparison with a reference four-component model. British Journal of Nutrition, 86, 45–52.

Geerling, B.J., Badart-Smook, A., Stockbrugger, R.W. and Brummer, R.J. (2000) Comprehensive nutritional status in recently diagnosed patients with inflammatory bowel disease compared with population controls. European Journal of Clinical Nutrition, 54, 514–521.

Gleeson, N.P. and Mercer, T.H. (1996) The utility of isokinetic dynamometry in the assessment of human muscle function. Sports Medicine, 21, 18–34.

Heymsfield, S.B., Arteaga, C., McManus, C. et al. (1983) Measurement of muscle mass in humans: Validity of the 24-hour urinary creatinine method. American Journal of Clinical Nutrition, 37, 478–494.

Heymsfield, S.B., Gallagher, D., Visser, M. et al. (1995) Measurement of skeletal muscle: Laboratory and epidemiological methods. The Journals of Gerontology Series A: Biological Sciences and Medical Sciences, 50, special issue, 23–29.

Heymsfield, S.B., Wang, Z., Baumgartner, R.N. and Ross, R. (1997) Human body composition: Advances in models and methods. Annual Review of Nutrition, 17, 527–558.

Hind, K., Oldroyd, B. and Truscott, J.G. (2011) In vivo precision of the GE Lunar iDXA densitometer for the measurement of total body composition and fat distribution in adults. European Journal of Clinical Nutrition, 65, 140–142.

Hull, H., He, Q., Thornton, J. et al. (2009) iDXA, Prodigy, and DPXL dual-energy X-ray absorptiometry whole-body scans: A cross-calibration study. Journal of Clinical Densitometry, 12, 95–102.

Jaffrin, M.Y. and Morel, H. (2008) Body fluid volumes measurements by impedance: A review of bioimpedance spectroscopy (BIS) and bioimpedance analysis (BIA) methods. Medical Engineering & Physics, 30, 1257–1269.

Jebb, S.A., Murgatroyd, P.R., Goldberg, G.R. et al. (1993) In vivo measurement of changes in body composition: Description of methods and their validation against 12-d continuous whole-body calorimetry. American Journal of Clinical Nutrition, 58, 455–462.

Jebb, S.A., Siervo, M., Murgatroyd, P.R. et al. (2007) Validity of the leg-to-leg bioimpedance to estimate changes in body fat during weight loss and regain in overweight women: A comparison with multi-compartment models. International Journal of Obesity (London), 31, 756–762.

Kawaguchi, Y., Fukumoto, S., Inaba, M. et al. (2011) Different impacts of neck circumference and visceral obesity on the severity of obstructive sleep apnea syndrome. Obesity (Silver Spring), 19, 276–282.

Mazess, R.B., Barden, H.S., Bisek, J.P. and Hanson, J. (1990) Dual-energy x-ray absorptiometry for total-body and regional bone-mineral and soft-tissue composition. American Journal of Clinical Nutrition, 51, 1106–1112.

Napolitano, A., Miller, S.R., Murgatroyd, P.R. et al. (2008) Validation of a quantitative magnetic resonance method for measuring human body composition. Obesity (Silver Spring), 16, 191–198.

Norman, K., Stobaus, N., Gonzalez, M.C. et al. (2011) Hand grip strength: Outcome predictor and marker of nutritional status. Clinical Nutrition, 30, 135–142.

Proctor, D.N., O'Brien, P.C., Atkinson, E.J. and Nair, K.S. (1999) Comparison of techniques to estimate total body skeletal muscle mass in people of different age groups. *American Journal of Physiology*, **277**, E489–E495.

Schoeller, D.A., Van Santen, E., Peterson, D.W. *et al.* (1980) Total body water measurement in humans with 18O and 2H labeled water. *American Journal of Clinical Nutrition*, **33**, 2686–2693.

Seoane, N. and Latham, M.C. (1971) Nutritional anthropometry in the identification of malnutrition in childhood. *Journal of Tropical Pediatrics and Environmental Child Health*, **17**, 98–104.

Silva, A.M., Heymsfield, S.B., Gallagher, D. *et al.* (2008) Evaluation of between-methods agreement of extracellular water measurements in adults and children. *American Journal of Clinical Nutrition*, **88**, 315–323.

Siri, W.E. (1956) The gross composition of the body. *Advances in Biological and Medical Physics*, **4**, 239–280.

Siri, W.E. (1961) Body composition from fluid spaces and density: Analysis of methods. In J. Brozek and A. Henschel (eds) *Techniques for Measuring Body Composition*. National Academy of Sciences, Washington, DC.

Swe Myint, K., Napolitano, A., Miller, S.R. *et al.* (2010) Quantitative magnetic resonance (QMR) for longitudinal evaluation of body composition changes with two dietary regimens. *Obesity (Silver Spring)*, **18**, 391–396.

Taylor, R., Price, T.B., Katz, L.D. *et al.* (1993) Direct measurement of change in muscle glycogen concentration after a mixed meal in normal subjects. *American Journal of Physiology*, **265**, E224–E229.

Wang, Z.M., Gallagher, D., Nelson, M.E. *et al.* (1996) Total-body skeletal muscle mass: Evaluation of 24-h urinary creatinine excretion by computerized axial tomography. *American Journal of Clinical Nutrition*, **63**, 863–869.

Watson, L.P.E., Raymond-Barker, P., Moran, C. *et al.* (2013) An approach to quantifying abnormalities in energy expenditure and lean mass in metabolic disease. *European Journal of Clinical Nutrition*, **68**, 234–240.

Wells, J.C., Fuller, N.J., Dewit, O. *et al.* (1999) Four-component model of body composition in children: Density and hydration of fat-free mass and comparison with simpler models. *American Journal of Clinical Nutrition*, **69**, 904–912.

Wells, J.C., Douros, I., Fuller, N.J. *et al.* (2000) Assessment of body volume using three-dimensional photonic scanning. *Annals of the New York Academy of Sciences*, **904**, 247–254.

Wells, J.C., Fuller, N.J., Wright, A. *et al.* (2003) Evaluation of air-displacement plethysmography in children aged 5–7 years using a three-component model of body composition. *British Journal of Nutrition*, **90**, 699–707.

Wells, J. C., Williams, J. E., Chomtho, S. *et al.* (2012) Body-composition reference data for simple and reference techniques and a 4-component model: A new UK reference child. *American Journal of Clinical Nutrition*, **96**, 1316–1326.

Wong, W.W., Sheng, H.P., Morkeberg, J.C. *et al.* (1989) Measurement of extracellular water volume by bromide ion chromatography. *American Journal of Clinical Nutrition*, **50**, 1290–1294.

Zdolsek, J.H., Lisander, B. and Hahn, R.G. (2005) Measuring the size of the extracellular fluid space using bromide, iohexol, and sodium dilution. *Anesthesia & Analgesia*, **101**, 1770–1777.

12
Energy Expenditure and Intake Methods

Klaas R Westerterp

Maastricht University

Key messages

- The human energy requirement is derived from measuring energy expenditure rather than calculating energy intake from reported food intake.
- Energy expenditure measurements are performed with direct calorimetry, based on the measurement of heat loss, or with indirect calorimetry, based on the measurement of oxygen consumption, carbon dioxide production and urine-nitrogen loss for energy production from carbohydrate, protein and fat.
- Heat loss matches total energy expenditure at rest, but can be up to 25% lower than total energy expenditure during exercise, due to the performance of external work.
- The main components of total energy expenditure are energy expenditure for maintenance or basal metabolic rate, the thermic effect of food or diet-induced energy expenditure, and the energy cost of physical activity or activity-induced energy expenditure.
- Basal metabolic rate generally is the largest component of total energy expenditure and is defined as energy expenditure at rest, awake, postabsorptive and in the thermoneutral zone. It is usually measured directly after waking up in the morning, where high-intensity exercise was prevented on the foregoing day, after a 10–12 hour fast, under a ventilated hood at a comfortable room temperature.
- Diet-induced energy expenditure is the energy expenditure for the intestinal absorption of nutrients, the initial steps of their metabolism and the storage of the absorbed but not immediately oxidised nutrients. When intake equals energy expenditure, diet-induced energy expenditure is around 10% of total energy expenditure for a mixed diet with 55 energy% carbohydrate, 15 energy% protein and 30 energy% fat.
- Activity-induced energy expenditure is the most variable component of total energy expenditure. Activity-induced energy expenditure can be calculated as 0.9 times total energy expenditure minus basal metabolic rate. Alternatively, the physical activity level of a subject is calculated by expressing total energy expenditure as a multiple of basal metabolic rate, where for the majority of the population the value ranges from 1.5 to 2.0.
- The main determinants of differences in total energy expenditure between individuals are body composition and physical activity, where the average woman has relatively more body fat and thus a lower expenditure than men with the same weight and physical activity.
- Changes in energy expenditure within individuals are mainly a function of physical activity, food intake and age. Energy restriction and increasing age are associated with a reduction of activity-induced energy expenditure.
- Reported energy intake is generally lower than habitual energy expenditure due to under-eating during diet reporting and not recording all foods consumed.

12.1 Introduction

Man is a heterotrophic organism, deriving its energy from organic compounds. Energy is provided by the oxidation of nutrients, being the carbohydrates, proteins and fats consumed, called the macronutrients. A fourth source of food energy that can sometimes make up a significant part of energy intake is alcohol. The oxidation of nutrients provides the energy necessary to synthesise adenosine triphosphate (ATP), which is used for metabolic work. Less than 50% of the potential energy available from the oxidation of nutrients is actually conserved in the phosphoanhydride bonds of ATP; the rest is lost as heat. Additionally, when ATP molecules provide energy for metabolic work by hydrolysis, most of the energy will be transformed into heat as well. Thus, energy expenditure can be assessed by measuring heat loss or, indirectly, by measuring gas exchange in

Nutrition Research Methodologies, First Edition. Edited by Julie A Lovegrove, Leanne Hodson, Sangita Sharma and Susan A Lanham-New.
© 2015 John Wiley & Sons, Ltd. Published 2015 by John Wiley & Sons, Ltd.
Companion Website: www.wiley.com/go/nutritionsociety

the oxidation of nutrients. The former method is named direct calorimetry, the latter indirect calorimetry.

Man is a homeothermic organism, maintaining an almost constant body temperature over a wide range of environmental temperatures. The metabolic requirements of a homeotherm are mainly a function of the body's surface area. The physiological explanation is that heat is lost via the body surface. The body surface is proportional to body mass to the power of 2/3. Thus, body mass is a determinant of metabolic requirement. Additional determinants are food intake, through the expenditure for food processing, and physical activity. Energy expenditure for maintenance, food processing and physical activity together largely explain the variation in daily energy expenditure within and between individuals.

Assessment of daily energy expenditure is the indicated method for the assessment of the energy requirement. Nowadays, energy expenditure can be accurately assessed with a calorimetric technique under daily living conditions over intervals of one or more weeks. As such, it has become the reference for the evaluation of methods to measure energy intake.

This chapter describes methods to measure energy expenditure, determinants of energy expenditure and the application of energy expenditure measurements for the evaluation of intake methods. The methods section includes techniques, methods to measure separate components of daily energy expenditure, and measuring substrate utilisation. The determinants section describes the subject characteristics involved, such as body composition, age and gender, and behavioural aspects including food intake and physical activity. Evaluation of intake methods is based on principles of energy requirement and techniques to assess energy homeostasis.

12.2 Measuring energy expenditure

History

The first measurements of energy expenditure, dating back to the early seventeenth century, were based on a balance technique. Sanctorius in 1614 demonstrated how a subject loses weight while seated in a chair suspended from a balance. He distinguished between sensible loss of weight in faeces and urine and insensible loss ascribed to insensible perspiration. Insensible perspiration was assumed to reflect energy expenditure. Now, we know that insensible loss is the sum of the weight of water vapour given off and the difference in weight of oxygen consumed and carbon dioxide produced for energy metabolism. The following calculation shows that insensible perspiration is more a reflection of water lost by evaporation than of energy expenditure. The

calculation is performed for a man with an average daily energy expenditure of 12 MJ/day, completely covered by glucose oxidation. The body produces energy from glucose by oxidation: 1 mol glucose ($C_6H_{12}O_6$) is oxidised with 6 mol oxygen (O_2) to 6 mol carbon dioxide (CO_2) and 6 mol water (H_2O):

$$C_6H_{12}O_6 + 6O_2 \rightarrow 6CO_2 + 6H_2O + energy$$

In grams, 180 g glucose (1 mol) oxidise with 192 g oxygen (6 mol = 6 × 32) to produce 264 g carbon dioxide (6 mol = 6 × 44), 108 g water (6 mol = 6 × 18) and energy. The heat of combustion of glucose is 2.8 MJ/mol. Thus, the energy expenditure of 12 MJ/day is covered by the oxidation of about 4 mol glucose. The body weight change due to the difference between the weight of oxygen consumed and carbon dioxide produced is (4 × 192) − (4 × 264) = −288 grams/day. Water loss through breathing and evaporation via the skin is on average one-third to two-thirds of the average daily water turnover of 3 l/day, or 1000–2000 g/day depending on clothing, ambient temperature and humidity. Thus, water loss through evaporation makes up for the largest part and for a highly variable part of insensible perspiration.

The next step in the measurement of energy expenditure was a calorimeter, measuring the heat released by an organism. It assumes that all energy provided by the oxidation of nutrients is eventually transformed into heat. Current techniques for the measurement of energy expenditure are based on the determination of oxygen consumed and carbon dioxide produced for energy metabolism. Measuring energy expenditure based on heat release is named direct calorimetry, to distinguish it from measurements based on gas exchange, named indirect calorimetry. Indirect calorimetry, including the simultaneous determination of oxygen consumption, carbon dioxide production and nitrogen loss in urine, can also be used to estimate the contribution of carbohydrate, protein and fat to energy production.

Direct calorimetry

There are several ways to measure the heat release of an organism to quantify energy expenditure. In Paris in 1780, Lavoisier placed a guinea pig in a wire cage surrounded by chunks of ice. As the ice melted from the animal's body heat, the water collected below in a container, which could be weighed. The amount of melted water allowed calculation of the heat production, 334 J/g. The calorimeter was adiabatic in that the outer space around the ice cavity surrounding the cage was packed with snow to maintain a constant temperature around the inner shell, which was filled with ice. The days when these measurements could be made were limited by the mild winters in Paris at a time when ice machines had not yet been invented. Later developments were an airflow calorimeter and a water-flow calorimeter.

An airflow calorimeter consists of a temperature-insulated ventilated space, for instance a room to house a subject. The temperature change of air flowing through the room multiplied by its mass flow rate and specific heat gives the rate of heat loss from the subject. The change in water vapour content of the air stream is measured to determine additional evaporative heat loss. A recent development of a water-flow calorimeter is a suit calorimeter. The suit calorimeter was developed from a device needed to cool astronauts while they are active outside their spacecraft. The subject is dressed in a close-fitting elastic undergarment, which carries a network of small plastic tubing over the entire body surface, except for the face, fingers and soles of the feet (Figure 12.1). Water circulated through the tubing carries heat from the skin, which is measured as the product of the mass flow of water and the change in temperature across the suit. Layers of insulating garments limit the exchange of heat with the environment. Evaporative heat loss is calculated from insensible perspiration; that is, body weight change corrected for intake and output of solids and liquids, and for the mass difference between estimated oxygen intake and carbon dioxide output.

Indirect calorimetry

In indirect calorimetry the energy production is calculated from oxygen consumption, carbon dioxide production and urine-nitrogen loss. The basis of the calculation is the gaseous exchange and energy release from the metabolised carbohydrate, fat and protein. As already described, 1 mol glucose is oxidised with 6 mol oxygen to 6 mol carbon dioxide and 6 mol water and produces 2.8 MJ energy. A similar equation exists for fat oxidation. Protein oxidation results in carbon dioxide, water and compounds of nitrogen (e.g. urea and creatinine), where the latter is excreted in the urine. The resulting three equations with three unknowns can be solved for energy expenditure (E):

$$E = a \times \text{oxygen consumption} + b \times \text{carbon dioxide production} + c \times \text{urine} - \text{nitrogen loss}$$

Examples of equations for the calculation of energy production derived from these figures are the Weir equation and the Brouwer equation.

$$\text{Weir equation}(1948): E(kJ)$$
$$= 16.32 \text{ oxygen consumption}(l)$$
$$+ 4.60 \text{ carbon dioxide production}(l)$$
$$- 2.17 \text{ urine} - \text{nitrogen}(g)$$

(a)

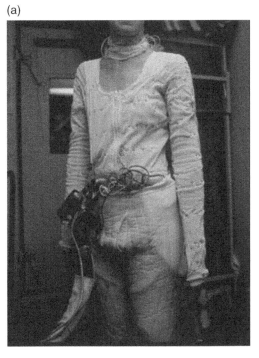

(b)

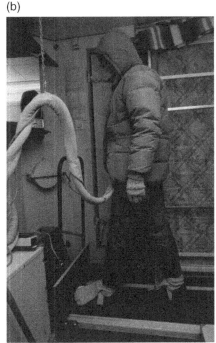

Figure 12.1 A subject in a suit calorimeter: (a) an elastic undergarment carrying a network of plastic tubing over the entire body and connected with a circulation pump (b) with insulating garments during a measurement walking on a treadmill.

$$\text{Brouwer equation} (1957): E (kJ)$$
$$= 16.20 \, \text{oxygen consumption} (l)$$
$$+ 5.00 \, \text{carbon dioxide production} (l)$$
$$- 0.15 \, \text{urine} - \text{nitrogen} (g)$$

Differences in the coefficients are caused by differences in assumptions on gaseous exchange and energy release from the metabolised carbohydrate, fat and protein. The contribution of measured urine-nitrogen loss to calculated energy production, the so-called protein correction, is only small. In the case of a normal protein oxidation of 10–15% of daily energy production, the protein correction for the calculation of E is smaller than 1%. Usually, urine-nitrogen is only measured when information on the contribution of carbohydrate, fat and protein to energy production is required. For calculating the energy production the protein correction is often neglected.

Current techniques utilising indirect calorimetry for the measurement of energy expenditure in man are a face mask or ventilated hood; a respiration chamber; and the doubly labelled water method. A typical example of a ventilated-hood system is an open canopy. It is used to measure resting energy expenditure and energy expenditure for food processing or diet-induced energy expenditure. The subject lies with his or her head enclosed in a plastic canopy, sealed off by plastic straps around the neck (Figure 12.2). Air is sucked through the canopy with a pump and blown into a mixing chamber, where a sample is taken for analysis. Measurements taken are those of the airflow and of the oxygen and carbon dioxide concentrations of the air flowing in and out. The most common device to measure the airflow is a dry gas meter comparable to that used to measure heating gas consumption at home. The oxygen and carbon dioxide concentrations are commonly measured with a paramagnetic oxygen analyser and an infrared carbon dioxide analyser respectively. The airflow is adjusted to keep differences in oxygen and carbon dioxide concentrations between inlet and outlet within a range of 0.5 to 1.0%. For adults this means airflow rates around 50 l/min.

A respiration chamber is an airtight room, which is ventilated with fresh air. Basically the difference between a respiration chamber and a ventilated-hood system is size. In a respiration chamber the subject is fully enclosed instead of enclosing the head only, allowing physical activity depending on the size of the chamber. With both methods, the airflow rate and the oxygen and carbon dioxide concentration difference between inlet and outlet air are measured in the same way. The flow rate to keep differences for oxygen and carbon dioxide concentrations between inlet and outlet air in the range of 0.5–1.0% is slightly higher in the respiration chamber than in the ventilated-hood system, as in the chamber subjects never lie down over the full length of an observation interval. In a sedentary adult a typical flow rate is 50–100 l/min, while in exercising subjects the flow has to be increased to over 100 l/min. In the latter situation one has to choose a compromise for

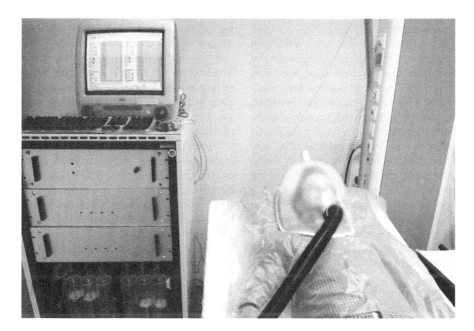

Figure 12.2 A ventilated hood.

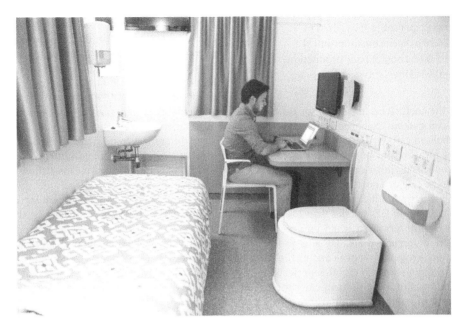

Figure 12.3 Respiration chamber.

the flow rate when measurements are to be continued over 24 hours including active and inactive intervals. During exercise bouts the 1% carbon dioxide level should not be surpassed for long periods. During resting bouts, like an overnight sleep, the level should not fall too far below the optimal measuring range of 0.5–1.0%. Changing the flow rate during an observation interval reduces the accuracy of the measurements due to the response time of the system.

A normal-size respiration chamber has a volume of 10–30 m³ and is equipped with a bed, toilet, washbasin and communication facilities like telephone, radio, television, and internet. Essentially it is a hotel room (Figure 12.3). The experimenter sets the room temperature. Food and drink are delivered through an air lock according to the experimental design. Physical activity is often monitored with a radar system to know when and how often subjects are physically active. A respiration chamber can be equipped with a cycle ergometer or a treadmill to perform standardised work loads. A respiration chamber has a much longer response time than a ventilated hood. Though the flow rate in both systems is comparable, the volume of a respiration chamber is more than 20 times the volume of a ventilated hood. Consequently, the minimum length of an observation period in a respiration chamber is of the order of 5–10 hours.

The doubly labelled water method for the measurement of energy expenditure is an innovative variant on indirect calorimetry. It is based on the discovery that oxygen in respiratory carbon dioxide is in isotopic equilibrium with the oxygen in body water. The technique involves enriching the body water with an isotope of oxygen and an isotope of hydrogen and then determining the washout kinetics of both isotopes. Most of the oxygen isotope is lost as water, but some is also lost as carbon dioxide, because CO_2 in body fluids is in isotopic equilibrium with body water due to exchange in the bicarbonate pools. The hydrogen isotope is lost as water only. Thus, the washout for the oxygen isotope is faster than for the hydrogen isotope, and the difference represents the CO_2 production. The isotopes of choice are the stable, heavy isotopes of oxygen and hydrogen, oxygen-18 (^{18}O) and deuterium (^2H), since these avoid the need to use radioactivity and can be used safely. Both isotopes naturally occur in drinking water and thus in body water. Oxygen-18 (^{18}O) has eight protons and ten neutrons instead of the eight protons and eight neutrons found in normal oxygen (^{16}O). Deuterium (^2H) has one proton and one neutron instead of one neutron for normal hydrogen (^1H). 'Normal' water consists largely of the lighter isotopes ^1H and ^{16}O; the natural abundance for ^2H is about 150 parts per million (ppm) and for ^{18}O 2000 ppm. Enriching the body water with doubly labelled water ($^2H_2{}^{18}O$) for the measurement of energy expenditure implies an increase of the background levels as mentioned, with 200–300 ppm for ^{18}O and with 100–150 ppm for ^2H. The CO_2 production, calculated from the subsequent difference in elimination between the two isotopes, is a measure of metabolism (Figure 12.4).

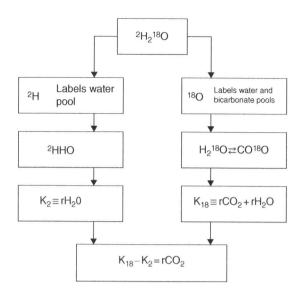

Figure 12.4 The principle of measurement of carbon dioxide (CO_2) production with doubly labelled water ($^2H_2^{18}O$). After administration of water labelled with heavy oxygen (^{18}O) and heavy hydrogen (^2H), the two isotopes mix with the body water, where ^{18}O exchanges with CO_2 in the bicarbonate pools as well. Thus, the elimination rate of ^2H (K_2) is a measure for water loss (rH_2O) and the elimination rate of ^{18}O (K_{18}) is a measure for rH_2O plus carbon dioxide production (rCO_2), and $rCO_2 = K_{18} - K_2$.

In practice, the observation duration is set by the biological half-life of the oxygen isotope as a function of the level of energy expenditure. The minimum observation duration is about 3 days in subjects with a high energy turnover, such as premature infants or endurance athletes. The maximum duration is 30 days or about 4 weeks in elderly (sedentary) subjects. An observation starts by collecting a baseline sample. Then a weighed isotope dose is administered, usually a mixture of 10% ^{18}O and 5% ^2H in water. For a 70 kg adult, between 100 g and 150 g water would be used. Subsequently the isotopes equilibrate with the body water and the initial sample is collected. The equilibration time is dependent on body size and metabolic rate. For an adult the equilibration time would be between 4 and 8 hours. During equilibration the subject usually does not consume any food or drink. After collecting the initial sample the subject performs routines according to the instructions of the experimenter, for instance to continue with 'daily life'. Longer observation periods are covered with multiple doses, where a subsequent dose is taken immediately after collecting the last sample of the foregoing dose. Body water samples (blood, saliva or urine) are collected at regular intervals until the end of the observation period.

There are different sampling protocols; that is, the multipoint versus the two-point method. The ideal protocol is a combination of both, taking two independent samples at the start, the midpoint and the end of the observation period. Thus an independent comparison can be made within one run, calculating carbon dioxide production from the first samples and the second samples over the first half and the second half of the observation interval. Validation studies, comparing the method with respirometry, have shown that estimates of CO_2 production based on the doubly labelled water method elicit an accuracy of 1–3% and a precision of 2–8%. The method requires high-precision isotope ratio mass spectrometry in order to utilise low amounts of the very expensive ^{18}O isotope.

The doubly labelled water method gives precise and accurate information on CO_2 production. Converting carbon dioxide production to energy expenditure needs information on the energy equivalent of CO_2, which can be calculated with additional information on the substrate mixture being oxidised. One option is the calculation of the energy equivalent from the macronutrient composition of the diet. In energy balance, substrate intake and substrate utilisation are assumed to be identical. Doubly labelled water provides an excellent method to measure energy expenditure in unrestrained humans in their normal surroundings over a time period of 1–4 weeks.

Comparing direct calorimetry with indirect calorimetry

With indirect calorimetry, the energy expenditure is calculated from gaseous exchange. The result is the total energy expenditure of the body for heat production and work output. With direct calorimetry, one measures heat loss only. At rest, total energy expenditure is converted to heat. During physical activity, there is work output as well. The proportion of energy expenditure for external work is the work efficiency.

An experiment was conducted to assess work efficiency by simultaneous assessment of total energy expenditure with indirect calorimetry and heat loss with direct calorimetry. Subjects were normal-weight 20–25-year-old adults, five women and five men. The experiment started with an overnight stay for the measurement of resting energy expenditure, followed by a 6-hour exercise session (walking on a treadmill and cycling with an ergometer). Gaseous exchange was measured in a respiration chamber; heat loss was measured with a suit calorimeter.

At rest, indirect calorimetry assessed energy expenditure-matched heat loss as measured with direct calorimetry (Figure 12.5). Resting energy expenditure was on average 100 watt, typical for a young adult. During physical activity, heat loss was systematically lower than indirect calorimetry-assessed energy expenditure. The difference increased with walking speed and cycling load. During cycling, indirect calorimetry-assessed energy expenditure

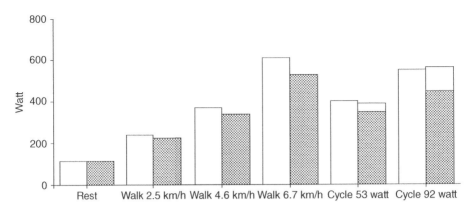

Figure 12.5 Indirect calorimetry assessed energy expenditure (left bar open) and direct calorimetry assessed heat loss (right bar stippled), at rest and during walking and cycling. When power output during cycling is added to heat loss, the sum matches indirect calorimetry assessed energy.

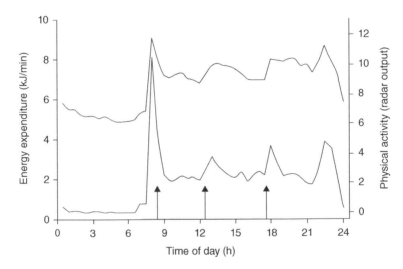

Figure 12.6 Energy expenditure (upper line) and physical activity (lower line) as measured over a 24-hour interval in a respiration chamber. Arrows denote meal times. Data are the average of 37 subjects, 17 women and 20 men, age 20–35 years and body mass index 20–30 kg/m².

matched the sum of heat loss and power output. The work efficiency during cycling, power output divided by energy expenditure, was in the range of 15–25%.

In conclusion, at present the state of the art is assessing total energy expenditure with indirect calorimetry. Direct calorimetry measures heat loss only. Body heat loss matches total energy expenditure at rest, but can be up to 25% lower than total energy expenditure during endurance exercise, without temporary heat storage.

Daily energy expenditure and its components

Daily energy expenditure consists of four components: sleeping metabolic rate (SMR), energy cost of arousal, thermic effect of food or diet-induced energy expenditure

(DEE), and energy cost of physical activity or activity-induced energy expenditure (AEE). Sometimes daily energy expenditure is divided into three components, taking sleeping metabolic rate and the energy cost of arousal together as energy expenditure for maintenance or basal metabolic rate (BMR). BMR usually is the main component of daily energy expenditure.

The variation of energy expenditure throughout a day is presented in Figure 12.6. Overnight, there generally is no food intake and, when one sleeps quietly, there is no physical activity. Energy expenditure gradually decreases to a daily minimum before increasing again at awakening and getting up. Then the increase is primarily caused by activity-induced energy expenditure and subsequently by diet-induced energy expenditure as soon as one has breakfast. Thus, variation in energy expenditure throughout the day is a function of body size and body composition as determinants of SMR and BMR, physical activity as a determinant of AEE and food intake as a determinant of DEE.

The indicated method for the measurement of SMR is a respiration chamber, for BMR a ventilated hood, and DEE can be measured in a respiration chamber or with a ventilated hood, as explained in the subsequent sections. Activity-induced energy expenditure can be measured under standardised conditions, as in a respiration chamber, or under free-living conditions with the doubly labelled water method. For the latter, the measurement of total energy with doubly labelled water is combined with a measurement of BMR under a ventilated hood; alternatively, BMR is estimated with a prediction equation based on the height, weight, age and gender of the subject.

Measuring sleeping metabolic rate and basal metabolic rate

The basal metabolic rate is defined as the daily rate of energy expenditure to maintain and preserve the integrity of vital functions. The measurement of basal metabolic rate must meet four conditions: the subject is awake; is measured in a thermoneutral environment to avoid heat production for the maintenance of body temperature; is fasted long enough to eliminate DEE; and is at rest to eliminate AEE. For the measurement of sleeping metabolic rate, subjects must be asleep and meet the remaining three conditions for the measurement of BMR.

To perform accurate measurement of BMR, one usually adopts an in-patient protocol. A subject stays overnight in the research facility where food intake and physical activity are strictly controlled, and BMR is measured directly after waking up in the morning. A 10–12-hour fast before BMR measurement is the accepted procedure to eliminate DEE. Thus, when BMR is measured at 7.00 am, subjects should be fasted from about 8.00 pm the day before. High-intensity exercise should be prevented on the day before BMR measurement. An out-patient protocol, where subjects are transported by car or public transport to the laboratory after spending the night at home, produces sufficiently reproducible results when subjects are carefully instructed and behave accordingly.

A typical protocol for BMR measurement with a ventilated-hood system takes 30 minutes. To eliminate effects of subject habituation to the testing procedure, the respiratory measurements over the first 10 minutes are discarded and the following 20 minutes are used to calculate BMR. The criterion for the chosen time interval is the reproducibility of the calculated BMR value. Longer measurements tend to result in higher values because subjects become restless. The use of a mouthpiece or face

mask for the collection of respiratory gases is discouraged, as it introduces stress during breathing and results in an overestimate of the BMR value. Similarly, values are generally higher for subjects observed in a sitting position than for subjects in a more relaxed, supine position.

There are several options to define sleeping metabolic rate as measured in a respiration chamber. The minimum interval for the measurement of energy expenditure in a respiration chamber, set by chamber volume and ventilation rate, is around 30 minutes. Then sleeping metabolic rate is defined as the average value of six subsequent 30-minute intervals, with the lowest value or the lowest residual of the individual relationship between energy expenditure and physical activity as a measure of DEE (see also the next section on DEE). Both procedures generally result in the same time interval; that is, the last three hours of the night before waking up between 3.00 and 7.00 am (Figure 12.6).

BMR and SMR are usually compared between subjects by standardising both to an estimate of metabolic body size, where fat-free mass is the main predictor. The reliable way of comparing BMR or SMR data is by regression analysis. BMR or SMR should never be divided by the absolute fat-free mass value, since the relationship between energy expenditure and fat-free mass has an axis intercept that is significantly different from zero (Figure 12.7). Comparing SMR per kg fat-free mass between women and men, as presented in Figure 12.7, results in significantly different values of 0.143 ± 0.012 and 0.128 ± 0.080 MJ/kg ($p < 0.0001$), respectively. The smaller the fat-free mass, the higher the SMR/kg, and thus the SMR per kg fat-free mass is on average higher in women, who have a lower fat-free mass compared to men.

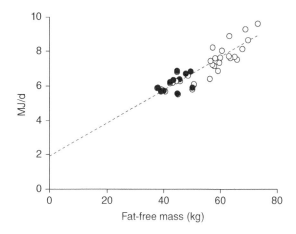

Figure 12.7 Sleeping metabolic rate plotted as a function of fat-free mass for 17 women (closed dots) and 20 men (open dots), age 20–35 years and body mass index 20–30 kg/m², with the calculated linear regression line.

When fat-free mass and gender are included as covariates in a regression analysis, gender does not come out as a significant contributor to the explained variation.

In conclusion, basal metabolic rate or sleeping metabolic rate measurements should meet the conditions of subjects being awake or asleep, respectively, and being postabsorptive, at rest and in the thermoneutral zone. Measured values can be compared between subjects in a regression analysis with fat-free mass and fat mass as covariates.

Measuring diet-induced energy expenditure

Diet-induced energy expenditure is the energy expenditure for the intestinal absorption of nutrients, the initial steps of their metabolism and the storage of the absorbed but not immediately oxidised nutrients. It is measured as the increase in energy expenditure above the basal fasting level after consumption of a meal, defined as the increase in energy expenditure above the basal fasting level divided by the energy content of the food ingested, and commonly expressed as a percentage.

The experimental design of most studies on DEE is a measurement of resting energy expenditure before and after a test meal, with a ventilated-hood system. The observation is started after an overnight fast, where subjects refrain from eating after the last meal at 8.00 pm at the latest. Thus, with observations starting between 8.00 and 9.00 am the next morning, the fasting interval is at least 12 hours. Postprandial measurements are made for several hours and subjects have to remain stationary, most often in a supine position, for the duration of the measurements. In some studies, measurements are for 30 minutes with 15-minute intervals, allowing for instance for sanitary activities.

The use of a respiration chamber to measure DEE has the advantage of reproducing more physiological conditions over a longer period of time while regular meals are consumed throughout the day. The DEE, as observed in a respiration chamber over 24 hours, has been evaluated in different ways:

1. As the difference in 24-hour energy expenditure between a day in the fed state and a day in the fasted state.
2. As the difference in daytime energy expenditure adjusted for the variability of spontaneous activity and basal metabolic rate.
3. As the difference in 24-hour energy expenditure adjusted for the variability of spontaneous activity and basal metabolic rate.

Reported intra-individual variability in DEE determined with ventilated-hood systems is 5–30%. Reported within-subject variability in DEE determined with a respiration chamber is 40–50%. The figures for the respiration chamber measurements are for the 24-hour DEE calculation as described under method 3, 24-hour energy expenditure adjusted for the variability of spontaneous activity and basal metabolic rate. Method 2, daytime energy expenditure adjusted for the variability of spontaneous activity and basal metabolic rate, resulted in an intra-individual variability of 125%.

The mean pattern of DEE throughout the day is presented in Figure 12.8. Data are from a study where DEE was calculated by plotting the residual of the individual relationship between energy expenditure and physical activity, as measured over 30-minute intervals from a 24-hour observation in a respiration chamber (Figure 12.8a), over time (Figure 12.8b). Subjects were the same 17 women and 20 men as depicted in Figures 12.6 and 12.7. The level of resting metabolic rate after waking up in the morning, and directly before the first meal, was defined as the basal metabolic rate. The resting metabolic rate did not return to the basal metabolic rate before lunch at 4 hours after breakfast, or before dinner at 5 hours after lunch. Overnight, basal metabolic rate was reached at 8–9 hours after dinner consumption.

Based on the amount of ATP required for the initial steps of metabolism and storage, the DEE is different for each nutrient. Reported DEE values for separate nutrients are 0–3% for fat, 5–10% for carbohydrate, 20–30% for protein and 10–30% for alcohol. In healthy subjects with a mixed diet, DEE represents about 10% of the total amount of energy ingested over 24 hours. Thus, when a subject is in energy balance, where intake equals expenditure, DEE is 10% of daily energy expenditure.

Measuring activity-induced energy expenditure

Activity-induced energy expenditure is the most variable component of daily energy expenditure. The indicated method for the measurement of AEE is the doubly labelled water method for the measurement of total energy expenditure (TEE) in combination with a measurement of basal metabolic rate under a ventilated hood, as described earlier. Then, AEE is calculated as TEE – (DEE + BMR) or $0.9 \times$ TEE – BMR, where DEE is estimated as 10% of TEE.

The doubly labelled water method is the gold standard for the validation of field methods of assessing physical activity. The indicated method for the assessment of habitual physical activity in daily life is a doubly labelled water validated accelerometer. Accelerometers can provide information about the total amount, the frequency, the intensity and the duration of physical activity.

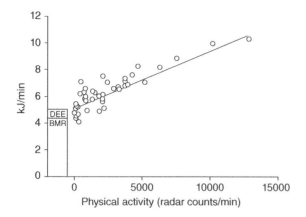

Figure 12.8a Energy expenditure over 30-minute intervals from a 24-hour observation in a respiration chamber, plotted as a function of physical activity measured with Doppler radar. Diet-induced energy expenditure (DEE) is calculated as the intercept of the linear regression line with the ordinate axis minus basal metabolic rate (BMR).

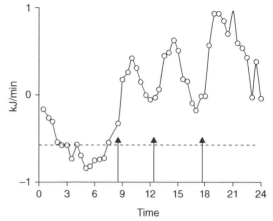

Figure 12.8b The mean pattern of DEE throughout the day, calculated by plotting the residual of the regression line as depicted in Figure 12.8a in time. Subjects were 17 women and 20 men as depicted in Figures 12.6 and 12.7, arrows denote meal times, and BMR is denoted by the dotted line.

However, validity studies should be interpreted with care. Results are based on a comparison between accelerometer output and doubly labelled water assessed TEE in a multiple regression analysis with subject characteristics as additional covariates. The separate contribution of accelerometer counts to the explained variation in TEE is often not presented and standard errors of agreement are large or not presented.

There are several methods to adjust TEE for differences in body size to compare the physical activity level between subjects. The most common method, as adopted by the Food and Agricultural Organization of the United Nations, the World Health Organization (WHO) and the United Nations University, is to express TEE as a multiple of BMR: physical activity level (PAL) = TEE/BMR. This assumes that variation in TEE is due to body size and physical activity, where the effect of body size is corrected for by expressing TEE as a multiple of BMR. Additionally, it assumes that the relationship between TEE and BMR has no significant intercept. The most sophisticated way to compare the physical activity level between subjects is a linear regression analysis. Then, the activity measure is the residual of the regression of TEE on BMR or SMR. Subjects with a positive residual have higher physical activity than the group average and subjects with a negative residual have lower physical activity than the group average. There was no difference between the two methods for a group of 37 subjects, where TEE plotted as a function of SMR has an intercept not significantly different from zero (Figure 12.9).

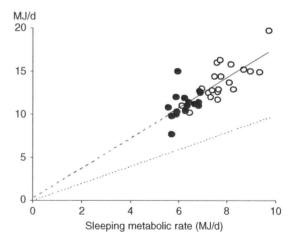

Figure 12.9 Total energy expenditure plotted as a function of sleeping metabolic rate with the calculated linear regression line. The lower dotted line denotes the minimum level of total energy expenditure, where total energy expenditure equals sleeping metabolic rate. Subjects were 17 women (closed dots) and 20 men (open dots), as depicted in Figure 12.8.

The common method to adjust AEE for differences in body size is by expressing AEE per kg body mass. This assumes that subjects weighing 100 kg spend twice as much energy for the same activities as subjects weighing 50 kg. However, not all daily activities are mass dependent. Normalising AEE by dividing by body mass to the exponent 1.0 might over-correct for body size in heavier subjects, making them appear less active. Thus, caution must be exercised when interpreting AEE data from individuals of markedly different body size. So far, physical activity level calculated as TEE divided by BMR or SMR, where BMR and SMR scale to metabolic body mass or body mass to the exponent 0.66 to 0.75, seems to be the best compromise.

The majority of the population has a physical activity level ranging from 1.5 to 2.0. The WHO defined an activity factor below 1.5 as inactive, between 1.5 and 2.0 as average to active and above 2.0 as very active. Studies to increase the physical activity level with exercise training repeatedly show an increase of the activity level to a value between 2.0 and maximally 2.5.

12.3 Determinants of energy expenditure

Differences in total energy expenditure between individuals are mainly a function of differences in body composition and physical activity, where body composition determines SMR and BMR and physical activity determines AEE. For a typical group of young adults, TEE ranged from 7.9 to 19.7 MJ/day, a more than two-fold difference between the lowest and the highest values (Figure 12.9). The lowest value was for a woman weighing 62.2 kg with a PAL value of 1.4. The highest value was for a man weighing 100.0 kg with a PAL value of 2.2. Women generally have a lower fat-free mass than men, due to a lower weight in combination with a higher body fat percentage. Thus, total energy expenditure is generally lower in women than in men unless a higher physical activity level compensates for the difference in maintenance metabolism. For the subject group depicted in Figures 12.6–12.9, the average values for TEE and PAL were 11.2 MJ/day and 1.76 for the women and 13.7 MJ/day and 1.74 for the men, respectively.

Changes in energy expenditure within individuals are mainly a function of physical activity, food intake and age. The physical activity level typically ranges between 1.5 and 2.0, where training programmes can induce an increase. Subjects over age 50 tend to compensate for training activity with a decrease of physical activity in the non-training time. A similar compensation mechanism occurs in young adults when a training programme is combined with energy restriction. Energy restriction results in a reduction of energy expenditure by a reduction of maintenance metabolism or BMR, DEE and AEE. In the classic Minnesota experiment, young men with a maintenance requirement of 14.6 MJ/day were restricted to 6.6 MJ/day for 24 weeks. They reached energy balance at the end of the experiment, where 58% of the total energy saving could be ascribed to a reduction of AEE, of which 40% was for a reduced body weight and 60% for a reduced physical activity. Studies on the effectiveness of diet-plus-exercise interventions versus diet-only interventions for weight loss show that it is difficult to overcome a diet-induced reduction of physical activity with exercise training. Physical activity gradually increases from early age to adulthood and decreases again in old age. At 1 year of age, when children start to walk, about 20% of TEE is accounted for by physical activity equivalent to a PAL value of 1.4. The fraction increases to adult values of about 33% or a PAL value of 1.75 at age 15 years, soon after reproductive age is reached. After age 15, AEE remains on average at a constant level, to decrease gradually after age 50. Subjects at age 90 are again spending 20% of TEE for physical activity, as at the age of 1 year when they started to walk. Thus, it seems that AEE is highest at reproductive age.

The upper limit of total energy expenditure is reached in endurance athletes. In professional endurance athletes like participants of the three-week Tour de France cycle race, doubly labelled water measured PAL values ranged from 3.5 to 5.5, twice the upper limit in the general population. Subjects maintained energy balance, as body weight and body composition did not change during the race. Endurance athletes are a select subject group with an increased fat-free mass through predisposition and long-term exercise training. Additionally, athletes performing at a high level of energy expenditure have learned to ingest large amounts of food and incorporate a significant amount of carbohydrate-rich drink into the diet.

12.4 Evaluation of intake methods

Energy expenditure is a function of body size and physical activity. Since the application of the doubly labelled water technique for measurement of total energy expenditure in free-living humans, we know that energy expenditure increases with body weight. Before, energy expenditure was derived from reported intake, resulting in the opposite conclusion. Figure 12.10 shows a typical example of reported intake and measured expenditure in the same subjects, with a body weight range from 51–103 kg for women and 59–141 kg for men. Reported intake is independent of body weight in women, while in men reported intake is significantly lower in heavier subjects ($p < 0.05$). In both genders, measured expenditure is significantly higher than reported intake ($p < 0.001$) and is significantly higher in heavier subjects ($p < 0.001$). Heavier subjects tend to show more under-reporting of food intake than lean subjects, as shown by the higher degree of misreporting in subjects with a higher body mass index. When reported intake is expressed as a multiple of estimated basal metabolic rate, this food intake-derived physical

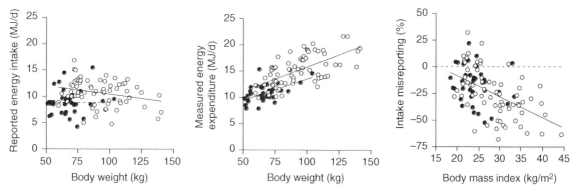

Figure 12.10 Reported energy intake as measured with a 7-day food record (left) and measured energy expenditure as measured simultaneously with doubly labelled water (middle) in the same subjects, plotted as a function of body weight for women (closed dots) and men (open dots), with the linear regression lines when there was a significant relation. Additionally, intake misreporting, calculated as (reported energy intake – measured energy expenditure) / measured energy expenditure, is plotted as a function of body mass index (right).

activity measure is significantly lower in subjects with a higher body mass index. Reported intake as a multiple of basal metabolic rate is often lower than the theoretical minimum of 1, especially in overweight and obese subjects.

The ratio of energy intake (EI) to BMR is often used to recognise under-reporting. Then, a cut-off limit for EI/BMR is set at a minimum PAL value, often a value of 1.3. However, cut-off limits do not take variation in individual PAL values into account. A subject with a reported intake of 10 MJ/day and a PAL value of 1.4 could be a correct reporter, where the energy expenditure and thus the intake of the same subject should be more than 14 MJ/day when the PAL value is 2.0. Thus, to validate reported energy intake, one should use a combination of BMR and physical activity. Basal metabolic rate can be measured or estimated with an equation from the literature, based on the height, weight, age and gender of the subject. Physical activity can be measured with a doubly labelled water validated accelerometer for movement registration.

Under-reporting of habitual intake can be explained by under-recording and/or under-eating. Comparing reported food intake and water intake with energy expenditure and water loss, as measured with doubly labelled water, separates the two errors. In healthy individuals, water balance is preserved and is therefore an independent indicator for under-recording. The recording precision of water intake is assumed to be representative for total food recording. Under-eating during food recording is monitored by measurement of body weight changes over the recording interval.

Under-reporting of food intake seems to be more of a concern for specific food items, which are generally considered 'bad for health'. An example is the inverse relation between fat intake and obesity entitled the 'American

paradox'. In the adult population the prevalence of overweight has increased and at the same time reported energy intake and %energy from fat have decreased. This might be due to lower physical activity and higher consumption of low-energy foods, but under-reporting has also increased. Combining the results of studies showing selective under-reporting of fat intake, the reported decrease in energy and fat intake seems to be doubtful.

References and further reading

Bonomi, A.G. and Westerterp, K.R. (2012) Advances in physical activity monitoring and lifestyle interventions in obesity – a review. *International Journal of Obesity*, **36**, 167–177.

Butte, N.F., Ekelund, U. and Westerterp, K.R. (2012) Assessing physical activity using wearable monitors: Measures of physical activity. Medicine & Science in Sports & Exercise, **44**, S5–S12.

Heitmann, B.L., Westerterp, K.R., Loos, R.J. *et al.* (2012) Obesity: Lessons from evolution and the environment. *Obesity Reviews*, **13**, 910–922.

Plasqui, G., Bonomi, A.G. and Westerterp, K.R. (2013) Daily physical activity assessment with accelerometers: New insights and validation studies. *Obesity Reviews*, **14**, 451–462.

Speakman, J.R. (1997) *Doubly Labeled Water, Theory and Practice.* Chapman and Hall, London.

Thomas, D.M., Bouchard, C., Church, T. *et al.* (2012) Why do individuals not lose more weight from an exercise intervention at a defined dose? An energy balance analysis. *Obesity Reviews*, **13**, 835–847.

Westerterp, K.R. (2009) Assessment of physical activity: A critical appraisal. *European Journal of Applied Physiology*, **105**, 823–828.

Westerterp, K.R. (2010) Physical activity, food intake and body weight regulation: Insights from doubly labeled water studies. *Nutrition Reviews*, **68**, 148–154.

Westerterp, K.R. (2013) *Energy Balance in Motion.* Springer, Heidelberg.

Westerterp, K.R. and Goris, A.H.C. (2002) Validity of the assessment of dietary intake: Problems of misreporting. *Current Opinion in Clinical Nutrition and Metabolic Care*, **5**, 489–493.

13
Application of 'Omics' Technologies

Helen M Roche,[1] Baukje de Roos[2] and Lorraine Brennan[1]

[1] University College Dublin
[2] University of Aberdeen

Key messages

- With the advent and continual advancement of state-of-the-art 'omics' technologies, it is now possible to investigate the dynamic, two-way interaction between nutrition and the human genome, which determines gene and/or protein expression and the consequent metabolic response.
- Genomics refers to gene-sequencing approaches to determine the total genetic information, or the genome, of a cell or an organism. In very simple terms, nutrigenomics attempts to explore the synergy between DNA sequence and nutritional exposure with a view to identifying gene–nutrient interactions.
- Transcriptomic approaches allow measurement of multiple mRNA transcripts simultaneously, with a view to understanding the interactions and co-expression patterns between numerous genes. This comprehensive approach can facilitate

the characterisation of multiple gene expression responses or a 'transcriptional signature' to an acute metabolic challenge and/or chronic nutritional intervention.
- Proteomics is a tool to identify and quantitate the proteins – enzymes, structural proteins and cell signalling proteins – that are regulated by certain dietary interventions.
- Proteomics can help to elucidate mechanisms whereby food components influence health or disease processes, or it could help to identify specific protein biomarkers to diagnose disease.
- Metabolomics is a tool to identify and quantify small molecules called metabolites.
- Metabolomics can be used in nutrition research for analysis of molecular mechanisms in dietary interventions; determination of biomarkers of dietary intake; and analysis of diet-related diseases.

13.1 An introduction to 'omics' technologies: Comprehensive tools to advance nutrition research

An individual's nutritional phenotype represents a complex interaction between the human genome and environmental factors during that individual's lifetime. With the advent and continual advancement of state-of-the-art 'omics' technologies, it is now possible to investigate the dynamic, two-way interaction between nutrition and the human genome, which determines gene and/or protein expression and the consequent metabolic response, the combination of which is reflected in an individual's health status. High-throughput molecular 'omics' technologies, defining the genome, epigenome, transcriptome, proteome and metabolome, are providing an

unprecedented opportunity to advance our understanding of the molecular effects of nutrition on health and common diet-related diseases.

This chapter will explain the basic principles relating to each technology platform, and thus explore the potential for high-throughput genomic, transcriptomic, proteomic and metabolomic technologies within human nutrition research. Every technology has great potential to advance the state of the art; however, it also needs to be acknowledged that each also has its limitations. It is important to note that these tools are best used in conjunction with strong nutritional/biochemical/physiological biomarkers of health and disease, with a view to using 'omics' technologies to gain a further understanding of the molecular processes wherein nutritional status and/or interventions contribute to that state.

Nutrition Research Methodologies, First Edition. Edited by Julie A Lovegrove, Leanne Hodson, Sangita Sharma and Susan A Lanham-New.
© 2015 John Wiley & Sons, Ltd. Published 2015 by John Wiley & Sons, Ltd.
Companion Website: www.wiley.com/go/nutritionsociety

13.2 What is genomics and why is it an important technology?

Genomics refers to gene-sequencing approaches to determine the total genetic information, or *genome*, of a cell or an organism. In very simple terms, genomics attempts to explore the deoxyribonucleic acid (DNA) sequence, or the precise order of the four bases – adenine, guanine, cytosine and thymine – in a nucleotide or strand of DNA within the genome. Genomics includes any method or technology that is used to determine the order; the common methods include genotyping arrays or 'BeadChip' technologies. The advent of very powerful genomic technologies has made it dramatically easier and very cheap to sequence DNA, so that it is now possible to determine complete genome sequences relatively easily. The expression of each gene when translated leads to the formation of a protein, which together with many other proteins that are coded by other genes forms tissues, organs and systems, and these combined constitute the whole organism. As illustrated in Figure 13.1, the flow of genetic information from the genome, transcriptome and proteome is reflected in the metabolome, and both nutrient and non-nutrient food components can interact at each level to affect the relationship between the human genome, nutrition and health.

Genetic polymorphisms are different forms of the same allele in the population. The 'normal' allele is known as the *wild-type allele*, whereas the variant is known as the polymorphic or mutant allele. A polymorphism differs from a mutation because it occurs in a population at a frequency greater than 1%. Alleles with frequencies less than 1% are considered as a recurrent mutation. The Human Genome Project demonstrated that the human genome is almost identical (99.9%) between individuals. The remaining 0.1% variation is principally accounted for by *single nucleotide polymorphisms* (SNPs). These common forms of inherited genetic variation involve a single base change in the DNA and account for almost 90% of variation between individuals. It is estimated that each of our genes contains approximately 10 variations or SNPs in its code from the standard gene. Important terminology related to genomics and nutrigenetics is presented in Box 13.1.

It is very important to note that not all polymorphisms have a functional impact. SNPs can occur in both the coding and the, more abundant, non-coding regions of the human genome. In addition, a single base change in a coding region of a gene does not necessarily alter gene function or the resultant amino acid sequence. Functional SNPs are those that may alter the amino acid sequence or a transcription-factor binding element.

DNA variants in several genes can interact with numerous environmental factors, including nutritional status, to determine several common, *polygenic*, diet-related diseases, including cardiovascular disease (CVD), obesity, type 2 diabetes (T2D), some cancers and so on. The research challenge lies in understanding how the combination genetic variation(s) determine cellular

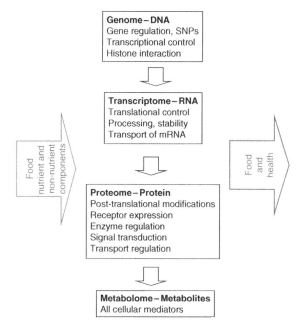

Figure 13.1 The health effects of nutrient and non-nutrient food components may be regulated via specific molecular interactions with the genome, transcriptome, proteome and/or metabolome.
Adapted from Roche, H.M. (2006) Nutrigenomics – new approaches for human nutrition research. *Journal of the Science of Food and Agriculture*, **86**, 1156–1163.

Box 13.1 Important terminology related to genomics

- The *genome* of an organism is the total number of genes that make up a cell or organism.
- Each diploid cell contains two copies of each gene; the individual copies of the gene are called *alleles*. Therefore an individual can carry the same or different alleles of every gene.
- The term *genotype* refers to the two alleles present at one gene locus.
- *Homozygous* individuals carry two identical alleles of a particular gene, whereas *heterozygotes* have two different alleles of a particular gene.
- The term *haplotype* describes a cluster of alleles that occur together on a DNA segment and/or are inherited together.
- *Genetic linkage* is the tendency for alleles close together to be transmitted or inherited together through meiosis.

homeostasis, whole-body metabolism and health, because each SNP makes a relatively small contribution. This complexity is in stark contrast to the more unusual, but very profound, *monogenic* conditions such as phenylketonuria (PKU) or familial hypercholesterolaemia, which are attributable to a single genetic defect that interacts with nutritional status. In the case of PKU, the defective gene for the hepatic enzyme phenylalanine hydroxylase (PAH) interacts with the amino acid phenylalanine to cause disease unless that amino acid is removed from the diet to maintain health.

More recently, *copy number variation* (CNV) has been identified as another common form of genetic variation. It is estimated that about 0.4% of the human genome differs with respect to CNV. As yet it has not been associated with susceptibility or resistance to diet-related diseases, but it is possible that this type of genetic variation may also be linked to nutrition and health.

In addition, alterations in DNA structure without changes in the underlying gene, nucleotide or DNA sequence, referred to as *epigenetics*, can also have important functional effects. Epigenetic modifications alter gene expression due to mechanisms beyond DNA sequence modifications. The molecular basis of this is complex, but it involves modifications including DNA methylation, DNA acetylation and histone modification. These changes in DNA structure cause the activation/deactivation of gene expression, thereby affecting the subsequent transcriptome, proteome and metabolome (as illustrated in Figure 13.1) without changing the DNA sequence.

Epigenetics will be dealt with in greater detail in Chapter 14, but briefly, DNA methylation refers to the addition of methyl groups to the *CpG islands* in the promoter regions of DNA and is associated with gene inactivation, which in turn affects transcriptional activity. Importantly, epigenetic modifications remain through cell division for the duration of the cells' life and can also be passed on to future generations, a process known as transgenerational epigenetic inheritance of functional DNA variation, where the genes express themselves differently despite being identical from a sequence perspective. Changes in DNA methylation are a potential molecular mechanism through which diet and lifestyle interventions mediate their effects on the transcriptome. Initial research showed that global DNA *hypermethylation*, and/or conversely *hypomethylation*, was implicated in the development and progression of cancer. From the nutritional perspective, folate status can affect DNA methylation, which in turn can affect gene expression through mechanisms that are being actively researched. Within the context of type 2 diabetes, it has been shown that family history is associated with differences in the DNA methylation status of important cell signalling and metabolic genes in skeletal muscle and adipose tissue. Furthermore, the DNA methylation status is modifiable by diet and exercise interventions, wherein the methylation state may modify the degree to which DNA can be transcribed into ribonucleic acid (RNA), thus affecting the transcriptome, and subsequent proteome and metabolome.

Genomics: Experimental approaches to identify gene–nutrient interactions

The term *nutrigenetics* focuses on investigating the relationship between common genetic variations or polymorphisms (or epigenetic modifications) and the nutritional environment. Such gene–nutrient combinations may determine an individual's nutrient requirements, their metabolic response and/or their responsiveness to a nutritional intervention, all of which may predispose an individual to a lesser or greater risk of developing a diet-related disease. Personalised nutrition approaches sometimes focus on the effect of genetic variation in response to dietary change, because some polymorphisms or epigenetic states may determine an individual's response and/or the therapeutic efficacy of a dietary intervention, which may in turn determine the outcome of certain disease states.

The *candidate gene approach* has been traditional for identifying the genes involved in a diet-related condition. The candidate genes can be identified according to biological function and/or linkage studies. Each subject with and without the disease (case and control groups) donates a DNA sample, the sequence of which is determined using an appropriate sequencing or array platform. Then association tests are carried out for significant differences in the allele frequencies of the SNPs of interest. If one variant of the allele is more frequent in the 'at-risk' patient group compared to a healthy control population, then the SNP is 'associated' with the disease. This candidate gene approach can be used within a case-control and/or prospective study design. While there have been a number of studies published using this approach, and interesting research has shown different interactions between different-risk SNPs and nutritional status. Nevertheless, it is important to note that overall there has been limited success from candidate gene studies, in terms of defining the genetic determinants of diet-related diseases. This limitation reflects the fact that a number of metabolic pathways with several candidate genes are often involved in diet-related disease and metabolic responses.

Furthermore, it is important to be aware of the potential limitations of gene association studies. Firstly, it is essential to replicate any potential finding in an independent cohort, as too often positive results in one cohort have not been replicated in subsequent studies. The main reasons for this are inadequate statistical power, multiple hypothesis testing, population stratification, publication bias and phenotypic differences. It is becoming increasingly evident that the identification of true genetic association in common multifactorial conditions, such as obesity, T2D or cancers, requires large studies consisting of thousands rather than hundreds of subjects. In addition, it is desirable to demonstrate a *functional effect* of a given SNP. For example, if a polymorphism introduces a missense change in the coding region of the peroxisome proliferator activator receptor gamma (PPARγ) gene, it probably represents a functional variant. Alternatively, functional assays may show greater or lesser activity of the protein arising from the gene. As an example, it has been shown that the Pro12Ala polymorphism in the transcription factor PPARγ gene was associated with less DNA-binding affinity and reduced transcriptional activity. Lastly, the absence of large single-gene effects and the detection of multiple small effects accentuate the need for the study of larger populations in order to identify reliably the size of the effect that we now expect for complex diseases.

Positional cloning involves mapping the susceptibility/causative loci purely on their chromosomal location, using multigenerational pedigrees and/or a large number of sibling pairs. This allows identification of genes without any prior knowledge of biological function or the disease mechanism. Linkage and linkage disequilibrium (LD) analysis relies on the fact that genes with similar chromosome positions will only rarely be separated during genetic recombination, so that susceptibility to causative genes can be localised by search for genetic markers that co-segregate with disease. However, to date this approach has identified relatively few candidate genes relevant to diet-related diseases. One of the earliest significant linkage peaks was at chromosome 2q37.3, which led to the identification of Calpain 10 (*CAPN10*) as a new putative diabetes gene. The authors implicated an A to G polymorphism in intron 3 of the gene encoding *CAPN10* with a greater risk of T2D. Subsequent to this initial report, several groups showed modest associations between *CAPN10* polymorphisms and metabolic phenotypes associated with T2D. Nevertheless, other groups have failed to show a relationship between *CAPN10* and metabolic traits indicative of T2D. The lack of a firm gene–phenotype relationship arising from a gene, identified using a positional cloning approach, may be due to a number of causes of inconsistency in association studies, including population-specific patterns of LD, population-specific environmental triggers and gene–gene or gene–nutrient interactions.

Genome-wide association studies (GWAS) focus on determining the prevalence of several (thousands of) SNPs simultaneously. The principle is similar for the candidate gene approach, with GWAS comparing the DNA of groups of cases versus control subjects. The DNA sequence of the cases and controls is determined using SNP arrays to determine whether the frequency of gene variant(s) is greater in the population with the condition versus controls. The associated SNPs are then considered to mark a region of the human genome that influences disease risk. GWAS goes beyond the candidate gene approach, which is limited to one or a few genetic regions based on prior knowledge and research bias. GWAS investigates the entire genome, thus it has the opportunity to identify novel genetic determinants. Again this approach has limitations, as while GWAS can identify new SNPs in DNA that are associated with a disease, it cannot specify which genes are causal. The potential limitations of GWAS relate to optimal study design. Sufficient numbers of accurately phenotyped cases and controls, adequate measures to control and correct for multiple testing to avoid the generation of false positive results and control for population stratification are important design issues that need to be addressed at the outset of a new study.

Next-generation sequencing (NGS) and high-throughput sequencing are technologies that have the capability greatly to enhance efficiency, producing thousands or millions of sequences at once. High-throughput sequencing technologies are intended to lower the cost of DNA sequencing compared to standard methods. NGS achieves high-throughput sequencing by completing the sequencing process of multiple DNA fragments that overlap in parallel or simultaneously. Then the final DNA sequence is reassembled by collating the DNA sequence information from the multiple overlapping DNA fragment sequences.

13.3 Transcriptomics: Quantification of multiple-gene mRNA expression

Transcriptomic approaches allow measurement of multiple messenger RNA (mRNA) transcripts (typically about 30 000) or gene expression profiles simultaneously, circumventing the limitations of single-transcript analyses such as reverse transcription polymerase chain reaction (RT-PCR) or northern blotting. DNA microarrays are useful tools for understanding the interactions and co-expression patterns between numerous genes at the transcriptional level. In general, the expression of large numbers of genes (i.e. an expression profile) changes when environmental conditions, such as nutrient exposure or nutritional status, are altered. Therefore, this comprehensive approach can facilitate the characterisation of multiple or global gene expression in response to an acute metabolic challenge and/or a chronic nutritional intervention. Transcriptomic analyses are also extremely valuable in terms of understanding the wide gene expression profile that contributes to the metabolic perturbations in diet-related pathologies. Thus, transcriptomic experiments not only allow the scientist to analyse genes that are known to be involved in a nutritional response or disease, but also allow measurement of the effect on many new genes for which no involvement in the disease has previously been described; and/or novel candidates that reflect a nutritional state or metabolic intervention for which the function is as yet unknown; or genes that were otherwise not known to be involved in nutrition. This helps the researcher to escape the trap of the literature or preconceived hypothesis bias and to focus on novel markers and molecular processes related to their area of nutrition research.

Since the initial description of microarrays, the application of transcriptomics has been astounding in terms of progressing our understanding of nutrition and health. Initial studies examined transcriptional responses in healthy versus unhealthy populations, the results of which have progressed our understanding of the molecular mechanisms of diet-related diseases. For example, elegant microarray studies identified the central role of PPARγ co-activator 1a (PGC-1a) and oxidative phosphorylation gene sets in the onset of T2D. More recently, nutrition research studies have used transcriptomics as a tool to attain more knowledge on novel functional and molecular effects of dietary challenges and/or nutritional interventions, with a view to deepening our understanding underpinning the physiological and metabolic responses related to the role of nutrition in human health.

Microarrays: Study design and technical issues to be appreciated

As with all experiments, sufficient sample numbers are ultimately important. Microarrays are very expensive, therefore the challenge is to ensure that the experiment includes sufficient biological replicates within budgetary constraints. As a rule of thumb, cell culture experiments require n = 5 samples per treatment group; animal experiments n = 10 per treatment group; and human samples at least n = 20 per treatment group. As human samples tend to display greater biological variation, the last estimate is dependent on the magnitude of the expected effect on the transcriptome and power calculations should be performed for each individual study. A typical transcriptome experimental flow chart is depicted in

Figure 13.2. Performance of a typical microarray experiment requires the isolation of sufficient quantities of highly pure and high-quality RNA to avoid any bias or failure of chip hybridisation. RNA is extracted from the tissue, quantified and the quality assessed. The RNA integrity number (RIN) is a measure of RNA quality that ranges from 0–10 (poor–excellent); as a rule of thumb the RIN should be at least 8. If the RNA is not of sufficiently high quality, then the sample(s) should be re-extracted to attain good-quality starting material. Where sufficient volumes of high-quality mRNA are purified, these RNA samples may be used to create complementary DNA (cDNA) for amplification using polymerase chain reaction (PCR). The PCR-amplified cDNA is then fluorescently labelled and used for microarray hybridisation.

Two types of microarray are in common use today: oligonucleotide microarrays and cDNA arrays. As oligonucleotide microarrays are the most common, for simplicity we shall confine our discussions to this type of array. A number of excellent reviews are available that describe both types of array in more detail (see References and further reading). Oligonucleotide arrays rely on the hybridisation of short 15bp regions of DNA from the 5′ region of the transcript to a complementary 15bp 'probe' randomly distributed across the chip. For each transcript being analysed, a set of approximately 10 such probes is located across the chip; for each probe in the probe set, a corresponding 'mismatch' probe is also found on the chip. The mismatch probes have a single-base mismatch compared to the perfect-match probe and are used to assess the level of background binding to the chip. After the complementary DNA strands have bound to the chip, the level of fluorescence at each probe location is measured in a purpose-designed scanner. Following scanning, the data produced should be ready for analysis.

Analysis of the spot intensities for a particular chip is a complicated process and requires evaluation of the intensities of all probes in a probe set as compared to the background staining level. At the most basic level, this is performed by subtracting the mismatch intensities from the perfect-match intensities for each probe in the probe set (i.e. probe signal minus probe background) and obtaining the mean intensity based on the corrected values. In this way each transcript can be given a value that roughly corresponds to its abundance within the sample. However, researchers must also account for differences in staining and hybridisation across microarray chips and mismatch binding levels that can exceed perfect-match binding levels. For this reason, more mathematically advanced approaches to microarray analysis have been developed, with algorithms such as robust multiarray average (RMA) and GC-corrected RMA (GCRMA)

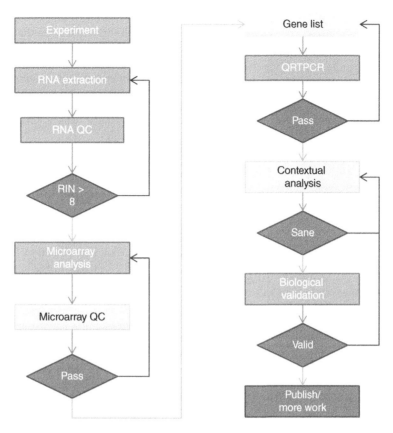

Figure 13.2 The experimental plan for a typical microarray experiment. Adapted from Morine, M.J., O'Brien, C. and Roche, H.M. (2008) Personalised nutrition: Transcriptomic signatures that have identified key features of metabolic syndrome. *Proceedings of the Nutrition Society*, **67**, 4, 395–403.

achieving widespread use and acceptance as methods suitable for the detection of biologically relevant transcript-level changes. By applying such methods to the analysis of microarray data, it is possible to discover which transcripts (if any) are differentially expressed at a statistically significant level between two conditions and to generate a gene list, a list of differentially expressed transcripts. At this stage it is common to validate the gene list, wherein the expression of a few targets that were significant – that is, quantitative RT-PCR assays – are conducted for a select number of genes that were significantly up- and downregulated to ensure that the results of the two gene expression methodologies agree.

Analysing data from a transcriptomic study

Depending on the results of the experiment, DNA microarrays will provide expression profiles of numerous known and unknown genes that will be up- or downregulated in response to a nutritional intervention or in different tissues at various stages of a diet-related disease. The generation of a gene list is normally one of the first-round approaches to examining transcriptomic data. Figure 13.3 illustrates the enormous amount of data that needs to be analysed in a more meaningful way. A simple list of up- and downregulated genes gives no conceptual understanding of the biological meaning of an experiment. While bioinformatic tools will be discussed in greater deal in Chapter 16, a brief overview of the approaches that might be used will be discussed here.

Very often in nutritional studies the magnitude of the gene expression profiles is modest. Arrays were first used in the cancer field, where the magnitude of the change in up- or downregulated genes was enormous; and within this context only the genes that were differentially regulated by at least two- or threefold were considered important. However, in nutritional studies the effect of an intervention or the difference between two nutritional states can be much more subtle. To overcome this limitation, it is possible to investigate the effect of those genes from the list of well-characterised biological context

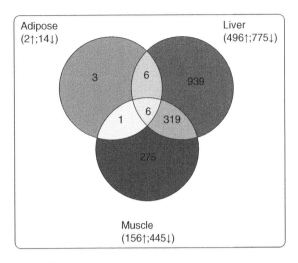

Figure 13.3 Number of genes within single gene lists from a transcriptomic study. Reprinted from Morine, M.J., McMonagle, J., Toomey, S. *et al.* (2010) Bi-directional gene set enrichment and canonical correlation analysis identify key diet-sensitive pathways and biomarkers of metabolic syndrome. *Bioinformatics*, **11**, 499. © BioMed Central.

processes such as signalling or metabolic pathways, or according to cellular location. A number of tools allow the visualisation of gene-list data in the context of biological pathways. Pathway databases such as the Kyoto Encyclopaedia of Genes and Genomes (KEGG) are very useful. KEGG is a bioinformatics resource that can be mined to identify groups of transcripts that are statistically over-represented in a gene list. In a similar approach, gene ontology (GO) classifications are routinely used to examine lists of differentially expressed transcripts to ascertain which functions are most over-represented among those genes on the gene list. The GO classifications, for example, will categorise gene lists according to cellular location or function. Gene-set enrichment analysis (GSEA) is another way to integrate gene sets based on biological function, chromosomal location or co-regulated genes. In many cases, a variety of biological databases are used to annotate a gene list, so as to identify significant effects on enzymatic activity, transcription regulation, cell signalling and so on. These bioinformatic approaches allow the investigator to explore the effect of nutrients on metabolic or biochemical pathways with a view to elaborating to more complex network analysis. These approaches allow the integration of genes that are functionally related to each other and facilitate characterisation of a 'transcriptomic signature' that describes the effect of a nutrient or metabolic state of a cell or tissue.

In concert with the growing availability of data from biological studies, bioinformatics software is continually advancing to incorporate an increasingly broad range of data. This will further facilitate the researcher in determining the effect of an intervention on the transcriptome. Indeed, the full use of the data set cannot be achieved without elaborate bioinformatic analysis that encompasses pathway and network analysis as well as other tools, such as clustering analysis and principal component analysis, which integrate multiple gene expression profiles.

13.4 What is proteomics and why is it an important technology?

Proteomics is the large-scale study of proteins, confirming the presence (or absence) of the protein and providing a direct measure of its quantity. The total complement of proteins in a cell type or biofluid at a single time is known as its proteome. The proteome of a cell or biofluid will vary with time and depend on the requirements, or stresses, that a cell or organism undergoes.

Proteins are essential parts of living organisms that participate in virtually every process within cells, a snapshot of which is presented in Figure 13.4. Many proteins are *enzymes*, which catalyse thousands of biochemical reactions that are vital to sustain life. Enzymes are highly selective catalysts that greatly accelerate both the rate and specificity of metabolic reactions. However, they also modulate processes such as DNA replication, DNA repair and transcription. Since enzymes are selective for their substrates and accelerate only specific reactions, the set of enzymes made in a cell determines which metabolic pathways occur in that cell.

Another set of proteins, *structural proteins*, confer stiffness and rigidity to cell components. Most structural proteins are fibrous proteins: for example, collagen and elastin are critical components of connective tissue such as cartilage, and keratin is found in hard or filamentous structures such as hair and nails. Some globular proteins, for example actin and tubulin, can polymerise to form long and stiff fibres that make up the cytoskeleton, which allows the cell to maintain its shape and size. Other proteins with structural functions are motor proteins, such as myosin, kinesin and dynein, which are capable of generating mechanical forces. These proteins are crucial for the cellular motility of single-celled organisms, but they also generate the forces that are necessary for muscle contraction, and they play an essential role in intra-cellular transport.

Last but not least, many proteins are involved in the processes of *cell signalling, signal transduction* and *ligand binding*. Some of these are extracellular proteins that transmit a signal from the cell in which they were synthesised to other tissues. Others are membrane proteins

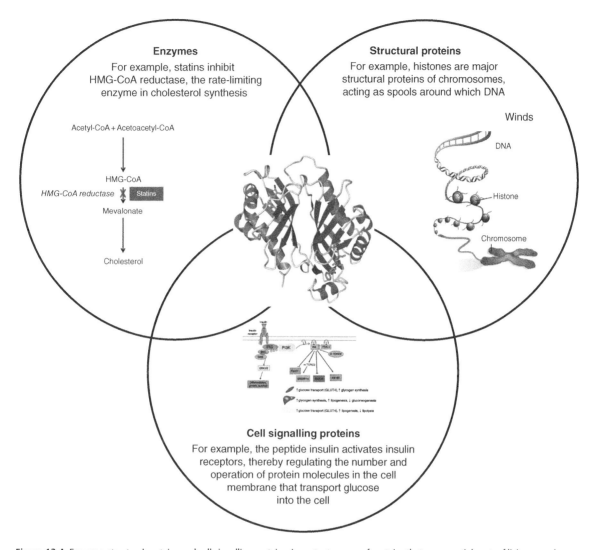

Figure 13.4 Enzymes, structural proteins and cell signalling proteins: important groups of proteins that are essential parts of living organisms.

that can act as a receptor and bind to signalling molecules in order to induce a biochemical response in the cell; or they are ligand transport proteins, such as haemoglobin, that bind particular small molecules, like oxygen, and transport them to other locations in the body. These proteins must have a high binding affinity when their ligand is present in high concentrations, but must also release the ligand when it is present at low concentrations in the target tissues.

A major advantage of proteomics is that it measures the functional product (protein) of gene expression in cells, tissues and biofluids, and allows the identification of modifications that may relate to the activation or inactivation of proteins. Indeed, proteome analysis of tissues or biofluids can enable the discovery of the mechanisms

whereby food components influence health or disease processes; it could also help to identify specific protein biomarkers to diagnose disease.

Proteomics: Moving on from transcriptomics

During protein biosynthesis, genes encoded in DNA are first transcribed into pre- mRNA by proteins such as RNA polymerase. Most organisms then process the pre-mRNA using various forms of post-transcriptional modification to form the mature mRNA. This in turn is used as a template for protein synthesis by the ribosome. During protein synthesis, or shortly thereafter, the residues in a protein are often chemically modified post-translationally. Many of these post-translational modifications are critical to the protein's function. The covalent addition of a chemical group to proteins alters the physical and chemical properties of the protein, resulting in differential folding, stability, activity state, cellular location and dynamic interactions with other proteins.

One such modification is phosphorylation, which happens to many enzymes and structural proteins that play a role in cell signalling processes. During phosphorylation, serine/threonine kinases mediate the addition of a phosphate to particular amino acids, most commonly serine and threonine. This causes the protein to become a target for binding to a distinct set of other proteins that will recognise the phosphorylated domain. Because protein phosphorylation is one of the most-studied protein modifications, many proteomic studies determine phosphorylated proteins in a particular cell or tissue type under particular circumstances. This may provide insights, for example, into the signalling pathways that are active.

Proteins can also undergo ubiquitination, where enzymes called E3 ubiquitin ligases attach the small protein ubiquitin to certain protein substrates. Knowledge about which proteins are poly-ubiquitinated by which ligases can help us to understand how protein pathways are regulated. Therefore, many proteomic studies assess ubiquitinated proteins in a particular cell or tissue type under particular circumstances.

In addition to phosphorylation and ubiquitination, proteins can be subjected to, for example, methylation, acetylation, glycosylation, oxidation and nitrosylation – there are over 200 known types of post-translational modifications that are present on at least 80% of eukaryotic proteins. Some proteins may undergo all of these modifications in time-dependent combinations.

When we take the extensive processes of post-transcriptional and post-translational modifications into account, it is not surprising to learn that the outcomes of transcriptomic and functional proteomic studies often do not correlate very well. Indeed, mRNA is not always translated into protein, and an mRNA produced in abundance may be degraded rapidly or translated inefficiently, resulting in a small amount of protein. Furthermore, as already mentioned, many proteins undergo post-translational modifications that profoundly affect the activity of the resulting proteins. For example, some proteins are not active until they become phosphorylated; or proteins may form complexes with other proteins or RNA molecules, and only function in the presence of these other molecules. In addition, the protein degradation rate could also play an important role in protein content. Proteomics measures the functional product (protein) of gene expression in cells,

tissues and biofluids, and allows the identification of modifications that may relate to the activation or inactivation of proteins. Therefore, this technology may give us a better understanding of the functioning of an organism compared to transcriptomics.

The human proteome is estimated to contain between 20 000 and 25 000 non-redundant proteins. The number of unique protein species is likely to increase by between 50 000 and 500 000 due to RNA splicing and proteolysis events, and when post-translational modifications are also considered, the total number of unique human proteins is estimated to range in the low millions. This illustrates the potential complexity in the cell proteome when studying protein structure and function.

Application of proteomics in nutrition studies

To perform proteomic analysis, a protein must be purified from other cellular components. This process usually starts with cell lysis, in which the membrane of a cell is disrupted and the internal contents of the cell are released into a solution known as 'lysate'. This mixture can be purified using ultracentrifugation, which fractionates the various cellular components into fractions containing soluble proteins; membrane lipids and proteins; cellular organelles; and nucleic acids. The use of different buffers also enhances the separation of various cellular fractions. For example, a Tris-based buffer containing protease inhibitors is often used to obtain cytosolic proteins, whereas the extraction of membrane proteins requires the addition of the chaotrophe urea and thiourea (to disrupt hydrogen and hydrophobic bonds), the reductant DTT (breaks disulphide bridges for denaturing proteins), the detergent CHAPS (disrupt membranes, solubilises lipids and delipidates proteins bound to vesicles or membranes), ampholytes (aids protein solubilisation and helps in the precipitation of nucleic acids during centrifugation) and protease inhibitors.

There are two major approaches in proteomics, top-down and bottom-up, as illustrated in Figure 13.5. Top-down proteomics involves separating intact proteins from complex tissue or biofluid homogenates using traditional separation techniques, such as 2D gel electrophoresis. This is a method for the separation and identification of proteins in a sample by displacement into two dimensions: isoelectric focusing is used in the first dimension to separate proteins by their charge, and SDS-PAGE is used in the second dimension to separate proteins by their molecular weight. As the separation of a sample takes place over a larger area, it increases the resolution of each component, allowing the investigation

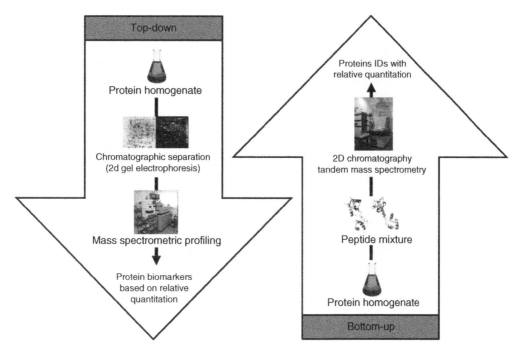

Figure 13.5 Top-down and bottom-up – the two major approaches in proteomics.

of global protein expression and the determination of differential protein expression. 2D gel electrophoresis is then followed by differential expression analysis using gel imaging platforms. The spots representing proteins that are differentially regulated are then identified using mass spectrometry. In nutrition research, 2D gel electrophoresis is still the most widely used proteomics approach, enabling the identification of proteins that relate to glucose and fatty acid metabolism as well as pathways involving oxidative stress, anti-oxidant defence mechanisms and redox status. While this method is one of the most labour intensive available, it actually yields a physical separation of intact polypeptides, providing information about molecular weight and iso-electric point, parameters that can be used to narrow down the identification of the protein. It also retains information on post-translational modifications, which are postulated to be relevant in many diseases and other biological processes. A recent advance is the introduction of difference gel electrophoresis (DIGE) technology, allowing direct quantitative comparison of differentially labelled protein samples using cyanine fluorescent dyes prior to electrophoresis. When absolute protein variation between two or three samples is the primary target, this method is more reproducible and accurate and not limited by distortion due to gel-to-gel variation, but it is costly and automation is difficult.

The bottom-up approach to protein profiling, also called 'shotgun proteomics', involves direct digestion of a protein homogenate using a proteolytic enzyme, such as trypsin. This cleaves the peptide at well-defined sites to create a complex peptide mixture. Digested samples can then be analysed on platforms consisting of liquid chromatography and tandem mass spectrometry. Shotgun proteomics can now be combined with stable isotope labelling to allow for the quantification of changes in expression levels of hundreds to thousands of proteins in a single experiment. The most commonly adopted approaches include isotope-coded affinity tags (ICAT) and isobaric tags for relative and absolute quantitation (iTRAQ). Quantification is based on relative changes in the levels of labelled peptides that may be common to a family of proteins, with differential regulation or abundance, and thus quantification experiments can sometimes lead to ambiguous or conflicting results.

Most proteomics techniques have difficulty with the detection of differential regulation of low-abundant but often clinically relevant proteins. Proteomic studies have to date revealed at maximum 50% of the predicted proteins in prokaryotic organisms and only 10% in higher organisms, with the numbers for quantified proteins being even smaller. Many proteomics methods also have difficulty finding post-translational modifications, as they are usually present at too low a concentration, therefore often only the unmodified version will be observed.

The increased quality and sensitivity of a new generation of mass spectrometers have already accelerated developments in detection and identification in the proteomics field. Hopefully future advances in mass spectrometry technology should further facilitate the accurate quantitative measurement of proteins and their post-translational modifications from complex biological samples, especially those that are present in low abundance. Until then, the success of proteomics in nutrition research will largely depend on the introduction and adaptation of more targeted, sensitive and quantitative approaches, such as chemical proteomics, multi-analyte profiling and multiple reaction monitoring.

Design and execution of proteomics studies

The actual use of the proteomics technique in dietary intervention trials is still very limited. This is probably due largely to the high costs of analysis, as well as challenges that come with the application of the technology. For example, high relative levels of biological and analytical variability in protein levels may sometimes mask subtle effects due to dietary interventions. Therefore, good experimental design should consider the impact of different sources of analytical variation originating from protein separation, staining, image acquisition and processing steps, and optimise standard operating procedures. The design should also consider the impact of different sources of biological variation that originate from environmental or genetic factors. This includes running sufficient replicates to ensure that the design has sufficient statistical power, sampling from a 'homogenous' population, and the inclusion of both baseline and end-value samples. Generally, biological variability is significantly lower in cellular proteomes compared with proteomics obtained from biofluids. Therefore, proteomics offers a valuable tool to study the cellular mechanisms of food compounds in target organs or blood cells such as liver, platelets and peripheral blood mononuclear cells (PBMC).

Several statistical and bioinformatics tools are available to help with the exploration and interpretation of proteomics results. For example, the use of boxplots and hierarchical clustering of samples and protein spots can help to identify outliers objectively or indicate the presence of an effect between groups. Principal component analysis is another approach to identify treatment effects. Furthermore, the combination of proteomics results with *in silico* network analysis will provide better insights into pathways that are activated by dietary compounds, as well as regulatory protein 'hubs' that are crucial for the regulation of these pathways. Both these regulatory protein hubs and the downstream products of the metabolic routes that are regulated by such hubs are expected to be likely biomarker candidates.

As for all studies that apply 'omics' technologies, proteomics studies need to consider the standardisation of interventions (diets and ingredients) and study populations, and because of high between-subject variability follow the double-blinded, placebo-controlled crossover design. The standardisation initiative in the proteomics community, MIAPE (Minimum Information About a Proteomics Experiment), provides guidelines on the minimal information needed and best-practice rules that should be applied for any nutritional intervention study.

13.5 Metabolomics and lipidomics

Introduction and overview of approach

Metabolomics refers to the comprehensive study of small molecules or metabolites present in biological samples, with the aim of studying alterations in metabolism under different conditions or physiological states. The complete complement of metabolites present in a sample is referred to as the metabolome. The study of metabolites reveals useful biological information, as the metabolites represent biological endpoints and are now implicated in the development of a number of human diseases.

The two main analytical approaches employed in metabolomics are nuclear magnetic resonance (NMR) spectroscopy and mass spectroscopy (MS). These techniques both have their advantages and disadvantages and at present there is no single analytical technique capable of analysing the complete metabolome in a single sample simultaneously. Therefore, in order to obtain comprehensive coverage of the metabolome it is necessary to use multiple platforms for data acquisition, further details of which are described by German, Hammock and Watkins (2005). NMR-based techniques have high reproducibility and little between-lab variation, but suffer from lower sensitivity. Even though they require higher sample volume, such techniques are not destructive and the sample can be reused for other analyses. GC-MS is best suited to volatile metabolites and to increase the volatility the samples are often derivitised. Examples of molecules routinely analysed using this approach include fatty acids, organic acids and sugars.

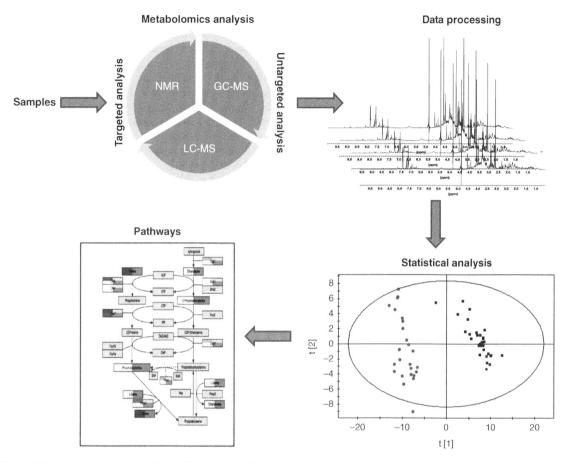

Figure 13.6 An overview of the steps involved in a metabolomics study.

LC-based techniques are sensitive and suited to soluble and lipophilic molecules. It should be noted that analysis of the lipids (a subclass of metabolites) is often referred to as lipidomics. Analysis of the diverse range of lipids is achieved through LC-MS–based techniques. For the purpose of this chapter we encompass lipid analysis in the term metabolomics.

Depending on the research question, the data can be acquired in a targeted or non-targeted manner. In hypothesis-free studies such as disease biomarker identification, non-targeted metabolomics is usually performed and data can be acquired using NMR, GC-MS and LC-MS–based techniques. Using this approach, a holistic overview of the metabolic alterations occurring under different conditions can be obtained. In general, the data obtained are semi-quantitative, as absolute concentration calculations require the use of multiple internal standards. When specific research hypotheses are to be tested, a targeted metabolomics approach measuring a defined series of metabolites quantitatively is the method of choice. Techniques commonly used in this type of data analysis are NMR, GC-MS, LC-MS/MS and flow injection-MS/MS.

A metabolomics study will perform the following steps: sample preparation; data acquisition; statistical analysis; and pathway mapping. The workflow in a typical metabolomics study is depicted in Figure 13.6. Sample preparation depends on the sample type, metabolite class to be analysed and platform to be used. Metabolomics can be performed on a range of samples and commonly used samples in nutrition research include saliva, urine, blood and biopsy samples such as adipose tissue.

The human metabolic profile or the metabolome is influenced by a number of phenotypical, physiological and external factors. Numerous studies have been carried out to assess these factors in humans. Clear evidence exists for the impact of BMI, age and gender on the metabolomic profile. Additionally, diurnal variation is known to alter metabolite levels. Other sources of variation include the impact of food constituents. To minimise the impact of these factors, careful consideration needs to be given to study design, and if possible standardisation of the diet 24 hours prior to sample collection should be implemented.

Data analysis

Metabolomic platforms generate large amounts of data that need to be analysed using multivariate strategies. While many statistical methods are available, some of the most commonly used methods include principal component analysis (PCA), partial least squares discriminant analysis (PLS-DA) and orthogonal partial least squares discriminant analysis (O-PLS-DA).

PCA is an unsupervised technique that allows visualisation of the data. Using this approach it is possible to identify inherent groupings of samples as a result of a similar metabolite composition. Supervised techniques, such as PLS-DA and O-PLS-DA, require a priori knowledge of the class membership and are used to identify metabolites that differ between groups of samples, such as treated versus placebo. When using supervised techniques it is imperative to validate any models developed. Approaches for validation include cross-validation, where samples are left out and their class membership is predicted. Permutation testing can also be employed, where randomly assigned class labels are used, and the predictability of the working model is compared to these data.

While the statistical tools mentioned are commonly used in the field, other approaches are also emerging. An example of one of these tools is a method for performing PCA with covariates (PPCCA; Nyamundanda, Brennan and Gormley 2010). PPCCA incorporates covariates into the model and facilitates joint modelling of metabolomic data and covariates, allowing inclusion of variation due to the covariates. This method has great potential use within the metabolomics field and is extremely important when studying human metabolism, as a number of phenotypical factors are known to have an impact on the metabolic profile. Examples of other statistical tools include random forests (RF), support vector machines (SVM) and artificial neural networks (ANN; Boccard, Veuthey and Rudaz 2010; Sugimoto *et al.* 2012).

Applications of metabolomics in nutrition research

The applications of metabolomics in nutrition research have expanded rapidly in recent years. In general,

applications in the nutrition field can be divided into three categories: dietary intervention studies; dietary biomarker discovery studies; and diet-related disease studies. Application of metabolomics to dietary intervention studies enables one to study the mechanistic effects of the interventions and establish how the diets or food items have an impact on metabolic pathways. Applications in this area are likely to rise every year and current examples exist where metabolomics has been applied to interventions with tea, chocolate, cocoa, vitamins, fish and fish oils.

In the field of dietary biomarkers, metabolomics has the potential to make a significant impact. It is widely accepted that dietary biomarkers are necessary to improve dietary assessment methods. In recent years a number of studies have emerged demonstrating the utility of metabolomics for the identification of biomarkers of dietary intake. Identification of biomarkers can be performed by using specific acute interventions with certain foods or by searching for biomarkers in cohort studies where subjects have been classified into low and high consumers. The biofluids collected in either method can be analysed in an untargeted metabolomics approach where no prior hypothesis about potential markers exists. This has been useful in the identification of markers for citrus fruit and cruciferous vegetables. Alternatively, a targeted metabolomics analysis strategy can be employed if the metabolite markers of interest are known. Independent of which strategy is used for biomarker discovery, validation of the candidate biomarker is crucial. Optimal validation should be in the form of an independent intervention study with the specific foods of interest.

Application of metabolomics and the related field lipidomics (where a focus is on lipid metabolites) to diet-related diseases such as T2D has the potential to enhance our understanding of the underlying molecular mechanisms and help to design prevention strategies. Additionally, metabolomics studies in this field can also lead to the discovery of biomarkers of risk.

Metabolomics is without doubt a useful tool in nutrition-related research and will continue to make a significant impact. The integration of metabolomics (including lipidomic) data with genetic and proteomic data will provide a powerful approach to elucidating the mechanisms by which certain diets and foods exert their effects. Furthermore, such an integrative approach should enhance our understanding of diet-related diseases.

13.6 Perspectives for the future

'Omics' technologies represent huge opportunities to advance nutrition research in terms of technical capabilities to measure the genome, transcriptome proteome and metabolome more accurately. The challenge will be to develop and apply robust nutritional genomics research initiatives that are sensitive enough to take account of both human genetic heterogeneity and diverse nutrient exposure. If nutrigenomic approaches enhance our understanding of human nutrition at the molecular level, then it may be possible to apply a more targeted and effective personalised nutrition approach to attenuate the effect of risk factors associated with diet-related diseases. Indeed, it could be proposed that a personalised nutrition approach, based on the molecular phenotype that spans from genotype to metabotype, may improve our understanding of the role of nutrition in human health. The ultimate aim is to enhance the scientific evidence base and the effectiveness of dietary guidelines and nutritional recommendations to promote health.

Acknowledgements

BDR is funded by the Scottish Government's Rural and Environment Science and Analytical Services Division (RESAS); HMR is supported by the Science Foundation Ireland Principal Investigator Programme (11/PI/1119).

References and further reading

Boccard, J., Veuthey, J.L. and Rudaz, S. (2010) Knowledge discovery in metabolomics: An overview of MS data handling. *Journal of Separation Science*, 33, 3, 290–304.

De Roos, B. (2008) Proteomic analysis of human plasma and blood cells in nutritional studies: Development of biomarkers to aid disease prevention. *Expert Review of Proteomics*, 5, 819–826.

De Roos, B. (2009) Nutrition proteomics and biomarker discovery. *Expert Review of Proteomics*, 6, 349–351.

De Roos, B. and McArdle, H.J. (2008) Proteomics as a tool for the modelling of biological processes and biomarker development in nutrition research. *British Journal of Nutrition*, 99, Suppl 3, S66–71.

De Roos, B. and Romagnolo, D.F. (2012) Proteomic approaches to predict bioavailability of fatty acids and their influence on cancer and chronic disease prevention. *Journal of Nutrition*, 142, 1370S–1376S.

De Roos, B., Duthie, S.J., Polley, A.C. *et al.* (2008) Proteomic methodological recommendations for studies involving human plasma, platelets and peripheral blood mononuclear cell. *Journal of Proteome Research*, 7, 2280–2290.

German, J.B., Hammock, B.D. and Watkins, S.M. (2005) Metabolomics: Building on a century of biochemistry to guide human health. *Metabolomics*, 1, 1, 3–9.

Mandruzzato, S. (2007) Technological platforms for microarray gene expression profiling. *Advances in Experimental Medicine and Biology*, 593, 12–18.

Morine, M.J., O'Brien, C. and Roche, H.M. (2008) Personalised nutrition: Transcriptomic signatures that have identified key features of metabolic syndrome. *Proceedings of the Nutrition Society*, 67, 4, 395–403.

Nyamundanda, G., Brennan, L. and Gormley, I.C. (2010) Probabilistic principal component analysis for metabolomic data. *BMC Bioinformatics*, 11, 571.

Roche HM (2006) Nutrigenomics – new approaches for human nutrition research. *Journal of the Science of Food and Agriculture* 86:1156–1163.

Sievertzon, M., Nilsson, P. and Lundeberg, J. (2006) Improving reliability and performance of DNA microarrays. *Expert Review of Molecular Diagnostics*, 6, 3, 481–492.

Sugimoto, M., Kawakami, M., Robert, M. *et al.* (2012). Bioinformatics tools for mass spectrometry-based metabolomic data processing and analysis. *Current Bioinformatics*, 7, 1, 96–108.

14
Epigenetics

John C Mathers

Newcastle University

Key messages

- Each individual has a fixed genotype, but his or her phenotype (e.g. adiposity and health status) is plastic in response to environmental factors, including nutrition, and this phenotypic plasticity can be mediated by epigenetic mechanisms.
- Epigenetics can be defined as the study of the processes through which gene expression (and cellular phenotype) is regulated, that are heritable across cell generations and that do not involve changes in the DNA sequence.
- Epigenetic mechanisms help regulate expression of the particular consortium of genes that is appropriate for a given cell type in the specific circumstances under study.
- The main epigenetic marks include methylation of cytosine residues within DNA and the covalent addition of chemical groups

- (e.g. phosphate, methyl and acetyl groups) to specific amino acid residues in the N-terminal tails of the histones around which DNA is wrapped in the cell nucleus.
- Epigenetically important molecules include the proteins that can 'read' the epigenetic marks on DNA and on histones and use this information to switch on, or switch off, the corresponding gene.
- MicroRNA are small RNA that do not code for proteins but regulate mRNA through base pairing with complementary sequences within the target mRNA species.
- Several dietary factors, including micronutrients and other plant food-derived bioactive compounds, result in changes in epigenetic marks and molecules, some of which lead to alterations in gene expression.

14.1 Introduction: The human genome and the regulation of gene expression

The human nuclear genome contains over 3 billion base pairs (bp) and the information to direct the synthesis of approximately 20 000 proteins. In addition, each mitochondrion within the cell contains about 16 600 bp, which encode just 37 genes. That said, any given human cell expresses only a small proportion of all the genes encoded in the genome. Most cells express a common set of genes, known as house-keeping genes, which are needed for generic purposes such as nutrient transport and adenosine triphosphate (ATP) generation. However, different cell types, such as neurones or hepatocytes, express consortia of genes that are characteristic of that cell type (described as cellular differentiation) and allow the cell to carry out the specific functions of the relevant cell type within particular tissues, for instance brain or liver. In addition, cells express distinctive complements of genes

at different stages during development and in response to specific physiological states, for example epithelial cells in the breast during lactation. Cells also need to be able to respond appropriately to environmental factors such as dietary intake or exposure to chemical hazards. For all of these reasons, cells have evolved sophisticated, and dynamic, processes to ensure that the correct consortium of genes is expressed in a particular cell under the specific circumstances pertaining at that moment in time.

Expression of genes can be regulated at any stage, from initial copying of the information within deoxyribonucleic acid (DNA) to make messenger ribonucleic acid or mRNA (transcription), through processing of ribonucleic acid (RNA) species and synthesis of the encoded proteins (translation) to post-translational processing of proteins. However, the key stages in the regulation of expression are regulating the amount of mRNA that is produced from a particular gene and then regulating the translation of that mRNA into protein. Such regulation operates over

Nutrition Research Methodologies, First Edition. Edited by Julie A Lovegrove, Leanne Hodson, Sangita Sharma and Susan A Lanham-New.
© 2015 John Wiley & Sons, Ltd. Published 2015 by John Wiley & Sons, Ltd.
Companion Website: www.wiley.com/go/nutritionsociety

a very wide range of timescales. For example, some genes are expressed only during very early life (embryogenesis and fetal development) and then remain silent (switched off) during the rest of the life course. In contrast, expression of other genes is regulated over periods of minutes or hours, for instance genes in immune cells when exposed to an antigen and hepatocytes in response to feeding or fasting. Because of the criticality of ensuring that cells are equipped appropriately to carry out their function, it is not surprising that about 10% of all the proteins encoded in the human genome contain DNA-binding domains and are involved in regulating gene expression. Many of these proteins are transcription factors that, often in combination, provide relatively short-term regulation of gene expression. In addition, epigenetic processes exert further control over gene expression, which is essential for cell and tissue function and for health.

14.2 What is epigenetics?

In 1942, a decade before Crick and Watson discovered the structure of DNA and ushered in the era of molecular biology, C.H. Waddington coined the term 'epigenetics'. Originally, epigenetics was used to describe how genes might interact with their environment to produce a particular phenotype. Nowadays, it is usually understood to be the study of the processes through which gene expression (and cellular phenotype) is regulated, that are heritable across cell generations and that do not involve changes in the DNA sequence. These processes involve a complex consortium of epigenetic marks and molecules that act in consort.

14.3 Epigenetic marks and molecules

The main epigenetic marks include chemical modifications of the cytosine base within DNA (Figure 14.1) and post-translational modifications of histones. The main epigenetic mark on DNA in animals is the addition of a methyl group to the 5′position on cytosine residues when that cytosine is followed by a guanine – that is, a so-called CpG dinucleotide – to produce 5′methylcytosine (5mC). In addition, it has been discovered very recently that methylated cytosines in CpG dinucleotides can be further modified by oxidation to form hydroxymethylcytosine (5hmC; Figure 14.1). Relatively high concentrations of 5hmC are seen in the brain and in embryonic stem cells. The role of 5hmC is not well understood, but it appears that it may be an intermediate in the demethylation of 5mC; that is, an important part of the dynamic process through which methyl marks can be added to, and removed from, DNA.

Histones are the chief protein components of chromatin. Two of each of the core histones (H2A, H2B, H3 and H4) forms a globular protein complex around which 147 base pairs of DNA are wrapped in the nucleus, with a linker histone (H1) at each end locking the DNA in place. Protruding from the globular core are N-terminal protein 'tails' in which specific amino acid residues can be covalently modified by the addition of small chemical groups – that is, phosphate, methyl and acetyl groups – and by the addition of small regulatory proteins – that is, ubiquitin and SUMO (small ubiquitin-like modifier). These constitute the epigenetic 'marks' on histones. Epigenetic molecules fall into two groups. The first are the enzymes and other proteins that add or remove epigenetic marks and those that 'read' those marks to switch on, or switch off, expression of the corresponding gene. For example, this group of molecules includes DNA methyltransferase (DNMT) enzymes, which catalyse the addition of methyl groups to cytosines in DNA, and histone acetyl transferases (HATs) and histone deacetylases (HDACs), which catalyse the addition and removal, respectively, of acetyl groups on specific amino acids, for instance lysine, in histone tails. The second group of epigenetic molecules is composed of small RNAs (described as microRNA), which are typically 22 nucleotides long. These microRNA do not code for proteins, but regulate the expression of genes through base pairing with complementary sequences within the target mRNA species.

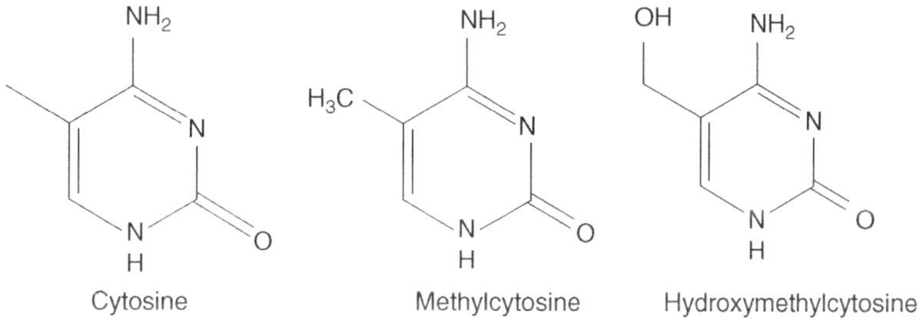

Figure 14.1 Cytosine and derivatives, which are the principle epigenetic marks on DNA.

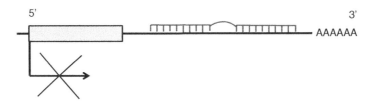

Figure 14.2 Binding of a microRNA molecule to a complementary sequence within a target mRNA species, causing gene silencing. The microRNA is shown in the centre. The box on the left represents the sequence within the mRNA that encodes the protein and the black cross indicates that binding of the microRNA to the 3′end of the mRNA transcript prevents translation of that protein.

In most cases, this binding to the 3′end of mRNA results in degradation of the target mRNA and, because this means that no protein is synthesised, the corresponding gene is effectively silenced (Figure 14.2). In mammals, there is only partial complementarity between the miRNA sequence and that of the corresponding mRNA. As a consequence, a given microRNA may have multiple mRNA targets and translation of a given mRNA may be regulated by a combination of microRNAs.

Epigenomics is the study of the totality of epigenetic marks and molecules within a cell or tissue, which is described as the epigenome. This is analogous to the terms genomics, transcriptomics, proteomics and metabolomics, which describe all the genes, mRNA species, proteins and metabolites, respectively, in a cell or other biological sample and are discussed in more detail in Chapter 13. Following the successful projects to map the human genome and to identify the genetic variants, such as single nucleotide polymorphisms (SNP) and copy number variants (CNV), in the human genome, there are now consortia attempting to map specific epigenomes. For example, the Human Epigenome Project (HEP) aims to identify, catalogue and interpret genome-wide DNA methylation patterns of all human genes in all major tissues (for details, see http://www.epigenome.org/).

14.4 Epigenetic regulation of gene expression

The genome of the fertilised human egg contains all the genetic information to direct development of the human adult, who contains over 200 different cell types, all of which contain exactly the same DNA but carry out distinctively different functions. Asymmetrical cell division leading to different cell types (cellular differentiation) occurs during embryogenesis and is very carefully orchestrated to ensure that each cell type expresses its characteristic complement of genes. This is achieved via chromatin, the DNA–nucleosome polymer, which is a dynamic molecule capable of existing in many configurations. The combination of epigenetic marks and molecules

(epigenome) determines the higher-order organisation of chromatin. Those chromatin domains that are highly compacted (known as heterochromatin) contain genes that are silenced, whereas the more open chromatin regions (known as euchromatin) allow access by the transcriptional machinery and gene expression.

In the same way that optimum health requires each of the body's organs and tissues to do its particular job efficiently in response to whatever challenge the body faces, so, at the cellular level, the proper function of each individual cell requires expression of the consortium of genes that is appropriate for that cell type, for instance an endothelial cell or an enterocyte, in its given environment. In addition, cells need to be able to respond correctly to changing conditions. For example, if we consume potentially hazardous chemicals (xenobiotics), hepatocytes may need to upregulate the expression of defence genes, such as those of the cytochrome P450 superfamily, to enable the body to detoxify those chemicals. Similarly, cells can save energy and other resources by shutting down the expression of genes that are not needed at that particular time. In summary, our genotype is fixed, but our phenotype is plastic and responds to life's experiences and exposures.

14.5 Nutrition and epigenetics

It is now established that several dietary factors, and other environmental exposures, result in changes in epigenetic marks and molecules, some of which lead to alterations in gene expression (see Table 14.1).

In many cases, the strongest evidence for the impact of nutrition on epigenetic regulation of gene expression comes from studies using model systems (mammalian cells and animal models), but there is growing evidence for similar effects from studies carried out in humans. This has led to the hypothesis that epigenetic processes are potentially important mechanisms through which dietary exposures and nutritional status may influence health. In particular, this is an attractive hypothesis for explaining how nutrition can have very long-term effects

Table 14.1 Examples of dietary factors and nutritional status that influence epigenetic marks (see McKay and Mathers 2011 for a detailed review).

Dietary factor	Epigenetic change
Folate and other methyl donors	Multiple effects on methylation of specific genes and on methylation and acetylation of histones
Butyrate	Extra butyrate increased acetylation of histones H3 and H4
Isoflavones	Isoflavone supplementation induced dose-dependent changes in methylation of genes in the mammary gland
Protein	Low protein intake during pregnancy caused reduced methylation of the promoters of several genes, including the glucocorticoid receptor (*GR*) and the peroxisomal proliferator-activated receptor alpha (*PPARα*) genes
Selenium	Supplemental selenium increased DNA methylation in the liver
Polyphenols	Polyphenols may alter patterns of DNA methylation by affecting expression of key enzymes, including DNMT
Obesity	Patterns of DNA methylation appear to be influenced by obesity and to predict responders to weight-loss interventions

on health. Because at least some epigenetic marks such as patterns of DNA methylation are copied from one cell generation to the next, altered DNA methylation caused by early-life nutrition could result in lifelong changes in gene expression, altered risk of disease and effects on life span. This is best illustrated by studies of the Agouti mouse. The coat colour of the offspring in this model is influenced by the supply of folate and other methyl donors provided to the dam during pregnancy (see Figure 14.3). Supplemented dams produce a higher proportion of offspring with darker (brown) coats rather than the predominantly yellow-coloured offspring of unsupplemented dams. This change in coat colour is due to altered expression of the *Agouti* gene caused by methylation of a regulatory region upstream of the gene. These effects of the maternal diet on DNA methylation are seen in every tissue of the body and the effects on coat colour endure throughout the animal's life. In this mouse model, maternal methyl donor supply affects not only coat colour but also other important phenotypical characteristics. For example, the 'yellow' mice tend to be fatter and more susceptible to obesity-related diseases such as type 2 diabetes than their brown litter mates. Interestingly, maternal exposure to genistein (an isoflavone from soybeans) and to bisphenol A (an industrial chemical used in production of polycarbonate plastics) results in similar changes in DNA methylation and in coat colour in Agouti mice, although neither genistein nor bisphenol A is a methyl donor.

These ideas are conceptualised in the 4Rs of nutritional epigenomics model (Mathers 2008), illustrated in Figure 14.4. In this model, exposure to specific dietary factors produces marks on the genome such as an altered pattern of DNA methylation; that is, the 'signal' is Received and Recorded. To have long term effects, there needs to be a mechanism through which evidence of that exposure is Remembered when the cell divides.

In the case of DNA methylation, this memory mechanism is the copying of patterns of DNA methylation from the parental strand of DNA to the daughter strand by the enzyme DNMT1, which occurs immediately after synthesis of the new (daughter) DNA strand during mitosis. Since at least some changes in DNA methylation (and other epigenetic marks) result in changes in gene expression, this is the mechanism through which the functional consequences of the original nutritional exposure are Revealed (Figure 14.4). Altered patterns of gene expression change cell function and such changes in cell function are the fundamental causes of altered phenotype, for instance health status. In summary, each individual has a fixed genotype, but his or her phenotype (e.g. adiposity and health status) is plastic in response to environmental factors, including nutrition, and this phenotypical plasticity is mediated, at least to some extent, by epigenetic mechanisms.

14.6 Measuring epigenetic marks and molecules – some basic concepts

Each individual has just one genome, the sequence of adenine (A), thymine (T), cytosine (C) and guanine (G) in his or her DNA that constitutes the unique pattern of genetic variants inherited at conception from his or her parents. This genome remains constant throughout the individual's life. In contrast, an individual's epigenome is much more complex, not only because it consists of a much wider range of epigenetic marks and molecules, but also because the epigenomes of different cells and tissues differ from each other; that is, an altered epigenome enables cellular differentiation during embryogenesis. In addition, unlike the static genome, the epigenome is dynamic, altering during growth and development and to facilitate changes in physiological

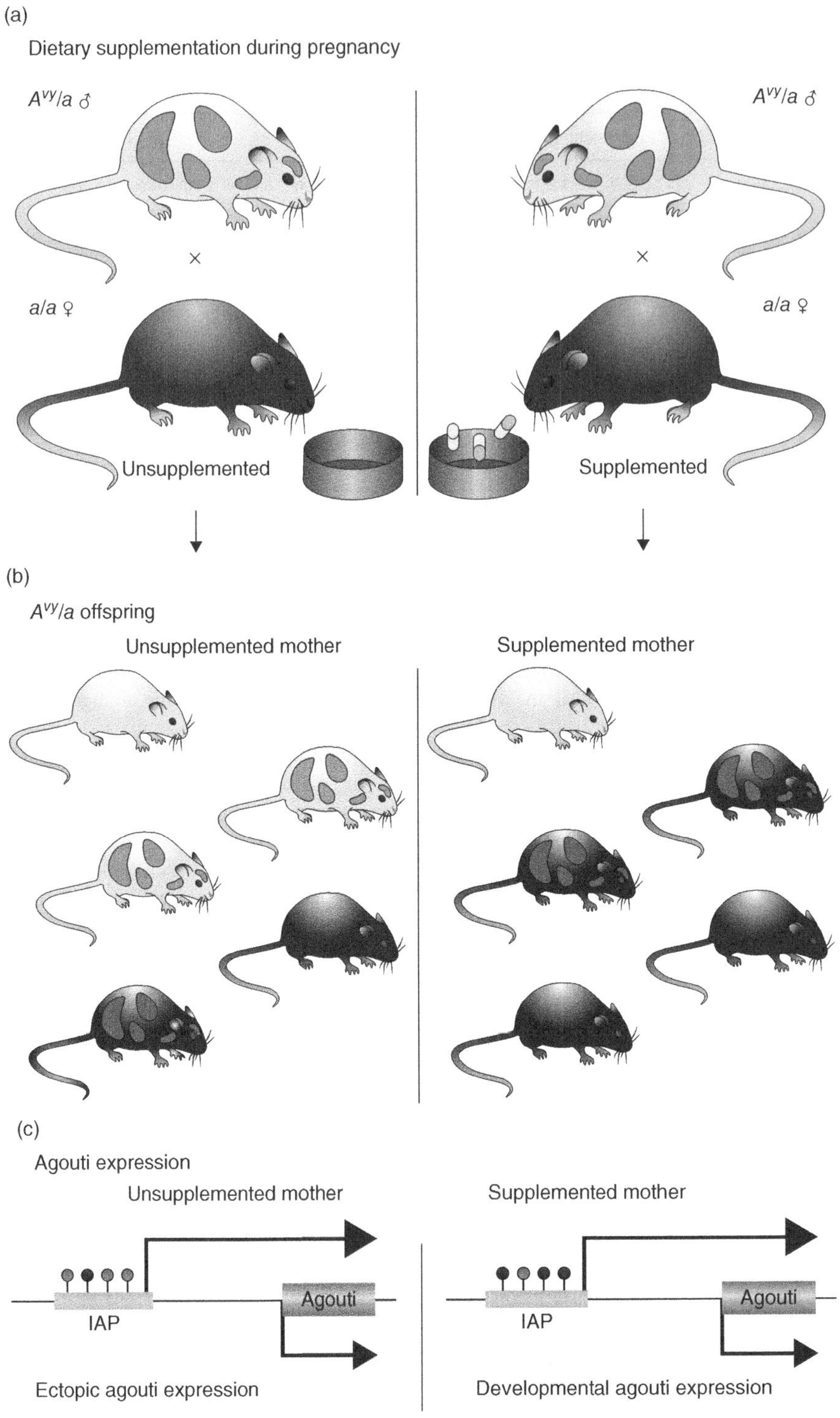

Figure 14.3 Maternal supplementation of Agouti mice with methyl donors (folate, betaine, vitamin B_{12} and choline ; Panel (a)) results in litters with a higher proportion of offspring with dark (brown) coats, whereas the offspring of the unsupplemented dams have predominantly yellow coats (Panel (b)). Panel (c) shows the molecular mechanism for this nutritionally induced phenotypical change. The pale grey bar represent the regulatory region (labelled IAP) upstream of the *Agouti* gene (shown on the right). Maternal supplementation results in greater methylation of DNA in the regulatory region, shown as black-filled circles above the IAP region. Reprinted by permission from Macmillan Publishers Ltd: Nat Rev Genet. Jirtle RL & Skinner MK. Environmental epigenomics and disease susceptibility, **8**(4):253-62, copyright 2007.

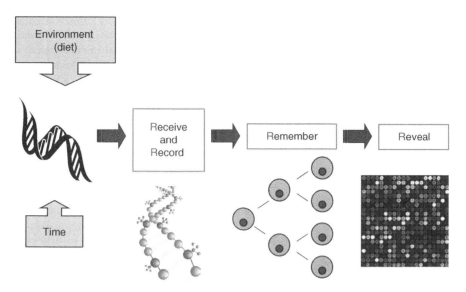

Figure 14.4 The 4 'Rs' of nutritional epigenomics. A conceptual model of the key processes through which altered epigenomic markings as a result of environmental (dietary) exposures are 'Received', 'Recorded', 'Remembered' and 'Revealed'. Mathers, J.C. (2008) Session 2: Personalised nutrition. Epigeneomics: A basis for understanding individual differences? *Proceedings of the Nutrition Society*, **67**, 4, 390–394.

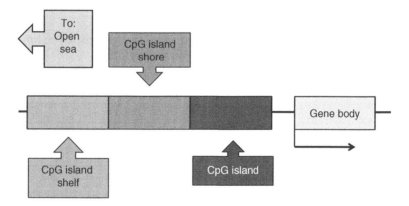

Figure 14.5 Cartoon of genomic locations (shown as boxes on the horizontal black line) of cytosine residues within CpG dinucleotides, which may become methylated and so influence expression of the corresponding gene (shown as the box on the right with a black arrow below it). Methylation within the gene body is known as intragenic methylation.

state, such as pregnancy. Furthermore, the epigenome appears to respond to a wide range of environmental exposures, including diet (see Figure 14.3 for an example). In consequence, our measurements of the epigenome will refer to the particular cell or tissue type assayed and the specific conditions under which the samples were collected.

As already noted, DNA is methylated at cytosine residues (5mC) within CpG dinucleotides. In most cases, methylation is associated with inactive (silenced) genes; it has been hypothesised that DNA methylation evolved as a host defence mechanism to silence 'foreign' sequences

(e.g. transposable elements and viral sequences) that have become incorporated into the (human) genome. Certainly, heterochromatin is rich in such foreign sequences and in these domains most CpGs are methylated. Conversely, in the promoter regions of the majority of human genes there are regions with unusually high densities of CpGs known as CpG islands. In expressed genes, such as house-keeping genes, the CpG islands are normally unmethylated. However, evidence is accumulating that methylation of genomic domains other than CpG islands, such as the CpG island 'shores', may also be important in providing longer-range regulation of gene

Table 14.2 Epigenetic marks on histone H3 with known effects on gene expression.

Description of histone H3 modification	Abbreviation	Effect on gene expression
Trimethylation of lysine 4	H3K4Me3	Active transcription
Trimethylation of lysine 36	H3K36Me3	Active transcription
Trimethylation of lysine 27	H3K27Me3	Gene silencing
Di and tri-methylation of lysine 9	H3K9Me2/3	Gene silencing

expression (Figure 14.5). While patterns of methylation within, or near, promoter regions may regulate gene expression, methylation within genes themselves (gene bodies – Figure 14.5), known as intragenic methylation, appears to regulate other important processes including splicing of mRNA, the initiation of transcription within genes and transcriptional elongation. This complexity in genomic location of these epigenetic methylation marks presents a challenge when designing assays for DNA methylation and also in the interpretation of the resulting data.

Many of the amino acid residues in histone tails can be chemically modified after the protein has been synthesised in the cell; that is, so-called post-translational modification. For example, histone H3 contains 19 lysine residues that can be methylated and, in each case, this can result in a mono-, di- or tri-methylated amino acid. Together with the other covalent modifications (see Section 14.3), this leads to very intricate patterns of epigenetic marks on histones and to the possibility of thousands of different patterns. To date, the relationship between each pattern and expression of the corresponding gene is only partly understood. Table 14.2 summarises some of the known relationships between histone marks and gene expression.

14.7 Methods for measuring DNA methylation

There are two main approaches for quantifying DNA methylation: those that quantify the total proportion of 5mC in the genome – often described as global DNA methylation – and those that measure methylation at defined genomic locations.

Measuring global DNA methylation by direct quantification of 5mC

This was the earliest approach for measuring global DNA methylation and involves three basic steps: isolation and purification of DNA from the cell or tissue of interest; hydrolysis of the DNA to release the constituent bases; and quantification of total cytosine (C) and of total 5mC in the hydrolysate. For reliable analyses, it is essential that the extracted DNA is purified, taking care to remove all RNA. In common with DNA, RNA contains cytosine residues and, therefore, contamination with RNA could lead to unreliable estimates of DNA methylation. Early approaches for the quantification of total C and of total 5mC in the DNA hydrolysate used high-performance liquid chromatography (HPLC) or high-performance capillary electrophoresis (HPCE) to separate the nucleotides by size. However, modern approaches are likely to couple a chromatographic approach with mass spectrometry (MS) to provide more sensitive measurements on smaller sample sizes. Some MS-based approaches can distinguish between 5mC and 5hmC and so yield estimates of both main cytosine modifications believed to be important in the epigenetic regulation of gene expression (Figure 14.1). The strengths of this method include very precise, and accurate, quantification of C, 5mC and, in some cases, 5hmC, but the approach is limited to those laboratories with access to relatively sophisticated, and expensive, chromatographic and MS instruments.

Indirect approaches for estimating global DNA methylation

Although direct estimation of the 5mC content of DNA remains the gold standard for global DNA methylation measurement, alternative approaches have been developed that are less demanding technically and make use of the less expensive equipment found commonly in laboratories undertaking molecular biological research. Several of these approaches take advantage of the finding that the treatment of DNA with bisulphite under alkaline conditions converts unmethylated cytosines to uracil (U), whereas methylated cytosines are stable under these conditions and remain as (methylated) cytosines (Figure 14.6). Following polymerase chain reaction (PCR) to amplify the amount of target material for assay, the presence of U in the unmethylated DNA strand leads to the insertion of an adenine (A) in the complementary strand. In contrast, with the methylated DNA, PCR amplification leads to insertion of a guanine (G) in the strand complementary to the originally methylated cytosine (see Figure 14.6 for an illustration).

PCR-based methods for the estimation of global DNA methylation include those that attempt to quantify the methylation of cytosine residues in major genome repeat elements such as LINE-1 (the long-interspersed nuclear element-1, a non-terminal repeat transposon). The human genome contains about 500 000 LINEs that make up about 17% of the total genomic sequence.

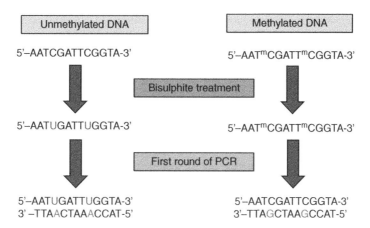

Figure 14.6 Illustration of the effect of bisulphite treatment of DNA to help distinguish between methylated and unmethylated cytosine residues in further analysis using sequencing approaches or methylation-sensitive enzymes.

In addition, there are over 1 million Alu sequences – so named because they were originally characterised by the action of the Alu (*Arthrobacter luteus*) restriction endonuclease – in the human genome, making up nearly 11% of the total genomic sequence, and these Alu sequences are another target for global DNA methylation assays. In practice, the extent of methylation at a few specific CpG sites within the repeat sequence is quantified for example by Pyrosequencing® (see later in this chapter) and the resulting data are used as estimates of global DNA methylation. These approaches have the advantage that they are relatively inexpensive and require only small amounts of DNA, making them suitable for human studies where for instance there may be large numbers of participants (hundreds or thousands) but only tiny amounts of DNA from blood samples or tissue biopsies. On the other hand, interpretation of the results from studies of methylation of repeat elements can be problematic. Firstly, the assay targets only one repeated element within the genome (albeit one that makes up a significant proportion of the total genomic sequence) and it is uncertain whether methylation of that element mirrors methylation across the genome. Given that, under normal circumstances, these repeat elements are heavily methylated as part of the cell defence mechanisms (see Section 14.6), the biological interpretation of changes in methylation of for instance LINE-1 or Alu in response to nutrition (or another environmental exposure) remains uncertain. However, reductions in LINE-1 methylation in response to ageing, or in diseases such as cancer, do appear to reflect the generalised hypomethylation of the genome seen in those conditions.

An alternative approach for quantification of global DNA methylation makes use of DNA-cutting enzymes – restriction endonucleases – that cut DNA at specific recognition nucleotide sequences, known as restriction sites. In some cases, these restriction endonucleases are sensitive to the methylation status of cytosine residues within the restriction site and do not cut when the DNA is methylated. This is particularly useful if it can be paired in an assay with another enzyme which cuts at the same genomic sequence but is insensitive to the methylation status. Such pairs of enzymes are known as isoschizomers. For example, the restriction enzymes HpaII and MspI are isoschizomers. Both recognise, and cut, the sequence 5'-CCGG-3' when it is unmethylated. However, when the second C (the C in the CpG dinucleotide) of the sequence is methylated, only the methylation-insensitive enzyme (MspI) cuts the DNA. This property is employed in the so-called luminometric methylation assay (LUMA) for global methylation, in which samples of the test DNA are cut separately by each of the two enzymes. The digestion ratio HpaII/MspI can be quantified by for instance, Pyrosequencing, and is inversely proportional to the methylation status of the DNA. In choosing isoschizomers for such an assay, more readily interpretable estimates of global DNA methylation will be obtained when the target nucleotide sequence is widely, and randomly, distributed across the genome. The LUMA assay requires only small amounts of DNA and can be carried out relatively quickly and at low cost, since it does not require bisulphite modification or other, relatively expensive, time-consuming preparation.

A major disadvantage of the LUMA assay, which it shares with all measures of global DNA methylation, is that it does not provide any information about where in the genome changes in methylation, detected by the assay, have occurred. Loss or gain of methylation from regions of heterochromatin is likely to have very different biological consequences from similar changes in euchromatin. For example, a nutritional intervention (or other exposure) might result in increases in methylation at some genomic locations that were counter-balanced by methylation losses at other loci. In such a circumstance, use of a global DNA assay could be very misleading since it might indicate 'no effect' whereas, in reality, there were changes in methylation across the genome, each of which might be biologically important but resulted in no net change in global DNA methylation. For these reasons, the results of assays that quantify methylation at specific, and known, genomic loci are (usually) easier to interpret.

Methylation of candidate genes

Often in nutritional research we have sufficient information about the problem under study to be able to identify specific genes whose methylation status (and, subsequently, expression status) is of particular interest. In such cases there are several approaches that can be used to characterise, and quantify, methylation of the target gene, and almost all take advantage of bisulphite modification of DNA to 'fix' the methylation status of methylated CpG sites in the original sample (Figure 14.6). One of the simplest approaches, which provides, essentially, a yes/no answer about methylation status, is methylation-specific PCR (MSP). In the MSP assay, two primer pairs are used. The first primer pair is designed to be methylated specific; that is, the primers will bind to, and amplify, only those target sequences that contain a C from the original 5-methylcytosine. The second primer pair is designed to complement (bind to and amplify) the target sequence when it contains a T resulting from an unmethylated cytosine in the original DNA sequence (see Figure 14.6 for a reminder of how bisulphite treatment of DNA 'fixes' the methylation status of CpG sites). Following separate PCR reactions with each of the two primer pairs, the products can be run on a gel. If there is a signal (DNA band on the gel) only in the lane from the primer pair designed to detect unmethylated cytosines then, within the limits of detection of the assay, one can conclude that the original DNA was not methylated at this locus. Often, however, there is a signal in both lanes, indicating that the test DNA sample contained a mixture of methylated and unmethylated sequences. The MSP approach cannot be used for quantification of the proportions of methylated/unmethylated sequences. The MethylLight assay is a modification of this approach that uses fluorescence-based real-time quantitative PCR (RT-qPCR) to provide a relatively high-throughput approach for methylation quantification at specific loci.

Another, more recently introduced approach takes advantage of the fact that the sequence within a given DNA domain affects the melting characteristics of double-stranded DNA. This assay is known as methylation sensitive high-resolution melting (MS-HRM). MS-HRM is a PCR-based assay in which methylation-insensitive primers are applied to bisulphite-modified DNA to amplify the region of interest and produce a product that contains a mixture of double-stranded DNA fragments from the originally methylated and unmethylated templates. Then a qPCR instrument is used to analyse the melting curves of this mixed product immediately after the initial PCR stage in a closed-tube system. The melting characteristics – the temperature range over which the DNA 'melts', meaning that the two complementary strands become separated – depends on whether there is an A–T pairing (from an originally unmethylated DNA domain) or a G–C pairing (from an originally methylated DNA domain) opposite each other in the DNA double strand. Analysis of the melting curves can provide a quantitative estimate of the methylation status of the target DNA locus.

Methods for quantifying methylation of multiple CpG sites within specific genomic loci

Although it is useful to have information about the methylation status of individual CpG sites, it is usually of more interest to be able to characterise methylation across several CpG sites within a given genomic locus. This can be achieved through various approaches, including direct sequencing of bisulphite-modified DNA. To identify the location of methylated CpG sites and to quantify the proportions of methylated versus unmethylated copies of the target sequence requires cloning of the PCR-amplified products before sequencing. Even with the use of kits, this is a relatively labour-intensive procedure and is unsuitable for high-throughput applications. Alternative approaches that give reliable quantification and higher throughput include Pyrosequencing and use of matrix-assisted laser desorption/ionisation–time-of-flight (MALDI-tof) mass spectrometry.

Pyrosequencing is a sequencing-by-synthesis approach that begins with PCR amplification of bisulphite-modified DNA. Then the quantitative composition of the region of interest is interrogated by adding the appropriate deoxribonucleotide triphosphates (dNTPs) one by one in the order in which they are expected to appear in the target sequence and the amount of dNTP incorporated is recorded. Pyrosequencing is highly quantitative and provides unambiguous estimates of the extent of methylation at specific CpG sites. In addition, it runs on a 96-well plate format and so is moderately high throughput. Its main limitation is that it is restricted to the interrogation of amplicons of up to 200 bp, so that for longer regions of interest two or more assays will need to be developed, with corresponding increases in costs.

Quantification of DNA methylation by MALDI-tof mass spectrometry is based on the principle that the base composition of DNA fragments can be predicted by estimating their mass. Application of this approach starts with bisulphite-modified DNA, in which the original methylation status of each cytosine residue has been 'fixed' (see Figure 14.6). PCR amplicons are then transcribed into RNA and cut (cleaved) by specific enzymes to produce specific RNA fragments. The masses of these fragments are determined by MALDI-tof mass spectrometry and the methylation status of the original DNA at each CpG site is estimated. This approach has the advantages that it can interrogate amplicons of up to 600 bp and is relatively high throughput. However, it is not as sensitive as Pyrosequencing and has lower precision.

Array-based approaches for investigating genome-wide DNA methylation

Array-based approaches are used widely in studies where the researcher wishes to examine methylation across the whole genome. This approach is analogous to microarray-based (also known as chip-based) studies for transcriptomics, which are described in detail in Chapter 13. Currently, popular arrays use bead-based technologies and can provide quantitative estimation of methylation at the individual CpG level of resolution for hundreds of thousands of CpG sites across the genome. Again, the researcher starts with bisulphite-modified DNA, which is interrogated using hundreds of thousands of pairs of small probes, each pair being complementary to the DNA domain containing the CpG site of interest. One member of each pair of probes detects bases corresponding to a methylated cytosine in the original DNA and the other member of the pair detects unmethylated cytosines. This approach has the advantage that it can provide simultaneous analysis of multiple CpG sites in the promoter regions and bodies of virtually all genes in a given genome. In addition, coverage can include domains such as CpG island shores (see Figure 14.5), but there are large numbers of CpG sites that are more remote from genes, which are usually absent from such arrays.

Next-generation sequencing for investigating genome-wide DNA methylation

Advances in genomic sequencing currently known as next-generation sequencing (NGS) offer the potential for low-cost assessment of all methylation marks across the whole genome. As noted in Chapter 13, NGS provides high-throughput sequencing by completing the sequencing process of multiple, overlapping DNA fragments simultaneously. Several variants of NGS are on offer that can sequence specific genomic domains, chromosomes or whole genomes at a tiny fraction of the cost of conventional (Sanger) sequencing and very much faster. NGS can be used to quantify methylation at a single CpG resolution and, as with most other approaches to DNA methylation assessment, the NGS-based approach starts with bisulphite-modified DNA (Figure 14.6). NGS produces very large data sets and the bioinformatics challenges in analysing and interpreting these complex data sets are a current limitation on the widespread use of the approach for nutritional research.

Measurement of hydroxymethylcytosine (5hmC)

One of the reasons that hydroxymethylcytosine (5hmC) in DNA was discovered only recently is that PCR-based approaches that start with bisulphite-modified DNA cannot distinguish between 5mC and 5hmC. However, if DNA is first oxidised to convert 5hmC to 5-formylcytosine (5fC), subsequent bisulphite treatment converts the 5fC to uracil. This makes it possible to quantify the amount of cytosine and of its two main epigenetically important derivatives (5mC and 5hmC) in DNA (Figure 14.1) using liquid chromatography–tandem mass spectrometry. In addition, this prior oxidation step forms the basis for quantitative mapping of 5hmC in genomic DNA at single-nucleotide resolution.

14.8 Detection of histone modifications

The post-translational modifications of histone that are involved in the regulation of gene expression include covalent additions of phosphate, methyl and acetyl groups to specific amino acid residues in histone tails. It has been proposed that the pattern of these marks represents a 'histone code', providing the information to determine whether the corresponding gene is switched on or is transcriptionally silent. However, to date the interpretation of the proposed code remains fragmentary. Table 14.2 gives some examples of histone marks known to be associated with gene expression, and Figure 14.7 illustrates how DNA methylation marks and marks on histones combine to silence gene expression.

Early attempts to investigate epigenetically important histone modifications were relatively crude and could provide, for example, estimates of the extent of acetylation of all the H3 histones in chromatin without providing any

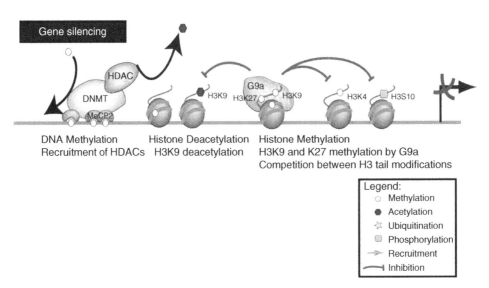

Figure 14.7 Epigenetic marks on histones combine with DNA methylation to silence gene expression. Republished with permission of Annual Reviews, Inc., from Dietary manipulation of histone structure and function, Delange B & Dashwood RH, Annu Rev Nutr, 2008(28):347–366; permission conveyed through Copyright Clearance Center, Inc. DNMT, DNA methyl transferase; G9a, histone-lysine N-methyltransferase (EHMT2); HDAC, histone deacetylase; MeCP2, methyl CpG binding protein 2.

information on where in the genome these acetylation marks are located. This is analogous to measurement of global DNA methylation and, while it can be useful as an overall measure of response to an exposure such as a dietary intervention, the biological consequences of such changes are difficult to interpret. If one is interested in links between histone marks and gene expression, then more sophisticated techniques that can interrogate candidate genes or larger chromatin domains become necessary.

Chromatin immunoprecipitation (ChiP)

Candidate gene-related approaches often use chromatin immunoprecipitation (ChiP), which can determine the specific location in the genome of histone modifications and, therefore, the likely target gene whose expression may be modified by those histone marks. ChiP is based on the principle that DNA and its associated histones can be bonded together (cross-linked) by, for instance, formaldehyde or ultraviolet treatment. When these DNA–protein complexes are sheared to generate fragments for analysis, the DNA and its histones remain together and can be immunoprecipitated ('pulled down') selectively, using antibodies that detect the histone modification of interest. The DNA fragments pulled down in this way can then be identified to determine the specific genes likely to be regulated by the histone modifications under study. ChiP-based approaches can be used to identify other proteins involved in the regulation of gene expression, such as transcription factors, since these are also pulled down during immunoprecipitation.

Genome-wide analysis of histone modifications using the ChiP-on-chip approach

ChiP-on-chip combines the ChiP approach for identifying specific histone modifications with the genome-wide array (or chip) approach to identify genes that are associated with the histone modifications of interest or other regulatory proteins. While it is a very powerful method for investigating the epigenetic regulation of gene expression, for instance in response to a dietary intervention, the ChiP-on-chip approach is relatively expensive and may not be able to provide the level of resolution desired. In addition, it depends on the availability of antibodies against the specific histone modification of interest and on that antibody being able to bind to its target when the protein is bound (cross-linked) to DNA. As with other genome-wide DNA and RNA analysis, array- (or chip-)based technologies are gradually being superseded by NGS-based approaches, so that ChiP followed by next-generation sequencing of the selected (pulled-down) DNA (so-called ChiP-seq) may become the approach of choice.

14.9 Quantification of microRNA

Although mRNA and other large RNA species have been known for many decades, the regulatory microRNA were not discovered until 1993. In part, this was because they are small (typically 22 nucleotides long) and so were discarded during the application of conventional protocols for RNA isolation and purification. All of the approaches for quantification of mRNA, including real-time, reverse transcription, qPCR for candidate-based approaches and microarrays (or chips) and next-generation sequencing for genome-wide approaches, are also applicable to the quantification of microRNA in biological samples. The task for genome-wide analysis of micro-RNA is considerably less than that for mRNA, because there is approximately an order of magnitude more mRNA (~20 000) than there are microRNA (~1000) in the human genome. Because of their relatively small size, microRNA are more stable in archived biological samples. For example, the isolation, purification and analysis of microRNA from formalin-fixed and paraffin-embedded tissue samples are relatively straightforward, so that such routinely prepared tissue samples are a good source of information about microRNA. Under the same archiving conditions mRNA become degraded, making their quantitative analysis problematic.

More recently, it has become apparent that there are single nucleotide polymorphisms (SNPs) in the genomic regions encoding microRNA. It is rare for these variants to appear in the 'seed region'; that is, within nucleotides 2–7 of the mature microRNA sequence that determines the specific mRNA to which the microRNA will bind. However, SNPs may affect microRNA function in other ways, including production of the primary transcript, during processing of this transcript to produce the mature microRNA or through effects on interactions between the microRNA and its target mRNA. As a consequence, future studies of microRNA may need to include candidate, or genome-wide, genotyping using the approaches described in Chapter 13 for other genetic variants.

14.10 Animal models for epigenetics research

As discussed in Chapter 18, judicious use of animal models can be very valuable in nutrition research for many reasons, including the ability to undertake lifelong, or multiple-generational, studies that would be unfeasible in humans; and highly controlled studies to collect biological samples that would be impractical and/or unethical in humans. In addition, modern molecular biological approaches, including genetic manipulations of the test organism, facilitate fundamental research on the molecular mechanisms through which nutrients, or other bioactive food components, influence cell function and, ultimately, health. Although much traditional nutrition research employing animal models used laboratory mammals, such as rats, mice and guinea pigs or farm animals such as chickens and pigs, modern molecular nutrition research has a much wider choice of animal models. Some of these, including the nematode worm *Caenorhabditis elegans* (*C. elegans*), the fruit fly *Drosophila melanogaster* and the zebrafish (*Danio rerio*), are of increasing interest for nutrition research because their biology is well understood, they are readily manipulated genetically, there is ready availability of molecular biological tools for their investigation and, importantly, they are relatively cheap and easy to keep in large numbers. In addition, their short life spans make them attractive models for studies of the life-course effects of nutritional, and other, manipulations.

A fundamental question to be considered before undertaking research in any model organism is whether the outcomes of that research will be interpretable in the context of one's real organism of interest, for example the human. From the epigenetics perspective, it is important to recognise that not all model organisms have the same epigenetic marks and molecules. Whereas histone modifications are epigenetic regulators in most organisms, there is no DNA methylation in some potentially useful animal models (Table 14.3).

It appears that DNA methylation is a very ancient mechanism used for genome defence and for the regulation of gene expression but, during the course of evolution, some organisms, notably many insects including *Drosophila*, have lost this genomic feature. This may be because there is some redundancy between DNA methylation and histone modifications in epigenetic

Table 14.3 Presence of epigenetic marks in model organisms.

Model organism	Common name	DNA methylation	Post-translational modification of histones
Saccharomyces cerevisiae	Budding yeast	No	Yes
Drosophila melanogaster	Fruit fly	No	Yes
Apis mellifera	Honey bee	Yes	Yes
Solenopsis invicta	Fire ant	Yes	Yes
Caenorhabditis elegans	Nematode worm	No	Yes
Danio rerio	Zebrafish	Yes	Yes
Mus musculus	Mouse	Yes	Yes

regulation. Interestingly, social insects, including fire ants and honey bees, have retained DNA methylation and in these animals changes in DNA methylation patterns are associated with altered phenotype. It may be that the greater complexities in responding appropriately to nutritional and other signals in these species (see Figure 14.4) require greater complexity in epigenetic regulation. In common with all mammals, the laboratory mouse (*Mus musculus*) combines both DNA methylation and histone modifications within its repertoire of epigenetic marks and molecules, and is a good model for epigenetic studies relevant to humans.

14.11 Applications of epigenetics-based approaches in future human nutrition research

Epigenetic mechanisms are a critical part of the complex regulatory machinery ensuring that cells express the appropriate complement of genes in given circumstances. In addition, epigenetic marks and molecules become disrupted during ageing and in the development of diseases, so that the study of epigenetics is now a central component of much health-related research. From the nutritionist's perspective, epigenetic processes are very attractive targets for understanding how nutritional status (e.g. obesity) and specific dietary exposures (e.g. micronutrients and bioactive components in plant foods) influence health throughout the life course.

Although there are some striking examples of the ways in which nutrition modulates phenotype via epigenetic mechanisms (e.g. the impact of maternal methyl donor supply during pregnancy in the Agouti mouse; see Section 14.5), epigenetics-based nutritional research is in its infancy. However, this research area looks set to grow rapidly as a core component of the expansion of

molecular nutrition research using 'omics' technologies (see Chapter 13). Because of their potential reversibility by environmental factors including food components, aberrant (or abnormal) epigenetic marks are important targets for nutritional interventions aimed at reducing disease risk and improving health and well-being. The growth of this research will be facilitated by the widespread availability, and increasing affordability, of the tools and technologies required to characterise and quantify epigenetic marks and molecules, including the bioinformatics tools to help interpret the resulting data.

Acknowledgements

Epigenetics-based research in my laboratory is supported by the Centre for Brain Ageing & Vitality, which is funded through the Lifelong Health and Wellbeing cross-council initiative by the MRC, BBSRC, EPSRC and ESRC, and by the BBSRC through grant BB/G007993/1.

References and further reading

Choi, S.-W. and Friso, S. (eds) (2009) *Nutrients and Epigenetics.* CRC Press, Boca Raton, FL.

Delage, B. and Dashwood, R.H. (2008) Dietary manipulation of histone structure and function. *Annual Review of Nutrition*, **28**, 347–366.

Jirtle, R.L. and Skinner, M.K. (2007) Environmental epigenomics and disease susceptibility. *Nature Reviews Genetics*, **8**, 4, 253–262.

Mathers, J.C. (2008) Session 2: Personalised nutrition. Epigenomics: A basis for understanding individual differences? *Proceedings of the Nutrition Society*, **67**, 4, 390–394.

McKay, J.A. and Mathers, J.C. (2011) Diet induced epigenetic changes and their implications for health. *Acta Physiologica*, **202**, 103–118.

Migheli, F., Stoccoro, A., Coppodè, F. *et al.* (2013) Comparison study of MS-HRM and pyrosequencing techniques for quantification of APC and CDKN2A gene methylation. *PloS One*, **8**, 1, e52501.

15
Nutrient–Gene Interactions

Anne Marie Minihane

Department of Nutrition, Norwich Medical School, University of East Anglia

Key messages

- Nutrigenetics is the interactive impact of genetic make-up and diet composition on health or risk of disease.
- This area of science does not involve the manipulation of the genetic code in any way, but simply the capture of genetic information and its use in disease risk prediction and the provision of lifestyle (and specifically dietary) advice.
- Over 99% of the genetic information between individuals is identical, with less than 1% variable, which determines an individual's risk of disease and response to their environment, including diet.

- Over 90% of genetic variability takes the form of common small changes to the DNA sequence, referred to as single-nucleotide polymorphisms (SNP).
- Candidate gene, GWAS and more recently DNA sequencing are examples of approaches used in nutrigenetic research.
- To date the majority of the genetic basis of the variability in disease risk and response to dietary change is unknown.

15.1 Introduction

There is some confusion within the scientific community regarding the terms nutrigenetics and nutrigenomics. *Nutrigenetics* refers to the impact of genetic variation (genotype) on the response to different diet constituents, whereas *nutrigenomics* is the effect of dietary components on the expression of genes. *Nutrigenomics* interactions are the focus of Chapter 13, with the current chapter providing an overview of the various types of genetic variation, scientific approaches and methodologies used to study nutrigenetic interactions, and what is currently known regarding the impact of genetic variability on the risk of disease and response to dietary change. The impact of genotype on the association between diet and disease is a complex one, with genetic variability influencing:

- Food intake and preferences
- The absorption, metabolism and elimination from the body of dietary constituents
- The impact of a particular tissue concentration of a dietary constituent on metabolism and overall health status

Our DNA (deoxyribonucleic acid) contains the information needed to synthesise all the proteins required for human development and function. The first draft of the majority of the sequence of the human genome was published in a *Nature* article entitled 'Initial sequencing and analysis of the human genome' in 2001, with the complete sequence available in 2004. This has subsequently led to the recognition that there is less than 1% genetic variation between individuals. When first published, the availability of the human genome sequence was considered to be a panacea, with genetic information predicted by many commentators to have a major impact on approaches used in the fields of medicine and overall public health. In nutrition it was thought that it would lead to the replacement of generic 'one size fits all' dietary guidelines with more efficacious, stratified dietary advice based in part on personal genetic information. However, this has not (as yet) transpired, with only a relatively small fraction of the estimated total genetic contribution to health and response to diet having been identified. This begs the critical question of whether our initial estimates of heredity (contribution of genotype to phenotype) are

Nutrition Research Methodologies, First Edition. Edited by Julie A Lovegrove, Leanne Hodson, Sangita Sharma and Susan A Lanham-New.
© 2015 John Wiley & Sons, Ltd. Published 2015 by John Wiley & Sons, Ltd.
Companion Website: www.wiley.com/go/nutritionsociety

inflated, or whether our current methods for the detection of genetic variation or the interpretation of the data have been insensitive or misleading in their approaches. The balance of evidence suggests the latter to be the case, as will be discussed in this chapter.

15.2 DNA and genetic variation

DNA and its discovery timeline

In plants and animals, DNA is organised into 23 pairs of chromosomes within the nucleus of the cell. One member of each pair is inherited from the mother and one from the father. Most DNA molecules are double-stranded helices of two long chains of repeating units called nucleotides. Each nucleotide consists of a sugar and phosphate group (which makes up the backbone of the chain) and a base attached to the sugar (Figure 15.1). The bases are adenine (A), thymine (T), guanine (G) and cytosine (C). Virtually every single cell in the body contains a complete copy of the approximately 3 billion DNA base pairs. A series of three bases encodes for a particular amino acid, with for example ACT, ACC, ACA and ACG coding for threonine, and ATG coding for methionine (Table 15.1).

DNA was first identified and isolated by Swiss physician and biologist Friedrich Miescher in 1871, with its

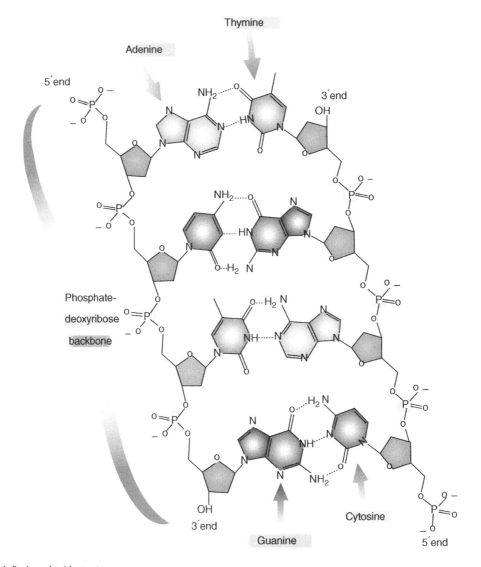

Figure 15.1 Basic nucleotide structure.

Table 15.1 DNA codon table.

	T		C		A		G		
T	TTT	Phe	TCT	Ser	TAT	Tyr	TGT	Cys	T
	TTC	Phe	TCC	Ser	TAC	Tyr	TGC	Cys	C
	TTA	Leu	TCA	Ser	TAA	**STOP**	TGA	**STOP**	A
	TTG	Leu	TCG	Ser	TAG	**STOP**	TGG	Trp	G
C	CTT	Leu	CCT	Pro	CAT	His	CGT	Arg	T
	CTC	Leu	CCC	Pro	CAC	His	CGC	Arg	C
	CTA	Leu	CCA	Pro	CAA	Gln	CGA	Arg	A
	CTG	Leu	CCG	Pro	CAG	Gln	CGG	Arg	G
A	ATT	Ile	ACT	Thr	AAT	Asn	AGT	Ser	T
	ATC	Ile	ACC	Thr	AAC	Asn	AGC	Ser	C
	ATA	Ile	ACA	Thr	AAA	Lys	AGA	Arg	A
	ATG	Met	ACG	Thr	AAG	Lys	AGG	Arg	G
G	GTT	Val	GCT	Ala	GAT	Asp	GGT	Gly	T
	GTC	Val	GCC	Ala	GAC	Asp	GGC	Gly	C
	GTA	Val	GCA	Ala	GAA	Glu	GGA	Gly	A
	GTG	Val	GCG	Ala	GAG	Glu	GGG	Gly	G

Ala, alanine; Arg, arginine; Asn, Asparagine, Asp, aspartic acid;; Cys, cysteine; Gln, glutamine; Glu, glutamic acid; His, histidine; Ile, isoleucine; Leu, leucine; Lys, lysine; Met, methionine; Phe, phenylalanine; Pro, proline; Ser, serine; Thr, threonine; Try, tryptophan; Tyr, tyrosine; Val, valine

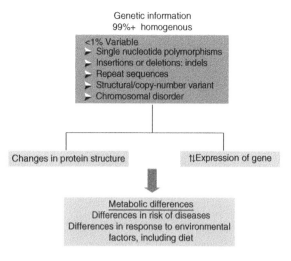

Figure 15.2 Genetic variation and its physiological impact.

double-helix structure discovered and published in 1953 by James Watson, Francis Crick and Rosalind Franklin. However, it was not until 2001 when the first output of the Human Genome Project (HGP) was published that information on the sequence of bases that make up DNA was available. The project was officially launched in 1990 through funding from the US National Institutes of Health (NIH) and Department of Energy, and resolved to sequence 95% of the DNA in human cells within 15 years. During the early years of the HGP, the UK's Wellcome Trust Sanger Institute became a major partner. In 2003, two years ahead of schedule, the HGP had achieved its major targets (http://ghr.nlm.nih.gov/handbook/hgp) as follows:

- *identify* all the approximately 20,000–25,000 genes (section of DNA which encodes a protein) in human DNA,
- *determine* the sequences of the 3 billion base pairs that make up human DNA,
- *store* this information in databases,
- *improve* tools for data analysis,
- *transfer* related technologies to the private sector, and
- *address* the ethical, legal, and social issues that may arise from the project.

In 2004 the almost complete (99.7%) sequence of human DNA was available.

DNA is divided into coding and non-coding regions, with coding regions constituting less than 2% of the total DNA, with the other 98% referred to as *junk DNA* with unknown biological function. However, unsurprisingly, it is becoming evident through initiatives such as the Encyclopaedia of DNA Elements (ENCODE) Consortium that a large proportion of this non-coding DNA does have essential roles.

Genetic variability

A mutation is the term used to describe a change in the base sequence and structure of DNA (Figure 15.2). Such mutations can be minor, with a change to only a single base in the DNA sequences referred to as a single-nucleotide polymorphism (SNP), right through to changes in the number of chromosomes. The functional consequence (penetrance) of the genotype varies between no detectable impact on phenotype, through to mutations with complete penetrance where all carriers of the mutation develop the trait or disease.

An SNP occurs every 100–300 bases and SNPs account for over 90% of all genetic variability. When a SNPs occur in the coding region of DNA, they may be silent, non-sense or missense (Figure 15.3). *Silent*, as the term suggests, has no impact on the amino acid sequence of the protein. A *non-sense* mutation results in a premature stop codon and a truncated and often non-functional protein. A *missense* SNP results in an amino acid change in the protein sequence, with the functional consequences dependent on where in the protein the amino acid change has occurred, and also on whether the physicochemical properties of the replacement amino acid are comparable to the original amino acid. Although with a few notable exceptions, such as sickle cell anaemia, SNPs rarely cause the disease, they may increase the risk, as

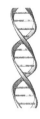
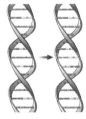

	Original		Silent	Non-sense	Missense
DNA codon	TCA		TCC	TAA	CCA
Amino acid	Serine		Serine	STOP	Proline

Figure 15.3 Categories of single-nucleotide polymorphisms (SNPs).

will be discussed later in this chapter. It is well known that SNPs in non-coding regions also have functional consequences, although the metabolic basis for this is less clear. A SNP in the gene promoter region may have an impact on the expression of the gene, whereas those in intergenic regions may affect the translation of the genetic code into a protein, for example by influencing mRNA stability or motility within the cell.

Structural variants, are operationally defined as genomic alterations (deletions, duplications, copy-number variants, insertions, inversions and translocations) that involve segments of DNA that are between 1 Kb and 3 MB, with smaller (<1 Kb) variations that involve DNA insertions or deletions referred to as INDELS. Repeat sequences are a length or nucleotide sequence that is repeated, with the consequences often dependent on the number of repeats.

Genetics and disease risk

Almost all diseases have some genetic component. A genetic disorder is where the genotype contributes to the aetiology of the disease. For the majority of cases of chronic age-related conditions such as cardiovascular diseases (CVD), Alzheimer's disease (AD) and osteoporosis, the greater part of the genetic risk is thought to be afforded by multiple low-penetrance SNPs and these disorders are therefore referred to as polygenic. However, a small percentage of the cases of such conditions are caused by high-penetrance single-gene defects (also referred to as Mendalian or monogenic disorders). For example, for AD, mutations in three genes, namely amyloid precursor protein, preselin-1 and preselin-2, have been linked to an early-onset (<60 years) monogenic form of the disorder, which accounts for less than 5% of all cases. In contrast,

the common *APOE4* genotype (20–25% of Caucasians) has been genetically linked to the late-onset form of the disease (>60 years). Individuals with two copies of the *APOE4 allele* (1–2% of the population) have a 50–90% chance of developing AD by age 85 years, with those with one copy having an approximately 45% chance, compared to a 20% chance in the general population. Furthermore, *APOE4* carriers develop AD about a decade earlier than non-*APOE4* individuals. However, being an *APOE4* carrier is neither necessary nor sufficient to cause the disease. Therefore, this form of AD is considered as polygenic and multifactorial.

To date, more than 6000 known single-gene (monogenic) disorders, including thalassemia, sickle cell anaemia, cystic fibrosis and Huntington's disease (HD), have been identified. The nature of the disease depends on the functions performed by the modified gene. The single-gene or monogenic disorders can be classified into three main categories: dominant, recessive and X-linked.

Monogenic autosomal-dominant disorders occur through the inheritance of a single copy of a defective gene (we have two copies of each gene, one from each parent) that is sufficient to 'over-ride' the functional gene. An example of such a disorder is HD, a neurodegenerative condition that leads to loss of muscle coordination and cognitive decline, with symptoms becoming apparent usually between the ages of 35 and 45 years. HD is an example of a trinucleotide repeat disorder. The Huntington (HTT) gene located on the short arm of chromosome 4 contains a sequence of three DNA bases – cytosine–adenine–guanine (CAG) – repeated multiple times. CAG is the three-letter genetic code (codon) for the amino acid glutamine, so a series results in the production of a chain of glutamine known as a polyglutamine tract (or polyQ tract). Normal individuals have fewer than 26 repeats, with individuals with 40 or more repeats suffering from HD. The presence of 36–39 repeats results in a reduced-penetrance form of the disease, with a much later onset and slower progression of symptoms. In some cases the onset may be so late that symptoms are not apparent.

For a monogenic autosomal-recessive condition to occur, both copies of the gene need to be defective. If just a single defective copy is present, the normal copy is sufficient to maintain function and the individual is usually an unaware carrier of the condition. Cystic fibrosis (CF) is an example of an autosomal-recessive disorder. About two-thirds of cases are caused by a deletion of three nucleotides in the cystic fibrosis transmemebrane conductance regulator (CFTR) gene on chromosome 7, which results in the loss of the amino acid phenylalanine at position 508 in the CFTR protein. However, there are thought to be up to 1500 other mutations that can result in CF. In X-linked disorders the defective gene lies on the X-sex chromosome. X-linked disorders are most common in males, as there is no second X chromosome carrying the normal copy to compensate. In males, therefore, a recessive gene can cause a genetic disorder. Duchenne muscular dystrophy is an example of an X-linked disorder.

In addition to monogenic and polygenic disorders, chromosomal and mitochondrial genetic disorders occur. In chromosomal disorders, as the name suggests, there is an alteration in the number of copies of a whole chromosome or a major chromosome section. For example, in Down's syndrome (trisomy 21) there are three copies of chromosome 21.

With the exception of genetic conditions that have a direct impact on the absorption or metabolism of dietary components, such as coeliac disease or phenylketonuria, often dietary change has a limited ability to affect the risk and severity of high-penetrance monogenic, chromosomal or mitochondrial genetic disorders. These conditions are also relatively rare and, although of significant consequence to the individual, only account for a small fraction of total population disease burden. For these reasons, the field of nutrigenetics over the last two decades has focused on the interactive impact of diet composition and common genotypes in determining phenotype, including the tissue status of diet-derived nutrients and non-nutrients, health status and risk of disease.

15.3 Research approaches used in nutrigenetic research

The majority of the nutrigenetics work conducted to date has taken a candidate gene approach (Figure 15.4). Although research tools developed in the last 10 years, such as genome-wide association studies (GWAS) and more recently sequencing techniques, have advanced knowledge of the genetic architecture of thousands of diseases, their contribution to nutrigenetics has been limited so far, as they generally do not capture dietary information on the participants included in the analysis.

Candidate gene approaches

Principles of the candidate gene approach
The candidate gene approach is hypothesis driven. Genotypes of interest are selected in candidate genes based on a priori knowledge of the gene's significant biological role in the phenotype under study. For identification of the 'disease allele' this approach usually uses a case-control design and asks the question: 'Is one allele of a candidate gene more frequently observed in those with the disease than in those who are disease free?' For nutrigenetic candidate gene studies, phenotypes such as disease risk indicators (e.g. plasma glucose, cholesterol etc. concentration, blood pressure or BMI) or nutrient status (e.g. plasma or tissue concentrations of dietary

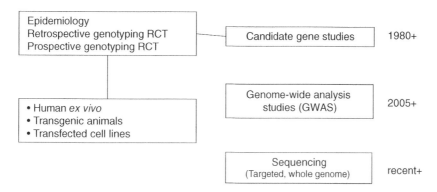

Figure 15.4 Research tools to identify common genotypes associated with disease risk and response to environment. RCT, randomised controlled trial.

nutrients or their metabolites) are often considered as a continuous variable. Much of the available candidate gene literature reporting on the impact of genotype on response to diet in human randomised controlled trials (RCTs) has taken a retrospective genotyping approach. As a result, due to a low number in the rarer allele genotype group, the studies are often underpowered to draw explicit conclusions. An approach where study participants are prospectively recruited and the genotype subgroups matched at baseline provides a much more rigorous design in candidate gene studies.

APOE genotype research as an example of the candidate gene approach

One of the most widely researched genotypes using the candidate gene approach is the *APOE* genotype, and its association with CVD and AD risk and its impact on the physiological response to altered dietary fat composition. Its selection is based on the known role of apolipoprotein E (apoE) in lipoprotein metabolism, which impacts on the plasma concentration of total-, LDL- and HDL-cholesterol and triglyceride levels. In the central nervous system the vast majority of lipid transport is mediated by apoE. In addition, apoE is an important determinant of amyloid protein metabolism, neurogenesis and neuronal and specifically synaptic function, dysregulation of which is a key pathological feature of AD.

In humans, the *APOE* gene is mapped to chromosome 19 in a cluster with *APOC1* and *APOC2*. Two missense SNPs in the *APOE* gene result in three specific apoE protein isoforms, namely apoE2, apoE3 and apoE4 (Table 15.2). The protein products differ in the amino acid present at residue 112 (rs429358) and 158 (rs7412) of the protein. ApoE2 contains 112 Cys/158 Cys, apoE3 112 Cys/158 Arg and apoE4 112 Arg/158 Arg. Although the amino acid alterations do not occur within the receptor-binding region (136–150 amino acids), the substitutions at positions 112 and 158 are known to have an impact on the salt bridge formation within the protein, which ultimately influences the receptor-binding activity, the lipoprotein 'preference' of the apoE protein

and their stabilities. Globally the *APOE* allelic distribution shows substantial variation, with an allele frequency of 60–90% for the wild-type ε3 allele. Approximately 65% of Caucasians are ε3/ε3, 19% ε3/ε4, 10% ε2/ε3, 4% ε2/ε4, 2% ε4/ε4 and 0.5–1% ε2/ε2.

As reviewed by Minihane in 2013, the *APOE* genotype was originally described as a genetic contributor to CVD, with *APOE4* carriers at increased risk. However, with ever larger meta-analysis it has become apparent that at a population level the impact on CVD risk is marginal and may only be relevant in subgroups with additional significant risk factors. For example, in both the Northwick Park (UK) and Framingham Offspring (US) cohorts, the risk of CVD was about twofold higher in smokers who were *E4* carriers versus wild-type *E3/E3*.

Perhaps the most consistent and consequential impact of the *APOE* genotype is on the risk of AD, as already described. Interestingly, when James D. Watson was presented with his genetic information, his being the first genome sequenced by next-generation sequence technologies (see later in this chapter), he elected not to know his *APOE* genotype.

The *APOE* genotype is also widely used as an example of the ethical, social, financial (e.g. health and life insurance) and practical issues associated with the more widespread use of predictive genetic testing for polygenic chronic conditions and the stratification or personalisation of lifestyle advice, including that on diet. The outputs from the Risk Evaluation and Education for Alzheimer's disease (REVEAL) study provide a comprehensive overview of this important aspect of nutrigenetics.

Furthermore, data are emerging to indicate that the *APOE* genotype is in part responsible for the variable responses of plasma lipids (total-, LDL-, and HDL-cholesterol and triglycerides), with *APOE4* carriers thought to be most responsive to the plasma cholesterol and triglyceride-modulating impact of total fat, cholesterol, saturated fat intakes and long-chain omega-3 PUFA (fish oil fatty acid) intakes. In the future, if current generic dietary fat recommendations, such as total fat and saturated fat of less than 33% and 10% of total energy for adults, are replaced with more stratified guidelines to suit the individual, it is likely that an individual's *APOE* genotype information may be used in the provision of such more personalised advice.

Methylenetetrahydrofolate reductase (MTHFR) genotype research as an example of the candidate gene approach

Methylenetetrahydrofolate reductase (MTHFR) is an enzyme important in folate/homocysteine metabolism. It provides a clear demonstration of how genetic information could be used to provide targeted dietary advice

Table 15.2 ApoE isoform amino acid differences and lipoprotein preferences.

Isoform	Amino acid 112	Amino acid 158	Lipoprotein preference
E2	Cys	Cys	HDL
E3	Cys	Arg	HDL
E4	Arg	Arg	VLDL, CM

Arg, arginine; CM, chylomicron; Cys, cysteine; HDL, high-density lipoprotein; VLDL, very low-density lipoprotein.

in an at-risk population subgroup. A homozygous mutant genotype (TT, rs1801133), which has a frequency of approximately 10% worldwide, is associated with reduced enzyme activity. It is emerging that the penetrance of the genotype is dependent on vitamin B status (folate, vitamins B2, B6 and B12), with adequate status likely to abrogate the negative physiological impact of this genotype on disease risk.

Genome-wide association studies (GWAS)

The candidate gene approach is limited by how much is understood about the biology of the phenotype of interest. For those with an incomplete understanding, important genes and variants in those genes will be overlooked. In contrast, GWAS are not hypothesis driven. The principles and relevance (to the nutrigenetic field) of the GWAS approach are outlined in Box 15.1.

Sets of nearby SNPs on the same chromosome are inherited together in blocks. This pattern of SNPs co-inherited on a DNA region is termed a *haplotype*. Although blocks may contain a large number of SNPs, a few SNPs are enough to identify the haplotype uniquely. The International HapMap is a map of these haplotype blocks and the specific SNPs that identify the haplotypes are called *tagging* SNPs. The International HapMap Project is an international collaboration open-access resource (http://hapmap.ncbi.nlm.nih.gov/). It officially started in 2002, with Phase I data published in 2005, Phase II in 2007 and Phase III in 2009. The project analysed DNA from populations of African, Asian and European ancestry, and included a total of 270 people from Nigeria (30 sets of samples from two parents and an adult child, termed trios), Japan (45 unrelated individuals), China (45 unrelated individuals) and US residents with northern and western European ancestry (30 trios).

In GWAS, *tagging* SNPs are quantified using commercially available SNP chips in a group of cases versus matched controls, in order to establish disease-associated variants. The advantage of this *tagging* SNP approach is that it precludes the need to quantify all SNPs in the human genome. Its disadvantages include the fact that it generally considers variants with a frequency of over 1–5%, and therefore will often miss rarer, but potentially high-penetrance genotypes and does not identify the functional SNP, which may or may not be the *tagging* SNP measured.

The first GWAS output, which included 50 cases and 50 controls, was published in 2005 and identified a polymorphism in complement H linked with age-related macular disease (ARMD). A landmark in the history of GWAS was the Wellcome Trust Case Control Consortium (WTCCC) study, the largest GWAS ever conducted at the time of its publication in 2007. The WTCCC included 14000 cases of seven common diseases (~2000 individuals for each of coronary heart disease, type 1 diabetes, type 2 diabetes, rheumatoid arthritis, Crohn's disease, bipolar disorder and hypertension) and 3000 shared controls. This study successfully identified a number of disease genotypes. In the last eight years GWAS has identified over 1600 variants associated with 250 traits and has had some success in identifying a large fraction of the genetic basis of particular phenotypes. For example, for ARMD five DNA regions have been identified that collectively explain 50% of the total heritability, with 25–30% of the genetic component of the plasma lipid profile explained. However, for the majority of polygenic traits the identified variants only account for a small proportion of the total estimated heritability, which varies from 20–80% depending on the phenotype of interest. For BMI and obesity, 32 individual loci have been identified (including FTO) and confirmed, but the effect size of each individual variant is small, and they collectively explain less than 5% of the heritability.

There are likely to be a number of reasons why GWAS has resulted in only modest capture of heritability. Firstly, although the gene variant may have been identified by GWAS, it may not have emerged as significant or its effect size may be underestimated for a number of reasons, which include:

- Use of stringent P-value (typically $P < 1 \times 10^{-8}$) to compensate for multiple testing (for the large number of SNPs measured).
- Imprecise phenotyping. For disease outcomes, patients in the 'case group' often present with a range of related conditions with variable genetic aetiology. For many outcomes, such as blood pressure, the precision of the measurement is problematic.
- Control group of questionable quality. Often an individual in the control group does not have a clinical diagnosis of the primary outcome but is a registered

---

Box 15.1 Outline of the GWAS research tool

- Typically takes a group of cases of a particular disease/condition and matched controls.
- Analyse 300,000 - 2×10^6 tagging SNPs that are correlated with (derived from HapMap) and provide information on 80–90% of common variation.
- Detects common variation (population frequency >5%), but far less for the low-frequency variants (0.01–5%) and virtually none for the rare variants (<0.01%).
- Does not identify functional genes or SNPs.
- Has identified over 1600 variants associated with 250 traits.
- Led to the identification of the fat mass and obesity-associated (FTO) gene.
- Generally no dietary data collected.

patient for an alternative condition, the risk of which may also be affected by the identified gene variants.

- True causal variants incompletely surveyed, as not in full linkage disequilibrium (LD) with *tagging* SNP.
- A number of causal variants may exist in the one locus, with only one *tagging* SNP chosen, which may result in an underestimation of the total heritability accounted for by that particular region.

Secondly, it is plausible and increasingly demonstrated that rarer, single-nucleotide changes or structural variants could make a significant contribution to *hidden variability*, with emerging next-generation genotyping technologies (see the next section) providing the analytical tools to capture these rare variants.

Thirdly, much of the missing genetic variation may be in the form of interactions, between allele pairs and between genotype and environmental (including diet composition) or physiological variables (see later in this chapter). These interactions are currently poorly understood.

Next-generation sequencing

Next-generation sequencing is becoming increasingly feasible and affordable. In the decade 2003–2013 the cost of sequencing an entire human genome reduced from approximately $40 million to $5k (http://www.genome.gov/sequencingcosts/). In contrast to the SNP chip/GWAS approach, this technology provides a complete map of an individual's genome, allowing the detection of less common variants. The 1000 Genomes Project, which will include over 1000 individuals from 14 populations, aims to capture all variants with less than 1% frequency and more than 0.1% in protein coding regions (exome). In 2012 this initiative provided a validated haplotype map of 38 million SNPs, 1.4 million short insertions and deletions, and more than 14 000 larger deletions in 1092 individuals. It is hoped that this and comparable comprehensive sequencing endeavours will detect much of the hidden heritability.

Impact of physiological variables on genotype–phenotype associations

Currently in genetic studies populations are considered as homogenous entities. It is becoming increasingly apparent that the penetrance of genotype is variable and, as a result, population genotype–phenotype associations often under- or overestimate the effect in subgroups.

As a simple example, if being a carrier of a particular variant increased disease risk by 50% in men but had no effect in women, then studying variant–disease association at a population (mixed-sex) level would provide an estimated increased risk of 25%, and be very

misleading as to the relative importance of the genotype in both sexes.

At this stage it is too early to say what the contribution of differential penetrance in population subgroups to the missing heritability is likely to be, but it is likely to be considerable. For biological processes with a known influence of sex, such as adiposity and plasma lipids, evidence of variable penetrance has indeed been reported. A number of publications suggest that common variants in genes such as the leptin receptor (LepR, Gln223Arg, rs1137101) and *APOA5* (−1131 T>C, rs662799) have an impact on fasting and postprandial triglycerides only in men. From a biological perspective this may be explained by the fact that in women, female hormones, which are known modulators of lipoprotein metabolism, may counteract the impact of the 'risky' variant. There is also evidence of racial/ethnic differences in the physiological impact of particular variants, as indicated by projects such as the Population Architecture using Genomics and Epidemiology (PAGE) Consortium (Fesinmeyer *et al.* 2012). In addition, LD patterns suggest that *tagging* SNPs used in GWAS for Europeans may not adequately capture the genetic variation in other ethnic groups. Apparent ethnic differences in genotype–phenotype associations from GWAS may also be in part attributable to differences in habitual diets between populations.

15.4 GWAS and next-generation sequencing in the study of nutrigenetic interactions

To date, the vast majority of our nutrigenetic knowledge has come from candidate gene approaches used in human epidemiological and RCTs. GWAS methodology and modelling do not lend themselves well to the direct study of genotype–diet–disease associations, in part due to the fact that the sample size needed would be enormous and that the collection of accurate dietary information from such a large number (often 100 000+ individuals) is logistically very difficult. An increasing number of GWAS studies have nutrient status (e.g. vitamin D and iron) as their primary endpoint. The output from GWAS has also informed the choice of variants for a more focused study of genotype–diet interactions in human epidemiology and intervention studies and in animal models. The identification of the *FTO* genotype by GWAS has led to a flurry of activity examining its impact on food intake, satiety and appetite and its interaction with macronutrient composition in determining BMI and risk of obesity. The relatively recent availability of GWAS data for cohorts for which participants have existing detailed dietary data, such as the Nurse's Health Study, Framingham

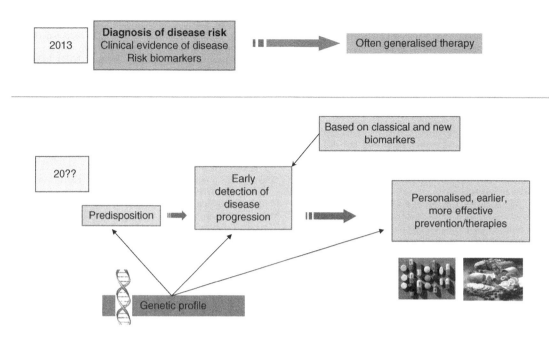

Figure 15.5 More widespread use of genetic profiling to predict disease risk and personalise lifestyle advice.

Heart Studies and EPIC, is likely to make a significant contribution to our nutrigenetic understanding in the near future.

15.5 Conclusions: The road ahead

With the availability of the human genome sequence (2001–04), it was expected that genetic profiling would by now be a key tool in disease prevention and therapeutics (Figure 15.5), allowing disease risk estimation prior to the appearance of any clinical symptoms and the stratification of lifestyle advice and drug use to maximise the impact of intervention on disease progression. Although there have been significant advances in the identification of the genetic basis for monogenic disorders over the last 10 years, and limited use of genetic information in the choice of medication and dosages (e.g. warfarin), the genetic basis for the majority of chronic age-related conditions is relatively unknown. Furthermore, there is insufficient nutrigenetic information currently to warrant the replacement of population-based dietary recommendations with stratified advice based on genotype. The future wider use of sequencing technology, the detailed and precise characterisation of study participants in genetic studies (including dietary data) and more sophisticated modelling of large genetic or other biomedical and lifestyle data sets will undoubtedly lead to the detection of variants of particular importance at a population or subgroup level. Many of the benefits of

genetics in medicine and overall public health remain to be realised and we have a long way to go. In the words of Winston Churchill, it feels like the 'end of the beginning' rather than the 'beginning of the end'.

References and further reading

1000 Genomes project, http://www.1000genomes.org/

Abecasis, G.R., Auton, A., Brooks, L.D. *et al.* (2012) An integrated map of genetic variation from 1,092 human genomes. *Nature*, **491**, 56–65.

Bush, W.S. and Moore, J.H. (2012) Chapter 11: Genome-wide association studies. *PLoS Computational Biology*, **8**, e1002822.

Corella, D. and Ordovas, J.M. (2009) Nutrigenomics in cardiovascular medicine. *Circulation: Cardiovascular Genetics*, **2**, 637–651.

Dunham, I., Kundaje, A., Aldred, S.F. *et al.* (2012) An integrated encyclopedia of DNA elements in the human genome. *Nature*, **489**, 57–74.

ENCODE Project Consortium (2004) The ENCODE (ENCyclopedia Of DNA Elements) Project. *Science*, **306**, 636–640.

Encyclopaedia of DNA elements (ENCODE),http://genome.ucsc.edu/ENCODE/

International HapMap Consortium (2003) The International HapMap Project. *Nature*, **426**, 789–796.

International HapMap Consortium (2005) A haplotype map of the human genome. *Nature*, **437**, 1299–1320.

Fenech, M., El-Sohemy, A., Cahill, L. *et al.* (2011) Nutrigenetics and nutrigenomics: Viewpoints on the current status and applications in nutrition research and practice. *Journal of Nutrigenetics and Nutrigenomics*, **4**, 69–89.

Fesinmeyer, M.D., North, K.E., Ritchie, M.D. *et al.* (2013) Genetic risk factors for BMI and obesity in an ethnically diverse population: Results from the Population Architecture using Genomics and Epidemiology (PAGE) Study. *Obesity*, **21**, 4.

HapMap International Project, http://hapmap.ncbi.nlm.nih.gov/

Human Genome Project, http://www.ornl.gov/sci/techresources/Human_Genome/medicine/pharma.shtml

Hurlimann, T., Stenne, R., Menuz, V. and Godard, B. (2011) Inclusion and exclusion in nutrigenetics clinical research: Ethical and scientific challenges. *Journal of Nutrigenetics and Nutrigenomics*, **4**, 322–343.

Lander, E.S. (2011) Initial impact of the sequencing of the human genome. *Nature*, **470**, 187–197.

Lander, E.S., Linton, L.M., Birren, B. *et al.* (2001) Initial sequencing and analysis of the human genome. *Nature*, **409**, 860–921.

Mahley, R.W., Weisgraber, K.H. and Huang, Y. (2006) Apolipoprotein E4: A causative factor and therapeutic target in neuropathology, including Alzheimer's disease. *Proceedings of the National Academy of Sciences*, **103**, 5644–5651.

Manolio, T.A., Collins, F.S., Cox, N.J. *et al.* (2009) Finding the missing heritability of complex diseases. *Nature*, **461**, 747–753.

Mccarthy, M.I., Abecasis, G.R., Cardon, L.R. *et al.* (2008) Genome-wide association studies for complex traits: Consensus, uncertainty and challenges. *Nature Reviews Genetics*, **9**, 356–369.

Minihane, A.M. (2013) The genetic contribution to disease risk and variability in response to diet: Where is the hidden heritability? *Proceedings of the Nutrition Society*, **72**, 40–47.

National Human Genome Research Institute (NIH), http://www.genome.gov/10000202

Rimbach, G. and Minihane, A.M. (2009) Nutrigenetics and personalised nutrition: How far have we progressed and are we likely to get there? *Proceedings of the Nutrition Society*, **68**, 162–172.

Risk Evaluation and Education for Alzheimer's Disease (REVEAL), http://www.genomes2people.org/reveal/

Roberts, J.S. and Uhlmann, W.R. (2013) Genetic susceptibility testing for neurodegenerative diseases: Ethical and practice issues. *Progress in Neurobiology*, **110**, 89–101.

Speliotes, E.K., Willer, C.J., Berndt, S.I. *et al.* (2010) Association analyses of 249,796 individuals reveal 18 new loci associated with body mass index. *Nature Genetics*, **42**, 937–948.

Wilson, C.P., Ward, M., Mcnulty, H. *et al.* (2012) Riboflavin offers a targeted strategy for managing hypertension in patients with the MTHFR 677TT genotype: A 4-y follow-up. *American Journal of Clinical Nutrition*, **95**, 766–772.

16

Data Analytical Methods for the Application of Systems Biology in Nutrition

Corrado Priami and Melissa J Morine

Department of Mathematics, University of Trento, and The Microsoft Research–University of Trento Centre for Computational and Systems Biology

Key messages

- Technological advancements in molecular data generation have transformed the field of nutrition, allowing researchers to study nutritional health at a remarkably fine scale.
- The sheer magnitude of high-throughput data presents the analytical challenge of identifying the key molecules that mediate the relationship between nutrition and health.
- Multivariate statistics encompasses a range of approaches for analysing high-throughput data, where the number of measured variables is considerably larger than the number of samples.
- Network analysis may aid in moving from large-scale, qualitative systems studied through correlation towards small-scale, quantitative mechanistic systems.
- Modelling the environmental interaction of molecular machinery makes models and analyses more realistic and amenable to prediction and control of 'real-world' systems behaviour.

16.1 Introduction

Technological advancements in the past decade have opened up vast avenues for systems-level understanding of nutritional health. In a field that developed from studies focusing on single nutrients and single genes, it is now commonplace in molecular nutrition to generate data sets containing tens of thousands, or even millions, of variables in a single assay. Although data analytical methods have progressed in the last decade, they have generally not followed the same pace as the technology for data generation. In particular, network analytical approaches have been mainly developed blindly with respect to the biological content of the available data. Indeed, some of the very same network analysis approaches have been proposed for molecular systems as well as social networks, for resource distribution networks as well as markets, simply because all these phenomena can be represented by graphs. A classic example is the search for hubs in networks by exploiting the topological features of the graphs. Although hubs are important, the functional meaning of graph elements might not always be related to topological characteristics. A major challenge for systems nutrition (SN) is in processing, analysis and interpretation of the growing body of available data by incorporating in the methods the idiosyncrasies of the biological systems of interest. SN and bioinformatics – which lie at the intersection of molecular biology, mathematics, engineering and computer science – comprise methods ranging from dynamic simulation to analysis of high-throughput (i.e. omic) data, with the goal of understanding nutrition-related systems at the molecular level (De Graaf *et al.* 2009). In this chapter we review the prevailing methods and achievements in bioinformatics and systems biology that have driven research in SN.

Nutrition Research Methodologies, First Edition. Edited by Julie A Lovegrove, Leanne Hodson, Sangita Sharma and Susan A Lanham-New.
© 2015 John Wiley & Sons, Ltd. Published 2015 by John Wiley & Sons, Ltd.
Companion Website: www.wiley.com/go/nutritionsociety

16.2 Gene set analysis

Gene set analysis has arguably become the most widely adopted method for high-throughput gene expression (i.e. transcriptomic) analysis. The general premise of gene set analysis (GSA) is to assign the genes in a high-throughput data set to functional categories, and then to test each category as a whole for significant differential expression. By abstracting gene-level information to the level of biological process, GSA has advantages both in terms of statistical power (by dramatically reducing the burden of multiple testing) and biological interpretability. The most commonly used functional categories (i.e. gene sets) are metabolic/signalling/regulatory pathways or Gene Ontology terms; however, in principle any functional grouping could be used. Other examples of gene sets that have been successfully applied in this context include cytobands, genes regulated by common micro-RNA (miRNA)/transcription factors, and pre-defined groups of disease genes, among others.

The common goal of any GSA algorithm is to identify coordinated changes in sets of functionally cohesive genes (defined a priori). However, there is a range of algorithms that have been developed for this purpose, and an even wider range of implementations available through standalone software, libraries for programming languages such as R or python, or via webservers (for an extensive list of tools see http://bioinformatics.ca/links_directory/category/expression/gene-set-analysis). The bioinformatics community has been so active in developing methods for GSA over the past 10 years that it has become a challenge simply to select the preferred method for use in analysis of a given data set. A 2009 survey by Huang et al. (2009a) identified 68 unique tools for GSA, and this number has only grown since then. Understanding and categorising the many GSA tools are challenging for end-users, and this may even be an obstacle for bioinformatics groups aiming to develop new approaches without replicating existing methods. There are, however, a smaller number of tools that tend to dominate the field, such as updated versions of the GSA algorithm proposed by Mootha et al. (2003; Subramanian et al. 2005), as well as the DAVID tool (Huang et al. 2009b), BiNGO (Maere et al. 2005), GoMiner (Zeeberg et al. 2003) and FatiGO (Al-Shahrour et al. 2004).

Statistical approaches to GSA

Despite the breadth of approaches to GSA, most methods can be broadly categorised as those based on over-representation; expression change scoring; or pathway topology. For an extended review of these approaches see Khatri et al. (2012).

Over-representation (OR) methods are the earliest examples of GSA. They are also arguably the simplest, and most broadly applicable across technological platforms. The general approach to OR proceeds as follows: first, a list of significantly regulated genes is determined from the microarray data using t-test, linear regression and so on, at a defined significance threshold. Next, the number of significant genes is counted both in the background list (often the entire microarray) and in each pre-defined gene set. Finally, each gene set is tested for significant enrichment with the genes of interest, typically using a test such as Fisher's exact, hypergeometric, chi-square or binomial. The strength of the OR enrichment approach is in its simplicity. Using only a list of significant genes as input (without the need for fold change values or other quantitative measurements), this approach can be easily applied across a range of technological platforms, such as microarray, ChIP-on-chip, SNP array and so on. However, this simple use of gene lists also implies that OR approaches consider highly significant genes as identical to marginally significant genes, thus ignoring a potentially informative dimension of the data. Furthermore, the use of a significance threshold to define the initial gene list may exclude potentially informative genes that miss this threshold. Although there are relatively widely accepted standards for p-value thresholds in transcriptomic analysis, gene lists are often chosen also on the basis of fold change, for which there are fewer standards and which may or may not reflect true biological importance.

Expression change scoring (ECS) approaches inherently consider expression data in the calculation of gene set enrichment, and do not impose pre-selection of a significant gene list. The best-known example of an ECS approach was proposed by Subramanian et al. (who coined the initialism GSEA, for gene set enrichment analysis), with the original methodology paper receiving over 4000 citations to date (Subramanian et al. 2005). Similar to OR methods, ECS approaches to GSA begin with calculation of differential expression scores for each gene in the data set. These raw gene-level statistics may be used, or they may be transformed using absolute values, square root or rank statistics to remove the distinction between up- and downregulated genes (Subramanian et al. 2005; Saxena et al. 2006; Morine et al. 2010). These gene-level scores are then aggregated to gene set–level statistics, and the significance of each gene set is typically determined by a permutation test, either permuting the class labels or the gene labels.

One drawback of OR and ECS approaches, when applied to pathway gene sets, is that they do not consider the connectivity patterns between genes in each pathway. To illustrate the relevance of this information, consider the case of a very large pathway for which gene expression data have been measured across two conditions. It may be the case that the condition-specific expression changes in the pathway are localised to one small subregion, or alternatively they may be distributed evenly throughout the pathway. Pathway topology (PT)-based approaches were developed in an effort to capture this information in GSA. Current implementations use an ECS or OR approach to determine gene-level changes, then combine this statistic with gene–gene expression correlations (or a similar statistic) within the pathway (Rahnenführer *et al.* 2004; Tarca *et al.* 2009). The clear advantage of this approach is that it explicitly models pathway connectivity structure, which is a step closer to an understanding of dynamic system behaviour. However, it should be noted that the precise connectivity structure for many pathways is still only partially known, particularly when considering tissue- and cell type–specific activity.

Interpretation of GSA results

In the case of OR, ECS and PT approaches, the typical outcome of GSA is a list of gene sets that are significantly responsive to a perturbation or correlated with a particular phenotype. Depending on the database of gene sets used, this list of significant gene sets can become very long, containing hundreds or even thousands of gene sets. In this case, the problem of the lack of interpretability of high-throughput data is not resolved, only reduced. Furthermore, the list of significant gene sets often contains redundancies in terms of gene content (for instance, in the case of multiple related signalling pathways with a core set of shared genes). For this reason, a number of tools and approaches have been developed to aid in the interpretation and prioritisation of GSA results.

One such method, developed by Alexa *et al.* (2006) for the use of Gene Ontology (GO) terms as gene sets, involves explicit consideration of the GO structure in calculating GSA p-values for GO terms. The GO database is a controlled vocabulary for representing biological processes, functions and cellular compartments. It is structured as a directed acyclic graph, wherein the lower (child) nodes represent more specific biological categories, and each node inherits the categories of its parents. The entire collection thus appears as a hierarchy with a strong dependency structure between the nodes, in the sense that the majority of genes in a given child node will also be found in its parent node. Because of this dependency structure, any assumption of independence of gene sets is not valid. The methods proposed by Alexa *et al.* (2006) address this lack of independence in two ways. The first approach (called *elim*) examines the GO hierarchy from the bottom up, testing each GO term for significant enrichment with the given list of significant genes, then removing those genes from the parent terms

if the tested child term is significantly enriched (essentially decorrelating the hierarchy). This approach favours the more specific child terms, which implicitly improves the interpretability of the results, as higher-level parent terms can become very broad in scope. In the second approach (called *weight*), significance scores of parent/child term pairs are compared, and the genes in the less significant term are downweighted. Although this second approach does not decorrelate the hierarchy, it enables local prioritisation among strongly dependent term pairs.

Another method for the interpretation and prioritisation of gene sets is called the leading-edge approach (Subramanian *et al.* 2007), which identifies gene sets containing the most highly scoring genes (i.e. the leading-edge subset). The implementation of this method allows for heatmap visualisation and calculation of correlation coefficients to assess the similarity between gene sets containing members of the leading-edge subset. Similar in concept to the approach of visualising the overlap between gene sets, the clueGO plugin (Bindea *et al.* 2009) for Cytoscape implements an OR approach to GSA and produces a network of enriched KEGG pathways of GO categories, wherein weighted links between gene sets represent the similarity between them, in terms of overlapping gene content.

The approaches already presented are relatively straightforward for the interpretation of data from simple study designs focusing on, for instance, a single nutrient/drug challenge or controls versus cases of a Mendelian disease. It is often the case in nutrition, however, that a researcher may be interested in the effects of a particular nutrient on a particular disease, and the high-throughput molecular changes that mediate the two. This complicates the interpretation of GSA results, because the gene sets that are most responsive to the nutritional intervention may not be those that are most strongly linked to the disease of interest (Morine *et al.* 2010). Furthermore, complex study designs involving multiple doses, time points and batches complicate the process of calculating a single statistic for each gene, as required by ECS approaches.

16.3 Multivariate analysis

Data sets produced in nutritional genomics studies are often of very high dimension. Human expression microarray platforms typically measure 20 000+ genes (with some platforms measuring exon-specific expression) and human SNP arrays may produce genotype data for as many as 5 million loci. Similarly, next-generation sequencing platforms produce billions of base pairs of data, either representing the whole genome or the expressed subset (i.e. exome sequencing or RNAseq).

Although proteomics and metabolomics platforms do not benefit from the same technical advantages of nucleotide-based platforms, these assays are constantly improving in sensitivity, producing data on thousands of proteins and metabolites. Clearly, each of these platforms offers a great opportunity for understanding nutritional processes with high precision, but the analysis and interpretation of these complex data structures have become a significant bottleneck in bioinformatics and systems biology (Palsson and Zengler 2010).

The simplest approach to identifying variables in a high-throughput data set that correlate with, for instance, a given phenotype response variable is to perform serialised bivariate analysis (such as linear or logistic regression), comparing each variable in the omic dataset to the response variable. Although straightforward and easily interpretable, this approach does not capture the correlation structure within the data set. Multivariate analysis incorporates a range of approaches for exploring the structure within and between multivariate datasets. A common underlying theme across many multivariate techniques is dimensionality reduction – that is, identifying informative low-dimensional representations of high-dimensional datasets. Although not all methods for multivariate analysis are covered in this chapter, Table 16.1 describes an extended list of approaches.

Cluster analysis

Cluster analysis is a widely used method for identifying groups of strongly correlated samples and/or variables in multivariate datasets. The most common methods for clustering methods, k-means and hierarchical clustering, are considered as unsupervised methods as they assume no prior knowledge of sample or variable classes. Hierarchical clustering does not assign observations to discrete clusters, but instead constructs a hierarchy of similarity, often visualised as a dendrogram. This can be

Table 16.1 Multivariate statistical approaches for analysis of high-throughput data.

Method/References	Description	Data input
Cluster analysis	Denotes a set of related methods for identifying either discrete or hierarchical clusters of samples/variables	Multivariate matrix of p variables for n samples
Principal component analysis	Identifies linear combinations of variables in a multivariate data set to represent a maximal amount of variance along a smaller number of dimensions	Multivariate matrix of p variables for n samples
Factor analysis	Similar to principal component analysis, but focuses on the covariance among the variables rather than the variance	Multivariate matrix of p variables for n samples
Multidimensional scaling	Similar to principal component analysis, but aims to conserve interpoint distances in the high-dimensional space by minimising a loss function	Multivariate matrix of p variables for n samples
Linear discriminant analysis	Identifies a linear function representing a linear decision boundary between classes of observations	Multivariate matrix of p variables for n samples, and discrete class vector of length n
Support vector machine	Identifies a hyperplane representing the (possibly non-linear) decision boundary between classes of observations	Multivariate matrix of dimension $n \times p$ and discrete class vector of length n
Random forest	Generates a set of classification/regression trees based on sampling (with replacement) of variables within the predictor data set, to produce ensemble classifier rules and measures of relative variable importance	Multivariate predictor matrix of dimension $n \times p$ and discrete/continuous class vector of length n
Canonical correlation analysis	Identifies maximally correlated latent variables determined from linear combination of p and q variables measured across n samples	Two multivariate matrices of dimension $n \times p$ and $n \times q$
Partial least squares regression	Identifies a regression model from a linear combination of p variables in X, in order to predict continuous response variable y (in the case of univariate response), or a linear combination of q variables in Y (in the case of multivariate response)	Multivariate predictor matrix of dimension $n \times p$ and continuous response matrix of dimension $n \times 1$ (univariate response) or $n \times q$ (multivariate response)
Partial least squares discriminant analysis	Same as partial least squares regression, but adapted to discrete response variables	Multivariate predictor matrix of dimension $n \times p$ and discrete response matrix of dimension $n \times 1$
Generalised canonical correlation analysis	Generalisation of canonical correlation analysis to model correlation structure across > 2 multivariate matrices	K multivariate matrices of dimension $n \times pk$

achieved either through agglomerative clustering (identifying similar observations and building the hierarchy from the bottom up) or divisive clustering (starting with the complete data set, and successively dividing it into nested subfractions). In either case, a similarity metric is required to define the similarity between observations quantitatively. Common similarity metrics include Euclidean, Manhattan and Mahalanobis distance. Apart from the similarity metric, a linkage criterion is also required in order to define the distance between clusters of observations. This may be the distance between the closest two observations between two groups (single-linkage clustering); the farthest two observations (maximum linkage clustering); or the distance between the centroid of the two groups (average linkage clustering). Given the simplicity and speed of hierarchical clustering, it is generally worthwhile to apply multiple similarity and linkage metrics to examine the structure of the data fully and identify observations that may strongly influence the clustering result.

Unlike hierarchical clustering, k-means clustering produces a discrete assignment of observations to clusters. The algorithm for k-means clustering generally proceeds by selecting k initial cluster centres and assigning each observation to the closest centre. Once each observation has been assigned, new cluster centres are calculated and each observation is assigned again to its closest cluster; in this step, some observations will change cluster while others will remain the same. The step of cluster centre calculation and observation reassignment is repeated until no observation changes cluster. In the application of k-means clustering, it is typical to run the algorithm across a range of values of k, and assess the goodness of fit of each result to the data using a diagnostic such as the elbow method, an information criterion method such as Akaike's Information Criterion, or the Gaussian approach proposed by Hamerly and Elkan (2003).

Principal component analysis

The best-known approach to dimensionality reduction is principal component analysis (PCA), first proposed by Karl Pearson (Pearson 1901), which identifies linear combinations of the variables in a multivariate data set that represent the variance structure in a smaller number of latent, orthogonal vectors. To illustrate with a simple example, consider a transcriptomic data set containing expression measurements for a large number of genes across a group of individuals. It may be the case that a subset of the genes displays strong correlation with each other, and thus could be represented by a composite (latent) variable that captures a large amount of the variance in these genes. The orthogonal transformation imposed by PCA is such that the first latent vector (first

principal component) accounts for the largest amount of variability in the data set, with each successive component accounting for less variability and being uncorrelated to the rest (i.e. due to the orthogonality constraint). Plotting the samples in this low-dimensional space (on the first two principal components, for example) may reveal an informative grouping structure across the samples, such as grouping by dietary treatment, phenotype, gender and so on.

Canonical correlation analysis

As it is increasingly common to measure more than one omics data type on a given set of samples, methods for exploring correlation structure within and between two multivariate data sets are essential for efficient analysis and clear interpretation of these large data sets. Canonical correlation analysis (CCA), originally proposed by Hotelling (1936), uses a latent variable approach to identify low-dimensional correlations between two sets of continuous variables – that is, by identifying maximally correlated pairs of latent variables. CCA accepts as input two matrices, X of dimension $n \times p$ and Y of dimension $n \times q$, both measured on the same n samples. The specific aim of CCA is to identify H pairs of loading vectors a_h and b_h of dimension p and q, respectively, that solve the objective function

$$\underset{a_h' a_h = 1,\, b_h' b_h = 1}{\arg\ max}\ cor\left(Xa_h, Yb_h\right), h=1,\dots,H,$$

where h is the chosen dimension of the solution, and the n-dimensional latent variables Xa_h and Yb_h denote the canonical variates. Analogous to PCA, the first dimension will represent the most strongly correlated canonical variates, with successive dimensions being progressively less correlated. Also similar to PCA, each pair of canonical variates is orthogonal to each other pair, which aids in the interpretability of CCA results as the variables represented on each dimension will be largely non-redundant (i.e. each dimension captures a unique subset of the data).

A fundamental limitation of CCA when applied to cases where $p+q>>n$ (as is the case with high-throughput data) is that the solution of the objective function requires calculation of the inverse of the covariance matrices XX' and YY', which are singular in the case of $p+q>>n$ and thus lead to non-unique solutions of the canonical variates. Because of this, a number of authors have proposed methods for penalising the covariance matrices to allow for reliable matrix inversion. A penalised version of CCA using a combination of ridge regression (also known as Tikhonov regularisation) and lasso (least absolute shrinkage and selection operator) shrinkage (Tibshirani 1996) was proposed by Waaijenborg and

Zwinderman (2009). Briefly, ridge regression obtains non-singular covariance matrices XX' and YY' by imposing a weighting penalty on the diagonal of the covariance matrices, wherein highly correlated pairs of variables receive similar weights. Lasso shrinkage imposes an additional penalty that shrinks variables with low explanatory power to zero, and thus can be viewed as a variable-selection procedure.

Partial least squares regression

Partial least squares (PLS) regression aims to model the relationship between two data sets in a regression context, where one data set is considered as a predictor and the other as a response (Wold *et al.* 1984). An example of where this could be appropriate in nutritional genomics is the analysis of multivariate dietary intake data (predictor) and transcriptomic data (response), as in Morine *et al.* (2011). As with CCA, PLS takes as input two matrices, X of dimension $n \times p$ and Y of dimension $n \times q$. Although there are a number of variants of PLS, the general approach seeks a decomposition of X and Y with p- and q-dimensional loading vectors to optimise the objective function

$$\arg_{a_h' a_h = 1, b_h' b_h = 1} \max \; cov\left(X_{h-1}a_h, Yb_h\right), h = 1, \ldots, H.$$

Note that the PLS algorithm seeks to maximise the covariance as opposed to correlation between the n-dimensional latent vectors, and performs the calculation based on the residual matrix X_{h-1} as opposed to X, as with CCA. An attractive feature of PLS is that it does not require inversion of the covariance matrices and thus it can be applied in the case of p+q>>n. However, penalised versions of PLS have been proposed, using lasso or ridge in order to facilitate variable selection simultaneously with dimensionality reduction (Kim-Anh *et al.* 2008).

In addition to variation in the algorithm for PLS objective function optimisation (with NIPALS and SIMPLS being the most common; Alin 2009), a number of extensions to PLS have been proposed to facilitate its applicability to various data forms, such as canonical mode PLS (Lê Cao *et al.* 2009) and PLS discriminant analysis (Lê Cao *et al.* 2011).

16.4 Network inference

Network inference complements the component-centric approach in which a gene or a protein of interest is fixed, and then local interactions with the selected gene or protein are identified by possibly fixing a distance for transitive interactions. Although this approach has been and still is very successful in identifying relevant

pathways, it is time-consuming and needs lot of work and literature searching to produce new knowledge. Furthermore, it rarely identifies cross-talk between pathways and typically reflects the canonical pathways stored in the available databases. The environmental effects (mainly diet) on molecular processes are thus neglected, and high-throughput assays for observing thousands of variables simultaneously are not considered in these approaches. Complementing the component-centric approach with computational methods that explore omics data could lead to the identification of interaction networks that provide a comprehensive view of the biological processes of interest, including their interactions with the reference environment.

A main issue in network inference is the validation of the outcome of the procedure. Indeed, the noise in the measurements and the stochastic nature of many biological processes (e.g. gene expression) make identification of the physical interactions very difficult.

Algorithmic approaches to infer the network structure of large-scale, and often multi-omic, experimental data have recently emerged. The main algorithms are grouped into classifier-based and reverse engineering from steady-state and/or time-series data of perturbation experiments. We start by looking at classifier-based algorithms.

A classifier is an algorithm that predicts m>0 response variables from n>0 predictor variables. Classifiers can be either supervised or unsupervised. Supervised classifiers use a set of known cases to train the algorithm, while unsupervised classifiers have no a priori knowledge of how to perform, like in cluster analysis. Both approaches have been applied to omics datasets.

Reverse-engineering algorithms are further grouped in physical approaches that aim to rebuild causal networks and influence approaches that aim to rebuild association networks. The former approach usually adopts sequence data and ribonucleic acid (RNA) expression to identify transcription factors and their deoxyribonucleic acid (DNA) binding sites, so that the inferred interactions are physical interactions between transcription factors (TFs) and promoters. The influence approach generalises the notion of interaction, including genes, proteins and metabolites and also linking nodes of the network when indirect interactions exist. This method relies on measurements of transcript concentrations in response to perturbation experiments. The goal is to compute correlation coefficients between elements of the network, fixing a threshold and adding a link for those coefficients over the threshold. An alternative solution is based on the notion of mutual information, which captures non-linear relations between random variables. Influence or association networks have practical utility for identifying functional modules; predicting the behaviour of the system following perturbations; and identifying real physical interactions by integrating the gene network with additional information from sequence data and other experimental data.

Network inference has recently been extended to cope with the reconstruction of metabolic and protein–protein interaction networks from both steady-state and time-series data of metabolite and protein concentrations.

Table 16.2 reports the most used network inference tools, the input data they are able to manage, the network type they infer and the method on which they are based.

The general statistical measures that are commonly used to assess the performance of the inference methods are sensitivity, specificity and accuracy, obtained by comparing the inferred network with the corresponding true network. Specifically, sensitivity is the frequency of correct identifications made by the model (i.e. the ratio between true positives and the sum of true positives and false positives), specificity is the frequency of identifications that should be made by the model (i.e. the ratio between true positives and the sum of true positives and false negatives) and accuracy is the fraction of correct predictions made by the model (i.e. the sum of true positives and true negatives over total predictions).

Another strategy to assess performance is related to the biological relevance of the inferred network, relying on enrichment analysis with ontology databases or pathway databases. A classical measure is the functional congruence of clusters of co-expressed genes (Datta and Datta 2006).

Network inference in systems nutrition can serve as a basis to identify the context in which a specific study is performed, allowing for a holistic view of the phenomena that can interact with those of interest. A further application of these methods is the definition of the interactions among metabolites, proteins, genes and micronutrients to identify signatures of specific biological processes and associated biomarkers, starting from experimental data. An example is in Zampetaki *et al.* (2010), where the authors infer an miRNA coexpression network to identify a signature of type 2 diabetes. Signatures can be related to biomarkers, as happens in the last example, or also to the identification of master regulator nodes in functional networks, as is the case for Piao *et al.* (2012), where the authors identify master transcriptional regulators in active regulatory networks involved in diabetes progression in Goto-Kakizaki rats.

For extensive reviews on network inference we refer readers to Bansal *et al.* (2007), De Smet and Marchal (2010), Lecca and Priami (2012) and Marbach *et al.* (2012).

16.5 Network analysis

Molecular networks are fundamental constructs in systems biology as they represent all details of a biological system of interest, albeit at different levels of granularity and complexity depending on the method of network

Table 16.2 Network inference software tools.

Tool/Reference	Input data	Network type	Method
Aracne (Margolin *et al.* 2006)	Microarray expression profiles (static data)	Gene regulatory network	Reverse engineering
Bandaru, Bansal and Nemenman (2011)	Metabolic profiling data (steady-state data)	Metabolic network	Reverse engineering
Bellomo *et al.* (2008)	Metabolite concentration (steady-state data)	Metabolic network	Classifier
Inferelator (Bonneau *et al.* 2006)	Gene expression data (static data)	Gene regulatory network	Reverse engineering
Çakır *et al.* (2009)	Metabolome data (steady-state data)	Metabolic network	Classifier
De Matos Simoes, Tripathi and Emmert-Streib (2012)	Gene expression data (static data)	Gene regulatory network	Reverse engineering
Lecca *et al.* (2012)	Concentration data (time series)	Metabolic, protein–protein and signalling networks	Reverse engineering
Lee *et al.* (2008)	Metabolite concentration (steady-state data)	Metabolic network	Classifier
Panteris *et al.* (2007)	Gene expression data (static data)	Gene regulatory networks	Classifier
Schmidt *et al.* (2011)	Metabolite concentration (time series)	Metabolic network	Reverse engineering
SEBINI (Taylor and Singhal 2009)	Heterogeneous data sets (protein sequence, gene expression)	Metabolic, protein–protein, gene regulatory and signalling networks	Reverse engineering
Vert, Qiu and Noble (2007)	Heterogeneous data sets (protein sequence, gene expression)	Gene regulatory, metabolic and protein–protein networks	Classifier
Yamanishi *et al.* (2008)	Genomic data and chemical information	Enzyme network	Classifier

reconstruction and the goal of the analysis. Apart from inferred networks, it is possible to use networks of experimentally validated interactions as the basis for the analysis of high-throughput data. The most common network types in bioinformatics analyses are metabolic (enzyme–metabolite metabolic interactions), protein–protein (complex formation and signal transduction interactions) and regulatory (transcription factor–gene interactions). These three networks are often analysed separately, although in reality the elements of each network type are interlinked in a common system. For instance, metabolic enzymes produce metabolites, which in turn may activate signalling cascades, which may activate gene regulatory interactions.

A fundamentally attractive feature of network analysis as an alternative to pathway analysis of high-throughput data is that global networks inherently consider the overlap and cross-talk between different canonical pathways. Analysis of omic data in the context of global networks is difficult, however, due to the considerable size of global interaction networks. For instance, the I2D database (http://ophid.uto ronto.ca), which assembles protein interaction data from multiple databases such as BIND, IntAct, BioGrid and others, contained 173 338 human protein interactions as of February 2013. While such a network could be used in an analysis as it is, it is important to consider that the interactions in databases such as this are identified using both experimental and computational (e.g. prediction through homology) approaches, and these global interaction databases tend to contain a (possibly high) fraction of false positive interactions (Mahdavi and Lin 2007). Moreover, human global interaction networks contain any reaction that could presumably occur in humans, and thus are not specific to tissues, cellular compartment or conditions. Identification of tissue- and cellular compartment–specific and otherwise quality-scored global interaction networks has been the subject of recent work (Guan *et al.* 2012; Magger *et al.* 2012; Schaefer *et al.* 2012), which provides a stronger basis for high-quality interaction networks that are specific to the biological system of interest.

Analysis of high-throughput data in the context of an interaction network requires some objective identification of the specific regions of the global network that are most strongly correlated with the covariate(s) of interest. Such an analysis begins with identification of a starting network as already described, then weighting the nodes and/or edges of the network based on available high-throughput data. This approach is most often applied to transcriptomic data, but in principle could be extended to any high-throughput platform (e.g. proteomic, metabolomics) for which variables in the data set can be quantified and mapped to the nodes in the network.

A well-known computational approach to analysis of high-throughput data in an interaction network is the jActiveModules algorithm (Ideker *et al.* 2002). With this approach, expression data are first analysed to identify p-values for the significance of the comparison of interest. These p-values are then converted to Z-scores and mapped to nodes in the network. Identification of the maximum scoring subnetwork then proceeds using a heuristic approach based on simulated annealing. A starting subnetwork is selected then, iteratively, nodes are added or removed and the subnetwork is rescored until a locally optimum solution is identified. The significance of the subnetwork is determined by randomly sampling subnetworks of the same size, and calculating an expected enrichment score. A related approach, GXNA (Nacu *et al.* 2007), presented improvements in speed and accuracy over jActiveModules, as well as a modification to the significance calculation to account for the non-independence of individual gene p-values.

An alternative approach proposed by Guo *et al.* (2007) emphasised edge-based scoring as the primary measure of activity in a subnetwork. Similar to previous work, these researchers implemented an approach based on simulated annealing to identify high-scoring subnetworks, but the score for a given subnetwork is determined by the sum of covariances between each node pair. The emphasis on edge-based scoring has strong biological justification, given that protein interactions are not static entities, but rather occur in a cell type-, tissue- and condition-specific manner (Jansen, Greenbaum and Gerstein 2002; Han *et al.* 2004; Rahnenführer *et al.* 2004). By measuring activity based on node pair covariance, edge-based methods place importance on the coordination of activity (possibly condition specific) in a subnetwork rather than the activity of any individual element, which is in line with the fundamental meaning of an interaction network. Another edge-based approach was recently proposed by Morine *et al.* (2011) and applied to a directed metabolic network. With this approach a highly coexpressed subnetwork is first identified, using Akaike's Information Criterion to determine coexpressed node pairs. Given a set of significant genes or nodes, paths are then traced from each significant node, taking into consideration the metabolic feasibility of each identified path from a biochemical standpoint.

A selection of available methods for the identification of active subnetworks is presented in Table 16.3, and is also reviewed by Wu, Zhao and Chen (2009).

16.6 Network simulation

Data analysis and influence/association network inference are mainly based on the correlation of observed quantities and on the localisation into subsystems (tissue, organ, subcellular compartment) of the relevant events.

Table 16.3 Methods for identification of active subnetworks.

Method/References	Description
Heinz (Dittrich *et al.* 2008)	Identifies high-scoring subnetworks using an approach based on the prize-collecting Steiner tree problem
Guo *et al.* (2007)	Implements an edge-based scoring of identified subnetworks, based on covariance of node pairs
jActiveModules (Ideker *et al.* 2002)	Heuristic approach to active subnetwork identification, starting with a seed subnetwork and adding/removing nodes to identify a locally optimum high-scoring network
Morine *et al.* (2011)	Identifies coexpressed paths in a metabolic network, taking into consideration the metabolic feasibility of identified paths
GXNA (Nacu *et al.* 2007)	Similar to jActiveModules, including algorithmic improvements and consideration of non-independence of individual genes
Scott *et al.* (2006)	Aims to find high-scoring paths from specific start and end points, then assembles identified paths into a high-scoring subnetwork
NetSearch (Steffen *et al.* 2002)	Identifies high-scoring paths from a given membrane protein to a given transcription factor
ILP (Zhao *et al.* 2008)	Uses an integer linear programming approach to identify high-scoring paths from a given start and end node

These approaches are suitable to answer *what* and *where* something happens. To improve our knowledge of the systems we need to answer *why* it happens, thus building on top of correlation a causation model. Starting from the networks identified with the previously described methods, we move down to the mechanistic details of relevant data-driven identified modules through functional annotation strategies. The next step is to map the modules of interest into a formal representation that is suitable for simulation.

The most common formalism to represent the dynamic behaviour of biological systems is based on differential equations, dates back to the 1960s and earlier to Schrödinger, has its roots in Newton's physics and was already used in the early twentieth century by Volterra to model rhythmical biological phenomena. Equation-based modelling represents system attributes by variables and describes system behaviour with a set of equations relating these variables over time. This modelling approach has been dealt with in many excellent reviews and books (Choi 2010).

An alternative formalism mainly used in the representation of biochemical reactions is based on the notion of rewriting a term (a quantity or a structure) into another on the fulfilment of a firing condition. Rewriting systems represent the dynamics of a system by replacing at each step some part of the initial representation with a new one until no more replacements are possible or a terminating condition is met by the configuration reached. We can have either term-rewriting (for textual representations) or graph-rewriting (for graphical representations). P-systems are a major example of this approach (Paun 2005; Gheorghe, Krasnogor and Camara 2008). Petri nets and their firing mechanism can also be viewed as a rewriting approach (Heiner, Gilbert and Donaldson 2008; Koch, Reisig and Schreiber 2011). Software tools (the so-called rule-based approach) have also been developed to implement the dynamics of biological systems. There are extensive reviews of these methods in Hlavacek *et al.* (2006) and Kholodenko, Yagge and Kolch (2012).

Computing has greatly influenced the way in which biological systems can be represented for computer simulation of their dynamics. Automata-based modelling represents the dynamics of systems by a set of states connected by arcs that represent the transitions between states and are triggered by input signals. An input trace determines a travel among the states, identifying the final state as the result of the computation. A more recent approach is algorithmic modelling (Priami 2009, 2010), which describes the algorithms executed by the system through programming language technologies (Priami and Quaglia 2004); the dynamics is described by the execution of the algorithms on a computer or a network of computers. Since the early work on stochastic pi-calculus (Priami 1995, 2002), many formalisms have been developed, including BioAmbients (Regev and Panina 2004), Kappa (Danos 2004), BioPEPA (Ciocchetta and Hillston 2009), Beta binders (Priami and Quaglia 2004) and BlenX (Dematté, Priami and Romanel 2008); their connection with ODE has also been studied (Cardelli 2009; Palmisano, Mura and Priami 2009). For a survey on language abstractions for biology, see Guerriero *et al.* (2009).

The methods described so far are quantitative, in that they need kinetic parameters to simulate the behaviour of systems. On the opposite side we have purely qualitative models such as statecharts (Efroni, Harel and Cohen 2003), which do however highlight interesting properties of systems that are invariant with respect to kinetics. In between there are Boolean networks (Xiao 2009) in which the firing of events is guarded by Boolean formulas.

Many software tools have been developed to support these modelling formalisms. The main difference between the tools is determined by the simulation algorithm adopted: deterministic, stochastic or hybrid. A simulation

Table 16.4 Parameter inference software tools.

Tool/Reference	Input	Method
Boys, Wilkinson and Kirkwood (2007)	Time-series data, reaction-based stochastic model	Bayesian inference
Goel, Chou and Voit (2008)	Time-series data, models of generalised mass action law of metabolic systems	Dynamic flux estimation
KInfer (Lecca *et al.* 2010)	Time-series data, reaction-based/ODE model	Probabilistic, generative model of the variations in reactant concentrations approximated by finite differences
Poovathingal and Gunawan (2010)	Time-series data, biochemical model	Maximum likelihood and density function distance to minimise the distance measures between model predictions and experimental data
Reinker, Altman and Timmer (2006)	Molecule count measured with errors at discrete time points, biochemical reactions	Approximate maximum likelihood and singular value decomposition likelihood
Rodriguez-Fernandez, Mendes and Banga (2006)	Time-series data, biochemical model	Hybrid stochastic–deterministic global optimisation
Sugimoto, Kikuchi and Tomita (2005)	Time-series data	Genetic algorithm
Tian *et al.* (2007)	Time-series data, stochastic differential equation model	Simulated maximum likelihood
BioBayes (Vyshemirsky and Girolami 2008)	Time-series data, ODE model	Bayesian parameter estimation and model ranking
SBML-PET (Zi and Klipp 2006)	Time-series data, SBML/ODE models	Stochastic ranking evolution strategy, i.e. a (μ, λ)-ES evolutionary optimisation algorithm that uses stochastic ranking as the constraint handling technique
PET (Zwolak, Tyson and Watson 2001)	Time-series data, ODE model	Parameter fitting with local and global strategies

algorithm is deterministic if it always produces the same outcome once the parameters and the input are fixed. A simulation algorithm that produces different outcomes with fixed parameters and input is either non-deterministic (if we cannot associate probabilities to different outcomes) or stochastic (if we can associate probabilities to different outcomes). A hybrid algorithm manages part of the system as deterministic and part of the system as stochastic. The most common stochastic simulation algorithm was designed by Gillespie (1977) and then adapted and optimised to specific modelling formalisms.

A main issue in developing dynamic models is the identification of the right parameters to drive the simulations. Some kinetics is available through databases like Brenda or SABIO-RK and distributed in the biochemical literature, but most parameters are unknown – particularly in human systems. Often the model is non-linear and no general analytical result exists to estimate its parameters. Therefore, non-linear optimisation techniques are needed where a measure of the distance between model predictions and experimental data is used as the optimality criterion to be minimised. Convergence to local solutions if standard local methods are used, very flat objective functions in the neighbourhood of the solution, over-determined models, badly scaled model functions or non-differentiable terms in the systems dynamics may increase the complexity of parameter inference. Traditional gradient-based methods, such as Levenberg–Marquardt or Gauss–Newton, may fail to identify the global solution and may converge to a local minimum even when a better solution exists just a small distance away.

This why there is a community effort in developing software tools that help modellers to infer the parameters needed by the model from a variety of different data sets. Table 16.4 reports some of the most common tools for parameter estimation with references, input and methods implemented.

A good review of parameter-estimation methods is Chou and Voit (2009). For extensive reviews on network simulation we refer readers to Morine and Priami (in press) and Dror *et al.* (2012); for the application of modelling and simulation in systems nutrition see De Graaf *et al.* (2009). For a comprehensive review of software tools for systems biology that could be applied to systems nutrition as well, see Ghosh *et al.* (2011).

16.7 Databases

Systems-level understanding of nutritional processes at a molecular scale requires a range of data types – for functional annotation of gene lists, identification of kinetic parameters, mining of previously identified disease genes or collection of publically available data sets for meta-analysis. Many public databases have been built recently to accommodate the huge amount of data continuously being produced. In this section we mention some of the most used databases, connecting them with the main methods that we have presented in this chapter.

Identification of the relevant functional modules to be exploited for simulating the mechanistic behaviour of the system is the first step in building a suitable model. The first step in this computational process is the identification of the universe (this may refer to sets of pathways, but for our purposes we refer to the global interaction network) from which we start pruning the irrelevant interactions and nodes. For this, interaction databases like Biocarta, Kegg, HMDB, HPRD, I2D, NCI-Nature pathway, OpenBEL, innateDB, Reactome, Stringdb and Wikipathways are fundamental. Identification of functional modules requires experimental data to connect the selection to biological data, thus experimental data repositories are extremely useful (e.g. arrayexpress, clinicaltrial.gov, GEO). After the identification of modules, it is necessary to assess their biological significance and for this it is useful to refer to ontologies like Gene Ontology.

After module identification, we can move towards simulation. A curated reference database for dynamic models is BioModels; SBML models for KEGG and the CellML repository can also be of help. Simulations are driven by quantities that govern the speed and probability of biochemical interactions. The enzyme kinetics is of fundamental importance here. The most relevant databases that can be used to collect these data are Brenda and SABIO-RK. The ultimate usage of simulations is to perform what-if analysis of systems by perturbing them and predicting their behaviour. In this step, collections of molecules like drugs and processes like diseases that can highly affect the fate of the system are useful. Relevant databases for this are drugbank, CTD and OMIM.

For extensive surveys on reference databases useful for systems nutrition and data analysis and simulation we refer readers to Attwood *et al.* (2011), Brazas *et al.* (2011), Bolser *et al.* (2012) and Galperin and Fernández-Suárez (2012).

16.8 Conclusions and moving forward

With the sheer magnitude of data produced on high-throughput platforms, it could be tempting to believe that a high-throughput dataset inherently contains the answer to a given nutritional question. However, of course this is not the case. Apart from the important challenge of defining appropriate data analytical strategies, additional analytical obstacles may be encountered

in the case of insufficient phenotyping, oversimplified or otherwise inappropriate study design, and little (or no) measurement of the environmental background. This is particularly problematic in the field of human nutritional genomics, which is often concerned with complex phenotypes (such as type 2 diabetes mellitus, T2DM) that are predicated by the interplay between genetic background and diverse environmental variables (including, notably, diet and activity level). Even considering the relatively simple example of comparing the liver tissue transcriptomes of individuals with T2DM to healthy controls, there would almost certainly be considerable phenotypical variation among the cases, as well as the controls. That is, the group of individuals categorised as T2DM may exhibit substantial variance in, for example, inflammatory status and anthropomorphic characteristics, among many others. This variation would be reflected in the transcriptomic data, but could not be properly modelled (and would thus be considered as 'noise') if these variables were not measured. Staying with this same example, habitual diet and activity level have substantial effects on hepatic transcriptome and T2DM-related characteristics. And while it is standard practice to take clinical samples following an 8-hour overnight fast, the previous days may have been characterised by fasting, chronic overeating, marathon running or a particularly traumatic event. This information cannot easily be measured on a chip as with expression data, but it is equally important in understanding the basis of variance in a given high-throughput data set.

Of course, this is not to say that these environmental variables are never measured. Certainly, the nutrition community is at the forefront in terms of awareness of the importance of environmental variables. However, there is more work to be done on comprehensively defining what to measure, how to measure and, importantly, how to promote sharing of these data in public databases along with any high-throughput data that are made available. Even in the case of studies on mice and other non-human model species, there may be considerable variation in the environmental conditions within and between studies (e.g. in diet, light cycle, humidity and interactions with other animals). In the case of human studies, data sharing raises the important issue of participant anonymity, particularly in the light of the recent identification of study participant identities based only on publicly available genetic, genealogical and demographic data (Gymrek *et al.* 2013). In any case, sharing of phenotype and environment data greatly enhances the power of meta-analyses of high-throughput data. Due in part to the recent editorial requirements of many scientific journals, there is a great deal of publically available high-throughput data (in particular transcriptomic). These data are in principle a valuable resource for performing meta-analyses with very high sample sizes, but without adequate metadata on each sample it becomes difficult or even impossible to extract a meaningful signal related to a dietary component or phenotype of interest.

Data collection, annotation and sharing are, however, merely the prerequisites to creating an analytical environment in which to study nutritional-related biological processes. Data analytical methods are sometimes applied blindly to the available data and no particular feature of the biological process under investigation is considered. An effort to provide guidelines on how to apply methods and how to integrate them with functional aspects of the biological processes is a necessary step forward to improve our understanding of nutrition. For instance, the topological properties of global networks are relevant, but their biological meaning must be interpreted in context, since the topology of a condition-specific network is likely to differ from that of the global network. To overcome this limitation of current approaches, identification of networks specific to the biological process of interest, followed by network modularisation to identify functional subnetworks (which can then serve as the framework for simulation studies), seems to be a very promising approach. Subnetwork identification is thus a way of linking the correlation-based analysis of biological systems with simulation-based analysis so that the static and dynamic properties of nutritional mechanisms can be merged to enhance our comprehension and our capacity for control.

References and further reading

Alexa, A., Rahnenführer, J. and Lengauer, T. (2006) Improved scoring of functional groups from gene expression data by decorrelating GO graph structure. *Bioinformatics*, **22**, 13, 1600–1607. Available at http://www.ncbi.nlm.nih.gov/pubmed/16606683 (accessed February 2013).

Alin, A. (2009) Comparison of PLS algorithms when number of objects is much larger than number of variables. *Statistical Papers*, **50**, 4, 711–720. Available at http://www.springerlink.com/index/10.1007/s00362-009-0251-7 (accessed February 2013).

Al-Shahrour, F., Díaz-Uriarte, R. and Dopazo, J. (2004) FatiGO: A web tool for finding significant associations of Gene Ontology terms with groups of genes. *Bioinformatics*, **20**, 4, 578–580. Available at http://www.ncbi.nlm.nih.gov/pubmed/14990455 (accessed February 2013).

Attwood, T.K., Gisel, A., Eriksson, N.-E. and Bongcam-Rudloff, E. (2011) Concepts, historical milestones and the central place of bioinformatics in modern biology: A European perspective. In M.A. Mahdavi (ed.) *Bioinformatics: Trends and Methodologies*. InTech, Croatia.

Bandaru, P., Bansal, M. and Nemenman, I. (2011) Mass conservation and inference of metabolic networks from high-throughput mass spectrometry data. *Journal of Computational Biology*, **18**, 2, 147–154. Available at http://arxiv.org/abs/1007.0986 (accessed June 2014).

Bansal, M., Belcastro, V., Ambesi-Impiombato, A. and di Bernardo, D. (2007) How to infer gene networks from expression profiles. *Molecular Systems Biology*, **3**, 78, 78. Available at http://www.ncbi.nlm.nih.gov/pubmed/17299415 (accessed June 2014).

Bellomo, D., de Ridder, D., Rossell, S. *et al.* (2008) Identifying the regulatory structure of metabolic networks: A constrained optimization approach. In *Proceedings of the 14th Annual Conference of the Advanced School for Computing and Imaging*. pp. 250–257.

Bindea, G., Mlecnik, B., Hackl, H. *et al.* (2009) ClueGO: A Cytoscape plug-in to decipher functionally grouped gene ontology and pathway annotation networks. *Bioinformatics*, **25**, 8, 1091–1093. Available at http://www.pubmedcentral.nih.gov/articlerender.fcgi?artid=2666812&tool=pmcentrez&rendertype=abstract (accessed November 2012).

Bolser, D.M., Chibon, P.Y., Palopoli, N. *et al.* (2012) MetaBase: The wiki-database of biological databases. *Nucleic Acids Research*, **40**, Database issue, D1250–1254. Available at http://www.ncbi.nlm.nih.gov/pubmed/22139927 (accessed June 2014).

Bonneau, R., Reiss, D.J., Shannon, P. *et al.* (2006) The Inferelator: An algorithm for learning parsimonious regulatory networks from systems-biology data sets de novo. *Genome Biology*, **7**, 5, R36. Available at http://www.pubmedcentral.nih.gov/articlerender.fcgi?artid=1779511&tool=pmcentrez&rendertype=abstract (accessed June 2014).

Boys, R.J., Wilkinson, D.J. and Kirkwood, T.B.L. (2007) Bayesian inference for a discretely observed stochastic kinetic model. *Statistics and Computing*, **18**, 2, 125–135. Available at http://www.springerlink.com/index/10.1007/s11222-007-9043-x (accessed June 2014).

Brazas, M.D., Yim, D.S., Yamada, J.T. and Ouellette, B.F.F. (2011) The 2011 bioinformatics links directory update: More resources, tools and databases and features to empower the bioinformatics community. *Nucleic Acids Research*, **39**, Web Server issue, W3–W7. Available at http://www.pubmedcentral.nih.gov/articlerender.fcgi?artid=3125814&tool=pmcentrez&rendertype=abstract (accessed June 2014).

Çakır, T., Hendriks, M.M., Westerhuis, J.A. and Smilde, A.K. (2009) Metabolic network discovery through reverse engineering of metabolome data. *Metabolomics*, **5**, 3, 318–329. Available at http://www.ncbi.nlm.nih.gov/pubmed/19718266 (accessed June 2014).

Cardelli, L. (2009) Artificial biochemistry. In A. Condon, D. Harel, J.N. Kok *et al.* (eds) *Algorithmic Bioprocesses*, Springer, Berlin, pp. 429–462. Available at http://www.springerlink.com/index/v178180h87770671.pdf (accessed June 2014).

Choi, S. (2010) *Systems Biology for Signaling Networks*. Springer, Berlin.

Chou, I. and Voit, E., 2009. Recent developments in parameter estimation and structure identification of biochemical and genomic. *Mathematical Biosciences*, **219**, 2, 57–83. Available at http://www.ncbi.nlm.nih.gov/pubmed/19327372 (accessed June 2014).

Ciocchetta, F. and Hillston, J. (2009) Bio-PEPA: A framework for the modelling and analysis of biological systems. *Theoretical Computer Science*, **410**, 33–34, 3065–3084.

Danos, V. (2004) Formal molecular biology. *Theoretical Computer Science*, **325**, 1, 69–110.

Datta, S. and Datta, S. (2006) Methods for evaluating clustering algorithms for gene expression data using a reference set of functional classes. *BMC Bioinformatics*, **7**, 1, 397. Available at http://www.ncbi.nlm.nih.gov/pubmed/16945146 (accessed June 2014).

De Graaf, A.A., Freidig, A.P., De Roos, B. *et al.* (2009) Nutritional systems biology modeling: From molecular mechanisms to physiology. *PLoS Computational Biology*, **5**, 11, p.e1000554. Available at http://www.pubmedcentral.nih.gov/articlerender.fcgi?artid=2777333&tool=pmcentrez&rendertype=abstract (accessed June 2011).

De Matos Simoes, R., Tripathi, S. and Emmert-Streib, F. (2012) Organizational structure and the periphery of the gene regulatory network in B-cell lymphoma. *BMC Systems Biology*, **6**, 1, 38. Available at http://www.biomedcentral.com/1752-0509/6/38 (accessed June 2014).

Dematté, L., Priami, C. and Romanel, A. (2008) The BlenX language: A tutorial. In M. Bernardo, P. Degano and G. Zavattaro (eds) *Formal Methods for Computational Systems Biology*. Springer, Berlin, pp. 313–365.

De Smet, R. and Marchal, K. (2010) Advantages and limitations of current network inference methods. *Nature Reviews Microbiology*, **8**, 10, 717–729. Available at http://www.ncbi.nlm.nih.gov/pubmed/20805835 (accessed June 2014).

Dittrich, M.T., Klau, G.W., Rosenwald, A. *et al.* (2008) Identifying functional modules in protein–protein interaction networks: An integrated exact approach. *Bioinformatics*, **24**, 13, i223–i231. Available at http://bioinformatics.oxfordjournals.org/content/24/13/i223.full (accessed June 2014).

Dror, R.O., Dirks, R.M., Grossman, J.P. *et al.* (2012) Biomolecular simulation: A computational microscope for molecular biology. *Annual Review of Biophysics*, **41**, 429–452. Available at http://www.ncbi.nlm.nih.gov/pubmed/22577825 (accessed January 2013).

Efroni, S., Harel, D. and Cohen, I.R. (2003) Toward rigorous comprehension of biological complexity: Modeling, execution, and visualization of thymic T-cell maturation. *Genome Research*, **13**, 11, 2485–2497. Available at http://www.pubmedcentral.nih.gov/articlerender.fcgi?artid=403768&tool=pmcentrez&rendertype=abstract (accessed February 2013).

Galperin, M.Y. and Fernández-Suárez, X.M. (2012) The 2012 nucleic acids research database issue and the online molecular biology database collection. *Nucleic Acids Research*, **40**, Database issue, D1–8. Available at http://www.pubmedcentral.nih.gov/articlerender.fcgi?artid=3245068&tool=pmcentrez&rendertype=abstract (accessed February 2013).

Gheorghe, M., Krasnogor, N. and Camara, M. (2008) P systems applications to systems biology. *BioSystems*, **91**, 3, 435–437. Available at http://www.ncbi.nlm.nih.gov/pubmed/17728056 (accessed February 2013).

Ghosh, S., Matsuoka, Y., Asai, Y. *et al.* (2011) Software for systems biology: From tools to integrated platforms. *Nature Reviews Genetics*, **12**, 12, 821–832. Available at http://www.nature.com/doifinder/10.1038/nrg3096 (accessed June 2014).

Gillespie, D.T. (1977) Exact stochastic simulation of coupled chemical reactions. *Journal of Physical Chemistry*, **81**, 25, 2340–2361.

Goel, G., Chou, I.-C. and Voit, E.O. (2008) System estimation from metabolic time-series data. *Bioinformatics*, **24**, 21, 2505–2511. Available at http://www.ncbi.nlm.nih.gov/pubmed/18772153 (accessed June 2014).

Guan, Y., Gorenshteyn, B., Burmeister, M. *et al.* (2012) Tissue-specific functional networks for prioritizing phenotype and disease genes. *PLoS Computational Biology*, **8**, 9, p.e1002694. Available at http://www.ncbi.nlm.nih.gov/pubmed/23028291 (accessed October 2012).

Guerriero, M.L., Prandi, D., Priami, C. *et al.* (2009) Process calculi abstractions for biology. In A. Condon, D. Harel, J.N. Kok *et al.* (eds) *Algorithmic Bioprocesses*. Springer, Berlin, pp. 463–486.

Guo, Z., Li, Y., Gong, X. *et al.* (2007) Edge-based scoring and searching method for identifying condition-responsive protein-protein interaction sub-network. *Bioinformatics*, **23**, 16, 2121–2128. Available at http://bioinformatics.oxfordjournals.org/content/23/16/2121.long (accessed June 2014).

Gymrek, M., McGuire, A.L., Golan, D. *et al.* (2013) Identifying personal genomes by surname inference. *Science*, **339**, 6117, 321–324. Available at http://www.ncbi.nlm.nih.gov/pubmed/23329047 (accessed February 2013).

Hamerly, G. and Elkan, C. (2003) Learning the k in k-means. In *Proceedings of the Seventeenth Annual Conference on Neural Information Processing Systems*, pp. 281–288.

Han, J.J., Bertin, N., Hao, T. *et al.* (2004) Evidence for dynamically organized modularity in the yeast protein–protein interaction network. *Nature*, **430**, July, 88–93.

Heiner, M., Gilbert, D. and Donaldson, R. (2008) Petri nets for systems and synthetic biology. In M. Bernardo, P. Degano and G. Zavattaro (eds) *Formal Methods for Computational Systems Biology*. Springer, Berlin, pp. 313–365.

Hlavacek, W.S., Faeder, J.R., Blinov, M.L. *et al.* (2006) Rules for modeling signal-transduction systems. *Science: Signal Transduction Knowledge Environment*, **2006**, 344, re6. Available at http://www.ncbi.nlm.nih.gov/pubmed/16849649 (accessed June 2014).

Hotelling, H. (1936) Relations between two sets of variates. *Biometrika*, **28**, 3/4, 321–377. Available at http://www.jstor.org.eproxy.ucd.ie/stable/2333955 (accessed October 2009).

Huang, D.W., Sherman, B.T. and Lempicki, R.A. (2009a) Bioinformatics enrichment tools: Paths toward the comprehensive functional analysis of large gene lists. *Nucleic Acids Research*, **37**, 1, 1–13. Available at http://www.pubmedcentral.nih.gov/articlerender.fcgi?artid=2615629&tool=pmcentrez&rendertype=abstract (accessed February 2013).

Huang, D.W., Sherman, B.T. and Lempicki, R.A. (2009b) Systematic and integrative analysis of large gene lists using DAVID bioinformatics resources. *Nature Protocols*, **4**, 1, 44–57. Available at http://www.ncbi.nlm.nih.gov/pubmed/19131956 (accessed February 2013).

Ideker, T., Ozier, O., Schwikowski, B., and Siegel, A.F. (2002) Discovering regulatory and signalling circuits in molecular interaction networks. *Bioinformatics*, **18**, Suppl 1, S233–240. Available at http://bioinformatics.oxfordjournals.org/content/18/suppl_1/S233.short (accessed June 2014).

Jansen, R., Greenbaum, D. and Gerstein, M. (2002) Relating whole-genome expression data with protein-protein interactions. *Genome Research*, **12**, 1, 37–46. Available at http://www.pubmedcentral.nih.gov/articlerender.fcgi?artid=155252&tool=pmcentrez&rendertype=abstract (accessed February 2013).

Khatri, P., Sirota, M. and Butte, A.J. (2012) Ten years of pathway analysis: Current approaches and outstanding challenges. *PLoS Computational Biology*, **8**, 2, p.e1002375. Available at http://www.pubmedcentral.nih.gov/articlerender.fcgi?artid=3285573&tool=pmcentrez&rendertype=abstract (accessed February 2013).

Kholodenko, B., Yaffe, M.B. and Kolch, W. (2012) Computational approaches for analyzing information flow in biological networks. *Science Signaling*, **5**, 220, re1. Available at http://stke.sciencemag.org/cgi/doi/10.1126/scisignal.2002961 (accessed June 2014).

Koch, I., Reisig, W. and Schreiber, F. (eds) (2011. *Modeling in Systems Biology: The Petri Net Approach*, 16th edn, Springer, Berlin.

Lê Cao, K.-A., Boitard, S. and Besse, P. (2011) Sparse PLS discriminant analysis: Biologically relevant feature selection and graphical displays for multiclass problems. *BMC Bioinformatics*, **12**, 1, 253. Available at http://www.pubmedcentral.nih.gov/articlerender.fcgi?artid=3133555&tool=pmcentrez&rendertype=abstract (accessed February 2013).

Lê Cao, K.-A., Rossouw, D., Robert-Granié, C. and Besse, P. (2008). A sparse PLS for variable selection when integrating omics data. *Statistical Applications in Genetics and Molecular Biology*, **7**, 1, 35.

Lê Cao, K.-A., Martin, P.G.P., Robert-Granié, C. and Besse, P. (2009) Sparse canonical methods for biological data integration: Application to a cross-platform study. *BMC Bioinformatics*, **10**, 34. Available at http://www.pubmedcentral.nih.gov/articlerender.fcgi?artid=2640358&tool=pmcentrez&rendertype=abstract (accessed March 2012).

Lecca, P. and Priami, C. (2012) Biological network inference for drug discovery. *Drug Discovery Today*, **18**, 5–6, 256–264. Available at http://www.ncbi.nlm.nih.gov/pubmed/23147668 (accessed June 2014).

Lecca, P., Palmisano, A., Ihekwaba, A. and Priami, C. (2010) Calibration of dynamic models of biological systems with KInfer. *European Biophysics Journal*, **39**, 6, 1019–1039. Available at http://www.ncbi.nlm.nih.gov/pubmed/19669750 (accessed February 2013).

Lecca, P., Morpurgo, D., Fantaccini, G. *et al.* (2012) Inferring biochemical reaction pathways: The case of the gemcitabine pharmacokinetics. *BMC Systems Biology*, **6**, 1, 51. Available at http://www.ncbi.nlm.nih.gov/pubmed/22640931 (accessed June 2014).

Lee, E., Chuang, H.Y., Kim, J.W. *et al.* (2008) Inferring pathway activity toward precise disease classification. *PLoS Computational Biology*, **4**, 11, e1000217. Available at http://www.ncbi.nlm.nih.gov/pubmed/18989396 (accessed June 2014).

Maere, S., Heymans, K. and Kuiper, M. (2005) BiNGO: A Cytoscape plugin to assess overrepresentation of gene ontology categories in biological networks. *Bioinformatics*, **21**, 16, 3448–3449. Available at http://www.ncbi.nlm.nih.gov/pubmed/15972284 (accessed February 2013).

Magger, O., Waldman, Y.Y., Ruppin, E. and Sharan, R. (2012) Enhancing the prioritization of disease-causing genes through tissue specific protein interaction networks. *PLoS Computational Biology*, **8**, 9, p.e1002690. Available at http://www.ncbi.nlm.nih.gov/pubmed/23028288 (accessed October 2012).

Mahdavi, M.A. and Lin, Y.-H. (2007) False positive reduction in protein-protein interaction predictions using gene ontology annotations. *BMC Bioinformatics*, **8**, 262. Available at http://www.pubmedcentral.nih.gov/articlerender.fcgi?artid=1941744&tool=pmcentrez&rendertype=abstract (accessed February 2013).

Marbach, D., Costello, J.C., Küffner, R. *et al.* (2012) Wisdom of crowds for robust gene network inference. *Nature Methods*, **9**, 8, 796–804. Available at http://www.ncbi.nlm.nih.gov/pubmed/22796662 (accessed June 2014).

Margolin, A.A., Nemenman, I., Basso, K. *et al.* (2006) ARACNE: An algorithm for the reconstruction of gene regulatory networks in a mammalian cellular context. *BMC Bioinformatics*, **7**, Suppl 1, S7. Available at http://arxiv.org/abs/q-bio/0410037 (accessed June 2014).

Mootha, V.K., Lindgren, C.M., Eriksson, K.F. *et al.* (2003) PGC-1alpha-responsive genes involved in oxidative phosphorylation are coordinately downregulated in human diabetes. *Nature Genetics*, **34**, 3, 267–273. Available at http://www.ncbi.nlm.nih.gov/pubmed/12808457 (accessed June 2014).

Morine, M.J. and Priami, C. (in press) *Analysis of Biological Systems*, Imperial College Press, London.

Morine, M.J., McMonagle, J., Toomey, S. *et al.* (2010) Bi-directional gene set enrichment and canonical correlation analysis identify key diet-sensitive pathways and biomarkers of metabolic syndrome. *BMC Bioinformatics*, **11**, 499.

Morine, M.J., Tierney, A.C., van Ommen, B. *et al.* (2011) Transcriptomic coordination in the human metabolic network reveals links between n-3 fat intake, adipose tissue gene expression and metabolic health. *PLoS Computational Biology*, **7**, 11, p.e1002223. Available at http://www.pubmedcentral.nih.gov/articlerender.fcgi?artid=3207936&tool=pmcentrez&rendertype=abstract (accessed April 2012).

Nacu, S., Critchley-Thorne, R., Lee, P., Holmes, S. (2007) Gene expression network analysis and applications to immunology. *Bioinformatics*, **23**, 7, 850–858. Available at http://www.ncbi.nlm.nih.gov/pubmed/17267429 (accessed June 2014).

Palmisano, A., Mura, I. and Priami, C. (2009) From ODES to language-based, executable models of biological systems. *Pacific Symposium on Biocomputing*, **250**, 239–250. Available at http://www.ncbi.nlm.nih.gov/pubmed/19209705 (accessed June 2014).

Palsson, B. and Zengler, K. (2010) The challenges of integrating multi-omic data sets. *Nature Chemical Biology*, **6**, 11, 787–789. Available at http://www.ncbi.nlm.nih.gov/pubmed/20976870 (accessed June 2014).

Panteris, E., Swift, S., Payne, A., Liu, X. (2007) Mining pathway signatures from microarray data and relevant biological knowledge. *Journal of Biomedical Informatics*, **40**, 6, 698–706. Available at http://www.ncbi.nlm.nih.gov/pubmed/17395545 (accessed June 2014).

Paun, G. (2005) Membrane computing: Main ideas, basic results, applications. In M. Gheorghe (ed.) *Molecular Computational Models: Unconventional Approaches*. IGI Global, Hershey, PA, pp. 1–31.

Pearson, K. (1901) On lines and planes of closest fit to systems of points in space. *Philosophical Magazine*, **2**, 6, 559–572.

Piao, G., Saito, S., Sun, Y. *et al.* (2012) A computational procedure for identifying master regulator candidates: A case study on diabetes progression in Goto-Kakizaki rats. *BMC Systems Biology*, **6**, Suppl 1, S2. Available at http://www.pubmedcentral.nih.gov/articlerender.fcgi?artid=3403593&tool=pmcentrez&rendertype=abstract (accessed February 2013).

Poovathingal, S.K. and Gunawan, R. (2010) Global parameter estimation methods for stochastic biochemical systems. *BMC Bioinformatics*, **11**, 1, 414. Available at http://www.pubmedcentral.nih.gov/articlerender.fcgi?artid=2928803&tool=pmcentrez&rendertype=abstract (accessed June 2014).

Priami, C. (1995) Stochastic pi-calculus. *The Computer Journal*, **38**, 7, 578–589.

Priami, C. (2002) Language-based performance prediction for distributed and mobile systems. *Information and Computation*, **175**, 2, 119–145. Available at http://linkinghub.elsevier.com/retrieve/pii/S089054010093058X (accessed February 2013).

Priami, C. (2009) Algorithmic systems biology. *Communications of the ACM*, **52**, 5, 80.

Priami, C. (2010) Algorithmic systems biology: An opportunity for computer science. In G. Rozenburg, T. Back and J. Kok (eds) *Handbook of Natural Computing*. Springer, Berlin.

Priami, C. and Quaglia, P. (2004) Modelling the dynamics of biosystems. *Briefings in Bioinformatics*, **5**, 3, 259–269. Available at http://www.ncbi.nlm.nih.gov/pubmed/15383212 (accessed June 2014).

Rahnenführer, J., Domingues, F.S., Maydt, J. and Lengauer, T. (2004) Calculating the statistical significance of changes in pathway activity from gene expression data. *Statistical Applications in Genetics and Molecular Biology*, **3**, 1, 16.

Regev, A. and Panina, E.M. (2004) BioAmbients: An abstraction for biological compartments. *Theoretical Computer Science*, **325**, 1, 141–167.

Reinker, S., Altman, R.M. and Timmer, J. (2006) Parameter estimation in stochastic biochemical reactions. *Systems Biology*, **153**, 4, 168–178.

Rodriguez-Fernandez, M., Mendes, P. and Banga, J.R. (2006) A hybrid approach for efficient and robust parameter estimation in biochemical pathways. *Bio Systems*, **83**, 2–3, 248–265. Available at http://www.ncbi.nlm.nih.gov/pubmed/16236429 (accessed June 2014).

Saxena, V., Orgill, D. and Kohane, I. (2006) Absolute enrichment: Gene set enrichment analysis for homeostatic systems. *Nucleic Acids Research*, **34**, 22, p.e151. Available at http://nar.oxfordjournals.org/cgi/content/abstract/34/22/e151 (accessed September 2009).

Schaefer, M.H., Fontaine, J.-F., Vinayagam, A. *et al.* (2012) HIPPIE: Integrating protein interaction networks with experiment based quality scores. *PloS One*, **7**, 2, e31826. Available at http://www.pubmedcentral.nih.gov/articlerender.fcgi?artid=3279424&tool=pmcentrez&rendertype=abstract (accessed February 2013).

Schmidt, M.D., Vallabhajosyula, R.R., Jenkins, J.W. *et al.* (2011) Automated refinement and inference of analytical models for metabolic networks. *Physical Biology*, **8**, 5, 055011. Available at http://www.ncbi.nlm.nih.gov/pubmed/21832805 (accessed June 2014).

Scott, J., Ideker, T., Karp, R.M. and Sharan, R. (2006) Efficient algorithms for detecting signaling pathways in protein interaction networks. *Journal of Computational Biology*, **13**, 2, 133–144. Available at http://www.ncbi.nlm.nih.gov/pubmed/16597231 (accessed June 2014).

Steffen, M., Petti, A., Aach, J. *et al.* (2002) Automated modelling of signal transduction networks. *BMC Bioinformatics*, **3**, 34. Available at http://www.pubmedcentral.nih.gov/articlerender.fcgi?artid=137599&tool=pmcentrez&rendertype=abstract (accessed June 2014).

Subramanian, A., Tamayo, P., Mootha, V.K. *et al.* (2005) Gene set enrichment analysis: A knowledge-based approach for interpreting genome-wide expression profiles. *Proceedings of the National Academy of Sciences of the United States of America*, **102**, 43, 15545–15550.

Subramanian, A., Kuehn, H., Gould, J. *et al.* (2007) GSEA-P: A desktop application for gene set enrichment analysis. *Bioinformatics*, **23**, 23, 3251–3253. Available at http://www.ncbi.nlm.nih.gov/pubmed/17644558 (accessed February 2013).

Sugimoto, M., Kikuchi, S. and Tomita, M. (2005) Reverse engineering of biochemical equations from time-course data by means of genetic programming. *Bio Systems*, **80**, 2, 155–164. Available at http://www.ncbi.nlm.nih.gov/pubmed/15823414 (accessed June 2014).

Tarca, A.L., Draghici, S., Khatri, P. *et al.* (2009) A novel signaling pathway impact analysis. *Bioinformatics*, **25**, 1, 75–82. Available at http://www.pubmedcentral.nih.gov/articlerender.fcgi?artid=2732297&tool=pmcentrez&rendertype=abstract (accessed February 2013).

Taylor, R. and Singhal, M. (2009) Biological network inference and analysis using SEBINI and CABIN. *Methods in Molecular Biology*, **541**, 551–576. Available at http://www.ncbi.nlm.nih.gov/pubmed/19381531 (accessed June 2014).

Tian, T., Xu, S., Gao, J. and Burrage, K. (2007) Simulated maximum likelihood method for estimating kinetic rates in gene expression. *Bioinformatics*, **23**, 1, 84–91. Available at http://eprints.gla.ac.uk/25339/ (accessed June 2014).

Tibshirani, R. (1996) Regression shrinkage and selection via the lasso. *Journal of the Royal Statistical Society. Series B (Methodological)*, **58**, 1, 267–288.

Vert, J.-P., Qiu, J. and Noble, W.S. (2007) A new pairwise kernel for biological network inference with support vector machines.

BMC Bioinformatics, **8**, Suppl 10, S8. Available at http://eprints.pascal-network.org/archive/00003244/ (accessed June 2014).

Vyshemirsky, V. and Girolami, M. (2008) BioBayes: A software package for Bayesian inference in systems biology. *Bioinformatics*, **24**, 17, 1933–1934. Available at http://discovery.ucl.ac.uk/1339729/ (accessed June 2014).

Waaijenborg, S. and Zwinderman, A.H. (2009) Correlating multiple SNPs and multiple disease phenotypes: Penalized non-linear canonical correlation analysis. *Bioinformatics*, **25**, 21, 2764–2771. Available at http://bioinformatics.oxfordjournals.org/cgi/content/abstract/25/21/2764 (accessed June 2010).

Wold, S., Ruhe, A., Wold, H. and Dunn, W. (1984) The collinearity problem in linear regression: The partial least squares (PLS) approach to generalized inverses. *SIAM Journal on Scientific and Statistical Computing*, **5**, 3, 735–743.

Wu, Z., Zhao, X. and Chen, L. (2009) Identifying responsive functional modules from protein-protein interaction network. *Molecules and Cells*, **27**, 3, 271–277.

Xiao, Y. (2009) A tutorial on analysis and simulation of boolean gene regulatory network models. *Current Genomics*, **10**, 7, 511–25. Available at: http://www.pubmedcentral.nih.gov/articlerender.fcgi?artid=2808677&tool=pmcentrez&rendertype=abstract (accessed June 2014).

Yamanishi, Y., Araki, M., Gutteridge, A. *et al.* (2008) Prediction of drug–target interaction networks from the integration of chemical and genomic spaces. *Bioinformatics*, **24**, 13, i232–i240. Available at http://www.ncbi.nlm.nih.gov/pubmed/18586719 (accessed June 2014).

Zampetaki, A., Kiechl, S., Drozdov, I. *et al.* (2010) Plasma microRNA profiling reveals loss of endothelial miR-126 and other microRNAs in type 2 diabetes. *Circulation Research*, **107**, 6, 810–817. Available at http://www.ncbi.nlm.nih.gov/pubmed/20651284 (accessed June 2014).

Zeeberg, B.R., Feng, W., Wang, G. *et al.* (2003) GoMiner: A resource for biological interpretation of genomic and proteomic data. *Genome Biology*, **4**, 4, R28. Available at http://www.pubmedcentral.nih.gov/articlerender.fcgi?artid=154579&tool=pmcentrez&rendertype=abstract (accessed June 2014).

Zhao, X.-M., Wang, R.-S., Chen, L. and Aihara, K. (2008) Uncovering signal transduction networks from high-throughput data by integer linear programming. *Nucleic Acids Research*, **36**, 9, e48. Available at http://www.pubmedcentral.nih.gov/articlerender.fcgi?artid=2396433&tool=pmcentrez&rendertype=abstract (accessed February 2013).

Zi, Z. and Klipp, E. (2006) SBML-PET: A Systems Biology Markup Language-based parameter estimation tool. *Bioinformatics*, **22**, 21, 2704–2705. Available at: http://www.ncbi.nlm.nih.gov/pubmed/16926221 (accessed June 2014).

Zwolak, J., Tyson, J. and Watson, L. (2001) Estimating rate constants in cell cycle models. In A. Tentner (ed.) *Proceedings of High Performance Constants in Cell Cycle Models*. ASTC, San Diego, CA, pp. 53–57.

17
Stable Isotopes in Nutrition Research

Margot Umpleby and Barbara A Fielding

University of Surrey

Key messages

- Stable isotope tracers can be used to measure the absorption and metabolism of macronutrients, vitamins, dietary minerals and trace elements.
- Mathematical modelling allows stable isotope tracer studies to give quantitative (kinetic) data on fluxes of metabolites through different compartments (pools) in the body.
- Stable isotopes of water can be used to be measure body composition and total energy expenditure.
- The natural variation of stable isotopes in nutrients and the environment can give information on the food sources of animals and humans (past and present).
- Stable isotopes can be used to study metabolism in cellular models.

17.1 Introduction

Stable isotopes have been used to study metabolism since the 1930s, when Shoenheimer and Rittenberg fed linseed oil labelled with deuterium to mice and showed that 33% of the deuterium-labelled fatty acids appeared in adipose tissue. The lack of availability of stable isotopes and the cost of the mass spectrometers needed for their measurement did not lead to widespread use. Because there was a plentiful supply of radioisotopes that could be easily measured by scintillation counters, this led to their use instead for the study of metabolism and nutrition in humans. The concern about the health hazards of radioisotopes, the development of more affordable mass spectrometers and the lack of availability of some suitable radioisotopes – for instance, for nitrogen the only available radioisotope has a half-life of 10 minutes – led to the greater use of stable isotopes in the late 1960s and early 1970s. Today in the UK, metabolic tracer studies almost exclusively use stable isotopes, although many of the techniques that are used were developed using radioactive tracers.

Certain elements are composed of atoms that are chemically identical but of a slightly different weight due to different numbers of neutrons. These are termed isotopes. The most abundant isotopes of the major elements

in the biological environment, hydrogen (H), carbon (C), nitrogen (N) and oxygen (O), are ^1H, ^{12}C, ^{14}N and ^{16}O and are by definition stable, but there are other stable isotopes of these elements that are much less abundant (0.02–1.1%); that is, ^2H, ^{13}C, ^{15}N and ^{18}O. For the purposes of this chapter, the term 'stable isotope' will refer to the less abundant stable isotopes. The substitution of one of these less abundant isotopes for the more common form in a molecule, known as 'labelling', creates a 'tracer' that has the same chemical properties as the original molecule, known as the tracee. Isotopic enrichment is expressed as the tracer:tracee ratio (TTR), corrected for the baseline TTR or as atom % excess (APE) or mole % excess (MPE).

$$\%APE = \left(tracer/tracer + tracee \right)_{post\,dose} - \left(tracer/tracer + tracee \right)_{baseline} \times 100$$

The standard nomenclature for a stable isotope tracer gives the isotope and the number of the atoms substituted with the isotope; thus, $[^2H_7]$glucose indicates the presence of seven atoms of ^2H, and $[U-^{13}C]$glucose indicates that every carbon has been replaced by a stable isotope (this is known as 'uniformly labelled'). The stable isotope of ^2H is called deuterium and a common nomenclature for this is D, for example $[^2H_2]$ glucose is shown as D_2 glucose.

Nutrition Research Methodologies, First Edition. Edited by Julie A Lovegrove, Leanne Hodson, Sangita Sharma and Susan A Lanham-New.
© 2015 John Wiley & Sons, Ltd. Published 2015 by John Wiley & Sons, Ltd.
Companion Website: www.wiley.com/go/nutritionsociety

Unlike radioactive isotopes, stable isotopes are not a source of ionising radiation. In the quantities administered they are safe and non-toxic and studies can be undertaken in humans, including pregnant women and children. Administration of a tracer either orally or intravenously enables the measurement of carbohydrate, lipid and protein metabolic pathways either qualitatively or quantitatively, depending on the methodology used. Tracers of vitamins can be used to study their absorption, metabolism and excretion. There are also less abundant stable isotopes of most of the major dietary minerals and the trace elements, and these can be used to study their absorption and kinetics.

The application of stable isotope tracers should induce only minor changes in the body's natural isotope ratios. Since there is a natural abundance of stable isotopes, any isotopic tracers that are administered will add to the existing background. Measuring the background levels is thus very important when undertaking stable isotope tracer studies. Because stable isotopes tracers have mass, it is important that the quantities used are low so that the concentration of the molecules (or elements) being measured is not significantly changed, as this could affect the kinetics of the tracee. Since measurement techniques are very sensitive, this requirement is usually satisfied.

17.2 Natural abundance

The natural abundance of stable isotopes has been of great interest to geochemists for many years and the development of the Isotope Ratio Mass Spectrometer (IRMS), initially used in the geochemistry field, has allowed natural abundance measurements to be feasible in nutrition research. The notation used to describe natural abundance comes from a system developed by geologists and is based on the difference in isotopic abundance of a sample compared with an international standard; for carbon this was initially PeeDee Belemnite (PDB), a rock formation that had a particularly high ^{13}C enrichment content. All measurements are normalised to the standard, so the output is a delta value ($\delta^{13}C\ ^0/_{00}$) or difference from the standard. On a practical note, a standard can be bought that has been verified against PDB in order to calibrate equipment. Natural abundance measurements are usually negative, because the ^{13}C enrichment is usually less than the standard. However, a simple formula can convert the delta value to a TTR, which is more easily understandable and from which APE and MPE can be calculated.

$$TTR\left(^{13}C/^{12}C\right)=\left(\delta^{13}C\ ^0/_{00}\ /1000\right)+1\times 0.0112372$$

Figure 17.1 shows the subtle differences in the isotopic abundance of stable isotopes within an environment. For example, the enrichment of ^{13}C in atmospheric CO_2 is higher than in fossil fuels. Marine plants have different isotopic signatures from terrestrial plants, fish are different from meat and so on. There are also small but significant differences between plants determined by the carbon fixation pathways used (the so-called C3 versus C4/CAM [Crassulacean acid metabolism] plants). Maize is a C4 plant and is isotopically enriched with ^{13}C, so should be avoided by volunteers prior to in vivo studies. An interesting point is that the difference in isotopic signature between the sugars in honey and cane or corn sugar can be used to detect the adulteration of honey with sugar. The same principle is also employed to detect adulteration in other foods.

Fractionation of different isotopes can occur in biological reactions. This is because the strength of a chemical bond is dependent on atomic mass, such that bond strength increases with the substitution of heavier isotopes. An example is pyruvate dehydrogenase, which produces acetyl CoA, which is depleted of ^{13}C relative to the precursor, pyruvate. Differences in the natural isotopic abundance of foodstuffs allow the habitual nutrition of animals and humans to be investigated; in addition, naturally enriched nutrients can be used to trace metabolism.

Habitual nutrition

With certain caveats, the isotopic analyses of tissues can indicate the relative contribution of C3 versus C4/CAM plants and C3 versus marine sources. For animals, this can distinguish between a grazer (C4) and a browser (C3). Using a combination of N and C isotopes can be more revealing, as carnivores have greater ^{15}N enrichment than non-meat-eaters. Dietary reconstruction using these techniques has been useful in ecology and paleontology and mathematical modelling can be employed to estimate dietary parameters. The natural abundance of ^{15}N enrichment has been used as an index of reduced nutrient intake. Isotopic signatures have been explored for use in studies of human nutrition and natural abundance measurements have the potential for distinguishing between meat versus fish, and the content of cane sugar and high-fructose corn syrup in the diet.

17.3 Measurement techniques

Measurement of stable isotopic tracers in a biological matrix (blood, expired air, urine, faeces, tissue etc.) requires an instrument that can quantitate either the

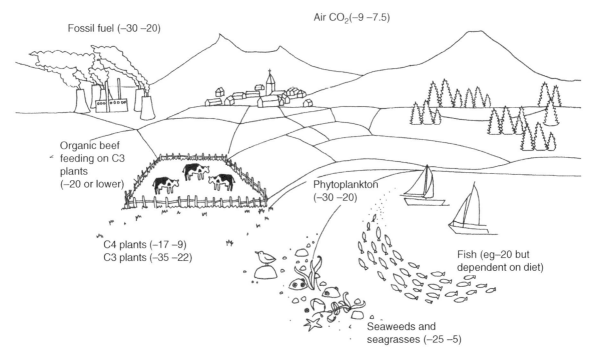

Fossil fuel (−30 −20)

Air CO$_2$(−9 −7.5)

Organic beef
feeding on C3
plants
(−20 or lower)

Phytoplankton
(−30 −20)

C4 plants (−17 −9)
C3 plants (−35 −22)

Fish (eg−20 but
dependent on diet)

Seaweeds and
seagrasses (−25 −5)

Figure 17.1 Range of carbon stable isotope natural abundance (in 'delta notation', see text for explanation) in environment and food sources. Photosynthesis favours the lighter ^{12}C over the heavier ^{13}C, so the carbon in the atmosphere contains more ^{13}C than it would if there were no plants. Fossil fuels are derived from plant material and are therefore low (delta value more negative) in ^{13}C enrichment. Redrawn from Mateo, M.A., Ferrio, J.P. and Araus, J.L. (2004) Isótopos estables en fisiología vegetal. In M.J. Reigosa, N. Pedrol and A. Sánchez (eds), La ecofisiología vegetal, una ciencia de síntesis, Paranimfo, Madrid, pp. 113–160.

isotopic element, for example ^{46}Ca, relative to the most abundant form of the element, or the tracer molecule, for example [1-^{13}C]palmitate, relative to the unlabelled molecule, in this case palmitate (i.e. the tracee). This is a major advantage of stable isotopes over radioactive isotopes, since both labelled and unlabelled molecules (or elements) are measured simultaneously with very high precision.

Instruments used are either nuclear magnetic resonance (NMR) or mass spectrometry (MS); the latter is often interfaced with an instrument that separates the tracee or molecule of interest, for instance gas chromatography (GC), liquid chromatography (LC) and so on. There are three components to a mass spectrometer: the ion source where the sample is ionised, the mass analyser that separates the ions and the detector (Figure 17.2). The mass analyser can be a magnetic mass analyser, a quadrupole mass analyser (or multiple quadrupoles, for example a linear series of three quadrupoles can be used, known as a triple quadrupole mass spectrometer), time-of-flight mass analyser, ion trap analyser or variations of these. Ions are separated according to their mass-to-charge ratio. There are different forms of ionisation depending on the phase (solid, liquid, gas) of the sample.

Examples include electron ionisation and chemical ionisation for gases, thermal ionisation for solids and electrospray ionisation for liquids.

An IRMS, which has a magnetic mass analyser, is set up to measure the isotopic enrichment of a gas. Samples must be processed before entering the ion source of the mass spectrometer, so that only a single chemical species enters at a time. This technique is used for measuring expired ^{13}CO$_2$ generated from the oxidation of a ^{13}C-labelled molecule and from this the oxidation rate can be inferred. Non-gaseous samples can be converted to simple gases by, for example, combustion or pyrolysis and the gas to be measured is purified by traps, filters, catalysts and/or chromatography. Because of the high sensitivity of this method it is used to measure very low enrichments of tracer molecules, such as LDL apolipoprotein B enrichment (Section 17.9), and is also used in natural abundance studies (Section 17.2).

GCMS is probably the most widely used method for measuring molecules labelled with a stable isotope. Their relatively small size, low cost and ease of use have made stable isotope tracer studies much more accessible. GCMS requires that the analytes first be derivatised, which can add considerable complexity to

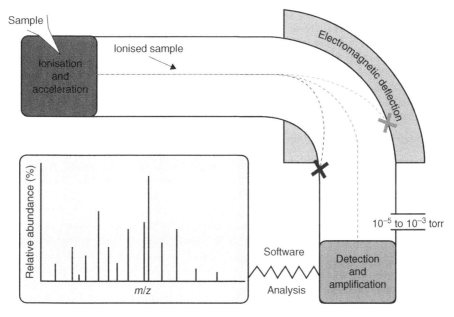

Figure 17.2 Diagram of a mass spectrometer with a magnetic mass analyser. A sample is injected; the molecules are ionised and accelerated, then separated by mass and charge by the mass analyser. Used with permission from Thermo Fisher Scientific.

the method. LCMS can measure many metabolites directly with limited sample preparation.

Tracers of minerals and trace elements are measured by thermal ionisation mass spectrometry or inductively coupled mass spectrometry. In the latter technique the sample is introduced through a nebuliser into high-temperature argon plasma, where it is volatilised and ionised.

17.4 Availability of tracers

The suppliers of stable isotopes of minerals and trace elements are limited. There are a larger number of suppliers of isotopically labelled molecules and the cost varies depending on the site of labelling and the number of labels. If a specifically labelled molecule is not listed by a supplier, they can often manufacture a small batch for a client, although this is costly. While stable isotopically labelled vitamins are also available, the supply of some can be intermittent. An alternative approach used by some researchers is to grow plants in a labelled medium containing ^{2}H or ^{15}N or in an atmosphere enriched with $^{13}CO_2$. This produces plants with intrinsically labelled nutrients, including vitamins or provitamins, which can be incorporated into a meal. Intrinsic labelling of animal-derived macronutrients has also been used. The degree of enrichment obtained is not necessarily very high, for example a relative ^{13}C enrichment of 1·4 APE

was successfully used in a physiological experiment in humans, in which peas were labelled. Infusion of a ^{13}C-labelled amino acid in cows has been employed to generate labelled milk proteins, which were used to assess protein digestion and absorption kinetics and the subsequent muscle protein synthetic response in humans.

17.5 Stable isotope tracer techniques

There are several different techniques and the choice of technique is dependent on the question to be answered.

Isotope dilution

The principle of this technique is that if a known amount of tracer is added to a biological system, sampling from the body pools where the tracer is mixed, and measurement of its dilution will provide a measure of the size of the body pool. This has been used for the measurement of body composition (Section 17.14). To measure the exchange between body pools or 'flux', the dynamic isotope dilution technique is used. This technique requires the tracee to be constant during the study; that is, in a steady state. The tracer is usually infused intravenously (iv) at a constant rate. It is assumed that the tracer is diluted in a single body pool, such as plasma. An isotopic steady state is reached with time, this being determined by the half-life of the tracee and the size of the tracee pool. At this point the tracer is lost from this pool at the same rate as the tracee. The dilution of the tracer by the tracee at an isotopic steady state is a measure of the rate of appearance (Ra) of the tracee into the pool, which in a steady state is equal to the rate of loss from the pool (also known as the flux; Figure 17.3).

$$Ra\,(mg/min) = Tracer\,infusion\,rate\,(mg/min)\,/\,TTR$$

In a steady state it is assumed that Ra = Rate of disappearance = flux. The metabolic clearance rate (MCR) of the tracee, a measure of the efficiency of the tracee removal, is calculated as

$$MCR\,(ml/min)$$
$$= Rd\,(mg/min)\,/\,tracee\,concentration\,(mg/ml)$$

If the pool size is large relative to the flux of the tracee, the duration of tracer infusion will be prolonged. To reduce this, a priming dose (PD) can be administered. The aim of the PD is to instantaneously label the total miscible pool of the tracee, to the level that would be achieved by an unprimed constant infusion. The appropriate priming dose is calculated as

$$PD\,(mg) = Tracee\,Pool\,size\,(mg)\,/\,Ra\,(mg/min)$$
$$\times\,Tracer\,Infusion\,rate\,(mg/min)$$

A bolus injection of the tracer rather than a constant infusion can also be used, although care should be given to ensure that the dose used does not disturb the steady state of the tracee. The tracer will decay exponentially with time and curve-fitting techniques are required. This method is usually combined with a mathematical model to describe the dynamics of the tracer. An exception to this is the use of labelled H_2O to measure total energy expenditure (Section 17.13). The isotope dilution technique can also be used in non-steady-state modelling. An isotopic steady state is achieved first with the tracer infusion and with the tracee also in a steady state. The steady state can then be disturbed, for instance with the infusion of a hormone, the subject exercising or

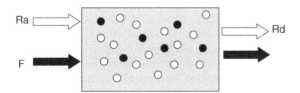

Figure 17.3 Schematic illustration of isotope dilution. Redrawn from Wolfe, R.W. (1992) Radioactive and Stable Isotope Tracers in Biomedicine: Principles and Practice of Kinetic Analysis, Wiley-Liss, New York. F, tracer infusion rate; Ra, rate of appearance; Rd, rate of appearance In an isotopic steady state Tracer/tracee = F/Ra. In a steady state Ra=Rd.

eating a meal. From the change in TTR and concentration with time, the change in the flux of the tracee can be determined using non-steady-state equations or mathematical modelling.

Oxidation rates using ^{13}C-labelled molecules

If a ^{13}C-labelled metabolite is administered, the appearance of ^{13}C in CO_2 can provide a measure of the oxidation rate of that metabolite. Expired air is collected in small bags or tubes and the $^{13}CO_2$ content is measured by IRMS. A measure of the CO_2 production rate is also needed to calculate the $^{13}CO_2$ expiry rate. This can be obtained using a gas analyser when collecting the samples. When combined with the isotope dilution technique, this can provide a quantitative measure of the tracee oxidation rate if a steady state of $^{13}CO_2$ is achieved.

The main consideration with this method is correction for any fixation of $^{13}CO_2$ in the body bicarbonate pool and other metabolic pathways. To measure fatty acid oxidation, loss of $^{13}CO_2$ in the Krebs cycle must be corrected for using an acetate recovery factor. This is estimated from a $^{13}C_2$-labelled acetate infusion in a separate study, which mimics the conditions employed for the determination of substrate oxidation.

When using ^{13}C-labelled tracers to measure oxidation rates if there is a change in the metabolic state during the study, care must be taken to ensure that any increase in $^{13}CO_2$ expiry rate is due to the oxidation of the tracer and not due to a change in the background enrichment. For example, the infusion of (unlabelled) dextrose, which is derived from corn starch, during a euglycaemic hyperglycaemic clamp will increase the $^{13}CO_2$ expiry rate, simply because the glucose infused has a higher natural abundance of ^{13}C than the body's glucose stores. This can compromise the results if the experimental protocol includes the measurement of $^{13}CO_2$ expiry rate from a ^{13}C-labelled stable isotope tracer such as [^{13}C]leucine. To overcome this, potato starch can be used, which has a natural abundance similar to the body's glucose stores.

The appearance of ^{13}C in CO_2 after administration of an oral ^{13}C-labelled tracer can be used to provide information about gastric emptying, oro-caecal transit time, gut bacterial overgrowth, fat and protein digestion, and clinically for the diagnosis of infection with Helicobacter pylori.

Dual isotope method

This technique is used for measuring oral absorption. A tracer of the molecule or element of interest is given orally with a meal and a tracer that is distinguishable from the oral tracer is given iv. This method has been used in the study of mineral absorption and cholesterol absorption. A modification is employed to measure postprandial glucose metabolism. Mathematical models are required to interpret the data.

Precursor product methods

This technique is used for measuring macromolecule synthesis rates. It is based on the assumption that the fractional rate of synthesis of a product can be measured if the TTR of the precursor is known and the TTR of the product is measured. If the absolute concentration of the product is also measured, then the absolute synthesis rate can be calculated. The difficulty with this method is that the TTR of the precursor is not always known. One approach to calculating this is using mass isotopomer distribution analysis (MIDA). This method determines the precursor enrichment from the pattern of labelling in the product (Section 17.11).

17.6 Trace elements/mineral absorption, body utilisation and turnover

Stable isotope studies of mineral and trace element metabolism have made a significant contribution to the quantification of their absorption and metabolism and have led to important dietary recommendations. Stable isotopes are available for most of the minerals necessary for mammalian life. The first studies using stable isotopes were in the 1960s. Methods for the measurement of mineral absorption and kinetics are now well established, especially for calcium. Stable isotope tracers are administered orally and/or iv, with the measurement of the tracers in blood, urine and faeces.

The standard method for assessing calcium absorption from a single meal is the dual tracer technique. A stable isotope of calcium is given orally with a meal and a second isotope is given iv as a short infusion over a few minutes. The isotopes used are usually ^{42}Ca, ^{44}Ca or ^{46}Ca, although both ^{43}Ca and ^{48}Ca can also be used. The oral tracer mixes with the central calcium pool and the iv tracer normalises for variations in the calcium pool mass between individuals. A urine collection is made for 24 hours after administration of the iv tracer and the isotopic enrichment of urine with the two tracers is measured. Fractional calcium absorption is calculated as the ratio of the oral to the iv tracer recovered in urine. Total calcium absorbed is calculated by multiplying the calcium intake by the fractional absorption. To calculate the kinetics of calcium metabolism after absorption, blood

samples are taken over an 8-hour period after administration of the iv tracer and the enrichment of the iv tracer is measured. When combined with a mathematical model, estimates of the deposition rate of calcium and the excretion of calcium can be determined.

The protocol for measuring magnesium absorption and kinetics uses the 2 stable isotopes of magnesium, ^{25}Mg and ^{24}Mg, and is very similar to the method for calcium, with the exception that the urine collection needs to be for 72 hours. The dual isotope technique, with ^{57}Fe and ^{58}Fe, is used for studies of iron absorption and iron incorporation into red blood cells. In this method only a blood sample is taken, usually 2 weeks post-dosing. Absorption studies using stable isotopes of zinc and copper require the oral administration of a stable isotope followed by a complete faecal collection for 10–12 days for zinc and 5–10 days for copper. The isotope enrichment in the faeces is a measure of the fraction of the oral dose absorbed. For copper, blood sampling at intervals over 72 hours after tracer administration can be used to identify abnormalities in copper metabolism. Stable isotopes of selenium and molybdenum have also been used to study the metabolism of these trace elements.

17.7 Using stable isotopes for studying vitamin absorption and metabolism

Stable isotope studies of vitamins have advanced the understanding of vitamin metabolism, body pool sizes and effect of food preparation and meal composition on bioavailability. This is too large a topic to cover extensively in this chapter, so just one example will be given, vitamin A. The most sensitive methods for the measurement of total body vitamin A pool size and vitamin A metabolism use stable isotopes. Deuterated or ^{13}C retinyl acetate or β-carotene tracers have been used. Studies investigating the bioavailability of vitamin A have either added a vitamin A tracer to a meal or used intrinsically labelled vitamin A, with blood sampling several hours after the meal and then at intervals over the next 3 days. Pool size is measured using the isotope dilution technique. The tracer is administered orally then after approximately 20 days, which allows the tracer to mix with endogenous vitamin A, a blood sample is taken to measure the serum TTR of vitamin A. Serum TTR is usually measured by GCMS for deuterated tracers and by GC-combustion IRMS for ^{13}C tracers. For intervention studies, for example the effect of specific diets, in the post-intervention study a different tracer is used to distinguish it from the first tracer, since the half-life of vitamin A is 140 days. For more information about using stable isotopes to study vitamins, see the review by Bluck (2009).

17.8 Protein metabolism

Muscle protein synthesis

Muscle protein synthesis can be measured by the incorporation of isotopically labelled amino acids into muscle protein, which can be sampled using a needle biopsy. This is a precursor product technique in which the labelled amino acid is infused iv at a constant rate for 8–10 hours and the enrichment of the tracer in muscle protein is measured in two biopsies, one taken after the precursor pool has reached a steady state and the other several hours later. Over this time period the tracer incorporation into muscle protein is assumed to be linear. [1-^{13}C] leucine is commonly used as the tracer.

One of the difficulties with the technique is obtaining an accurate measure of the isotopic enrichment of the immediate precursor pool for muscle protein synthesis, which is amino acid tRNA. Muscle tissue fluid leucine enrichment has been shown to be a good approximation of leucine tRNA enrichment. An alternative measurement of precursor enrichment is plasma α ketoisocaproate (KIC), which is formed by the deamination of leucine inside most cells. This occurs very rapidly and is released into plasma. The fractional synthesis rate (FSR) is calculated as

$$FSR\,(\%\,/\,hour) = \left(E_{tissue}(t_1) - E_{tissue}(t_2)\right) \times 100\,/\,E_{Precursor} \times \left(t_1 - t_2\right)$$

where E_{tissue} and $E_{Precursor}$ are the enrichment of muscle protein and the precursor pool respectively and t is time in hours.

Whole-body protein synthesis and protein breakdown

Whole-body protein turnover can be measured with an intravenous bolus or constant infusion of a tracer using the isotope dilution technique. This method generally uses a constant infusion of [1-^{13}C] leucine, an essential amino acid, as the amino acid tracer. It is based on the concept that, in a fasting state, dilution of the tracer with unlabelled leucine is a measure of the rate of appearance of leucine (Ra), which is assumed to be a measure of protein catabolism since leucine cannot be endogenously synthesised. During fasting – that is, the steady state – leucine Ra is equal to the rate of disappearance (Rd). When leucine is oxidised the ^{13}C is removed into the bicarbonate pool, where it is exhaled. Measurement of expired $^{13}CO_2$ together with a measure of the CO_2 production rate using a gas analyser and correction for loss in the bicarbonate pool provides a measure of the leucine oxidation rate. Since leucine has only two metabolic fates, oxidation or incorporation into protein, the latter

is calculated by subtracting the leucine oxidation rate from leucine Rd (Figure 17.4). Plasma αKIC TTR is measured rather than plasma leucine TTR, since this provides a better measure of the intracellular leucine TTR. If the bicarbonate pool is primed with a bolus of NaH$^{13}CO_3$, (see Section 17.5 for an explanation of priming) the measurement can be undertaken in 3 hours.

For fasting measurements this provides a simple, robust method, but the technique becomes more difficult during feeding. For parenteral feeding the infusion of leucine in the feed can be subtracted from the total Ra to calculate endogenous Ra (protein catabolism). With oral feeding an additional tracer needs to be added to the meal to determine the percentage of leucine removed by the liver. Intrinsic labelling of proteins can also be used to assess protein digestion and absorption kinetics (Section 17.4).

In the 1960s, [^{15}N] glycine was first used in humans to study protein metabolism. The technique employed, a modification of the isotope dilution technique, was known as an end product method. It is based on the concept that an infusion of a non-essential [^{15}N] amino acid tracer labels the metabolic pool of N in the body by the transamination reaction. The N in this pool is from protein intake or protein catabolism. N can leave this pool when incorporated into proteins (for protein synthesis) or when amino acids are degraded and excreted. The method assumes that in a steady state

Amino acid Intake + Protein Catabolism =
Protein synthesis + Urinary N excretion = N flux

Thus

Synthesis = N Flux – N Excretion

and

Catabolism = N Flux – Amino acid Intake

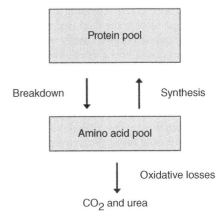

Figure 17.4 Simple model of protein turnover in the fasting state.

Excretion of [^{15}N] as urinary urea is assumed to be a measure of urinary N excretion. Flux is equal to the infusion rate of [^{15}N] glycine/urinary urea enrichment. Thus, all that was needed was a collection of multiple urine samples and the measurement of the enrichment of urinary urea. To satisfy the steady-state requirement subjects had to be fasting or given repeated meals (every 30 minutes).

There are several problems with the method. The measurement of urea enrichment by IRMS is difficult and the urea pool turns over very slowly, so a true plateau is not reached even with a constant infusion of [^{15}N] glycine for 30 hours. Despite this, the method can still have a role in measuring postprandial protein metabolism. [^{15}N] alanine has been shown to be a better tracer than [^{15}N] glycine, since transamination with alanine is a major route for nitrogen transfer to the liver. With alanine, urinary ammonia can be used as the endpoint and urinary ammonia reaches a plateau in a much shorter time.

Plasma proteins

The precursor product technique is also used to measure the synthesis of plasma proteins produced by the liver, such as albumin, fibrinogen, C reactive protein and the apolipoproteins (apo). The technique is identical to that already discussed, except that since plasma proteins are readily accessible, multiple blood samples can be taken to describe more accurately the incorporation of labelled amino acid into the protein. Deuterated or [^{13}C] leucine is usually used as the tracer. Studies are undertaken in a steady state, either fasting or with constant feeding. Over a 10-hour period the incorporation of tracer into albumin and fibrinogen is linear and FSR can be calculated as demonstrated earlier.

Plasma αKIC has been shown to provide a reasonable estimate of the precursor pool enrichment in liver. If the TTR for VLDL apoB100 is measured concurrently, the plateau value provides an alternative measure of the precursor pool enrichment (Section 17.9). The FSR is equal to the fractional catabolic rate (FCR), which can be converted to MCR by multiplying by plasma volume. Since plasma albumin and fibrinogen concentration can be measured, the absolute synthesis rate (ASR) can be calculated as

$$\text{ASR (mg/day/kg)} = \text{FSR (pools/day)} \times \text{Pool size (mg) / BW (kg)}$$

where

$$\text{Pool size} = \text{concentration (mg/l)} \times \text{Plasma volume (l)}$$

Recent studies have measured the synthesis and clearance of C reactive protein. This has a faster turnover than albumin and fibrinogen and a monoexponential equation is used to fit the tracer enrichment curve rather than a regression equation. The measurement of apolipoprotein flux will be discussed in the next section.

17.9 Lipoprotein metabolism

Two alternative approaches have been taken to measure lipoprotein metabolism using stable isotope techniques. One approach, which provides a measure of lipoprotein particle kinetics, is to label one of the apolipoprotein components with a labelled amino acid; the other is to label the triacylglycerol (TAG) component.

Apolipoprotein kinetics

For VLDL, apo B100 FCR and ASR can be measured following an iv constant infusion of a labelled amino acid tracer, as described earlier for plasma proteins. Linear regression or use of a monoexponential equation is inappropriate for calculating FSR and FCR, so mathematical modelling is used. A number of different model structures have been proposed.

An alternative approach is to administer the tracer as an intravenous bolus. If a bolus of tracer is used, the modelling can become more complicated. Because VLDL is metabolised to IDL and then LDL in the circulation and during this process apoB100 is retained within the lipoprotein, it is possible to describe this metabolic pathway if apoB100 is labelled. While VLDL and IDL apoB100 enrichment can be measured by GCMS, there is considerable dilution of the tracer by the large pool of LDL apoB100, necessitating the measurement of LDL enrichment by GC-combustion IRMS, which has a much higher sensitivity than GCMS. It is now recognised that there are two forms of VLDL: VLDL1, a large TAG-rich lipoprotein, and VLDL2, which has less TAG. VLDL2 is formed by two pathways, direct secretion from the liver and catabolism of VLDL1. Several studies have measured the kinetics of both VLDL1 and VLDL2 apoB100. One of the difficulties with the measurement of LDL particle kinetics is the slow turnover and the limited description of the LDL enrichment curve with a study performed on a single day. The use of an iv bolus of tracer is an alternative approach that enables LDL apoB100 enrichment to be measured over several days. This may give a more accurate measurement of LDL kinetics.

In studies where constant meal feeding is used to achieve a postprandial steady state, labelling of apoB48 can provide a measure of chylomicron particle kinetics. The methodology is identical to that described for VLDL apoB100.

HDL particle kinetics has been measured by labelling apoA1, the main protein component. All studies to date have used a constant infusion of labelled amino acid over the course of a single day. The slow turnover of HDL, which has a half-life of 5 days, means a very limited description of the enrichment curve is gained in this short space of time. In addition, apoA1, unlike apoB100, is not an integral part of HDL and can move from one particle to another. The iv bolus technique with measurement of enrichment over several days may be more appropriate.

TAG kinetics

The most widely used method for measuring TAG kinetics is an iv bolus of $[^2H_5]$ glycerol, with measurement of the rise and decline in enrichment of the tracer in TAG over 8–12 hours. Compartmental modelling is used to determine the FSR (and FCR), as already described for apoB100 kinetics. Total VLDL TAG or VLDL1 TAG and VLDL2 TAG kinetics can be measured (Figure 17.5). Some studies have used a constant infusion or injection of labelled palmitate to measure TAG kinetics, but recycling of non-esterified fatty acids (NEFA) can lead to an underestimation of the VLDL TAG synthesis rate.

A recent study has shown that an iv bolus of $[^2H_5]$ glycerol is also incorporated into TAG in chylomicrons and can be used to measure chylomicron TAG synthesis in a constant feeding study. This is the first time that the chylomicron TAG production rate has been quantified. One of the difficulties in measuring chylomicron TAG kinetics is the separation of chylomicron particles from VLDL particles. In this method an immunoaffinity technique was employed, which used three antibodies to apoB100 to separate VLDL and chylomicrons.

17.10 Cholesterol absorption and synthesis

Cholesterol may assimilate in the plasma from the diet or from *de novo* synthesis, and stable isotope tracers can be used to measure both. There are several methods to measure cholesterol absorption and the reader is referred to an excellent review by Matthan and Lichtenstein (2004). Of the stable isotope techniques, the dual isotope method is often used. An oral dose of $[^2H_5]$ cholesterol (or $[^2H_6]$ or $[^2H_7]$ cholesterol) in a meal and an intravenous injection of $[^{13}C_5]$ cholesterol (or $[^{13}C_6]$ or $[^{13}C_7]$ cholesterol) is administered on day 0, and on day 3 the plasma enrichment of the two tracers is measured. At this point it is assumed that the enrichment of the tracers in the plasma is stable. A limitation of this method is that cholesterol absorption would not necessarily be the same in 'real' food.

Cholesterol absorption is calculated as a percentage, as follows:

$$\% \text{ cholesterol absorption} = \text{plasma } [^2H_5] \text{ cholesterol TTR}/[^{13}C_5] \text{ cholesterol TTR} \times 100$$

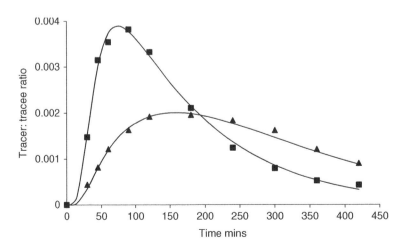

Figure 17.5 Typical curve fit of VLDL1 and VLDL2 glycerol enrichment using a modelling programme in a single subject. VLDL₁ shown as squares; VLDL₂ shown as triangles. The solid lines indicate the curve fit. From Sarac, I., Backhouse, K., Shojaee-Moradie, F. *et al.* (2012) Gender differences in VLDL1 and VLDL2 triglyceride kinetics and fatty acid kinetics in obese postmenopausal women and obese men. *Journal of Clinical Endocrinology & Metabolism*, **97**, 7, 2475–2481.

Cholesterol synthesis may be calculated using the same principle as the *de novo* synthesis of fatty acids described in the next section; that is, incorporation of a deuterium tracer into cholesterol. However, it has been shown that the plasma concentrations of some cholesterol precursors can be a good surrogate measure of cholesterol synthesis.

17.11 Fatty acid metabolism

Adipose tissue lipolysis

The Ra of non-esterified fatty acids (NEFA) is used to describe the flux of fatty acids into the blood from tissues, mainly peripheral adipose tissue. This is an index of whole-body adipose tissue lipolysis of stored TAG, since the bulk of plasma NEFA are assumed to arise from this route. A stable isotope tracer of a fatty acid salt, such as potassium palmitate, is complexed with human albumin to aid solubility and infused intravenously to achieve a steady state after approximately 30 minutes. Because the rate of infusion is known, the flux of fatty acids entering the plasma pool (using the principle of isotopic dilution, as described in Section 17.5) can be calculated. NEFA Ra can also be measured during the postprandial period, using non-steady-state equations. However, in the postprandial period, fatty acids hydrolysed from dietary fat (chylomicrons) directly enter the plasma pool, erroneously contributing to the measurement of NEFA Ra.

Because of re-esterification within adipose tissue, NEFA Ra is not entirely equivalent to adipose tissue lipolysis. Glycerol Ra measured with a constant infusion of $[^2H_5]$ glycerol provides a better measure of lipolysis, since the levels of glycerol kinase are very low so there is very little recycling within adipose tissue.

Nevertheless, a fatty acid tracer can be used to calculate the rate of disappearance of NEFA, a robust measurement of NEFA flux to tissues and organs. The choice of fatty acid tracer is an interesting point. Oleate is a good choice for a fatty acid tracer because of its good solubility, and it is the most common fatty acid in the plasma NEFA pool. However, it is quite expensive. Palmitate is almost universally used because it is cheaper (and is also a common fatty acid), but it has the disadvantage of being difficult to solubilise. Moreover, contamination with background palmitic acid during sample preparation can be an issue.

Adipose tissue fatty acid uptake

The combination of using stable isotope tracer techniques and arteriovenous difference allows very specific measurements across human adipose tissue *in vivo*.

Using a dual isotope technique, meal (exogenous) fatty acids can be traced by labelling with one isotope, for instance [U-^{13}C]palmitate, while exogenous fatty acids (iv infusion) can be traced simultaneously by labelling with another isotope, for instance [$^2H_2$]palmitate. This allows calculation of the rates of chylomicron-TAG hydrolysis by the enzyme lipoprotein lipase in adipose tissue. This is a specific measure of adipose tissue disposal of dietary fatty acids after a meal. The method also allows calculation of the flux of fatty acids that escape uptake into adipose tissue (the 'spillover' fraction), and estimates of the direct uptake of fatty acids from the plasma NEFA pool can also be made. For example:

$$\begin{aligned} &\text{Adipose tissue spillover of} \left[U\text{-}^{13}C\right] \text{palmitate, after ingestion} \\ &\text{of a meal containing} \left[U\text{-}^{13}C\right] \text{palmitate} \\ &= \text{non-esterified} \left[U\text{-}^{13}C\right] \text{palmitate} \left(\text{adipose venous blood}\right) \\ &\quad - \text{non-esterified} \left[U\text{-}^{13}C\right] \text{palmitate} \left(\text{arterial blood}\right) \\ &\quad \times \text{adipose tissue blood flow} \end{aligned}$$

Hepatic fatty acid synthesis (DNL)

The *de novo* synthesis of fatty acids (frequently referred to as *de novo* lipogenesis, DNL) requires the assembly of multiple units of acetyl CoA. The incorporation of isotopically labelled acetate into palmitate should enable the determination of DNL if the TTR of the precursor is known and the TTR of the product, palmitate, is measured. In this case, the plasma acetate TTR cannot be assumed to be the true precursor, since there are different pools of acetyl CoA in the liver used for different metabolic pathways. In order to estimate the true precursor TTR, the MIDA method has been used (Figure 17.6). This technique allows calculation of the precursor enrichment from the labelling pattern of the product, in this case palmitate. The frequency of double labelled relative to single labelled palmitate allows the calculation of the TTR of the precursor using an algorithm. Various algorithms have been published. The acetate tracer is administered as a constant iv infusion for 6–8 hours, with measurement of the enrichment of palmitate at the end of the infusion period. Studies can be done in the fasted or fed state; with the latter, hourly meals are given. If the infusion period was 6 hours, the fractional synthesis of palmitate would be determined as

$$\text{FSR}\left(\%/\text{hour}\right) = \left(E_{\text{palmitate}}\left(t_6\right) - E_{\text{palmitate}}\left(t_0\right)\right) \\ \times 100/E_{\text{Precursor}} \times \left(t_6 - t_0\right)$$

where $E_{\text{palmitate}}$ is the enrichment of palmitate at time 0 (before the tracer infusion) and 6 hours and $E_{\text{Precursor}}$ is the enrichment of the precursor pool at 6 hours.

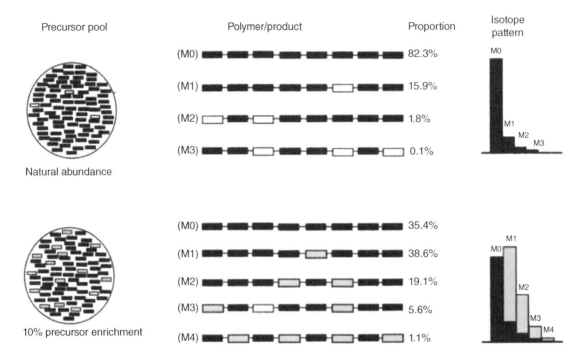

Figure 17.6 The principle of mass isotopomer distribution analysis for measuring the synthesis of polymers such as fatty acids. Natural abundance or 10% enrichment of the precursor subunits with tracer combine to make a polymer of 8 subunits. The distribution of the tracer – no tracer (M0), one tracer subunit (M1), 2 tracer subunits (M2) etc. – in the polymer is measured. The different masses of the polymer are mass isotopomers and from this pattern the precursor pool enrichment can be determined using a combinatorial probability model. Reproduced from Hellerstein, M.K. and Neese, R.A. (1999) Mass isotopomer distribution analysis at eight years: Theoretical, analytic, and experimental considerations. *American Journal of Physiology – Endocrinology and Metabolism,* **276,** E1146–E1170. © The American Physiological Society.

The process of *de novo* synthesis of fatty acids incorporates H from NADPH and H_2O and this can also be exploited to measure the synthesis rate. Orally administered ^2H_2O rapidly equilibrates with total body water and is incorporated into fatty acids during their synthesis, reaching a plateau of deuterium enrichment within 12 hours.

To measure hepatic palmitate synthesis, a baseline blood sample is taken prior to the administration of ^2H_2O to measure baseline TAG-palmitate enrichment by GCMS and plasma ^2H_2O enrichment by IRMS. The oral dose (3 g/kg body weight), which aims to produce 0.45% enrichment of body water, is given in the evening, half with the evening meal and half at 10 pm. Subjects drink only water (0.45% enriched), to prevent dilution of the labelled body water, until after a blood sample is taken the following morning for repeat measurements. If all TAG-NEFA is derived from DNL, the enrichment in TAG-palmitate will be equal to the enrichment of the plasma water and the maximum number of labelled H (n) that can be incorporated into the fatty acid:

$$\text{Maximum palmitate TTR} = \text{TTR}_{2H2O} \times n$$

Palmitate has 31 hydrogens that could potentially be labelled. However, not all hydrogens are equivalent. Seven H are directly from H_2O, 14 are from NADPH and 10 are from acetyl CoA. Complete equilibration with the labelled body water pool does not occur with the latter two pools. Using MIDA, it has been shown that the n value for palmitate is 21.

The proportion of TAG-palmitate derived from DNL is calculated from the ratio of the observed TAG-palmitate enrichment to the maximum palmitate enrichment (the theoretical enrichment if all TAG-palmitate is derived from DNL):

$$\%\text{DNL} = \text{TAG} - \text{palmitate TTR} / \text{maximum palmitate TTR} \times 100$$

If the total VLDL TAG synthesis rate is known, then the absolute rate of VLDL TAG synthesis from DNL is calculated as

$$\text{VLDL} - \text{TAG} \,(\text{i.e. palmitate}) \text{ synthesised via DNL per day} = \text{VLDL TAG production} / \text{day} \times \%\text{DNL} / 100$$

Fatty acid desaturation

There has recently been considerable interest in SCD-1, a delta 9 desaturase, the enzyme responsible for the desaturation of fatty acids – that is, 16:1 n-7 from 16:0 and 18:1 n-9 from 18:0 – produced as a direct result of DNL. This is important in nutrition because of the association between high sugar intake and increased DNL. SCD-1 also acts on dietary saturated fatty acids. Stable isotope tracers have been used to determine fatty acid desaturation in humans *in vivo*, giving an isotopic desaturation index, using ^{2}H or ^{13}C labelled substrates.

Figure 17.7 shows the hepatic SCD index calculated using an intravenous infusion of [U-^{13}C]palmitate. As shown in the figure, the ratio reaches a steady value at about 360 minutes after the start of the infusion. The ratio obtained by this method is considerably lower than the ratios calculated from non-isotopic measurement, probably reflecting fasting SCD activity rather than a 'long-term average' of SCD activity, with little dilution from dietary fatty acids. A limitation is that the isotopic ratio does not reflect the desaturation of newly synthesised 16:0. Both isotopic and non-isotopic ratios (e.g. 16:1 n-7/16:0) cannot account for the partitioning of fatty acids to pathways of oxidation/synthesis.

Hepatic fatty acid partitioning

The liver receives fatty acids from a number of endogenous and exogenous sources and using a combination of the techniques described in this chapter can allow the relative partitioning of the different sources to pathways of esterification and oxidation. A simple calculation can determine the proportion of fatty acids in VLDL TAG that arises from the systemic plasma NEFA pool, using a stable isotope tracer of palmitate. This assumes that palmitate is representative of all fatty acids (which is a reasonable if not completely valid assumption):

$$\text{\% Systemically derived VLDL palmitate} = \frac{\text{TTR of palmitate in the plasma NEFA pool}}{\text{TTR of palmitate tracer in VLDL TAG}} \times 100$$

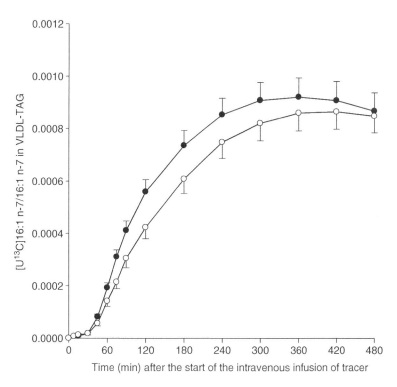

Figure 17.7 Product of desaturation of 16:0 *in vivo* in humans. The graph shows the appearance of [U^{13}C] tracer in 16:1 n-7 in VLDL-TAG after an intravenous infusion of [U^{13}C]16:0. Filled circles (●) represent VLDL1 TAG, open circles (○) represent VLDL2 TAG. The data points represent mean ± SEM in 56 healthy women. Reproduced from Hodson, L. and Fielding, B. (2013) Stearoyl-CoA desaturase: Rogue or innocent bystander? *Progress in Lipid Research*, **52**, 1, 15–42. © Elsevier.

With the inclusion of the relevant stable isotope tracers, this model can be expanded to calculate the production of VLDL TAG from endogenous systemic, DNL and dietary fatty acid sources.

17.12 Carbohydrate metabolism

Whole-body glucose flux can be studied using the isotope dilution technique. With a primed constant infusion of a glucose tracer, an isotopic steady state is achieved within 2 hours. The tracer of choice is often [6,6 ^{2}H$_2$] glucose, since this tracer is not recycled via the Cori cycle due to loss of deuterium during metabolism of glucose to three carbon products. An infusion of [6,6 ^{2}H$_2$] glucose is frequently combined with a euglycaemic low-dose hyperinsulinaemic clamp to enable calculation of the insulin sensitivity of the endogenous glucose production rate. An isotopic steady state is achieved first and then the insulin is infused at a dose that aims partially to suppress the endogenous glucose production rate. Glucose is clamped at 5 mmol/l. Since the glucose production rate will decrease during the study, non-steady-state modelling is needed, unless a new isotopic steady state is achieved, in which case steady-state modelling can be used.

For postprandial studies the dual isotope technique is used, with [U^{13}-C] glucose added to a meal and [6,6 ^{2}H$_2$] glucose infused intravenously, either as a constant infusion or as a variable infusion to match the predicted change in endogenous glucose production rate. Mathematical models are used to calculate the rate of meal glucose appearance, endogenous glucose production rate and glucose clearance rate.

An accurate measure of gluconeogenesis using stable isotopes has proved problematic and various methods have been investigated. The most robust method uses an oral drink of ^{2}H$_2$O (an identical protocol to the DNL ^{2}H$_2$O protocol). The deuterium enrichment of glucose on carbon 5 and plasma water enrichment are measured to calculate fractional gluconeogenesis. If a constant infusion rate of [6,6 ^{2}H$_2$] glucose is also given to calculate glucose flux, the absolute rate of gluconeogenesis can be calculated as the product of these two measurements.

17.13 Total energy expenditure (TEE) with doubly labelled water

The measurement of TEE is of key importance for understanding energy balance and has provided invaluable insight into the consequences of inadequate or excessive energy intake. TEE has three main components: basal metabolic rate, the thermic effect of food and physical activity. It can be calculated from oxygen consumption using a respiration chamber, but with this method physical activity is restricted, so this is not a measure of free-living TEE. The doubly labelled water method (H_2^{18}O and ^{2}H$_2$O), first applied in humans in the early 1980s by Schoeller, is now considered the gold standard method for measuring TEE in free-living humans. This method has revealed that obese individuals have a higher TEE than lean controls and that weight gain, in any individual (lean or obese), is associated with an increase in TEE. Body weight is a very strong predictor of TEE. Similarly, weight loss results in a decrease in TEE, due to both the change in weight and adaptive changes in energy efficiency.

The method provides a measurement of the CO_2 production rate, which can be converted to TEE. It is very easy to use and is non-invasive, but the H_2^{18}O is costly. The fundamental reaction underpinning this method is

$$CO_2 + H_2O \leftrightarrow \underset{\text{carbonic anhydrase}}{H_2CO_3} \leftrightarrow H^+ + HCO_3^-$$

which results in an equilibrium between oxygen in body water and CO_2. Oxygen atoms in H_2^{18}O will quickly label the CO_2 pool and will thus be eliminated from the body tbody solely as a function of water turnover. The difference between the elimination rates of the deuterium and the ^{18}O is thus a measure of the CO_2 production rate (rCO2).

The H_2^{18}O and ^{2}H$_2$O are administered orally then blood, urine or saliva samples are collected over 1–2 weeks, with the time of the dose and sample collection recorded accurately. The method also requires the collection of a pre-dose sample. The enrichment of the sample with ^{18}O and ^{2}H is measured by IRMS and plotted against time. From the decay curves the rate of elimination of ^{18}O and ^{2}H can be determined (Figure 17.8). The difference between the elimination rates of ^{2}H and O^{18} is a measure of CO_2 production. TEE can then be calculated from the CO_2 production rate and the respiratory quotient (RQ) using the de Weir equation:

$$\text{TEE}\left(\text{kcal/day}\right) = \left(3.941\,\text{rCO2}\left(\text{l/day}\right)/\text{RQ}\right) \\ + 1.106\,\text{rCO2}\left(\text{l/day}\right) \\ - 2.17\,\text{Urinary N}\left(\text{g/day}\right)$$

If the RQ is unknown, a measured food quotient provides a good alternative.

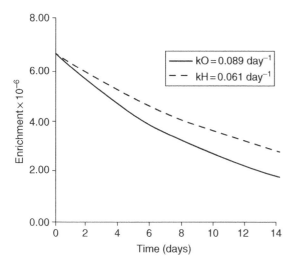

Figure 17.8 Schematic representation of the decline in ^2H_2O and $H_2^{18}O$. Reproduced from Wolfe, R.W. (1992) Radioactive and Stable Isotope Tracers in Biomedicine: Principles and Practice of Kinetic Analysis. Wiley-Liss, New York. k = rate parameter.

17.14 Body composition

Body composition can be measured from the dilution of orally administered labelled water (^2H_2O or $H_2^{18}O$) in body water. The method measures total body water (TBW) as an index of fat-free mass (FFM). It assumes that water occupies 73% of FFM. Subjects are studied fasting, a baseline sample of blood, urine or saliva is taken (t_0) to measure background enrichment, then the oral dose of labelled H_2O is given. After a 4-hour (t_4) equilibration period another sample is taken. TBW and FFM are calculated as

$$TBW(kg) = \text{dose of tracer}(g) / (TTR(t_4) - TTR(t_0)) \times 10^3$$
$$FFM(kg) = TBW(kg) / 0.73$$

17.15 Cellular models

Cellular models of nutrition have traditionally adopted radioactive tracers due to the sensitivity and ease of measuring radioactivity in samples. However, because of the difficult regulations imposed on the use of radionuclides, stable isotope tracers are a good alternative, especially as the amounts needed are very small in comparison to whole-body measurements. A particular advantage of using stable isotopes is of course that the tracers can be followed into specific molecules. For example, stable isotope tracers have been used to measure the uptake of glucose and fatty acids into adipocytes and to trace their metabolic fate. Substrate oxidation can be measured by labelling the substrate with ^{13}C or ^2H and measuring rates of appearance of $^{13}CO_2$ or ^2H_2O respectively.

17.16 Future perspectives

Stable isotope tracer techniques are often combined with sophisticated mathematical modelling techniques in order to derive multicompartmental models of metabolism. Systems biology is a rapidly evolving tool that uses experimental data from single pathways, cellular models and beyond to model *in vivo* metabolic pathways. The combination of stable isotope techniques in humans *in vivo* with systems biology provides an exciting challenge for our future understanding of nutritional metabolism in health and disease.

References and further reading

Abrams, S.A. (2008) Assessing mineral metabolism in children using stable isotopes. *Pediatric Blood & Cancer*, **50**, Suppl, 438–441.

Bickerton, A.S., Roberts, R., Fielding, B.A. *et al.* (2007) Preferential uptake of dietary fatty acids in adipose tissue and muscle in the postprandial period. *Diabetes*, **56**, 1, 168–176.

Bluck, L.J. (2009) Recent progress in stable isotope methods for assessing vitamin metabolism. *Current Opinion in Clinical Nutrition and Metabolic Care*, **12**, 495–500.

Collins, J.M., Neville, M.J., Pinnick, K.E. *et al.* (2011) De novo lipogenesis in the differentiating human adipocyte can provide all fatty acids necessary for maturation. *Journal of Lipid Research*, **52**, 9, 1683–1692.

Duggleby, S.L. and Waterlow, J.C. (2005) The end-product method of measuring whole-body protein turnover: A review of published results and a comparison with those obtained by leucine infusion. *British Journal of Nutrition*, **94**, 141–153.

Fielding, B. (2011) Tracing the fate of dietary fatty acids: Metabolic studies of postprandial lipaemia in human subjects, *Proceedings of the Nutrition Society*, **70**, 3, 342–350.

Hodson, L., Skeaff, C.M. and Fielding, B.A. (2008) Fatty acid composition of adipose tissue and blood in humans and its use as a biomarker of dietary intake. *Progress in Lipid Research*, **47**, 5, 348–380.

Hopkins, J.B. III and Ferguson, J.M. (2012) Estimating the diets of animals using stable isotopes and a comprehensive Bayesian mixing model. *PLoS One*, **7**, 1, e28478.

Korach-Andre, M., Roth, H., Barnoud, D. et al. (2004) Glucose appearance in the peripheral circulation and liver glucose output in men after a large 13C starch meal. *American Journal of Clinical Nutrition*, **80**, 4, 881–886.

Matthan, N.R. and Lichtenstein, A.H. (2004) Approaches to measuring cholesterol absorption in humans. *Atherosclerosis*, **174**, 2, 197–205.

Michener, R. and Lajtha, K. (eds) (2007) *Stable Isotopes in Ecology and Environmental Science*, 2nd edn, Wiley-Blackwell, Oxford.

Parks, E.J. and Hellerstein, M.K. (2006) Thematic review series: Patient-oriented research. Recent advances in liver triacylglycerol and fatty acid metabolism using stable isotope labeling techniques. *Journal of Lipid Research*, **47**, 1651–1660.

Rennie, M.J. (1999) An introduction to the use of tracers in nutrition and metabolism. *Proceedings of the Nutrition Society*, **58**, 935–944.

Schoeller, D.A. (1983) Energy expenditure from doubly labeled water: Some fundamental considerations in humans. *American Journal of Clinical Nutrition*, **38**, 999–1005.

Schoenheimer, R. (1937) The investigation of intermediary metabolism with the aid of heavy hydrogen. *Bulletin of the New York Academy of Medicine*, **13**, 272–295.

Schrauwen, P., van Aggel-Leijssen, D.P., van Marken Lichtenbelt, W.D. *et al.* (1998) Validation of the [1,2-^{13}C]acetate recovery factor for correction of [U-^{13}C]palmitate oxidation rates in humans. *Journal of Physiology*, **513**, 215–223.

Shojaee-Moradie, F., Ma, Y., Lou, S. *et al.* (2013) Prandial hypertriglyceridemia in metabolic syndrome is due to an overproduction of both chylomicron and VLDL triacylglycerol. *Diabetes*, **62**, 12, 4063–4069.

Wolfe, R.R. (1992) *Radioactive and Stable Isotope Tracers in Biomedicine: Principles and Practice of Kinetic Analysis*. Wiley-Liss, New York.

18
Animal Models in Nutrition Research

Andrew M Salter

University of Nottingham

Key messages

- Animal experimentation has made major contributions to our understanding of nutritional principles for over two centuries.
- Much of our early understanding of energy and nutrient requirements was initially derived from the results of animal experiments.
- In more recent years animals have been used extensively to explore the links between diet and the development of non-communicable diseases.
- While rats and mice are the most commonly used laboratory species, differences in physiology and metabolism between these and humans must be taken into account when interpreting results and other species may represent more appropriate models. While larger mammals such as pigs and primates show many physiological similarities to humans, ethical considerations and expense have restricted their use.

- Naturally occurring mutations, and more recently genetic manipulation, can often be used to explore the relationship between diet and chronic disease. However, it must be recognised that in humans, diseases such as cardiovascular disease, obesity, diabetes and cancer are multifactorial and it is unlikely that all genetic and lifestyle factors can be mimicked in any one animal model.
- Animal models have proved particularly useful in the study of the impact of diet throughout the lifecycle and have made major contributions to our understanding of the impact of maternal nutrition on subsequent disease risk in the offspring.
- Experiments in short-lived species (such as mice and rats) have suggested that restricting energy intakes can extend the life span. However, attempts to reproduce this in longer-lived primate species have produced conflicting results.

18.1 Introduction

The use of animals in research represents one of the most emotive topics on the scientific agenda. The population generally falls into two groups: those who on moral grounds oppose all animal experimentation; and those who support a well-controlled and regulated system that allows animal experimentation, but with strict consideration of animal welfare and the minimisation of pain and suffering. This is certainly not a new debate; in the UK the first legislation regulating the use of animals in experiments was introduced in 1876. A swell of public opinion against animal experimentation, which clearly caused suffering and pain to animals, led to a debate over the regulation of such procedures in Victorian England that included Charles Darwin himself. This resulted in the passing of the Cruelty to Animals Act 1835, which included a

system of licensing and inspection of laboratories and the requirement that experiments likely to cause pain and suffering were regulated and licensed by the Home Office. This legislation, which imposed fairly minimal penalties, was finally replaced by a much stricter system of licensing and regulation over a century later in the Animal (Scientific Procedures) Act 1986. More recently, a European Union Directive (2010/63/EU) has set minimum standards for the regulation and monitoring of animal experimentation across the EU. Around the world the specific nature of laws and guidelines relating to experimentation with animals varies substantially, but most seek to limit the amount of pain and suffering that can be inflicted on animals.

However, for a significant number of individuals such legislation is still not sufficient and they continue to call for a ban on animal experimentation. A frequently used argument is that no animal is a suitable model for

Nutrition Research Methodologies, First Edition. Edited by Julie A Lovegrove, Leanne Hodson, Sangita Sharma and Susan A Lanham-New.
© 2015 John Wiley & Sons, Ltd. Published 2015 by John Wiley & Sons, Ltd.
Companion Website: www.wiley.com/go/nutritionsociety

humans and thus all such experiments are fundamentally flawed. Scientists fully accept the limitations of animals as models of humans, but point to the valuable contribution that animal experiments have made to human health and well-being. The aim of this chapter is to guide the reader through some of the contributions that animal experimentation has made, and is making, to our understanding of human nutritional requirements and the impact of nutrition on lifelong health and well-being. It is also important to note that not all nutritional experiments on animals have been undertaken to model humans. The extensive and precise science of farm animal nutrition has made major contributions to the efficiency and capacity of animal agriculture, the benefits of which have played a major role in alleviating hunger and nutrient deficiencies in large parts of the world.

18.2 Ethics of animal experimentation

In all areas of science there are examples of badly designed experiments that, in hindsight, were never going to achieve the hoped-for outcomes. In most countries, where experiments directly involve human subjects there are processes in place to ensure, at the very least, that the potential to cause harm, suffering or loss of dignity is minimised and that the experiments are designed in such a way as to maximise the chances of testing the stated hypothesis. In human nutrition research this means that most interventions will be aimed at reducing disease risk or symptoms or,

at worst, looking at their impact on biomarkers of disease. When using an animal model, the scientist potentially has the opportunity to test an intervention that can cause illness, pain or even death. However, in many countries society demands, and often enshrines in law, an obligation that animal experimentation undergoes similar ethical review to that in humans. Central to such regulation is the process, first described by UK scientists William Russell and Rex Burch in 1959, of the 3Rs: replacement, reduction and refinement. In essence these can be defined as:

- **Replacement** of conscious, living vertebrates by non-sentient alternatives.
- **Reduction** in the number of animals needed to obtain information of a given amount and precision.
- **Refinement** of procedures to reduce to a minimum the incidence or severity of suffering experienced by those animals that have to be used.

It is probably fair to say that the widespread adoption of the principle of the 3Rs following a House of Lords Review on Animals in Scientific Procedures in 2002 has substantially improved the quality of animal experimental design, as well as addressing public concern. Through the adoption of such principles one might expect the number of animals used in experimentation to have reduced; however, as will be discussed later in this chapter, the development of techniques to genetically manipulate animals (predominantly mice), often to produce more relevant models of human disease, has in fact increased the total number of animals used. Figure 18.1 shows recent trends

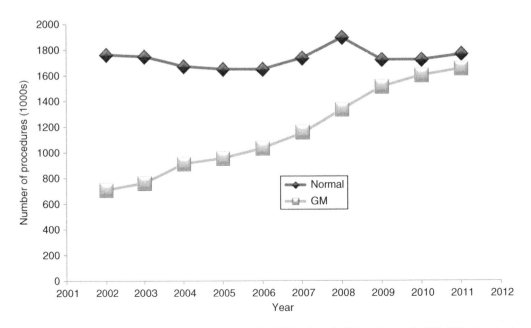

Figure 18.1 A comparison of the use of normal and genetically modified (GM) animals in biological research, 2002–2011. Redrawn from data obtained from Home Office (2012) *Statistics of Scientific Procedures on Living Animals. Great Britain 2011*. Stationery Office, London.

in the number of normal and genetically manipulated (GM) animals used in regulated procedures in the UK. It can be seen that over the period 2002–11 the number of normal animals used remained stable, while the use of GM animals has more than doubled. Of the GM animals used, 92% were mice and 67% were specifically used for breeding purposes. It is of note, however, that even including GM animals, the total of approximately 3.8 million procedures carried out in 2011 is substantially less than the peak in use of animals seen in the 1970s, when annual totals frequently exceeded 5 million.

18.3 Choosing the right species

Figure 18.2 shows the use of different species in regulated procedures in the UK in 2011. It can be seen that 71% of all animal experiments were carried out on mice. Approximately half of these were undertaken on normal animals, while the other half represented those either presenting with a genetic mutation or specifically genetically manipulated. Many people will be surprised at the relatively small proportion (7%) of rats used, the number of which fell from 510 000 in 2002 to 202 000 in 2011. This, however, probably does not reflect the use of these species in nutrition research. A crude PubMed search for the year 2011 using the search terms *rat/mouse and nutrition* yielded similar numbers of publications, 990 and 1124 for rat and mouse respectively. A search for *transgenic mouse and nutrition* yielded only 220.

Why is the rat such a popular species to study in terms of nutritional research? Pragmatically, rats are relatively cheap to buy, house and feed in carefully controlled environments, they are very compliant to changes in diet, they are omnivorous, will eat 'almost anything' and there are specific, well-defined genetic strains. Decades of research have carefully defined the nutritional requirements of rats and it is relatively easy to design an experimental diet that is guaranteed to meet those nutritional requirements while testing the effects of single components. However, there are some obvious disadvantages of this species. They are relatively short-lived and not particularly susceptible to some of the chronic diseases associated with ageing humans (particularly cardiovascular disease). Their gastrointestinal system varies in a number of significant ways to that of the human, including the presence of a well-developed caecum and the absence of a gall bladder. A number of important differences also exist in terms of metabolism, including relatively high rates of lipogenesis in adipose tissue and liver, high rates of hepatic cholesterol synthesis, but low levels of plasma cholesterol, almost all of which is normally carried in the high-density lipoprotein fraction. Perhaps most importantly, some of the very things that make the rat so attractive can potentially reduce its value as a model for humans. The human response to a particular nutrient, food or diet can be influenced by genetic polymorphisms, epigenetic changes in gene expression and the nature of the gut microflora, all things that we have sought to minimise by careful breeding and regulation of

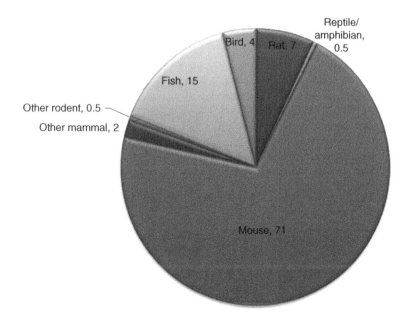

Figure 18.2 Percentage distribution of the use of different species in licensed procedures in the UK in 2011. Redrawn from data obtained from Home Office (2012) *Statistics of Scientific Procedures on Living Animals. Great Britain 2011*. Stationery Office, London.

experimental animal housing environments. Thus, while the rat may represent a useful model of the essentiality of specific nutrients in the diet, it may be less useful in predicting the impact of a specific dietary change on susceptibility to a chronic disease in humans. Nevertheless, as a tool for proof of principle they can be invaluable.

The mouse exhibits many of the strengths and weaknesses of the rat in modelling human nutrition. However, inbreeding in mice has produced a wide array of strains with different phenotypes and susceptibilities to disease, which have been used in understanding the interactions between genotypical, phenotypical and environmental (including dietary) influences on disease progression. More recently, the development of techniques for the genetic manipulation of mice has had a profound impact on laboratory animal experimentation. It is now possible to knock out or over-express specific genes in the whole body or in a tissue-specific way. Genes can be incorporated into the mouse genome from other species (including humans) that can specifically alter susceptibility to disease. While such technologies have made an immeasurable contribution to our understanding of the relationship between genetic and environmental influences on disease susceptibility and progression, they have also highlighted the 'polygenic' nature of many of the chronic diseases faced by the human race. In the vast majority of individuals, increased susceptibility to diet-induced diseases, including cardiovascular disease, diabetes and cancer, is the result of multiple gene polymorphisms rather than mutations at a single gene locus.

While mice and rats have been extensively used in modelling human nutrition, they are certainly not the only species that have made contributions to our understanding. Other small mammals, including rabbits, guinea pigs and hamsters, have also been shown to represent important models of specific aspects of the interactions between diet and disease. While these species can sometimes exhibit phenotypes that model important aspects of human biochemistry and physiology, their use has been hampered by the lack of 'molecular tools' that are widely available for the study of mice and rats.

Larger animal species have made important contributions to our understanding of nutritional principles. The understanding of the nutritional requirements of farm animals, primarily for the purposes of improving the efficiency of human food production, has made an immense contribution to the overall science of nutrition. The highly developed nature of the gastrointestinal tract and metabolism of ruminants, which allows them to exist on high-cellulose, plant-based diets, has limited their usefulness as a model of human nutrition and disease. However, the pig is frequently cited as an under-utilised model of human nutrition. This truly omnivorous species is relatively long-lived and displays many biochemical and physiological

similarities to humans that would make it particularly attractive for the study of the impact of nutrition on the chronic disease of ageing. However, their size and dietary intake make them an expensive choice of model that can generally only be studied by those institutions with specialist facilities. Other species that have historically made important contributions to our understanding of nutrition include cats, dogs and primates. Their use in animal experimentation is highly regulated and, except for very specific reasons, they are rarely used as models of human nutrition. The use of dogs in animal experimentation in the UK is now largely restricted to pharmaceutical safety testing, while the total number of cats used in regulated procedures in the UK in 2011 was only 235. One area where primates are yielding potentially interesting results in the USA is on the impact of 'calorie restriction' on longevity, which will be discussed later in this chapter.

The choice of species to be used in an experiment modelling human nutrition is vital, but experimental design is equally important. Factors that are perhaps most frequently overlooked in experimental design include the dose and the form in which a nutrient is delivered. For example, the beneficial effects of fruit and vegetables on human health are broadly accepted across the world. Numerous research groups have used animal experiments to attempt to identify specific phytonutrients that may contribute to their beneficial effects. However, such studies frequently use specific chemical entities extracted (often by extensive chemical processes) from plant material and fed at doses dramatically higher than found in natural diets, with little consideration of bioavailability or metabolism of the 'active' compound, either by the gut microflora or the host animal itself.

18.4 The role of animal models in the early years of nutritional science

From the seventeenth century onwards, animal experiments have been used to develop the basic principles on which modern nutritional science is based. It is not the aim of this chapter to try to document all of this history. However, some examples are presented of the way in which in these early animal experiments have shaped our understanding of such principles.

Animal experiments and energetics

Demonstrating a connection between combustion and life has been accredited to John Mayow of London in the seventeenth century, who showed that if a candle and an animal were placed in a confined, sealed space, both 'died' simultaneously. Laviosier, working in the late

1700s, went on to identify oxygen consumption and carbon dioxide production as the common factor in both the burning of the candle and the 'respiration' of the animal. He then developed the earliest whole-body calorimeter, which demonstrated that heat production by an animal was directly proportional to oxygen consumed. Subsequent work in the mid-nineteenth century by Regnault and Reiser, working in species as diverse as earthworms, frogs, rabbits and dogs, helped develop the principle of the respiratory quotient (RQ), which showed that the ratio of CO_2 produced to O_2 consumed varied depending on the nature of the food consumed. Around the same era, animal experiments indicated that carbohydrate, fat and protein were all potential 'metabolic fuels' that can provide energy for the body. This was encapsulated in Rubner's Isodynamic Law, which indicated that, on an energy-equivalent basis, carbohydrate, fat and protein (when adjusted for urea excretion) are interchangeable as fuel sources. However, it was not until the end of the nineteenth century, when Atwater and colleagues designed and built the first calorimeter that could accommodate human subjects, that it was generally accepted that this principle also applied to people.

Animal experiments and essential nutrients

The first half of the twentieth century is often regarded as the 'golden years' of nutritional science. It was certainly during this period that most of the nutrients essential for life were discovered. The major breakthrough came with a move from using natural foodstuffs to the use of purified diets in animal experiments. In 1913 McCollum reported the results of feeding rats diets containing casein, lard, lactose, minerals and starch. The results showed that while these animals could grow well for up to 14 weeks, they would then stop, or even lose weight. Adding an ether extract of egg or butterfat (but not cottonseed oil or olive oil) to the diet restored growth. It was concluded that such foods contained a lipid-soluble 'Factor A', deficiency of which was also shown to cause night blindness and xerophthalmia. This, of course, was the discovery of vitamin A, which was finally isolated from fish oil in 1939. The whole story was, however, complicated by the discovery that a highly coloured extract from leaves and carrots also appeared to relieve such symptoms; this was later found to be β-carotene, from which the active 'vitamin' could be derived. At a similar time it was shown that if even more highly purified casein and lactose were used in the diet, a deficiency in a water-soluble 'Factor B' resulted in the condition known as BeriBeri. The active factor was later identified as thiamin(e) or vitamin B1.

Thus began decades of research identifying a range of lipid- and water-soluble entities that we now recognise as vitamins. The same era saw the first suggestions that some polyunsaturated fatty acids were essential in the diet. Similarly, the observation that some sources of protein supported growth better than others led to the discovery of a group of 'essential' amino acids. Subsequent work has shown important differences between requirements for 'essential' nutrients between various animal species and humans. A classic example is the lack of requirement of rats for vitamin C (much of the early work on this vitamin was performed on the guinea pig). Similarly, differences in the activity of gut microflora, and the subsequent absorption of vitamins produced, can mean that animal requirements differ substantially to those of humans. Nevertheless, it is undeniable that animal experimentation in the first half of the twentieth century made a major contribution to our understanding of the essential nutrients.

18.5 Animal models of the interaction of nutrition and chronic disease

As countries become more economically stable, food availability and diversity tend to increase and malnutrition and nutrient deficiencies tend to become less common. As life span increases, however, people become more prone to chronic non-communicable diseases (NCDs), on which diet often has an impact. In the last 50–60 years there has been intense interest in the relationship between diet and the development of such diseases. Increasing recognition that dietary fat intake is associated with the development and progression of cardiovascular disease (CVD) led to the search for animal models that could be used to explore this relationship. This is an area where animal experimentation has made perhaps some of the most meaningful contributions to our understanding of the relationship between diet and disease, so this will be considered in some detail. More recently, the so-called epidemic of obesity and associated insulin resistance and type 2 diabetes has led to attempts to model this disease progression in many animal species. Possibly one of the most challenging areas has been the development of meaningful models of the impact of nutrition on cancer development. In the next few sections these areas are briefly explored.

Atherosclerotic cardiovascular disease

Atherosclerotic CVD appears to have been evident in human populations throughout history. It has impacts on all populations throughout the world, though with considerable variations in incidence and consequences.

As CVD morbidity and mortality increased dramatically in many 'developed' countries to a peak in the late 1960s and early 1970s, it became increasingly clear that it is a multifactorial disease with both genetic and lifestyle factors contributing to overall risk. Early animal studies demonstrated that the deposition of cholesterol in the artery wall was fundamental to the process of narrowing and loss of elasticity that defines 'atherosclerosis'. Human epidemiological studies showed a clear association between the amount and type of dietary fat consumed, the level of cholesterol in the blood and the risk of developing CVD. It was then recognised that not all cholesterol is equal, with that carried in the low-density lipoprotein (LDL) fraction promoting the progression of atherosclerosis, while that carried in high-density lipoprotein (HDL) is protective. The ability to model this disease process in an animal species has long been the aim of nutritional scientists. However, when considering the myriad other factors that influence the development of atherosclerosis and CVD, including hypertension, smoking, obesity, physical activity, ethnicity, sex and a range of genetic polymorphisms, it is perhaps not surprising that we have failed to find a model that recapitulates the whole disease process. Above all, we need to recognise that in humans, atherosclerosis is

a disease that normally develops over decades before resulting in a catastrophic clinical endpoint, such as a heart attack or a stroke, while in most animal species the process is modelled, at best, over a period of months.

'Normal' animal models

Animal species are often classified as 'LDL mammals' and 'HDL mammals', depending on the distribution of cholesterol between these lipoprotein fractions. Figure 18.3 shows that on a low-cholesterol diet (humans habitually consuming no more than 0.05 g cholesterol/100 g food), the majority of animal species carry most of their cholesterol in the HDL fraction. This is particularly true for mice and rats that frequently carry in excess of 80% of their plasma cholesterol in this fraction. By contrast, the guinea pig has very low levels of HDL and carries the vast majority of cholesterol in the LDL fraction. The hamster and the rabbit have a distribution of cholesterol between these two fractions that is closer to that of humans, though the total concentration of cholesterol is considerably lower. Of the species shown, the pig and the chimpanzee show a profile most similar to that of humans. Ethical and practical considerations exclude the use of the latter as a model in all but the most specialised facilities.

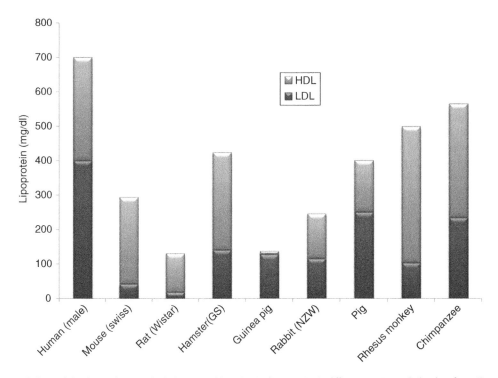

Figure 18.3 Cholesterol distribution between high-density and low-density lipoproteins in different species. Includes data from Chapman, J.M. (1986) Comparative analysis of mammalian plasma lipoproteins. In J.P. Segrests and J.J. Albers (eds) Methods in Enzymology. Academic Press, Waltham, MA, pp. 70–143.

In general, there is little evidence of any of these species developing atherosclerosis in the absence of a dietary challenge. One species that has been reported to develop atherosclerosis naturally are some breeds of pigeon; however, on a cholesterol-free diet even atherosclerosis-susceptible breeds still carry the majority of cholesterol in the HDL fraction. In most experimental species, atherosclerosis can only be induced by cholesterol feeding (often in combination with a diet rich in saturated or *trans* fatty acids). The amount of cholesterol required to induce atherosclerosis can vary considerably depending on the species or specific breed/strain. The earliest experiments, performed over a century ago, used rabbits typically fed between 1% and 3% (by weight) cholesterol. After several weeks of consuming such a diet, many rabbit strains develop severe hypercholesterolaemia with an accumulation of beta-migrating, very low-density lipoprotein (VLDL) particles, similar to those seen in humans suffering from type III (or remnant) hyperlipoproteinaemia. This is associated with the development of atherosclerotic lesions in the aortic arch and thoracic aorta (rather than in the abdominal aorta, which is more common in humans). While rabbits represent an important model of the development of early atherosclerotic lesions, the nature of the hyperlipidaemia is very different to that seen in most humans, which has limited the rabbit's usefulness as a model in which to study the impact of diet.

Rats are relatively resistant to diet-induced atherosclerosis and the response in mice is highly dependent on strain. Work by Paigen and co-workers in the 1980s showed wide variations in the susceptibility to atherosclerosis of inbred strains of mice fed on diets containing 15% fat, 1.25% cholesterol and 0.5% cholic acid. As in other models, the positioning of the lesions is somewhat different than that in humans, with lesions developing, at least initially, in the aortic root. Lesions in the actual coronary arteries are relatively rare and, in any case, can be difficult to study due to their small size. Lesions do not normally develop into the unstable atherosclerotic plaques frequently associated with the clinical outcomes in humans. Nevertheless, the variability in susceptibility to atherosclerosis between inbred mouse strains has proven an invaluable genetic resource for identifying candidate genes involved in the atherosclerotic process.

Cholesterol-fed guinea pigs and Golden Syrian hamsters have both been used as models of diet-induced atherosclerosis. Both show a significant rise in LDL cholesterol in response to cholesterol feeding that is modulated by a range of dietary factors, including the amount and type of fat, protein and carbohydrate, and over a sufficient length of time of cholesterol feeding they develop relatively simple aortic atherosclerotic lesions. In the 1980s, John Dietschy and colleagues performed a seminal series of studies on the hamster aimed at elucidating the impact of

different types of dietary fat on LDL metabolism. The hamster shows a number of advantages over the rat and mouse as a model of lipoprotein metabolism, including the production of 'human-like' VLDL that contains only apolipoprotein (apo) B100 (that of mice and rats contains B48 and B100) and having a hepatic cholesterol synthesis rate that more closely represents that of humans. These researchers' work clearly showed that dietary fatty acids work primarily by regulating the uptake of LDL particles following interaction with LDL receptors in the liver. Saturated and *trans* fatty acids act to reduce the expression of LDL receptors and thereby increase LDL cholesterol, while unsaturated fatty acids tend to increase hepatic LDL receptor expression and thereby speed the removal of LDL from the plasma. The molecular mechanisms underlying these effects remain a major area of research.

Larger animal species have also been used to study dietary-induced atherosclerosis. There is a considerable literature describing the impact of diet on lipoprotein metabolism and atherosclerosis in a range of new- and old-world primates. Rhesus monkeys have been the most extensively used, primarily due to their relatively small size and the ease with which they adapt to laboratory conditions. Cynomolgus and African green monkeys also develop lesions in their coronary arteries that are similar to those of humans, and wild-living baboons have been shown to develop aortic atherosclerotic lesions naturally. However, availability, expense, housing and ethical considerations have all limited the extensive use of such species in atherosclerosis research.

The pig has attracted considerable interest as an animal model of diet-induced atherosclerosis. It is large enough to allow non-invasive measurements of atherosclerosis, which has been shown to develop in the coronary arteries. It has a human-like lipoprotein profile and similarities in body size have made it useful for study of the impact of haemodynamics on the artery wall. Over a period of several months, pigs fed cholesterol/saturated fat-rich diets will develop LDL-based hypercholesterolaemia and foam cell-rich aortic lesions. A number of naturally occurring genetic models of hyperlipidaemia have been found in pigs and in these models, complicated coronary lesions occur, including the development of a fibrous cap and calcification of the plaque. While the size of the animal and similarities to human lipoprotein metabolism make it an attractive model of diet-induced atherosclerotic disease, the long-term housing and feeding of such animals can be prohibitively expensive and restrict its use to fairly specialised research facilities.

Genetically manipulated animal models
Over several decades of using animal models to study atherosclerosis, a number of naturally occurring genetic mutations have emerged that have been immensely valuable in progressing our understanding of the disease.

Considerable differences in the susceptibility of different inbred mouse strains have already been mentioned. Gene mutations in rabbits, most notably the Watanabe rabbit model of LDL receptor deficiency, and pigs have produced models with increased susceptibility to diet-induced atherosclerosis. However, the development of techniques to genetically manipulate animal species has certainly had the most profound effect in this field and, indeed, in virtually all aspects of animal experimentation. While techniques are rapidly developing for the genetic manipulation of many other species, to date it is the GM mouse that has had the biggest impact and the discussion here will be restricted to this species.

Two GM mouse models of atherosclerosis have dominated the scientific literature over the last two decades, namely the apoE$^{-/-}$ and LDLr$^{-/-}$ models. The apoE$^{-/-}$ model lacks apoE, a component of chylomicrons, VLDL and their remnant particles. As a result, the clearance of these lipoproteins is impaired and there is an accumulation of remnant particles in the plasma that is analogous to type III (remnant) hyperlipidaemia. These animals spontaneously develop lesions, but the process can be considerably accelerated by feeding high-fat, high-cholesterol diets. The complex lesions that develop in these mice bear considerable similarities to the advanced lesions seen in humans. A disadvantage of this strain, particularly when trying to model the impact of nutrients on lipoprotein metabolism and atherosclerosis, is the fact that the hypercholesterolaemia induced is largely associated with apoB48-enriched remnant particles rather than apoB100-containing LDL. ApoE also has a number of other physiological functions that affect macrophage biology, immune function and adipose tissue biology, all of which have the potential to influence the development of atherosclerosis and other physiological function. Thus, while this model's contribution to the understanding of the atherosclerotic process and the development of pharmaceuticals has been immense, its contribution to nutritional research has been more limited. A variation on the apoE$^{-/-}$ mouse is the apoE*3 Leiden mouse. This is a transgenic model expressing the dysfunction human apoE variant, apoE*3 Leiden. While on a normal diet plasma cholesterol is low and animals are essentially free of atherosclerosis (Figure 18.4a), atherosclerosis can be induced in proportion to the level of cholesterol/saturated fatty acids in the diet (Figure 18.4b). This model has the advantage that functions other than lipoprotein transport, associated with apoE, remain unaffected.

The LDLr$^{-/-}$ mouse is an animal model of familial hypercholesterolaemia, one of the most common single-gene defects occurring in human populations. It results in a complete absence (homozygote) or reduced (heterozygote) expression of LDL receptors and hence a decreased clearance of LDL from the circulation. In

(a)

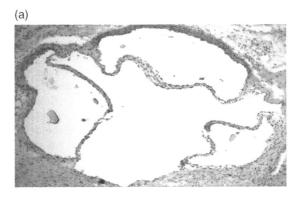

(b)

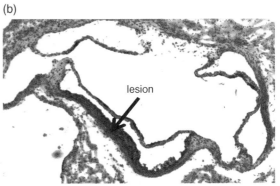

Figure 18.4 Development of aortic atherosclerosis in the apoE*3 Leiden mouse. Histological sections through the aorta of mice fed low fat chow (a) or a high saturated fat/high cholesterol diet (b). The presence of atherosclerotic lesions in the latter are indicated as the darker region which was stained with oil red O.

general, LDLr$^{-/-}$ animals are relatively resistant to atherosclerosis unless fed high-cholesterol/high-fat diets. In addition to an accumulation of LDL particles in the plasma, these animals also have raised VLDL cholesterol. A major disadvantage of this model for nutritional studies is that, as already discussed, dietary fatty acids, and perhaps other nutrients, may have a specific impact on plasma lipoprotein, and thereby atherosclerosis, through regulating the hepatic expression of the LDL receptor, the very protein knocked out in this model.

More recent years have seen the development of a wide range of knock-out and transgenic models of atherogenesis. Often using the background of the apoE$^{-/-}$ or LDLr$^{-/-}$, the specific ability of a particular protein to affect the development of atherosclerosis can be demonstrated by either knock-out, over-expression or humanising (inserting a human version) of a gene. This has made major contributions to our understanding of the inflammatory, immune and cellular aspects of the atherosclerotic process. As yet, however, it has still perhaps not presented us with the 'ideal' model on which to study the impact of diet.

Obesity and diabetes

Obesity represents the excessive accumulation of adipose tissue. This occurs when energy consumption exceeds energy expenditure. The ability to store excess energy as triacylglycerol in adipose tissue allows species to tolerate variations in food availability and, in general, the larger the store, the longer an animal can survive periods of deprivation. However, prolonged intake of energy in excess of that required can result in an inappropriately excessive accumulation of adipose tissue. In humans, obesity is frequently associated with increasing resistance to the actions of insulin. This then results in a range of metabolic abnormalities including hypertriglyceridaemia, reduced-plasma HDL, elevated blood pressure and raised fasting glucose levels. Together these have been termed the metabolic syndrome (Met Syn), which is closely associated with increased risk of developing type 2 diabetes and CVD. Over the past decade it has also been recognised that obesity and Met Syn are closely associated with the development of non-alcoholic fatty liver disease (NAFLD), which in some individuals can progress to steatohepatitis, cirrhosis, hepatocarcinoma and liver failure. Finding an animal model that recapitulates the progression of these metabolic failures has been an important goal of many nutritional scientists in recent years.

In most species studied there are inherent mechanisms to reduce food intake in response to prolonged overconsumption. It has been demonstrated across a wide range of species that increasing energy density of food will result in reduced intake. However, this is not always a precise response and can vary between species, strain and composition of the diet. The response to high-fat feeding is perhaps the most poorly regulated and, depending on the animal model used, switching to a high-fat diet can result in energy consumption increases of over 25% and the development of obesity. This is probably potentiated by the relative restriction on energy expenditure that normal animal housing imposes. Further increasing the palatability of food can increase excessive consumption. This is probably best illustrated by the so-called cafeteria diet. Experiments in the 1970s showed that obesity could be readily induced in rats fed a variety of palatable foods normally consumed by humans. Feeding foods such as cheese, chocolate, baked products and processed meat products, particularly when varied on a daily basis, resulted in large increases in daily energy intake and rapid weight gain compared to chow-fed animals. However, the major criticism of the cafeteria diet is that when using such a wide variety of foods it is difficult to monitor not only energy intake, but also macro- and micronutrient consumption, which could have an impact on the metabolic response to such diets. Furthermore, it can be very difficult to compare results between laboratories due to the variability in composition of the diets.

In addition to diet-induced models of obesity, a number of monogenetic mutations resulting in obesity have been discovered and have contributed immensely to our obesity research. One of the first to be discovered was the ob/ob mouse. Initially identified in the Jackson Laboratories in 1949, it took 50 years for the specific nature of the gene defect to be identified. Eventually this was shown to the result of a single base pair deletion in the leptin gene. Leptin, a protein produced by adipose tissue, plays an important role in regulating appetite. In its absence, the ob/ob mouse exhibits uncontrollable food intake, becomes severely obese and goes on to develop severe insulin resistance and ultimately type 2 diabetes (see Figure 18.5). The db/db mouse, discovered 17 years later, exhibits a similar phenotype, developing obesity by as early as 1 month of age and frank hyperglycaemia by 8 weeks. This was later shown to be a result of a mutation in the leptin receptor rather than leptin itself. The Zucker fatty rat (ZFR), first described in 1961, also

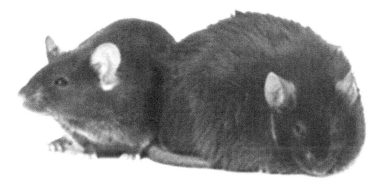

Figure 18.5 A comparison of an ob/ob and a wild-type mouse. Reproduced with permission from the Jackson Laboratory (http://jaxmice.jax.org/strain/000632.html).

carries a mutation in the leptin receptor that results in uncontrolled food intake, obesity and insulin resistance. While this original strain does not develop full-blown type 2 diabetes, a substrain, the Zucker diabetic fatty (ZDF) rat, was subsequently discovered that does.

Another commonly studied monogenic model of obesity is the Agouti lethal yellow mouse. Several mutations in the agouti gene have been discovered that result in ubiquitous expression of the agouti protein. In addition to becoming obese, the mice are characterised by a display of various coat colours. Agouti protein competes with alpha-melanocyte-stimulating protein, an anorexigenic factor (which normally reduces appetite) thereby increasing food intake. Obesity in this strain occurs in adult life, later than leptin/leptin receptor-deficient models, and also leads to the development of hypertension. These, and other monogenic models, have made an immense contribution to our understanding of the pathophysiology of obesity. However, the fact that they have a specific mutation resulting in dysregulation of appetite limits their use in nutritional experiments designed to look at the effects of specific diets and nutrients on food intake.

In addition to these monogenic models, a number of polygenic strains have been described. One with the most severe phenotype is the New Zealand obese (NZO) mouse. These animals demonstrate marked increases in food intake and develop obesity within the first 2 months of life. The males (but not females) are also susceptible to the development of type 2 diabetes. The specific natures of the metabolic perturbations in the strain remain to be fully established and, while they may be associated with leptin resistance, the mice have normal leptin and leptin receptors. It has also been observed that compared to other strains of mice they exhibit reduced levels of activity. In addition to spontaneously developing mutations, in recent years the ability to manipulate the expression of individual genes in the mouse has thus led to major developments in our understanding of the regulation of food intake and adipose tissue deposition.

Other species, including dogs, pigs and primates, have also been used in obesity research. As with cardiovascular research, the pig has attracted particular attention. Ironically, many commercial breeds of pigs have been bred over many generations specifically to reduce fat, and increase lean, deposition. However, a number of 'more primitive' breeds, including the Yucatan, Ossabaw and Gottingen mini-pig breeds, have been shown to be susceptible to obesity.

While an animal model of obesity may be valuable in studying the nutritional factors involved in the regulation of food intake and adiposity per se, many researchers are interested in studying the pathophysiological consequences of the obese state. Many of the animal models already described will develop some of the characteristics of the Met Syn and, as already alluded to, a number of monogenetic animal models of obesity progress to develop type 2 diabetes (this includes both ob/ob and db/db mice and the ZDF rat). These models also tend to develop some level of NAFLD, though this tends not to develop beyond relatively benign steatosis. However, a model that includes all aspect of Met Syn and the increased susceptibility to both CVD and diabetes has remained elusive. Crossing ob/ob or db/db mice with transgenic mice prone to athersclerosis (LDLr $^{-/-}$ or apoE$^{-/-}$) produces strains that are susceptible to dietary-induced obesity, insulin resistance and atherosclerosis, but the latter is in response to markedly elevated VLDL and/or LDL cholesterol rather than the low HDL cholesterol, hypertriglyceridaemia and hypertension associated with human Met Syn. The JCR:LA cp rat has shown considerable promise as a model of Met Syn. These animals, carrying a mutation in the leptin receptor, are obese, insulin resistant and develop spontaneous arterial lesions. Their susceptibility to atherosclerosis appears to be associated with an overproduction of both chylomicrons and VLDL. This strain has been used in a number of studies looking at the impact of diet on Met Syn, including a demonstration that both omega-3 PUFA and conjugated linoleic acid improve the hyperlipidaemia and reduce cardiovascular complications. The female Ossabaw mini-pig, when fed a high-fat, high-cholesterol diet, also develops many features of Met Syn including obesity, insulin resistance, elevated plasma triacylglycerol and hypertension and has been shown to develop coronary artery atherosclerosis. However, its limited availability to a small number of laboratories in the USA limits its use by the broader scientific community.

Cancer

Diet can have impacts on cancer in a number of ways. Nutrients, non-nutrient components of food and contaminants may either promote or protect against the development of tumours. The direct study of the impact of diet on cancer risk in humans is difficult, as there are no obvious 'safe' biomarkers that can be studied. Thus, while with CVD the impact of diet on risk factors such as plasma cholesterol or blood pressure can be studied without any long-term impact on the health of subjects, there are no analogous measures that can be taken when looking at cancer risk. We are largely dependent on epidemiological studies to demonstrate the impact of diet on cancer risk. Furthermore, cancer is not a homogenous disease and risk factors for development in particular anatomical sites will vary. Tissues of the gastrointestinal (GI) tract may be particularly vulnerable to dietary carcinogens, as these tissues are exposed to the highest concentrations of the compounds involved. For example, excessive alcohol consumption has been associated with increased risk of cancer throughout the GI tract. However, diet clearly has other, more systemic effects on the development of cancer. High energy intakes and associated obesity have been linked to a range of cancers, including those of the colon, kidney, gall bladder, breast, prostate and endometrium. Consumption of diets rich in fat and meat (particularly processed meat) have been associated with increased risk of a range of cancers. By contrast, diets rich in fruit and vegetables and high fibre intakes may be protective.

As with other NCDs, a number of animal models have been developed for studying the link between diet and cancer. Most commonly, this involves either using specific chemical agents to induce cancer or using xenografts (implanted rodent or human tumours) in rats or mice that are 'nude' (with an impaired immune system so they do not reject the transplant). Two common examples of chemicals used to induce cancers are 1,2-dimethylbenz(a)anthracene (DMBA), used to induce breast cancer, and 1.2-dimethylhydrazine (DMH), which induces colon cancer. In recent years, such models have been employed extensively to investigate the impact of different types of dietary fatty acid on cancer development and growth. Such experiments have suggested that, compared to saturated or monounsaturated fatty acids, omega-6 PUFA appear to promote tumour growth, while omega-3 PUFA and *trans* fatty acids (including conjugated linoleic acid, CLA) may be protective. How translatable these findings are to the development of cancer over the human life span remains to be established.

18.6 Animal models of nutrition through the lifecycle

Through manipulation of our environment in many parts of the world, humans have extended their life span long beyond that of other wild-living animals. Deaths from accidents, infectious diseases and starvation have been dramatically reduced in many 'developed countries'. Evolution, through natural selection, is largely 'interested' only in the reproductively active period of our lives. As we pass through this phase the human body undergoes a whole range of physical and metabolic changes that we associate with ageing. Is this process inevitable? Can we slow the ageing process? Does diet have an impact on the speed of the ageing process? Answering these questions in a species living frequently over 80 years is obviously difficult and, since the early twentieth century, scientists have used shorter-lived animal species to try to understand more about the ageing process.

More recently, we have come to recognise that health in later life is influenced by events very early in life. Thus,

metabolic insults *in utero*, or in the first months or years of life, may have an impact on our susceptibility to a range of non-communicable diseases and hence our ultimate life span. While early evidence for the 'developmental origins of health and disease' (DOHaD) hypothesis came from human epidemiological studies, animal models have been instrumental in providing biological plausibility for the theory and in elucidating potential mechanisms.

Models of the developmental origins of health and disease

The primary evidence that led to the DOHaD theory was generated from retrospective human epidemiological studies. Using birth records, the impact of weight at birth on subsequent health indicated that individuals born with a lower weight had higher blood pressure, a greater prevalence of type 2 diabetes and a greater risk of developing metabolic syndrome. Maternal nutrition is one factor that can give rise to low birth weight and the impact of maternal under-nutrition on the subsequent health of the offspring has been explored in a number of animal species, including rats, mice, guinea pigs, pigs, sheep and baboons. A large number of nutritional insults in pregnancy have been tested, including global nutrient restriction, low-protein diet and micronutrient (e.g. zinc) restriction. The most studied species is the rat, in which total food restriction or specifically protein restriction has been shown to induce hypertension, insulin resistance and hyperlipidaemia in the adult offspring. Strangely, over-nutrition and obesity in pregnant rats appear to result in a similar susceptibility to metabolic disease in the offspring. Thus, very different nutritional insults seem to produce a similar phenotype in adult offspring.

Many studies have subsequently been undertaken to try to elucidate the mechanisms underlying these effects. It has been suggested that remodelling of tissues during development, as a consequence of maternal nutritional status, leads to irreversible changes in organ structure (e.g. reduced nephron number in the kidneys) that ultimately result in the increased disease susceptibility in the offspring. Underlying these effects may be epigenetic changes in gene structure that permanently alter their expression. Such changes may include methylation of specific bases, with the DNA structure altering the way in which the expression of a specific gene is regulated. Studies in mice have demonstrated that changes in the methylation status of specific genes coding for transcription factors are involved in regulating metabolism. These changes may not only affect the immediate offspring but can possibly be passed on to subsequent generations. The potential for specific nutrients to regulate metabolism through epigenetic changes in gene structure represents one of the most exciting discoveries in modern nutritional science.

Animal models of ageing

The preceding sections have clearly indicated that diet can have an impact on life span by increasing, or decreasing, susceptibility to chronic disease. All other things being equal, a population at high risk of developing CVD or cancer is likely to have a lower mean life expectancy than one that is relatively protected from the disease. However, can nutrition have an impact on the ageing process per se, and can it affect maximum, as well as mean, life span?

Animals models have been used for over 75 years in exploring this process. In the 1930s McCay and co-workers showed that if rats were fed a nutritionally adequate, but energy-reduced, diet their average and maximum life span could be extended substantially, with the delay of a range of age-associated pathologies. In a number of rodent species (including rats, mice and hamsters), so-called caloric restriction (CR) has been shown to reduce the age-related development of cancer, obesity, diabetes, autoimmune disease, sarcopenia and CVD. In general, the more severe the caloric restriction, the greater the increase in life span (though below a certain level the energy restriction itself becomes life threatening) and the earlier the restriction starts in the life of the animal, the greater the effect. This was subsequently shown to be the case in a wide range of short-lived species, including flies, worms and even yeast.

However, can it be assumed that the same applies to longer-lived species, including humans? In order to answer this question a number of studies are underway in non-human primates. One species being studied is the Rhesus monkey, which has a median life span of approximately 26 years and a maximum life span of approximately 40 years. The University of Wisconsin-Madison study, which started in 1989, is looking at the impact of a 30% restricted energy intake from early adulthood (starting age 8–14 years). In 2009 these researchers reported that caloric restriction was associated with a reduction in the incidence of diabetes, cancer, cardiovascular disease and brain atrophy. Figure 18.6 shows that the restricted animals display fewer physical signs of ageing. Preliminary data also suggested a potential effect on life span, with 80% of CR animals surviving compared to 50% of control animals. Yet a similar study, conducted by the National Institute of Aging, recently reported that CR, initiated either in young, middle or old age, has so far failed to demonstrate an increase in life span. Thus, at the present time whether the benefits of CR can be extrapolated to longer-lived animals remains to be firmly established.

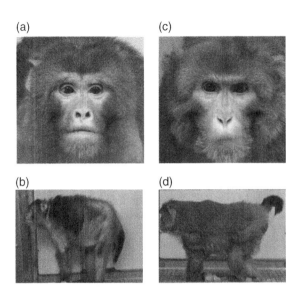

Figure 18.6 Impact of caloric restriction (CR) on signs of ageing in the Rhesus monkey. Animal appearance in old age. (a and b) Photographs of a typical control animal at 27.6 years of age (about the average life span). (c and d) Photographs of an age-matched animal on CR. From Colman, R.J., Anderson, R.M., Johnson, S.C. *et al.* (2009) Caloric restriction delays disease onset and mortality in Rhesus monkeys. *Science,* **325,** 201–204. Reprinted with permission from AAAS.

Animal models have also been used to try to understand the mechanisms by which CR works in shorter-lived animals, in the hope of identifying a target that could perhaps be subject to pharmaceutical intervention to increase the human life span. One theory is that at lower energy intake there is less oxidative metabolism, less production of free radicals and therefore less molecular/tissue damage, resulting in a slowing of the ageing process. However, a number of nutrient-sensitive proteins, including metabolic regulators and transcription factors, have potentially been implicated in longevity and it has been proposed that CR induces some form of metabolic reprogramming of the ageing process.

18.7 Conclusions

Health, disease and longevity are a function of a wide range of both genetic and lifestyle factors. Humans live a unique lifestyle that is almost impossible to model completely in any other animal species. In many populations, diet and physical activity have changed dramatically compared to their evolutionary past. Our ability to manipulate our environment is unique among animal species. However, our basic requirements for macro- and micronutrients are fundamentally similar to other animal species and there is little doubt that early animal experimentation has provided vast amounts of information about energy and nutrient requirements. In more recent decades we have become increasingly focused on the impact of nutrition on the development of NCDs and even the ageing process itself. No single animal species can mirror the impact of diet, and other lifestyle factors, on the aetiology of such diseases. Nevertheless, animal experimentation has been invaluable in testing hypotheses as to the impact of nutrients on risk factors for such diseases and pinpointing specific targets that may be useful in treatment and prevention. Our ability to manipulate the genetic make-up of animals by knocking out or over-expressing endogenous genes or inserting human genes into animals has refined such experimental work. It is, of course, equally important to recognise the limitations as well as the opportunities that such models provide to nutritional science. However, taken together with *in vitro* models and human epidemiological and intervention studies, appropriately designed and interpreted, animal model studies still have the potential to make major contributions to nutritional science. This chapter has highlighted a few of the many existing examples of such work.

References and further reading

Baker, D.H. (2008) Animal models in nutrition research. *Journal of Nutrition*, **138**, 391–396.

Bennen, A.C. and West, C.E. (eds) (1988) *Comparative Animal Nutrition 6: Use of Animal Models for Research in Human Nutrition*. Karger, Basel.

Carpenter, K.J. (2003) A short history of nutritional science: Part 3 (1912–1944). *Journal of Nutrition*, **133**, 3023–3032.

Chapman, J.M. (1986) Comparative analysis of mammalian plasma lipoproteins. In J.P. Segrests and J.J. Albers (eds) *Methods in Enzymology*. Academic Press, Waltham, MA, pp. 70–143.

Colman, R.J., Anderson, R.M., Johnson, S.C. *et al.* (2009) Caloric restriction delays disease onset and mortality in Rhesus monkeys. *Science*, **325**, 201–204.

Getz, G.S. and Reardon, C.A. (2012) Animal models of atherosclerosis. *Arteriosclerosis, Thrombosis, and Vascular Biology*, **32**, 1104–1115.

Home Office (2012) *Statistics of Scientific Procedures on Living Animals. Great Britain 2011*. Stationery Office, London.

Johnson, D.E. (2007) Contributions of animal nutrition research to nutritional principles: Energetics. *Journal of Nutrition*, **137**, 698–701.

Kennedy, A.J., Ellacott, K.J.L., King, V.L. and Hasty, A.H. Mouse models of the metabolic syndrome. *Disease Models & Mechanisms*, **3**, 156–166.

Lane-Petter, W. (1976) The ethics of animal experimentation. *Journal of Medical Ethics*, **2**, 3, 118–126.

Langley-Evans, S.C. (2013) Fetal programming of CVD and renal disease: Animal models and mechanistic considerations. *Proceedings of the Nutrition Society*, **72**, 3, 317–325.

Mattson, J.A., Roth, G.S., Beasley, T.M. *et al.* Impact of caloric restriction on health and survival in Rhesus monkeys from the NIA study. *Nature*, **489**, 318–322.

McMullen, S. and Mostyn, A. (2009) Animal models for the study of the developmental origins of health and disease. *Proceedings of the Nutrition Society*, **68**, 306–320.

Russell, J.C. and Proctor, S.D. (2006) Small animal models of cardiovascular disease: Tools for the study of the roles of metabolic syndrome, dyslipidemia and atherosclerosis. *Cardiovascular Pathology*, **15**, 318–330.

Sauer, L.A., Blask, D.E. and Dauchy, R.T. (2007) Dietary factors and growth and metabolism in experimental tumours. *Journal of Nutritional Biochemistry*, **18**, 637–649.

Spurlock, M.E. and Gabler, N.K. (2008) The development of porcine models of obesity and the metabolic syndrome. *Journal of Nutrition*, **138**, 2, 397–402.

Stylianou, I.M., Bauer, R.C., Reilly, M.P. and Rader, D.J. (2012) Genetic basis of atherosclerosis: Insights from mice and humans. *Circulation Research*, **110**, 337–355.

Varga, O., Harangi, M., Olsson, I.A.S. and Hansen, A.K. (2009) Contribution of animal models to the understanding of the metabolic syndrome. *Obesity Reviews*, **11**, 792–807.

19
Cellular Models in Nutrition Research

Kathleen M Botham

The Royal Veterinary College

Key messages

- Cellular models are crucial for the study of the way in which nutrition influences events at the cellular and molecular level, which causes changes in the functions of cells and tissues. They are used to investigate both how nutrients affect basic cell function to promote health and how they may act to prevent or retard disease.
- There are two main types of cultured cell model: primary cells, isolated directly from humans or animals and with a limited life in culture; and immortalised cell lines, derived from naturally occurring cancers or laboratory manipulation, which are able to divide indefinitely *in vitro*.
- Cells may be cultured in suspension (floating freely in the medium), but most mammalian cells are anchorage dependent and are grown or maintained on hydrophilic, negatively charged surfaces such as plastic tissue culture-treated dishes.
- Many analytical techniques are applicable to cellular models, but they are particularly suited to the investigation of cell behaviours such as proliferation, migration and motility, and for the study of the expression of specific proteins using immunocytochemistry.

- The modern techniques of confocal microscopy and flow cytometry play important roles in this area.
- The study of dynamic processes in living cells has been greatly aided by the discovery of biological fluorophores such as green fluorescent protein (GFP), which are used in conjunction with confocal or fluorescence microscopy.
- Cellular models have provided and continue to provide invaluable information that has helped in the current understanding of how nutrients influence the basic functions of cells in the normal animal, including cell proliferation, migration, differentiation, cell cycle, apoptosis, cell signalling pathways, gene expression, ion transport, secretion of hormones or other factors, enzyme activities and many more.
- Cellular models have made an important contribution to the understanding of the interactions between malnutrition and infection and also of the role of nutrients in metabolic diseases related to the Western lifestyle, such as obesity and diabetes, chronic degenerative diseases, such as cancer and heart disease, and neurodegenerative disorders, such as Alzheimer's disease.

19.1 Introduction: Why use cellular models in nutrition research?

The aim of nutrition research is to investigate the responses of the body to diet in order to determine optimal nutritional status in humans and animals – not only in the healthy adult, but at the various stages of development, including growth, reproduction and ageing – and also to study the relationship between diet and disease. It was first recognised in the late eighteenth century that, in addition to the deleterious effects of insufficient food in the diet (i.e. under-nutrition or starvation), components of the diet (which we now call nutrients) are necessary for the proper functioning of the physiological processes of the body and

for the prevention of disease. Since then, nutritionists have used intervention studies, in which human healthy subjects, patients or animals (see Chapter 3) are fed a particular food or dietary component and the effects on their physiology and metabolism are assessed, and epidemiological (or population) studies, which observe the patterns of dietary intake and their relationship to health and disease in defined populations (see Chapter 2). These approaches have been very successful and have led to great strides in the understanding of how nutrients influence health. However, if we are to comprehend fully the mechanisms by which nutrients affect physiological responses, it is essential to study the events occurring at the cellular and molecular level that lead to changes in the functions of

Nutrition Research Methodologies, First Edition. Edited by Julie A Lovegrove, Leanne Hodson, Sangita Sharma and Susan A Lanham-New.
© 2015 John Wiley & Sons, Ltd. Published 2015 by John Wiley & Sons, Ltd.
Companion Website: www.wiley.com/go/nutritionsociety

cells and tissues. Since the amount of information of this kind that can be obtained from epidemiological or intervention studies is limited, cellular models are widely used for these investigations. Together with the advances in scientific disciplines such as genetics and molecular biology that have occurred in the last few decades, such models have made it possible for scientists to dissect out the intracellular pathways by which cells alter their function in response to signals from their environment. The use of cellular models, therefore, is crucial for the further advancement of nutritional science.

For the purposes of this chapter, cellular models will be defined as those involving the use of primary cells (i.e. cells derived directly from humans or animals), immortalised cell lines, tissue microstructures (e.g. pancreatic islets), tissue explants and isolated perfused organs. These experimental systems are currently being used or have the potential to be used in many different aspects of nutrition research, including:

- Understanding how nutrients affect normal cells by influencing molecular mechanisms, nutrient–gene interactions (Chapter 15), cell signalling pathways, cell–cell interactions, cell function, enzyme activities and so on.
- Investigation of the bioavailability (i.e. the proportion of an ingested nutrient that is absorbed and available for use or storage within the body) of nutrients.
- Discovery of new nutrients and new functions for known nutrients.
- Study of the way in which nutrients may affect the initiation and progression of chronic diseases such as autoimmune disease, heart disease and cancer.
- Determination of the role of nutrients in modulating the development of obesity and interlinked metabolic conditions such as diabetes.
- Investigation of the interaction of nutrients with disease agents, including viruses, bacteria and prions (causal agents of neurological diseases such as Alzheimer's disease).

- Testing of the safety of food and food supplements. Cellular models enable compounds to be screened prior to animal trials, and thus help to minimise the use of animals in research.

19.2 Cellular models in *ex vivo* and *in vitro* experimental systems

Experimental systems may be described generally as *in vivo*, a Latin term meaning literally 'within the living', *ex vivo* ('outside the living') or *in vitro* ('in glass'); see Table 19.1.

- *In vivo* studies are those carried out using the whole animal, and intervention studies such as those described in Chapter 3 are examples that fall into this category.
- *Ex vivo* experiments are done using living tissue, but in a laboratory apparatus outside the organism where natural conditions are maintained as far as possible. *Ex vivo* techniques include isolated perfused organ systems, the use of tissue segments such as blood vessel rings or small sections of the intestine maintained in a suitable oxygenated medium, and other methods such as the chick chorioallantoic membrane assay, in which angiogenesis is measured on the membrane outside the chick embryo. Such experiments are by their nature time-limited to a few hours, up to a maximum of about 24 hours.
- *In vitro* studies are those that use isolated tissues, cells or components thereof (e.g. subcellular organelles or purified proteins), usually in culture dishes or test tubes. The dividing line between *ex vivo* and *in vitro* is not clearly defined and there is some overlap between the use of the two terms.

The advantage of using *ex vivo* or *in vitro* as compared to *in vivo* systems is that the immense complexity of the whole animal, which makes the study of particular cell and organ functions or responses extremely difficult, is simplified so that particular effects can be investigated

Table 19.1 *In vivo, ex vivo* and *in vitro* experimental systems.

System	Literal meaning	Type of experiment	Advantages	Disadvantages
In vivo	Within the living	Whole animal	Physiological conditions maintained throughout	Complexity makes interpretation of results difficult
Ex vivo	Outside the living	Perfused organs, tissue segments and explants maintained in the laboratory outside the organism	Enables specific tissue functions to be studied while retaining tissue architecture and extracellular matrix	Only short-term experiments possible Outside natural environment
In vitro	In glass	Isolated cells or cell components maintained in culture dishes or (subcellular organelles or proteins) used in test tubes	Enables the study of cell function at the molecular level	Interactions with other cells/ tissues excluded Outside natural environment

more easily. *Ex vivo* experiments have the additional advantage of retaining the tissue architecture, but the disadvantage that they are inherently short term, while *in vitro* experiments allow scientists to drill down to the molecular mechanisms that enable cells to function. The main disadvantage of both *ex vivo* and *in vitro* approaches is, of course, that the studies are done outside the natural environment of the tissues or cells, and thus great care needs to be taken in applying the results to the *in vivo* situation. In nutrition research, for example, nutrients producing a particular desirable response in cells in culture *in vitro* may fail to do so *in vivo* because they do not arrive at the target tissue in sufficient quantities or because they have adverse effects on other cell types.

Cellular models may be employed in *ex vivo* and *in vitro* systems, but by definition they are not used in studies *in vivo*.

19.3 Types of cellular models

Cultured cells

Cultured cell models can be divided into two general types, primary cells and immortalised cell lines (Table 19.2).

Primary cells

Primary cells are isolated directly from humans (mainly blood cells, but other cell types can also be obtained from biopsy samples) or experimental animals by gentle disruption of the target tissue in various ways that avoid destruction of cellular integrity (see later in this chapter). Some types of primary cells grow well in culture (e.g. fibroblasts), while others can be maintained for some days, but do not divide (e.g. hepatocytes).

Primary cells have the advantage that they usually retain the physiological features they demonstrate *in vivo*, the results obtained are generally relatively easy to interpret and they are cost effective, as much smaller amounts of reagents are required than for *in vivo* experiments. However, some specialised cell types tend to become dedifferentiated (i.e. lose their specialised functions) in culture: for example chondrocytes (the cells that produce cartilage proteins) do not retain the chondrocyte phenotype, but revert to fibroblast-like cells, and the expression of liver-specific genes is progressively lost in cultured hepatocytes. Strategies have been designed to limit dedifferentiation, but they have met with limited success. A more generally applicable disadvantage is that, with the exception of stem cells, all primary cells are only able to survive in culture for a limited time. After a certain number of cell divisions the cells become senescent and stop dividing. This phenomenon is termed the Hayflick limit, after the scientist who first observed that human fetal cells divide only 40–60 times before entering the senescence phase. The shortening of telomeres in the DNA of the cells is believed to be the reason why further cell division eventually becomes impossible. Stem cells have the ability to differentiate into different types of specialised cells and are found in embryonic tissue and in adults in bone marrow, adipose tissue and blood. They can divide indefinitely in culture as well as *in vivo*.

Immortalised cell lines

Unlike primary cells, immortalised cell lines are able to undergo unlimited cell division without becoming senescent. Immortalisation happens *in vivo* when cells mutate, become cancerous and proliferate in an uncontrolled way.

Table 19.2 Types of cellular models.

Model type	Origin	Advantages	Disadvantages
Primary cells	Isolated directly from animal tissue or human blood/biopsy samples	Retain *in vivo* physiology Relatively inexpensive	Limited life in culture (Hayflick limit) Extracellular matrix and tissue architecture lost May not divide in culture May lose tissue-specific function in culture
Immortalised cell lines	Cells derived from cancerous tumours or laboratory manipulation	Unlimited divisions in culture Unlimited quantity of genetically identical material available Relatively inexpensive	Often show significant differences from parent cell type Specialised tissue function may be lost No extracellular matrix or tissue architecture
Tissue explants	Small blocks of tissue from animals or human biopsy samples	Maintain tissue architecture and extracellular matrix Can be used to obtain cultures of primary cells	Limited amount of material available Often only short-term experiments possible
Isolated perfused organs	Directly from animals by cannulation of suitable blood vessels	Maintain whole organ with various cell types in natural tissue architecture	Complex experimental systems required Only relatively short-term experiments possible

Table 19.3 Some immortalised cell lines.

Name	Species	Origin	Cell type
HeLa	Human	Cervical carcinoma	Epithelial
THP-1	Human	Acute myeloid leukaemia	Monocytes/ macrophages*
HEK293	Human	Transformation of embryonic kidney cells using adenovirus	Kidney epithelial
CaCo-2	Human	Colorectal adenocarcinoma	Intestinal epithelial cells (enterocytes)
HepG2	Human	Hepatocellular carcinoma	Hepatocytes
MCF-7	Human	Breast adenocarcinoma	Mammary epithelial
CHO	Hamster	Chinese hamster ovary	Epithelial
RAW264.7	Mouse	Abelson murine leukaemia virus-induced tumour	Macrophages
McA-RH7777	Rat	Hepatoma	Hepatocytes
CV-1	African green monkey	Adult kidney cells transformed with Rous sarcoma virus	Fibroblasts
COS-7	African green monkey	CV-1 cells transformed with simian virus 40	Fibroblast-like

*Can be differentiated into macrophages by treatment with phorbol ester *in vitro*

Cancer cells cultured *in vitro* continue to divide indefinitely, and this makes them a useful tool for nutrition research. An example still widely used today is the HeLa cell line, which was originally derived from a human cervical cancer in 1951. More examples of immortalised cell lines are shown in Table 19.3.

In addition to obtaining cell lines from naturally occurring cancers, it is also possible to generate them in the laboratory by genetic manipulation (Figure 19.1). This can be done in a random way by treating cultured cells with a known mutagen, then selecting continuously dividing cells. More targeted approaches, however, aim to introduce into the cells genes for specific proteins that influence cell division using a recombinant virus vector, such as adenovirus or a retrovirus. Proteins that have been used effectively to transform primary cells into immortalised cell lines include telomerase, an enzyme that lengthens telomeres and thus enables cell division to continue indefinitely, and viral genes, which interfere with the normal cell cycle. For example, telomerase transfection has been used to immortalise primary human skin fibroblasts, retinal cells and endometrial stromal cells, and adenovirus technology was used to generate the human embryonic kidney (HEK) 293 cell line by the introduction of a viral gene for a protein that alters the cell cycle so that cell division is promoted. Antibody-producing B lymphocytes can also be transformed into cell lines by fusion with a cancerous B cell (myeloma) forming a hybridoma, a technique that is used for the production of monoclonal antibodies.

The use of immortalised cell lines in nutrition research has the advantage that, because they continue to divide in culture indefinitely, they provide an unlimited quantity of homogenous, genetically identical cells, and so it is possible to carry out large numbers of experiments easily and relatively cheaply. The disadvantage of this type of model, however, is that because mutation is required for immortality, the cells may show significant differences from the primary cells from which they were derived, and highly specialised functions may be lost. It is important, therefore, to be aware of these limitations when interpreting the results.

Tissue explants

An explant is a small block of tissue that is taken from an animal or human biopsy sample under sterile conditions and maintained in an artificial medium *ex vivo* or *in vitro* (Table 19.2). Explant culture has the advantage that the cell architecture and extracellular matrix remain intact in the tissue blocks, thus enabling their function to be studied in an environment that more closely resembles *in vivo* physiology than that in cultured isolated primary cells. Examples include the use of animal cartilage explants to study osteoarthritis and ileal tissue explants to study the function of intestinal cells. However, because of the difficulty of maintaining the viability of cells in the centre of the block, explants are of necessity very small (no more than a few millimetres long), so the amount of material that can be obtained is limited, and this technique is much less widely used than cell culture models in human and animal studies.

In addition to their use to study tissue function, cultured explants are also employed in the isolation of primary cells, which can then be grown on in the absence of the tissue block (see later in this chapter). Adipose tissue explants are commonly used in this way to provide adipocytes for the study of the causes of obesity.

Isolated perfused organs

Perfused organ systems use animal organs such as the liver and heart, which are isolated from the body and perfused through their physiological vascular system using an oxygenated perfusate, or even sometimes whole

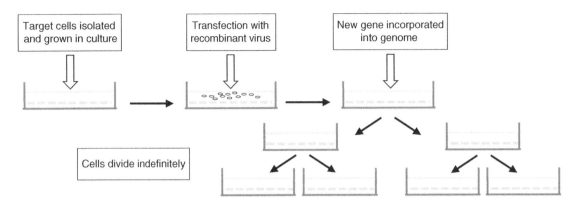

Figure 19.1 Generation of immortalised cell lines in the laboratory. Cells may be transfected with genes such as the Simian virus large T and small t tumour antigens (SV40T), which influence the cell cycle or the catalytic subunit of human telomerase reverse transcriptase (hTERT). The genes are incorporated into the genome and stably expressed, allowing unlimited cell division.

blood (Table 19.2). This has the advantage that a particular organ in its entirety, with its various cell types embedded in the natural tissue architecture, can be studied in the absence of the influence of other organs or factors such as hormones that circulate in the whole animal. The disadvantages are that perfusion systems are necessarily rather complex and the organ can only be kept alive for a limited time, usually some hours.

As well as the liver and heart, organs that are widely used in perfusion studies include the kidneys, lungs, intestine and blood vessels such as the aorta. Rodent such as rats, mice and guinea pigs are often employed as donors, but organs from larger species such as pigs and sheep have also been used successfully.

19.4 General approaches in nutrition research

Cellular models may be employed in *ex vivo* and *in vitro* systems, but by definition they are not used in studies *in vivo*. We can divide the experimental approaches involving cellular models that are likely to be used in nutrition research into two main types.

The first type resembles an intervention study, in that human volunteers (either healthy or after diagnosis of disease) or experimental animals (normal or disease models caused by mutation – e.g. the ob/ob obese mouse, a model for obesity and type II diabetes – or induced by chemicals/drugs – e.g. small doses of carbon tetrachloride used to induce liver disease – or diet – e.g. the use of a high-carbohydrate, high-fat diet to induce obesity) are given the test food or nutrient in the diet (or for acute studies in a test meal), and tissues are then taken for cell culture or organ perfusion (Figure 19.2). For obvious reasons, in experiments involving humans this approach

is mostly limited to blood cells, but sometimes cells can be isolated from biopsy samples (e.g. hepatocytes can be isolated from liver biopsy samples). Basic cell functions and their responses to external factors added to the cell medium or organ perfusate can then be investigated and the effects of the test nutrient on the cells/tissues determined by comparing the results with those observed in cells/tissues from subjects/animals given a control diet or test meal. In this way, information may be gained about how nutrients taken in the diet influence normal cell function and thus may have health benefits, and also about how they may protect against or retard disease processes.

The second, simpler approach is entirely *in vitro* and may involve isolated perfused organs, primary cells or immortalised cell lines (Figure 19.3). In this case the effects of a nutrient on cell/tissue function are assessed directly by adding it to the perfusate or cell culture medium of primary cells harvested from humans or experimental animals (either healthy or disease models, as earlier) or to cell lines. This type of study has the advantage of *in vitro* systems in being easy to use and providing large quantities of data relatively inexpensively, but the disadvantage that the normal physiological processes of digestion and absorption are bypassed, and thus any changes observed may not reflect what happens *in vivo*.

19.5 Cell culture methods

Cell isolation

For culture *in vitro*, most primary cells must first be released from the extracellular matrix with no, or minimal, damage to the plasma membrane, as otherwise they will not be able to survive. Leucocytes (white blood cells) are an important exception to this, as they can be isolated

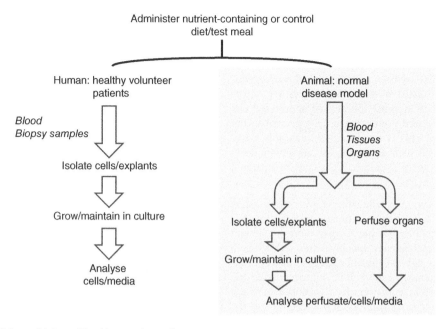

Figure 19.2 Cellular models in nutritional intervention studies.

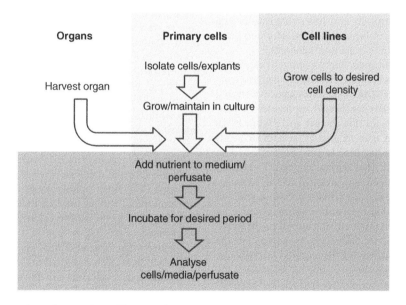

Figure 19.3 *In vitro* experimental systems in nutrition research.

directly from the blood. Enzymes such as collagenase, which attack the matrix protein collagen, or other general proteases such as trypsin or pronase are often used for the release of cells from tissues. The tissue is minced or gently homogenised before treatment with the enzymes. Perfusion of the organ with collagenase can also be used with highly vascularised tissues, and this approach has been very successful for the the isolation of hepatocytes from the liver. Since calcium ions play an important role in cell–cell adhesion in the tissues, a calcium chelator (an agent that binds to calcium ions) such as ethylenediaminetetraacetic acid (EDTA) is often used in conjunction with the proteases. An alternative method avoiding the use of enzymes that may damage the cell membrane is the use of tissue explant culture (see earlier). In this technique, single cells that grow out from a small piece of tissue maintained *ex vivo* are harvested, then grown and used in a culture system.

Once the cells have been released from the extracellular matrix or isolated from the blood, another step is often required to separate the desired specialised cell type from the mixed population usually present in the cell suspension. This is important, because just a few fast-growing cells such as fibroblasts can rapidly overgrow other cell types in culture. Cells may be separated on the basis of their:

- *Size and density*. Centrifugation exploits the differences in size and density of different cell types to separate them from each other. Larger, denser cells will form a pellet relatively quickly when centrifuged, while smaller, lighter cells will remain in the supernatant. The separation can often be improved by centrifuging the cells in density gradient, a solution in which the density increases from the top of the tube to the bottom.
- *Adherent properties*. Many mammalian cell types will adhere to a suitably treated (tissue culture-treated) plastic surface in culture, and this property can be used to separate strongly and less strongly adhering cells. It is also useful for the removal of blood cells, since hematopoietic cells are non-adherent.
- *Surface antigen expression*. Surface antigens expressed by specific cell types can be utilised in magnetic activated cell sorting (MACS) or fluorescence activated cell sorting (FACS), a specialised application of flow cytometry (see later in this chapter and Figure 19.4). The MACS system uses magnetic particles or beads carrying antibodies that bind to antigens expressed on the cells of interest. In a strong magnetic field, cells expressing the antigen stay attached to the particles, while non-expressing cells remain unbound and can be removed. Selection may be positive or negative, so that the desired cell type remains bound to the particles and can then be harvested (positive), or the unwanted cells bind, leaving the required cell type free in the solution (negative). In the FACS system, the antibody is linked to a fluorescent probe and the cells are passed singly through a laser beam, then given a positive or negative charge depending on whether they are fluorescent or not, and positive and negatively charged cells are separated by the application of an electric field.

Application of these techniques results in near homogenous preparation of specific primary cell types, which can then be grown or maintained in culture. Immortalised cell lines obtained either from naturally occurring cancers or by laboratory manipulation (see earlier) retain their viability when stored at $-80\,^\circ$C after freezing in liquid nitrogen, and thus can be recovered and grown up when required.

Cell culture

The techniques used for cell culture are similar for both primary cells and immortalised cell lines. The cells are placed in flasks or dishes and kept at the appropriate temperature in an incubator in which the atmosphere can be controlled. Typical conditions for mammalian cells are a temperature of $37\,^\circ$C and an atmosphere of 5% carbon dioxide/95% air. The culture medium generally consists of a mixture of salts, amino acids, vitamins, growth factors, antibiotics and antifungal agents at a defined pH (usually 7.4) with glucose as a fuel source, but the exact composition varies depending on the cell type under study. Table 19.4 shows the contents of a typical culture medium suitable for most types of cells. Media are also commonly supplemented with a small amount of animal serum (e.g. fetal calf serum) to provide a physiological profile of growth factors. In addition, a pH indicator such as phenol red is often included so that any pH changes can be detected.

Clearly, it is important to be sure that the cells used in culture are viable at the start and throughout the experiment. Typically, cell preparations with less than 90% viability are discarded. Viability may be assessed in a number of different ways. One of the most common is the Trypan blue exclusion test. Since the blue dye does not cross the membrane of intact cells, dead cells appear blue, while live cells remain colourless. Other membrane integrity tests include the use of propidium iodide, which can distinguish between normal, necrotic and apoptotic cells, and the assay of lactate dehydrogenase, an enzyme that leaks into the medium when the cell membrane is damaged. The spectrophotometric MTT assay, which measures the activity of enzymes that reduce the tetrazolium dye MTT to the purple-coloured formazan, is also widely used.

The two main types of culture system are suspension, where cells float freely in the culture medium, and adherent, where cells attach to a suitable surface, usually in a single layer. As indicated earlier, hematopoietic (blood) cells grow in suspension, but most animal tissue-derived cells are adherent, meaning that they attach, spread and grow when provided with a suitable hydrophilic, negatively charged surface. Plastic dishes that have been chemically treated to generate this kind of surface are, therefore, essential for most cell culture systems. They are termed tissue culture treated and are widely available commercially.

Cell suspensions obtained after the isolation of primary cells or the recovery of cell lines from storage

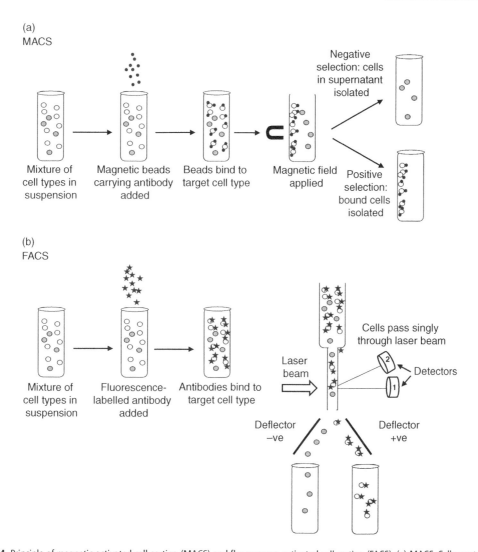

Figure 19.4 Principle of magnetic activated cell sorting (MACS) and fluorescence activated cell sorting (FACS). (a) MACS. Cells are treated with magnetic beads carrying antibodies, which bind to antigens on the cell surface. A strong magnetic field is applied and cells expressing the antigen stay attached to the particles, while non-expressing cells remain unbound and can be removed. In positive selection cell types that remain bound to the particles are harvested, while in negative selection the unwanted cells bind, leaving the required cell type free in the solution. (b) FACS. Cells are treated with a fluorescent antibody, passed singly through a laser beam, then given a positive or negative charge and separated by the application of an electric field. The detectors allow analytical data to be collected on the size and granularity (1) or fluorescence intensity (2) in the cells.

at −80 °C (see earlier) are seeded into dishes, where they either grow in suspension or attach to the surface. Cells in suspension maintain a rounded appearance, but on attachment they flatten and spread in a single layer. When this layer covers the entire surface it is called a confluent monolayer (Figure 19.5). At this stage cell-to-cell contact tends to inhibit further growth. In suspension cultures, cells will also reach a point where there are too many for the volume of medium available.

In addition, in both culture types the nutrients start to be used up and there may be an accumulation of debris from dead cells. Thus, if more cells are needed for the planned experiments, the culture will need to be passaged. This involves splitting the cells from one dish so that a small number are seeded into several new dishes in fresh medium (Figure 19.6). Cells in suspension are simply diluted with fresh medium, but adherent cells need to be released from the surface of the dish and resuspended.

Table 19.4 Contents of Dulbecco's modified Eagle's medium, one of the most common medium formulations, used for the culture of all types of cells. Antibiotics such as penicillin and streptomycin are also often added to inhibit bacterial growth.

Salts	Amino acids	Vitamins	Others
Calcium chloride	Arginine	Choline	Glucose
Ferric nitrate	Cystine	Folic acid	Pyruvic acid
Magnesium sulphate	Glycine	Myo-Inositol	Phenol red (if a pH
Potassium chloride	Histidine	Niacinamide	indicator is required)
Sodium bicarbonate	Isoleucine	Pantothenic acid	
Sodium chloride	Leucine	Pyridoxal	
Sodium monohydrogen	Lysine	Pyridoxine	
phosphate	Methionine	Riboflavin	
	Phenylalanine	Thiamine	
	Serine		
	Threonine		
	Tryptophan		
	Tyrosine		
	Valine		
	Glutamine		

(a)   (b)

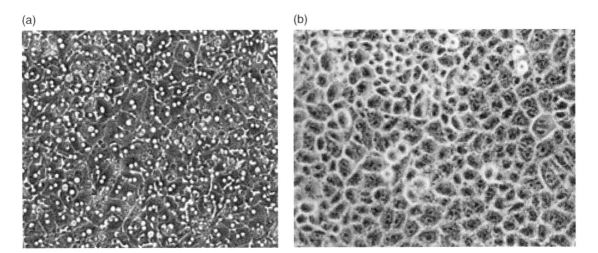

Figure 19.5 Cells in monolayer culture. Confluent monolayers of (a) Primary human hepatocytes. Reprinted from LeCluyse, E.L. (2011) Human hepatocyte culture systems for the in vitro evaluation of cytochrome P450 expression and regulation. European Journal of Pharmaceutical Sciences, 13, 343–368. Copyright 2001, with permission from Elsevier. (b) HeLa cells. Reprinted from Pickett, C.L. and Whitehouse, C.A. (1999) The cytolethal distending toxin family. Trends in Microbiology, 7, 292–397. Copyright 1999, with permission from Elsevier.

This is usually achieved using a protease, often trypsin, in combination with a calcium chelator such as EDTA.

Although, as already indicated, most animal cell types are anchorage dependent, for specialised studies, such as the investigation of proteins that are not expressed in the adherent form, they can sometimes be adapted for suspension systems. In general, however, adherent cell culture is the most widely used for nutrition research.

Adherent and suspension culture systems are compared in Table 19.5.

Adherent culture models

The most common type of adherent culture model used for nutritional studies is a monolayer culture of a single cell type grown or maintained in plastic tissue culture-treated dishes. In this system, cells are almost always

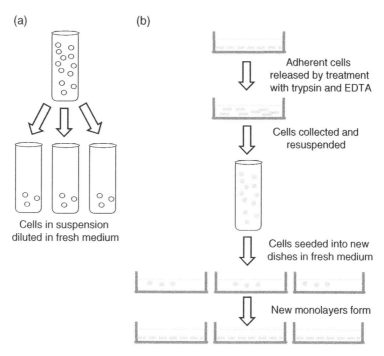

Figure 19.6 Cell passaging. (a) Suspension cell culture (b) adherent cell culture.

Table 19.5 Comparison of suspension and adherent cell culture systems.

	Suspension culture	Adherent culture
Cell types used	Cells that are non-adherent, such as hematopoietic cells Cells grown on microbeads Cells specially adapted for suspension culture	Most types of primary cells and immortalised cell lines
Cell origin	Isolated directly from blood	Primary cells released by enzymes such as collagenase or outgrowth from tissue explants Cell lines grown up from samples stored at −80 °C
Passaging	Culture diluted when cell density becomes too high to sustain optimum cell health	Required at regular intervals, cells are usually detached from the culture surface using an enzyme such as trypsin together with a calcium chelator
Culture vessel	Tissue culture treatment not necessary	Must be tissue culture treated or coated with a biological matrix
Applications	Research on hematopoietic cells Large-scale production of proteins such as monoclonal antibodies commercially	All types of cell biology research

used when they reach confluence, unless a parameter where this is not appropriate, such as cell proliferation, is under study. In the case of primary cells such as hepatocytes, which do not grow in culture, cell numbers that are likely to form a confluent monolayer are added to the dishes at the start of the experiment. Once the cells have adhered and formed a confluent monolayer, they are incubated for a defined time period, and both the medium and the cells can then be collected for analysis.

A typical experiment of this type is illustrated in Figure 19.7.

As well as this simplest form of adherent cell culture, however, a number of other, more complex systems have been developed (Table 19.6). These include:

- *Culture on a biological matrix* (e.g. collagen or gelatin). Coating tissue culture dishes with proteins that form part of the extracellular matrix (ECM), the structure that

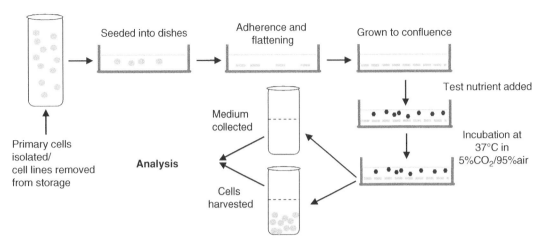

Figure 19.7 A typical experiment using monolayer cell culture in nutrition research.

Table 19.6 Adherent cell culture systems.

Culture system	Culture surface	Experimental conditions	Applications
Monolayer culture	Tissue culture-treated plastic (hydrophilic and negatively charged)	Confluent monolayer of a single cell type	Culture of most types of primary cells and cell lines
Monolayer culture on a biological matrix	Plastic coated with a protein such as collagen or gelatin, which forms a biological matrix for the cells	Confluent monolayer of a single cell type	Improved attachment, proliferation and differentiation in some cell types
Culture on microcarrier beads	Spherical particles 100–400 μm in diameter with hydrophilic and negatively charged surface coating	Beads kept in suspension by stirring or agitation	Studies requiring large numbers of cells Commercial production of cell products for research
Culture on membrane inserts	Porous membrane	Membrane inserted into well, allowing basolateral and apical cell surfaces to be exposed to medium in different compartments	Transport studies Cell migration studies Co-culture studies
Co-culture	Tissue culture-treated plastic Porous membrane	Two or more cell types cultured simultaneously	Study of cell–cell interactions
Culture under flow	Tissue culture-treated plastic or biological matrix	Cell medium passed over cells at flow rates that mimic those found in blood	Study of vascular cells under the stresses caused by blood flow *in vivo* Study of interactions between blood cells and vascular cells
3D culture	Synthetic or natural (e.g. collagen or fibronectin) hydrogels	3D culture in scaffold provided by hydrogel	Tissue engineering Tissue-regeneration studies

holds cells together in tissues, can improve factors including attachment, proliferation and differentiation for some cell types. Collagen, an ECM protein found in all tissues, and gelatin, a mixture of high molecular weight water-soluble proteins produced when collagen is hydro-lysed, are often used in this way. For example, the proliferation of primary human umbilical vein endothelial cells (HUVEC) has been found to be increased three- to fourfold when cultured on gelatin, as compared to tissue culture-coated dishes, and by 20% when cultured on collagen, as compared to gelatin-coated dishes (Figure 19.8).

• *Culture on microcarrier beads.* Microcarrier beads are spherical particles 100–400 μm in diameter with a surface coating suitable for the attachment of monolayers of adherent cells, which are kept in suspension by agitation or stirring of the culture vessel. The advantage of this system is the greatly increased surface area available for culture in a given volume of medium, and it is used for studies where large numbers of cells are required and for large-scale applications such as the commercial production of cell products for research.

• *Culture on membrane inserts.* Many cell types, particularly those that line body cavities (e.g. intestinal epithelial cells), have two distinct membrane domains with differential functions, the apical side, which faces the lumen, and the basolateral membrane, which forms the basal and lateral surfaces. Membrane inserts allow both membrane sides to be observed independently by culturing cells on porous membranes, which are then inserted into a well so that the two cell surfaces are exposed to the medium in separate compartments (Figure 19.9). When cultured in this system, epithelial cells form a polarised monolayer that mimics their *in vivo* function of acting as a barrier to the passage of certain molecules, thus facilitating the study of the transport of compounds through the epithelium. For example, the human intestinal epithelial cell line, CaCo-2, is commonly used in this way as a model for the absorption of nutrients or drugs in the intestine. In addition, the system is useful for assay of chemotaxis (the movement of cells towards chemoattractants), cell migration, and for co-culture of different cell types (see the next point). The use of membrane inserts for transport studies, cell migration assays and in co-culture in nutrition research are illustrated in Figure 19.10.

• *Co-culture of two (or more) cell types.* This is the culture of two or more cell types together for the study of cell–cell interactions. Since the physiological functions of cells are often regulated by substances released from other cell types, co-culture systems have the advantage that they are more representative of the situation *in vivo* than single cell types cultured in isolation. The different cell types may be cultured together in the same dish (e.g. interactions between hepatocytes and Kupffer cells during liver inflammation have been studied in this way), but membrane inserts (see earlier) are also often used. Cells may be cultured on either side of the membrane, or together on one side, or, if close cell-to-cell contact is not required, one type may be grown on the membrane and the other on the base of the insert (Figure 19.10). Examples of the use of co-culture systems include the provision of 'feeder' cell layers to provide factors such as cytokines, which affect the function of the other cell type; study of hormonal stimulation, including ligand–receptor interactions; and investigation of cell–cell communication.

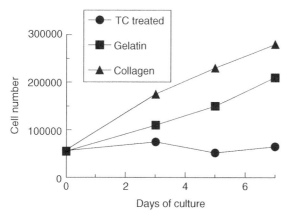

Figure 19.8 Effect of culture on a biological matrix on the proliferation of HUVEC. Proliferation of HUVEC when cultured on tissue culture (TC)-treated dishes, or dishes coated with gelatin or collagen. Data from www.colepalmer.com/TechLibraryArticle/70.

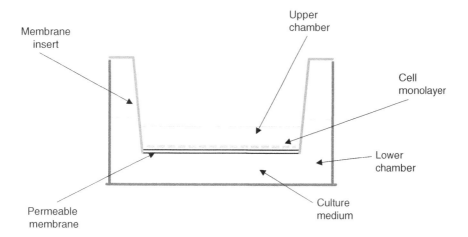

Figure 19.9 Cell culture on a membrane insert.

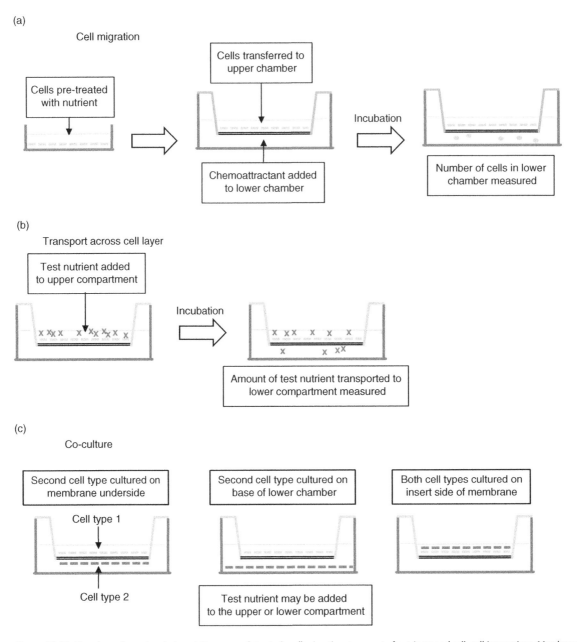

Figure 19.10 Use of membrane inserts in nutrition research to study cell migration, transport of nutrients and cell–cell interactions. Membrane inserts can be used to study the effects of nutrients on cell migration (a), the transport of nutrients across a cell layer such as the intestinal epithelium (b) and the influence of nutrients on cell–cell interactions using co-culture systems (c).

- *Culture under flow.* In physiological conditions, certain cell types, such as vascular endothelial cells that line blood vessels, are continuously exposed to the flow of blood. This causes stress, which has important effects on their function and behaviour. Since a static monolayer culture cannot reproduce this environment, systems have been devised to study these cells under flow conditions that mimic those found in arteries or veins. Figure 19.11 shows a typical apparatus that has been used for this purpose. The model can be employed to study the basic functions of endothelial cells and their responses to factors such as nutrients that may be present when they are subjected to the stresses that are found in blood vessels *in vivo*, and

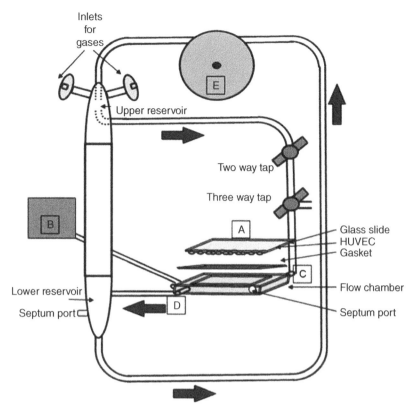

Figure 19.11 Cell culture under flow. (a) Flow chamber, silicon gasket and glass slide with attached confluent monolayer of endothelial cells (b) vacuum pump at the periphery of the chamber complex. The flow chamber has two slits through which flow medium enters and exits the channel (c, d). The flow rate is controlled by the peristaltic pump (e). Cell culture medium or diluted blood is recirculated from the reservoir to the inlet tubing onto the flow chamber and back into the reservoir (grey arrows). Reproduced from Macey, M., Wolf, S.I. and Lawson, C. (2010) Microparticle formation after exposure of blood to activated endothelium under flow. *Cytometry Part A*, **77A**, 761–768.

may also be used to investigate cell–cell interactions, such as the adhesion of leucocytes to the endothelium, which are important in the development of vascular diseases such as atherosclerosis.

- *Three-dimensional (3D) culture.* Monolayer cultures of cells can be considered to be two dimensional (2D), since in the conditions normally used the cells flatten to form a thin layer. Clearly, however, in their natural environment cells live and grow in three dimensions, and in recent years methods have been developed to reproduce similar conditions *in vitro*. These involve providing a gel that acts as a scaffold for the cells, rather like the ECM does *in vivo*. Both synthetic and natural (using proteins of the ECM such as collagen and fibronectin) hydrogels have been used with some success, but this technology is still in its infancy and the vast majority of experimental work with cultured cells is still done in conventional 2D systems.

19.6 *Ex vivo* methods

Isolated perfused organs

A number of organs, including the heart, kidney and liver, retain their functions for some hours when isolated from experimental animals and perfused via convenient blood vessels at 37 °C with a physiological medium containing of salts and nutrients and oxygenated with 95% oxygen/5% CO_2. In some systems oxygenated whole blood may be used as the perfusate. Basic functions and the responses of the tissue to factors such as test nutrients added to the system can be investigated by analysis of the perfusate and the tissue after the experiment. For example, the Langendorff heart perfusion model (Figure 19.12), in which the heart is kept beating for several hours after its removal from the body, is used extensively for studies of basic cardiac functions and pharmacological investigations. Reverse perfusion of the

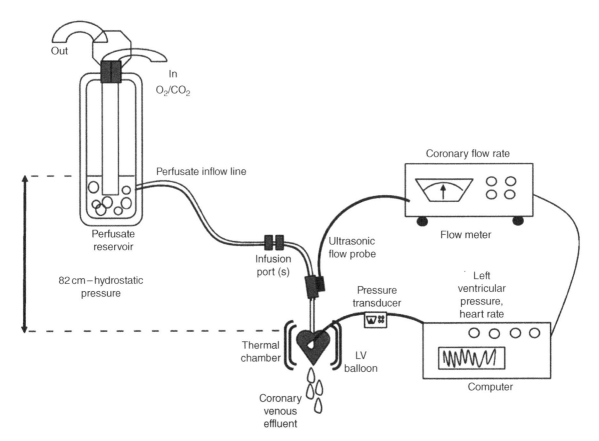

Figure 19.12 The Langendorff heart perfusion model. The perfusion solution enters the aorta via the aortic cannula, passing through a water-jacketed tubing system from a water-jacketed reservoir gassed with oxygen and carbon dioxide (95% and 5% respectively). The system keeps the level of the perfusion solution at a constant level, allowing retrograde perfusion at a constant hydrostatic pressure of 82 cm H_2O (for rat hearts). The perfusion solution flow rate, reflecting the flow rate in the coronary circulation, is recorded by a Doppler flow meter placed in the inflow line. Left ventricular systolic and diastolic pressures and heart rate are recorded by a pressure transducer connected to a small balloon placed in the left ventricle. Devices are connected to a computer, which allows the recording and analysis of data. Reprinted from Skrzypiec-Spring, M., Grotthus, B., Szelag, A. and Schulz, R. (2007) Isolated heart perfusion according to Langendorff: Still viable in the new millenium. *Journal of Pharmacological and Toxicological Methods*, **55**, 113–126. Copyright 2007, with permission from Elsevier.

organ via cannulation of the aorta causes the aortic valve to close and allows the perfusate to flow through the coronary blood system. This model is commonly used for the investigation of heart functions such as heart rate and contractile strength, and also of the responses to ischaemic injury.

Tissue segments, explants and microstructures

True perfusion involving blood vessel cannulation is often not necessary to keep small segments of tissue functioning for several hours if they are placed in an oxygenated physiological medium in an temperature-controlled organ bath. Blood vessel contraction and relaxation, for example, are commonly tested in such systems using rings of arterial tissue mounted on wires; and, of particular relevance to nutrition research, small segments of intestine (sometimes called gut sacs), flushed and often turned inside out (everted), are widely used to study the transport of molecules across the intestinal epithelium (Figure 19.13). Ion transport across epithelial cells can also be measured using an Ussing chamber (Figure 19.14). This consists of two halves that are clamped together around a sheet of intestinal mucosa (or a monolayer of epithelial cells), so that the apical and basolateral sides of the cells are separated. When both sides of the chamber are filled with the same physiological solution, a voltage change is generated by the

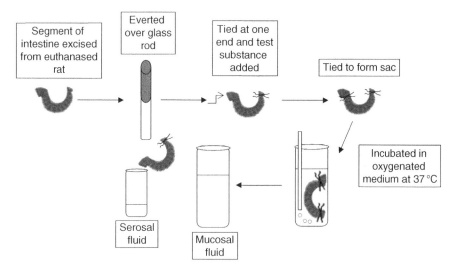

Figure 19.13 The rat everted gut sac model. Segments of intestine are excised from the rat and everted using a glass rod. They are then tied at one end, the test substance is introduced and the other end is tied to form a sac. The sacs are incubated in oxygenated physiological medium at 37°C for the desired period and the mucosal fluid (remaining in the incubation vessel) and the serosal fluid (from inside the sac) is collected for analysis.

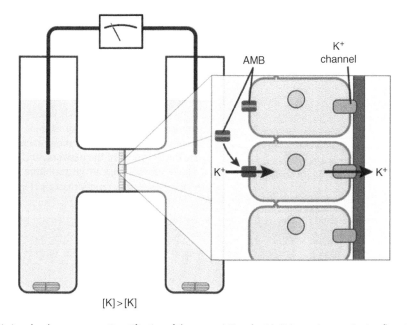

Figure 19.14 The Ussing chamber apparatus. Quantification of the permeability of epithelial monolayers using ion flow. Here, a monolayer of intestinal epithelial cells was used with the apical side facing a buffer containing a high concentration of K^+ and the basolateral side a low K^+ concentration. On addition of a permeabilising agent (amphotericin B, AMB) to the apical side, the concentration gradient drives K^+ through the cell layer and the resulting trans-epithelial current can be measured. Reprinted from Burgess, B.L., Cavigiolio, G., Fannucchi, M.V. *et al.* (2010) A phospholipid–apolipoprotein A-I nanoparticle containing amphotericin B as a drug delivery platform with cell membrane protective properties. *International Journal of Pharmaceutics*, **399**, 1–2, 148–155. Copyright 2010, with permission from Elsevier.

movement of ions across the cell layer, which can be used to measure their net transport very accurately.

When tissue explants are used to study the tissue function rather than as a source of isolated cells, the small tissue pieces are usually maintained on a collagen substratum, which helps the attachment of the tissue to the surface and also forms microchannels to allow the cells in the explant greater contact with the culture medium.

Another approach that falls somewhere in between isolated cell and tissue explant models is the isolation and culture of tissue microstructures consisting of functional groups of cells, which may include different cell types. An example of this that has been very successful is the use of islets of Langerhans (containing alpha, beta and delta cells, which secrete glucagen, insulin and somatostatin, respectively, as well as other cell types) from the pancreas to study the causes of diabetes. The pancreatic tissue is gently digested with collagenase, either by mincing or by perfusion *in situ* in the experimental animal, and the islets are then separated from non-islet tissue and single cells by density gradient centrifugation (Figure 19.15). The islets are cultured in

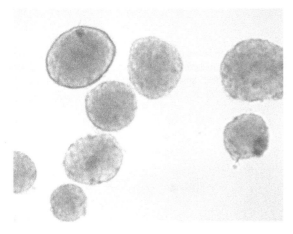

Figure 19.15 Isolated pancreatic islets in culture. Reprinted from Carter, J.D., Dula, S.N., Corbin, K.L. *et al.* (2009) A practical guide to rodent islet isolation and assessment. *Biological Procedures Online*, **11**, 1, 3–31. © BioMed Central.

suspension and glucose sensitivity has been reported to be retained for up to 7 days, although other changes in function may occur after 1–4 days.

The chick chorioallantoic membrane assay

A widely used experimental approach that falls between *in vivo* and *in vitro*, but does not fit well into the *ex vivo* categories described here, is the chick chorioallantoic membrane assay. The chorioallantoic membrane of a developing chick embryo is highly vascularised and the blood vessel network can be easily accessed for observation by cutting a window in the egg shell, making it a good model for the study of the growth of new blood vessels, termed angiogenesis. The natural process of angiogenesis enables wounds to heal and animals to reproduce. However, it is also essential for the growth of cancerous tumours and underlies the development of other disease conditions, such as age-related macular degeneration (causing blindness in the elderly), skin diseases and diabetic ulcers. The study of the processes regulating angiogenesis and substances that may influence it, therefore, is of vital importance for medical and nutrition research, and because it is relatively inexpensive and simple to carry out, the chick chorioallantoic assay is one of the most common methods used.

To prepare fertilised eggs for a typical experiment, the shell is cut away from the airspace at one end to expose the inner cell membrane, which lies on top of the chorioallantoic membrane. After infusion of saline the blood vessels in the chorioallantoic membrane become visible and the development of the network, and how it is affected by added substances, can be monitored and quantified by scoring using a stereomicroscope (Figure 19.16).

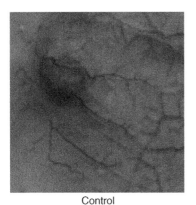
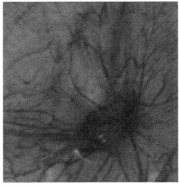
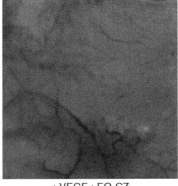

Control	+VEGF	+ VEGF + EO-CZ

Figure 19.16 Use of the chick chorioallantoic membrane assay to demonstrate the anti-angiogenesis effect of essential oil from Curcuma zedoaria (EO-CZ), a traditional Chinese herb. In the presence of vascular endothelial growth factor (VEGF), a positive control, angiogenesis is increased, but when EO-CZ is added the process is inhibited. Reprinted from Chen, W., Lu, Y., Gao, M. *et al.* (2011) Anti-angiogenesis effect of essential oil from Curcuma zedoaria in vitro and in vivo. *Journal of Ethnopharmacology*, **133**, 1, 220–226. Copyright 2011, with permission from Elsevier.

19.7 Analytical methods

In cell culture models, both medium and/or cells/tissues may be analysed by a wide variety of methods in general use, many of which are covered in other chapters in this book. 'Omics' technology such as genomics, proteomics and metabolomics (Chapters 13 and 16) may be applied; gene expression may be assessed using molecular biology techniques such as polymerase chain reaction (PCR) and immunoblotting (sometimes called Western blotting); and genes may be over-expressed or knocked out using transfection techniques or small interfering RNA (siRNA). Cell functions may be assessed by methods including the determination of the production of metabolites and/or enzyme activities, and the secretion of substances such as hormones, cytokines and so on. Cell models, however, are particularly suited to the investigation of cell behaviours such as proliferation, differentiation, apoptosis (programmed cell death), migration and motility, and are also widely used to study the regulation of expression of specific proteins and their subcellular location and transport using immunocytochemistry. Many of these studies, in turn, are dependent on visualisation of the cells (cell imaging) using microscopy.

Microscopy

Since Van Leeuwenhoek discovered cells in the late seventeenth century using the first practical microscope, microscopy has been a powerful technique in biological research. To overcome the magnification limitations of the light, or optical, microscope, the electron microscope was developed in the 1930s, providing the ability to see cell ultrastructure and even individual macromolecules. Fluorescence microscopy, which uses fluorescence to produce an image, became available in the early twentieth century. It was the development of confocal microscopy in the 1950s, however, that revolutionised cell and tissue imaging and enabled the production of the highly sophisticated pictures that we see today.

Light microscopy

Light microscopy has been used for observations of living cells for more than 300 years, and is still an important tool in the study of cells and tissue. The inverted microscope (Figure 19.17) in which the objectives are below the specimen under observation, while the light source and condenser are on top ('inverted' as compared to a conventional light microscope), is of particular value for cell culture models because it enables cells to be viewed in the bottom of cell culture dishes, rather than on a glass slide under a cover slip. In these conditions cells remain

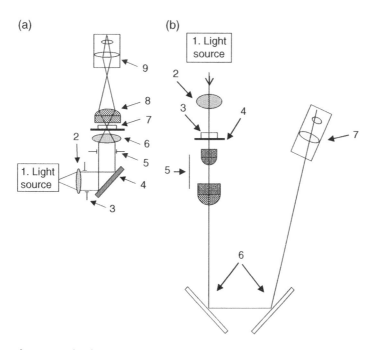

Figure 19.17 Comparison of conventional and inverted microscope systems. (a) Typical conventional microscope: 1. Light source; 2. Collecting lens; 3. Field diaphragm; 4. Mirror; 5. Iris diaphragm; 6. Condenser; 7. Sample; 8. Objective lens; 9. Eyepiece. (b) Inverted microscope; 1. Light source; 2. Condenser lens; 3. Sample; 4. Sample stage; 5. Objective lens; 6. Mirror; 7. Eyepiece.

alive over a much longer period. Phase contrast microscopy is a type of light microscopy in which the brightness of an image is altered according the phase shifts of light passing through a transparent object. This enables cells to be viewed without staining and is an important technique used for the observation of living cells (see later in this chapter).

Electron microscopy

In this system, a beam of electrons is used to produce very high magnifications (up to $\times 10\,000\,000$ compared to a maximum of about $\times 2000$ in a conventional light microscope). This resolution is sufficient to visualise individual macromolecules, and so it is an immensely powerful technique. Its drawback in relation to research with cell models, however, is that the specimen under observation needs to be in a vacuum, so it cannot be used to examine living cells.

Fluorescence microscopy

When materials emit light after excitation with light of a different wavelength, they are said to fluoresce. A fluorescence microscope takes advantage of this phenomenon to produce an image. The specimen is irradiated by light at an appropriate wavelength and the fluorescence can then be observed after passing the light through a series of filters. Some cell constituents (e.g. chlorophyll) fluoresce in their natural form, but normally a fluorescent probe is used (see later in this chapter).

Confocal microscopy

An important disadvantage of fluorescence microscopy is that because all of the specimen is fluorescing at the same time, there is always an unfocused background (or haze) in the image. Confocal microscopy overcomes this problem by using a pinhole to eliminate the out-of-focus

light so that, because of the small depth of field, the image is produced from a thin section of the sample (Figure 19.18). By scanning through a series of these thin sections, a clear 3D picture is built up. This system produces very high-quality images and is widely used for imaging in cell culture studies.

Immunocytochemistry and immunohistochemistry

Histochemistry is defined as the identification of chemical compounds in biological specimens and the study of their distribution, and traditionally employs histological staining or other imaging techniques in conjunction with microscopy. For example, hematoxylin and eosin (H&E) staining is very widely used to distinguish the cell nuclei, which is stained blue by hematoxylin, and the cell cytosol, which is stained pink by eosin (Figure 19.19). Immunohistochemistry is a refinement of this technique that uses the biological specificity of antibodies to detect particular proteins, providing information about their presence, subcellular location and movement within cells. This technique is widely used in studies with cellular models, but because in these systems the cells have almost always been removed from their extracellular matrix, in this case it is termed immunocytochemistry, rather than immunohistochemistry.

The essential principle of immunocytochemistry is the tagging of the protein of interest (the antigen) with a specific antibody, which is linked directly or indirectly to a fluorescent probe such as fluorescein isothiocyanate (FITC) or rhodamine. The sensitivity of the direct method is low, and indirect labelling in which the probe is attached to a secondary antibody, which binds to the immunoglobulin G (IgG) of the animal used to raise the

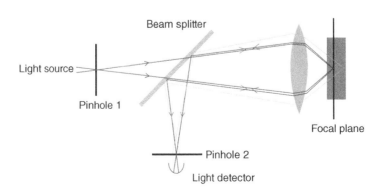

Figure 19.18 In confocal microscopy, a common focal plane for lightpaths for illumination and detection is achieved using two pinholes, each of which is the same distance from the sample. The light passes through a pinhole and is reflected by a beam splitter to the objective and sample. The emitted light from the sample passes through the beam splitter to the detection pinhole and the detector. This use of the pinholes means that light reaching the detector comes from a narrow focal plane. Thus, by scanning through a series of these thin sections a clear 3D image is produced.

(a)

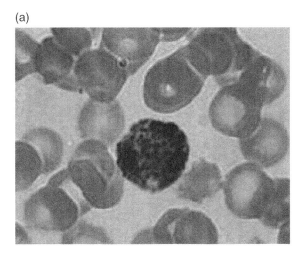

(b)

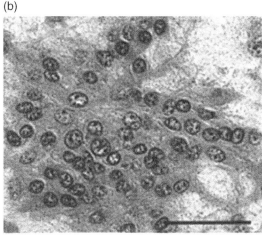

Figure 19.19 Hematoxylin and eosin (H&E) staining. Hematoxylin stains cell nuclei and other basophilic structures blue, while eosin stains eonosophilic structures pink or red. (a) The large dark cell in the centre is a basophilic granulocyte stained blue and so appears darker than the eosin-stained are eosinophilic erythrocytes. (b) A human adenoid cystic carcinoma cell line stained with H&E. The blue stained nuclei appear darker than the eosin-stained cell cytoplasm. (b) is reprinted with permission from Spandidos Publications. Tanaka, N., Urabe, K., Hashitani, S. *et al.* (2007) Establishment and characterization of a human adenoid cystic carcinoma cell line forming colonies cultured in collagen gel and transplantable in nude mice. *Oncology Reports*, **17**, 2, 335–340.

primary antibody, is more commonly used. For example, if the primary antibody was raised in a mouse, then the secondary antibody linked to the fluorescent probe would be anti-mouse IgG raised in another species, such as a rabbit or a sheep. Since more than one secondary antibody binds to the primary antibody the signal from the probe is amplified, increasing the sensitivity of the detection. Indirect labelling also avoids the potentially expensive and time-consuming process of producing a fluorescent-linked antibody for each specific protein under study, since antibodies to IgG from many species are widely available commercially. After treatment with the antibodies, cell images are generated using fluorescence or confocal microscopy (see later in this chapter). A typical experiment using confocal microscopy is shown in Figure 19.20. Interpretation of the image is often assisted by using a different stain to delineate the cell or a prominent subcellular organelle (counterstaining): for example, 4′,6-diamidino-2-phenylindole (DAPI) is commonly used to stain the cell nucleus blue (Figure 19.21). Two (or more) proteins can also be studied simultaneously using fluorescence of different colours, allowing investigation of their co-localisation or other interactions in processes such as endocytosis.

Live cell imaging

For immunocytochemistry studies, cells need to be attached to a solid support and permeabilised to allow the antibodies and fluorescent probes to enter the cells. In addition, chemical fluorophores such as FITC can cause phototoxicity and are prone to photobleaching, which affects the stability of the image. In order to be useful for live cell imaging, a fluorescent probe must be able to enter the cell without damaging its structural integrity, be specifically targeted to a molecule or organelle and be detectable while the cell is alive. In recent years, therefore, a number of chemical probes have been developed that meet these criteria, including the application of nanotechnology using quantum dots. In addition, biological fluorophores such as green fluorescent protein (GFP) have emerged that have greatly aided the study of dynamic processes within living cells.

Chemical fluorescent probes for live cell imaging

Examples of chemical probes that can be used with live cells include Indo-1 (2-[4-(bis(carboxymethyl)amino)-3-[2-[2-(bis(carboxymethyl) amino)- 5-methylphenoxy] ethoxy] phenyl]-1H-indole-6-carboxylic acid), which fluoresces when bound to calcium ions; linear fluorescence resonance energy transfer (FRET) and oligonucleotide (ODN) probes, used to monitor the expression of specific RNAs; and lipophilic probes such as DiI (alkyl-3,3,3′,3′-tetramethylindocarbocyanine) and DiD (1,1′-dioctadecyl-3,3,3′,3′-tetramethylindo-dicarbocyanine perchlorate), which label cell membranes. Dynamic cell processes such as endocytosis can also be investigated by linking the molecule under study to a non-toxic probe such as DiI or DiD, which is able to enter intact cells.

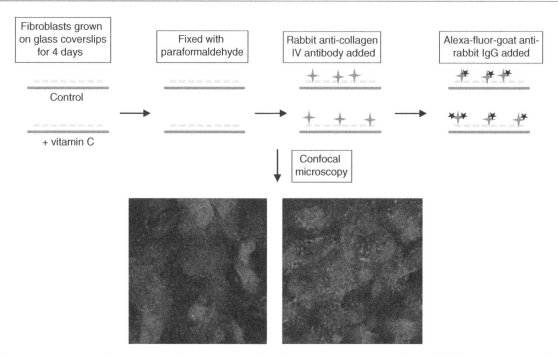

Figure 19.20 Immunocytochemistry: a typical experiment using confocal microscopy. Primary mouse embryonic fibroblasts were grown on glass coverslips for 4 days in the presence or absence of 20 mM vitamin C. Cells were fixed with 4% paraformaldehyde then treated with rabbit anti-collagen IV antibody followed by Alexa Fluor® 488–labelled goat anti-rabbit immunoglobulin G. A confocal microscope with ×63 objective lens was used to capture images, which show that intracellular collagen levels are increased after incubation with vitamin C. Reproduced from Kuo, S.M., Burl, L.R. and Hu, Z. (2012) Cellular phenotype-dependent and independent effects of vitamin C on the renewal and gene expression of mouse embryonic fibroblasts. PLOS One, **7**, 3, e32957.

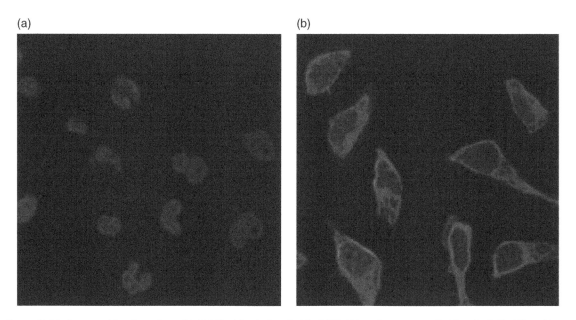

Figure 19.21 Counterstaining the nucleus with 4′,6-diamidino-2-phenylindole (DAPI). HeLa cells were treated with anti-tubulin followed by an Alexa fluor–labelled secondary antibody and counterstained with DAPI. (a) DAPI staining only, in the image, the blue-stained nuclei appear medium grey on the dark background. (b) Tubulin and DAPI, the pink-stained tubulin in the cell cytosol can now be seen as lighter grey areas around the nuclei. Reprinted from Park, J., Lammers, F., Herr, W. and Song, J.-J. (2012) HCF-1 self-association via an interdigitated Fn3 structure facilitates transcriptional regulatory complex formation. Proceedings of the National Academy of Sciences, **109**, 43, 17430–17435.

Quantum dots

Quantum dots are an example of how the new science of nanotechnology can be used to further research on living cells. These nanoparticles are semiconductors of 2–10 nm in diameter (a width of only 50 atoms on average). They fluoresce when excited by laser light and produce a brighter signal, which lasts longer than those produced by conventional fluorophores. These properties enable them to be used to study events inside living cells at the molecular level, including protein expression, trafficking and interactions with other molecules. This technique is in its infancy, but potentially in the future it may provide the ability to track drugs and nutrients as they enter cells and move through subcellular compartments.

Green fluorescent protein

Green fluorescent protein (GFP) is a natural protein found in marine organisms that fluoresces bright green when irradiated with light of wavelengths in the blue to ultraviolet part of the spectrum. It was cloned from the jellyfish *Aequora victoria* in the 1990s and has proved to be an invaluable tool in studies with cellular models. The gene for GFP can be introduced into cells by transfection, either by itself or fused to the gene for the protein of interest so that the protein is always expressed with GFP and is effectively tagged with a fluorescent label inside the living cell. The expression, subcellular location and movement of the protein can then be followed in real time using fluorescence or confocal microscopy. Since the cloning of the original GFP, a number of mutant forms of the protein have been developed to improve its fluorescence and stability, and colour variations such as yellow, blue and cyan fluorescent proteins have also been produced (Figure 19.22).

All the approaches described above depend on the culture of cells in a way that allows them to be viewed by an optical, fluorescence or confocal microscope. Live cell imaging culture chambers specially designed for this purpose enable cells to be viewed at high resolution while maintaining the conditions needed for normal cell processes to continue for many hours or even days. The simplest systems involve cells on a microscope slide under a sealed coverslip, while more complex chambers enable the temperature, atmosphere (gas composition and humidity), pH and culture medium to be controlled and also allow perfusion of the cells during the experiment. Using these techniques, digital videos can be obtained to show cell division (Figure 19.23) or the movement of proteins or organelles within cells (using fluorescent probes), for example the translocation of transcription factors to the nucleus, and the movement (or motility) of cells (using optical microscopes) in processes including the migration of neural axons to synapses and wound healing, in which cells such as fibroblasts or endothelial cells migrate to fill the space when a confluent monolayer is scratched. Modern computer software programs enable the data collected from these studies to be quantified and analysed in many different ways.

Flow cytometry

Although flow cytometry does not provide images of cells, it is nevertheless a powerful and versatile technique that is widely used with cell culture models. A flow cytometer measures cell characteristics as they flow in a culture medium through a laser beam. Cells are usually treated with a fluorescent probe and as they pass through the beam they scatter the light and fluoresce. The scattered and fluorescent light is then diverted to appropriate detectors using beam splitters and filters and computer analysis is used to provide information about subpopulations of cells, such as different types of white blood cells in blood or those expressing a particular surface antigen (Figure 19.24). Characteristics that can be measured in this system include cell size, granularity and internal complexity and relative fluorescence intensity.

One of the most common applications of flow cytometry is to determine the proportion of cells in a population that express surface or internally expressed antigens. As well as providing valuable information about the presence of particular proteins on or within cells, this is useful for the evaluation of a wide range of parameters, including cell viability, proliferation, necrosis, apoptosis, oncosis (ischaemic cell death), senescence and differentiation. In addition, flow cytometry can be employed to measure DNA and RNA content, calcium flux, membrane potential and the generation of reactive oxygen species in cells, and is also used for cell sorting by FACS (see earlier in this chapter).

19.8 Cellular models in basic nutrition research

An understanding of how nutrients influence the basic functions of cell in the normal animal is crucial for the optimisation of nutritional status, and cellular models have provided invaluable information that has helped to build the current consensus. The effects of nutrients on numerous and diverse cell functions, including cell proliferation, migration, differentiation, cell cycle, apoptosis, cell signalling pathways, gene expression, ion transport, secretion of hormones or other factors, enzyme

(a)

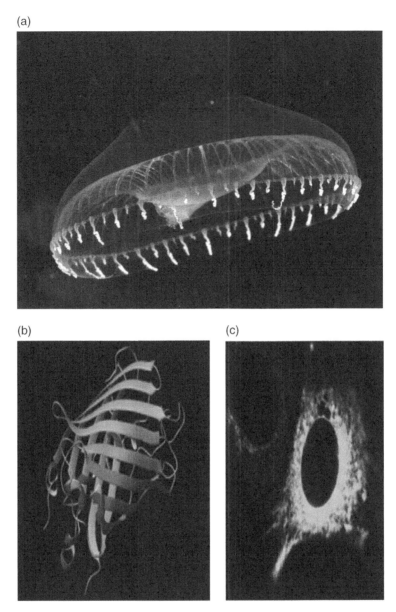

(b)   (c)

Figure 19.22 Green fluorescent protein (GFP). (a) The jellyfish Aequora victoria, which expresses GFP naturally. (b) Molecular model of GFP structure. (c) Mouse myoblasts transfected with a plasmid containing the gene for SPCA2 (a Ca^{2+} ATPase enzyme) linked to the gene for GFP. (a) http://en.wikipedia.org/wiki/File:Aequorea4.jpg, © Sierra Blakeley (b) Structure protein data bank (1EMA), http://www.rcsb.org/pdb/index.html (c) Reproduced from Pestov, N.B., Dmitriev, R.I., Kostina, M.B. *et al.* (2012) Structural evolution and tissue-specific expression of tetrapod-specific second isoform of secretory pathway Ca(2+)-ATPase. Biochemical and Biophysical Research Communications, **417**, 4, 1298–1303, with permission.

| −43 | −37 | −34 | −1.6 | 0 | 1.6 | 4.8 | 6.4 | 10 | 29 min |

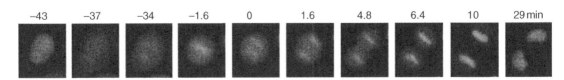

Figure 19.23 Live cell imaging. Images from a time-lapse video of an HeLa cell showing cell division. Cells were maintained in a microscope stage incubator at 37°C in a humidified atmosphere of 5% CO_2 throughout the experiment. Reprinted by permission from Macmillan Publishers Ltd: Schmitz, M.H., Held, M., Janssens, V. *et al.* (2010) Live-cell imaging RNAi screen identifies PP2A-B55alpha and importin-beta1 as key mitotic exit regulators in human cells. Nature Cell Biology, **12**, 9, 886–893, copyright 2010.

(a)

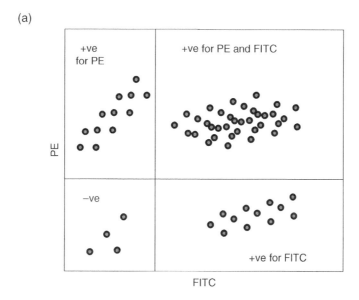

(b)

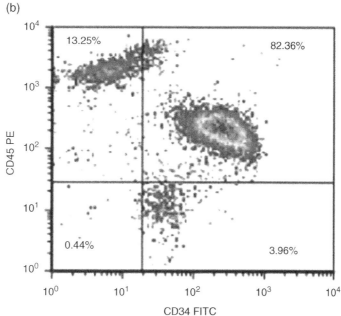

Figure 19.24 Flow cytometry. (a) Diagram showing flow cytometry dot plot of cells expressing two surface antigens labelled with either phycoerythrin (PE) or fluorescein isothiocyanate FITC). Lower left quadrant, cells −ve for both labels; top left quadrant, cells +ve for PE; lower right quadrant, cells +ve for FITC; top right quadrant, cells +ve for both labels. (b) Flow cytometry dot plot showing expression of CD45 (PE label) and CD34 (FITC label) on human B cells. Reproduced from www.lifelinecelltech.com/product-specs/spc-hbc.asp.

activities and many more have been studied using these methods. Some examples include:

- *Mechanisms of action of vitamin D.* Experiments using the Ussing chamber (see earlier in this chapter), everted gut sacs, intestinal cell lines such as CaCo-2, cultured kidney tubules and bone cells such as chondrocytes and osteoblasts have been used to help identify the proteins (such as receptors and proton pumps) and cell signalling pathways involved in the effects of 1,25 dihydroxy vitamin D3 (or calcitriol), the active form of vitamin D3 (cholecalciferol) in the body, on bone and mineral homeostasis.

- *Liver lipid metabolism.* The liver has a central role in processing dietary lipids. One of its major functions in this respect is to secrete very low-density lipoprotein (VLDL), which carries triacylglycerols to the tissues and is also the precursor of low-density lipoprotein (LDL), the major blood cholesterol carrier in humans. Studies with the isolated perfused rat liver and both primary isolated hepatocytes from humans and rodents as well as liver cell lines, including human HepG2 and rat McA-RH7777 cells, have made an important contribution to knowledge about the mechanisms by which saturated and polyunsaturated fats in the diet regulate hepatic VLDL secretion.

- *The multiple functions of retinoids.* Retinoids are compounds related to vitamin A, of which retinyl esters and plant carotenoids such as β-carotene (which gives carrots their orange colour) occur naturally in foodstuffs and are nutrients required for health. After conversion to the active forms in the body, retinoids function in multiple processes including vision, gene transcription, cell differentiation, reproduction and skin maintenance. Determination of the role of these compounds in many of these functions has been facilitated by cellular models such as cultured Müller cells (glial cells of the retina) and retinal rod photoreceptor cells for the study of retinoids in vision; cultured keratinocytes for mechanisms by which skin health is maintained; and embryonic stem cells for investigation of functions in differentiation and reproduction.

Knowledge of the bioavailability of a nutrient is clearly of great importance for nutrition research, as altering the amount of a component in the diet will have no effect on the body unless the amount reaching the bloodstream is also changed. Bioavailability is influenced by a number of factors. Nutrients in food are contained in a matrix, which may be altered by how it is cooked or prepared, and this influences the amount of nutrient available for absorption in the intestine. For example, the bioavailability of the red tomato pigment lycopene, a micronutrient with antioxidant properties, is higher after processing into products such as tomato purée or ketchup than in the raw fruit. In addition, individual compounds, even in their free form, differ in their absorbability by intestinal epithelial cells. *Ex vivo* and *in vitro* methods of assessing bioavailability using cellular models are often more convenient, less expensive and allow better control of experimental variables than whole animal studies. Although rat everted gut sacs mimic physiological conditions more closely than isolated cell systems and give higher rates of transport, the most common *in vitro* model currently employed is monolayers of the human intestinal epithelial cell line, CaCo-2, in the Ussing chamber or grown on membrane inserts (see earlier in this chapter).

In addition to the traditional categories of nutrients, including carbohydrates, proteins and amino acids, fats, vitamins and minerals, in the past few decades it has been recognised that many substances produced by plants and present in small quantities in common foods such as fruit and vegetables are beneficial to health, and can be classed as micronutrients. Cultured cell models have made a major contribution to the discovery that a number of compounds belonging to groups such as flavonoids (e.g. catechins and quercitin found in green tea; anthocyanins, the red, blue or purple pigments found in berries), polyphenols (e.g. oleuropein derivatives found in virgin olive oil; resveratrol found in red wine) and carotenoids (e.g. lycopene, the red pigment in tomatoes) have antioxidant, anti-allergenic and/or anti-inflammatory properties. There are, however, thousands of such compounds produced by plants, many of which may prove beneficial, and cellular models provide convenient and relatively inexpensive methods to test their potential prior to more complex and costly intervention trials in animals and, ultimately, human subjects.

19.9 Cellular models in research on the role of nutrition in disease

As well as the deficiency diseases caused by a lack of particular nutrients in the diet, malnutrition is closely linked with infectious diseases in the under-nourished, causing poor growth, increased susceptibility to infection and increased mortality. Nutritionally acquired immunodeficiency syndrome (NAIDS) is the most common cause of immunodeficiency in the world and affects more than 100 million people, most of them children. Diseases related to poor nutrition, however, are not always due to lack of food. In the last three decades there has been a rise in the incidence of obesity and other related metabolic disorders such as insulin resistance and type 2 diabetes mellitus – mainly in developed countries, but increasingly also in the developing world – which is so large that it has to be compared to an epidemic. Modern diets rich in processed food, high in fat and low in vegetables and fruit are a major factor in this explosive increase. In addition, it has become evident in the past decades that good nutrition has a role in the prevention or retardation of the development of chronic diseases such as cancer, heart disease and neurogenerative disorders (e.g. Alzheimer's disease and Parkinson's disease). Clearly, therefore, research into the interactions between nutrients and the development of these various diseases is of vital importance, and cellular models provide valuable research tools to aid in these investigations.

Infectious disease

Malnutrition is linked to infectious disease in a downward spiral in which weight loss, depressed immune responses and low growth (in children) caused by too little food in the diet increase susceptibility to infection, and diarrhoea and fever caused by infection lead to reduced absorption of nutrients, loss of appetite and increased demand for energy and micronutrients (Figure 19.25), thus aggravating the under-nutrition. This synergistic relationship between nutrition and infection is influenced by a number of factors, including:

- Reduced capacity to form antibodies
- Decreased phagocytic activity of macrophages
- Reduced production of substances that protect against infection (e.g. cytokines) in response to bacterial toxins such as lipopolysaccharide
- Reduced inflammatory response
- Delayed wound healing and collagen formation
- Altered intestinal flora
- Changes in endocrine activity

Lack of sufficient protein in the diet is known to be closely associated with these changes, but micronutrient deficiencies also play a significant role. Cellular models have made an important contribution to the understanding of many of these interactions between malnutrition and infection. For example, reduced phagocytic activity, decreased secretion of inflammatory cytokines such as

tumour necrosis factor -α (TNF-α, produced to protect against bacterial toxins) and suppressed translocation to the nucleus of nuclear factor-κB (NF-κB, a transcription factor that mediates inflammatory responses) during protein deprivation or starvation have been demonstrated using monolayer cultures of primary rodent peritoneal and alveolar macrophages and murine macrophage cell lines. In addition, delayed wound healing in malnourished individuals has been shown to involve reduced fibroblast proliferation, decreased collagen synthesis and dysfunction of B and T lymphocytes in cultured cell models.

Metabolic diseases

Obesity is the most common metabolic disorder in the developed world. Its increasing prevalence is due to over-consumption of food high in fat and sugar and low levels of physical exercise, leading to the formation of excess adipose tissue in the body. Obese individuals are predisposed to other metabolic disorders including insulin resistance and type 2 diabetes (as well as to hypertension, heart disease and cancer); extensive epidemiological studies indicate that these conditions are also related to nutrition, since diets rich in fruit, vegetables and fibre protect against their development.

Adipose tissue is not only the main energy reservoir in the body, storing fatty acids in the form of triacylglycerols and mobilising them when required, but is now recognised as an endocrine organ that has important roles in energy balance, appetite regulation, sensitivity of tissues to insulin and inflammatory responses. Because of the part played by excess adiposity in metabolic diseases, an understanding of the mechanisms regulating the way in which adipose tissue develops and expands is paramount, and adipocyte cell models have proved to be a powerful tool for the study of these processes. Figure 19.26 illustrates the difference between healthy and obese adipose tissue.

Unlike most adult tissues, adipose tissue contains stem cell adipocyte precursors, enabling adipose tissue

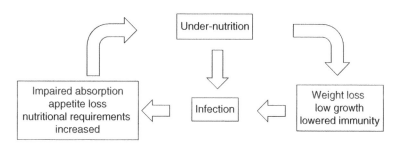

Figure 19.25 The nutrition–infection cycle.

(a)　　　　　　　　　　　　　　　　　　　(b)

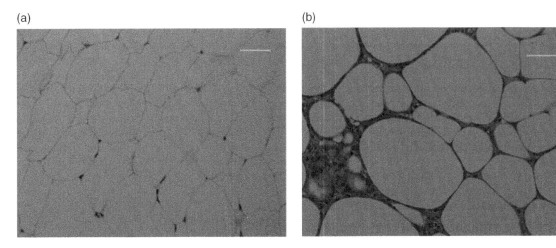

Figure 19.26 Comparison of adipose tissue in normal and genetically obese (ob/ob) mice. (a) Healthy epididymal fat pad tissue from a normal mouse with densely packed, hexagonal adipocytes and limited immune cell infiltration. (b) Epididymal fat pad tissue from an ob/ob mouse containing a high level of immune cell infiltration and enhanced ECM (dark areas). Scale bars: 50 μm. Reprinted with permission of American Society for Clinical Investigation, from Sun, K., Kusminski, C.M. and Scherer, P.E. (2011) Adipose tissue remodelling and obesity. Journal of Clinical Investigation, **121**, 6, 2094–2101; permission conveyed through Copyright Clearance Center, Inc.

to expand via the formation of new fat cells at any stage of life. The ability of pre-adipocytes to differentiate into mature adipocytes *in vitro* in the appropriate culture conditions has provided a marvellous cellular model for investigation of the processes involved in adipocyte differentiation. Tissue from both humans and experimental animals can be studied in this way, and this system has made a major contribution to knowledge about the influence of nutrition in this area over the past 20 years.

In addition to adipocyte cell models, the use of isolated pancreatic islets in culture (see earlier in this chapter and Figure 19.15), a technique developed by Paul Lacey in the late 1960s, has been important in the investigation of the cellular and molecular mechanisms regulating insulin secretion by β-cells and the interactions between α-, β- and γ-cells in the islets, how they are disturbed in type 2 diabetes and how the effects of the disease may be modulated by nutrients. Isolated primary hepatocytes, hepatocyte cell lines and, to a more limited extent, the isolated perfused liver are other *in vitro* and *ex vivo* models that have been widely used in studying the links between nutrition and metabolic diseases. Monolayer cultures of primary rat hepatocytes and the hepatoma cell lines HepG2 (human) and McA-RH7777 (rat), as well as the perfused rat liver, have been used to investigate, for example, the action of insulin on liver cells and the dysfunctions in lipid metabolism associated with obesity and type 2 diabetes, and how they are influenced by nutrients such as glucose, fructose, fatty acids and

micronutrients such as flavonoids and polyphenols found in fruit and vegetables.

Chronic degenerative diseases

It is now clearly established that poor nutrition is a factor in the development of chronic diseases such as heart disease, cancer and neurodegenerative diseases, and it has been suggested that a properly balanced diet is crucial for the retardation or prevention of all major chronic degenerative diseases that start to be apparent in middle age.

Heart disease

Early studies on the relationship between nutrition and cardiovascular disease focused on the role of different types of fatty acids in the diet (i.e. saturated or unsaturated), but more recently the emphasis of much research has shifted to the role of ω-3 polyunsaturated fatty acids (found in oily fish) and micronutrients such as vitamins, carotenoids, flavonoids and polyphenols from fruit and vegetables. Atherosclerosis, a condition in which lipid is deposited in the artery wall causing narrowing of the arteries, is a major cause of cardiovascular disease and is closely interlinked with the diet. Dysfunction of the vascular endothelium is followed by invasion of the vessel wall by monocytes, differentiation into macrophages and the generation of lipid-engorged macrophage foam cells. The accumulation of foam cells together with the proliferation and migration of vascular smooth muscle cells

(VSMC) to form a fibrous cap results in the formation of atherosclerotic lesions. The influence of nutrition on these early events has been extensively studied using cultured cell models of all the various cell types involved. Examples include:

- The investigation of endothelial function using blood vessel rings in organ bath experiments (see earlier in this chapter) and monolayer cultures of primary endothelial cells such as HUVEC, porcine pulmonary and human aortic endothelial cells.
- The use of primary human monocytes and the human monocyte cell line THP-1 in suspension culture to evaluate monocyte activation and chemotaxis.
- The study of macrophage foam cell formation using monolayer cultures of human monocyte-derived macrophages (HMDM), macrophages derived from the THP-1 cell line and the murine macrophage cell line J774.
- Proliferation and cell migration experiments using monolayer cultures of human aortic, porcine pulmonary artery and rat embryonic aorta VSMC.

In addition to the studies indicated using a single cell type *in vitro*, co-cultures of cells such as endothelial cells and monocytes, in static conditions or using a flow system (see earlier in this chapter), or endothelial cells and VSMC enable the investigation of cell–cell interactions in atherosclerosis development.

Cancer

The ability of cancerous cells to grow indefinitely in culture makes cellular culture models particularly useful for the study of the role of nutrition in cancer, and about 4700 papers in which cultured cells have been used for this purpose have been published since 2000. In comparison, cultured cell models have been employed in the investigation of the role of nutrients in atherosclerosis in about 300 studies in the same period. Some of the main diseases studied in this way are breast, liver and colorectal cancers, but prostate and pancreatic cancers and leukaemia are also well represented.

Neurodegenerative diseases

Since the discovery that low-level inflammation caused by oxidative stress is implicated in neurodegenerative conditions such as Alzheimer's disease, which progressively cause cognitive decline leading to dementia in old age, research into how nutrition may help to alleviate and delay the onset of these disorders has focused on the effects of micronutrients from plants such as polyphenols, flavonoids and anthocyanins, which are known to have antioxidant activity. Various cell types in culture, such as the murine BV-2 microglial cell line, the rat neuronal cell line PC12, human SH-SY5Y neuroblastoma

cells and primary rat hippocampal neuronal cells, have been used to study the effects of such compounds on the signalling pathways that mediate inflammatory responses and oxidative stress in the brain.

Parkinson's disease results from a progressive loss of neurons that respond to the neurotransmitter dopamine in the brain. As in Alzheimer's disease, oxidative stress is believed to play a part in the damage caused, thus plant-derived micronutrients with antioxidant activity may potentially be of benefit. As yet there have only been a few studies in this area using cultured cell models, but experiments with primary mouse cortical neurones and human neuroblastoma SH-SY5Y cells have demonstrated that polyphenols such as caffeic acid, tyrosol and oxyresveratrol protect the cells against the detrimental effects of oxidative stress.

19.10 Future directions

Methods for cell culture and live cell imaging are improving all the time and becoming more and more sophisticated. Since conventional 2D culture systems do not reproduce the anatomy and physiology of living tissues very well, culture in 3D, where cells are grown in an ECM that mimics that found *in vivo*, is likely to become more prevalent. In addition, the application of nanotechnology to live cell imaging using quantum dots provides the exciting potential to follow the progress of nutrients through cells and study their interactions with subcellular structures. Powerful modern analytical 'omics' techniques, particularly metabolomics, which provide a sensitive measure of both genotypical and phenotypical effects, also increase the value of cellular models for investigation of the effects of nutrients at the cellular and molecular levels. In the future, therefore, cellular models are likely to become increasingly important for basic nutrition research and that into the relationship between diet and disease.

References and further reading

Carter, J.D., Dula, S.B., Corbin, K.L. *et al.* (2009) A practical guide to rodent islet isolation and assessment. *Biological Procedures Online*, **11**, 1, 3–31.

Dzik-Jurasz, A.S.K. (2003) Molecular imaging in vivo: An introduction. *British Journal of Radiology*, **76**, S98–S109.

Gesta, S., Lolmede, K., Daviaud, D. *et al.* (2003) Culture of human adipose tissue explants lead to profound alteration of adipose gene expression. *Hormone and Metabolic Research*, **35**, 3, 158–163.

Katona, P. and Katona-Apte, J. (2008) The interaction between nutrition and infection. *Clinical Practice*, **46**, 1582–1588.

Lambrinoudaki, I., Ceasu, I., Depypere, H. *et al.* (2013) EMAS position statement: Diet and health in midlife and beyond. *Maturitas*, **74**, 99–104.

Rothman, S.S. (2002) *Lessons from the Living Cell: The Culture of Science and the Limits of Reductionism*. McGraw-Hill, New York.

Skrzypiec-Spring, M., Grotthus, B., Szelag, A. and Schulz, R. (2007) Isolated heart perfusion according to Langendorff: Still viable in the new millenium. *Journal of Pharmacological Toxicology Methods*, **55**, 113–126.

Srinivas, P.R., Philbert, M., Vu, T.Q. *et al.* (2010) Nanotecnology research: Applications in nutritional sciences. *Journal of Nutrition*, **140**, 119–124.

Sun, K., Kusminski, C.M. and Scherer, P.E. (2011) Adipose tissue remodelling and obesity. *Journal of Clinical Investigation*, **121**, 2094–2101.

20
Translation of Nutrition Research

Judith Buttriss

British Nutrition Foundation

Key messages

- To be effective and of value, the communication of nutrition principles should be based on robust evidence and be in a form that is relevant, accessible and understood by the intended audience.
- The internet and social media have transformed the options for communicating nutrition information.
- The approaches taken should be tailored to the topic and intended audience.

- Legislation shapes the information that can be communicated in some contexts.
- Nutrition research and policy shape public health communications and the agenda for the food industry.

20.1 Importance of the translation of nutrition science

To be of real use in a public health context, the findings of individual nutrition studies need to be rigorously assessed, considered in the context of the wider peer-reviewed literature and transformed into guidance that can steer individuals and those who advise them (e.g. health professionals and educators) towards healthier diets and lifestyles. To be effective and of value, the communication of nutrition principles should be based on robust evidence, set in the context of everyday life, consistent, timely, repeated over time to increase understanding and adoption, and in a form that will be relevant, accessible and understood by the target audience.

The benefit of getting this right is considerable. In the UK, for example, two-thirds of adults and almost a third of children are overweight or obese, and ill health associated with obesity and overweight is costing the NHS more than £5 billion each year. Furthermore, poor nutrition has a role to play in the aetiology of a number of chronic diseases, including cardiovascular disease (CVD), type 2 diabetes and some cancers, as well as conditions such as anaemia and dental caries.

Communication channels

A large European survey of 16 000 people (age 15 years and over) conducted in 2003 showed that advice from health professionals was an important source of information, but the media was also of considerable importance (Figure 20.1). Over the past decade or so, media channels have become more diverse and in just a couple of decades, information exchange has been transformed by the internet. While this development brings with it massive opportunities for knowledge transfer, it also has its challenges, not least the fact that new research is in the public domain almost instantaneously, sometimes before it has even been peer reviewed, and to the untrained eye in broader terms it is often not clear what is good science and what is flawed opinion.

Internet usage

The impact and reach of the internet are now huge. Worldwide in 2012 there were over 2.4 billion internet users (www.internetworldstats.com/stats.htm) and the penetration in different parts of the world is shown in Figure 20.2.

Nutrition Research Methodologies, First Edition. Edited by Julie A Lovegrove, Leanne Hodson, Sangita Sharma and Susan A Lanham-New.
© 2015 John Wiley & Sons, Ltd. Published 2015 by John Wiley & Sons, Ltd.
Companion Website: www.wiley.com/go/nutritionsociety

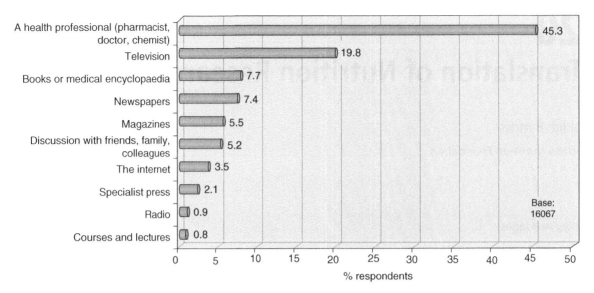

Figure 20.1 European Union citizens and sources of information about health. Reprinted from European Opinion Research Group, *European Union Citizens and Sources of Information about Health*, March 2003. © European Union, 1995–2014.

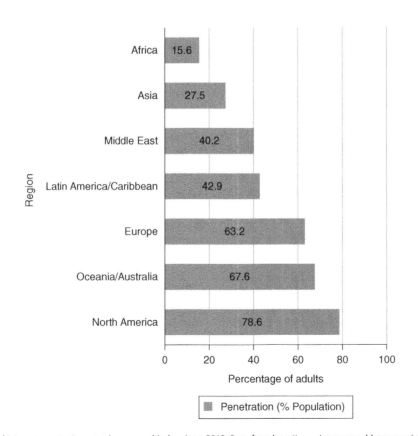

Figure 20.2 World internet penetration rates by geographical regions, 2012. Data from http://www.internetworldstats.com/stats.htm.

In Great Britain in 2012, according to the Office of National Statistics, 80% of households had internet access, almost exclusively via broadband, compared to less than 10% in 1998, and 67% of adults used a computer every day. The highest internet usage was in London (88% of adults) and the lowest in Northern Ireland (77% of adults), with all regions showing an increase since 2011. Men (87%) were slightly more likely to use the internet than women (83%), and 15% of adults had never used it. Figure 20.3 shows usage by different age groups.

The nature of internet usage in Britain is shown in Table 20.1, which reveals that the most common use is finding out about goods and services (77%), followed by social networking (57%) and using services related to travel and accommodation (57%). Use of social media

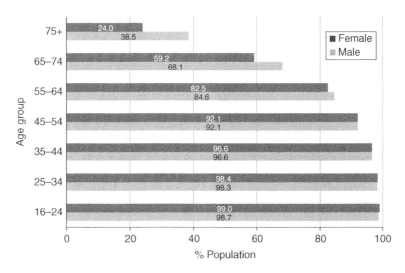

Figure 20.3 Internet users by age group and sex, 2012. Data from Office for National Statistics licensed under the Open Government Licence v.1.0, http://www.ons.gov.uk/ons/rel/rdit2/internet-access-quarterly-update/2012-q3/stb-iaqu.html.

Table 20.1 Internet activities by age group and sex, 2012. Data from Office for National Statistics licensed under the Open Government Licence v.1.0, http://www.ons.gov.uk/ons/rel/rdit2/internet-access—households-and-individuals/2012-part-2/stb-ia-2012part2.html.

	16–24	25–34	35–44	45–54	55–64	65+	Men	Women	% All
Sending/receiving emails	83	87	87	77	69	41	74	72	73
Finding information about goods and services	71	83	81	74	66	34	69	65	67
Buying goods or services over the internet	79	87	84	72	61	32	68	67	67
Social networking, for example Facebook or Twitter	87	78	62	40	24	10	48	48	48
Internet banking	43	69	65	52	43	18	51	44	47
Reading or downloading online news, newspapers or news magazines	58	66	59	49	38	20	51	44	47
Using services related to travel or travel-related accommodation	41	57	55	51	42	22	47	41	44
Playing or downloading games, images, films or music	67	60	46	36	27	12	43	37	40
Listening to web radio or watching web television	56	55	48	37	27	12	44	32	38
Uploading self-created content, for example text, photos, music, videos etc.	60	50	45	32	22	11	36	35	35
Posting messages to chat sites, blogs, forums or instant messaging	60	56	41	28	18	7	35	32	33
Telephoning or making video calls over the internet	45	49	40	31	23	11	33	31	32
Selling goods or services, for example on eBay	27	36	31	22	15	5	24	20	22
Making a medical appointment	7	15	12	12	11	4	11	9	10
Creating websites or blogs	16	11	7	5	1	1	7	6	6

Base: Adults (aged 16+) in Great Britain.

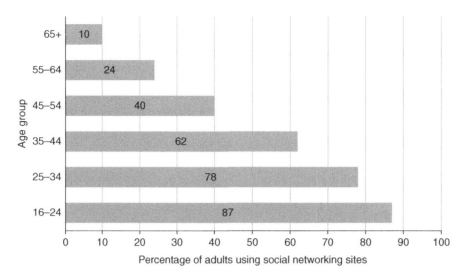

Figure 20.4 Social networking by age group in the UK, 2012. Data from Office for National Statistics licensed under the Open Government Licence v.1.0, http://www.ons.gov.uk/ons/rel/rdit2/internet-access---households-and-individuals/2012-part-2/stb-ia-2012part2.html.

was slightly more common in women (60%) than men (54%), and was almost universal in 16–24-year-olds (91%) and also commonplace in 25–34-year-olds (76%). The internet is used to search for health-related information by 42% of adults (51% of 25–34-year-olds).

Social media

A major change has been the escalating use of social media, especially among younger people. In 2012, 48% of all adults, irrespective of gender, used a social networking site, with a third of all adults having accessed sites through their mobile phone.

Social networking was the most popular internet activity in 16–24-year-olds, with 87% having used a social networking site in 2012. This was the first time that emailing had not been the most popular internet activity in any population group. However, social networking is not exclusively used by younger age groups (Figure 20.4). An EC-funded project (www.foodrisc.org) has compared food crisis coverage by social and traditional media routes and has found some interesting differences that would be worthy of further consideration by researchers.

20.2 Integration of different approaches to support effective communication

At the British Nutrition Foundation (BNF), a variety of different approaches are used, often in combination, to disseminate the findings of research projects to others in

the nutrition field and to communicate with school children, their teachers, health professionals and the general public. These approaches range from 'traditional' published reports and peer-reviewed papers and conferences to websites, internet-based resources for schools, interactive eSeminars and social media approaches. The various case studies in this section illustrate different approaches to knowledge transfer and communication.

Sustainability of the food supply

These days it is important to be mindful of the challenges faced in the identification of a 'diet fit for the future' – a healthy, sustainable, affordable yet environmentally low-impact way of feeding the world's population now and in the light of its projected rise from the current 7 billion to over 9 billion by 2050. An unprecedented confluence of pressures has been described whereby a growing and in some cases increasingly prosperous global population, alongside increasing demand for limited resources and the urgent need to address environmental challenges such as climate change and changing weather patterns, means that food security is seriously and increasingly threatened. Much of the discussion has focused on greenhouse gas (GHG) emissions associated with food production and the contribution from meat production and dairying has been highlighted. These protein-rich foods are features of Western-style diets and as such make a substantial contribution to the intakes of a wide range of essential nutrients. It is therefore important to understand the impact on overall dietary patterns and associated nutrient intakes if consumption levels fall, as well as the impact from a sustainability standpoint. From a nutritional perspective, the initial knee-jerk reaction of simply eating less meat is already being replaced by a more sophisticated debate that is now considering whether a healthy diet, as currently framed by food-based dietary guidelines, can also be a sustainable dietary pattern now and in the future.

There are some important questions that need to be addressed in order for a clearer picture to emerge. For example, it is as yet uncertain which dietary choices consumers would make if their consumption of these foods were to be reduced, what effect these choices would have on their health and on the sustainability of the food supply, and which groups of the population or individuals within households would be most vulnerable, recognising that there are demographic changes already underway associated with an ageing population. Recent surveys from the UK's Global Food Security programme and the consumer organisation Which? suggest that consumers are open to receiving more information about the options and trade-offs faced in meeting the challenges of feeding the global population now and in the future.

Dietary surveys and modelling, using food composition databases linked to reference nutrient intakes, have an essential part to play in determining both the impact of the types of change in diet that are likely to be necessary if food security is to be achieved for future decades, and how the nutrient needs of a growing global population can best be met from the resources available. The BNF contributed to the debate through various articles and a themed issue of the journal *Nutrition Bulletin*.

The role of nutrition in early development

It has been recognised for some time that there are periods of fetal and early-life development when the balance of nutrients is particularly important – these are the 'critical windows' in an offspring's development during which his or her future health and development may be 'programmed'. To explore the potential for nutrition during early life to shape future health, a BNF Task Force was established under the chairmanship of Professor Tom Sanders, which reported in May 2013 (*Nutrition and Development: Short- and Long-Term Consequences for Health*). The Task Force considered the effect of nutrition on the development of the various organ systems and also the extent to which current recommendations about nutrition in pregnancy and during early life are being followed by the population in the UK and elsewhere. A key finding was that there is now unequivocal evidence of the biological link between the health status of women and conditions such as obesity, type 2 diabetes and cardiovascular disease in their children in later life. Almost half of women of child-bearing age in England are

overweight or obese and this can affect the environment in the womb, the baby's birth weight and subsequent health in early life and on into adulthood. Maternal obesity increases the risk of complications in pregnancy, including pre-eclampsia, which can result in a small, growth-retarded baby. Evidence suggests that poor fetal growth, especially if followed by accelerated growth in infancy, may be associated with long-term adverse consequences for health. Poor fetal growth may also affect kidney development, making offspring more sensitive to the blood pressure-raising effect of salt and therefore increasing their risk of cardiovascular disease in later life. Obese women are also more likely to have gestational diabetes, which increases the fuel supply to the baby. This can increase the likelihood of the baby having a very high birth weight and developing obesity. It also predisposes the child to developing type 2 diabetes in later life.

Communications activities associated with the conference to launch the report stressed the food industry's responsibility in shaping the food supply. They also emphasised the critical role of health professionals in alerting women to the risks – to both themselves and their babies – associated with being obese during pregnancy, as well as supporting women planning a pregnancy and after the birth in establishing and maintaining a healthy weight. To help with this, a website-based four-week planner for women of child-bearing age was produced and promoted via media activity, alongside website-based meal planners and tips on healthy eating and physical activity for women planning a pregnancy, as well as for those who have recently had a baby and want to get their figure back (http://www.nutrition.org.uk/healthyliving/healthylifeplanner). To help midwives keep up to date on the importance of good nutrition, an online training course was produced with the Royal College of Midwives. To reach women directly there is a Nutrition4Baby section to the BNF website, which uses social media routes to deliver information on a weekly basis to women during their pregnancy. The press information was picked up by breakfast television and national and regional newspapers, as well as trade and health professional publications. The headlines generated focused on the risks of maternal obesity.

Folic acid

Neural tube defects (NTD, e.g. spina bifida and anencephaly) annually affect an estimated 320 000 newborns worldwide (4500 affected pregnancies per year in Europe) and folic acid supplementation and fortification of the maternal diet during the peri-conceptional period form an effective primary prevention strategy. In the UK, all women of child-bearing age are advised to take a daily supplement of 400 µg of folic acid and to consume a folate-rich diet. Nevertheless, compliance is generally poor – one UK study showed that less than 55% of women reported ever taking a folic acid supplement and uptake of the advice is adversely affected by lower education level and socioeconomic group. Furthermore, many pregnancies are unplanned. Countries such as Canada that have mandated folic acid fortification of wheat flour as a means of delivering the nutrient report an average 46% reduction in NTD-affected birth prevalence (see Table 20.2 for other examples).

Folic acid fortification of bread flour was introduced in the USA in 1998 and more than 70 countries around the world have followed suit, but to date no European country has taken this step. The science supporting peri-conceptional use of folic acid as a preventative measure for NTD was reviewed some years ago by the Scientific Advisory Committee on Nutrition (SACN), which recommended fortification of flour in the UK. In making this recommendation, SACN noted a concern about the risk of folic acid supplementation masking B12 deficiency and its sequelae in some groups (e.g. older people), by ameliorating the anaemia that B12 deficiency produces but allowing neurological damage to progress. There has also been concern that folic acid fortification could cause cancer and investigation of this has delayed a decision about its use in the UK. Folate is necessary for gene stability and so can be expected to protect against cancer in healthy individuals. However, it is also important for cell replication throughout life and there have been suggestions that in individuals with early cancer, folic acid supplementation may, over time, promote cancer growth and proliferation. Three meta-analyses have been published over the past couple of years, the most recent in early 2013 by Vollset and colleagues, and a decision on fortification from the UK's Chief Medical Officer is expected in early 2015. Recognising the challenges already experienced in encouraging women of child-bearing age to comply with advice on folic acid supplementation (despite promotional campaigns targeting health professionals and women) and also the reality that peri-conceptional usage is lowest in at-risk groups such as teenagers, low-income groups and obese women, folic acid fortification of commonly consumed foods may be the most efficient way to increase folate status in such women.

The role of nutrition in healthy ageing

The 2011 census revealed that 16.4% of the population of England and Wales (1 in 6 people) is now over the age of 65 years, the highest percentage ever recorded (http://www.ons.gov.uk/ons/rel/census/2011-census/population-and-household-estimates-for-england-and-wales/index.html), making this a large and expanding population group. Furthermore, in 2011 there were 430 000 residents in England and Wales aged at least 90 years, compared with 340 000 in 2001 and just 13 000 in 1911. People over the age of 65 are very heterogeneous in terms of their health and their needs. The improvement in life expectancy in the UK, which has been increasing by around 2 years per decade, is being matched in many other parts of the world (Figure 20.5) even where poverty is rife, but crucially, increases in healthy life expectancy are not keeping pace, either in the UK or elsewhere. We are living longer, but much of this extra time is being spent in ill health (Figure 20.6). This demographic trend poses many challenges for society and our healthcare systems.

To investigate the potential of diet and lifestyle to improve healthy life expectancy, in 2005 BNF established a Task Force on nutrition and healthy ageing, under the chairmanship of Professor John Mathers, the report of which was published in 2009. The genes we inherit at conception set the trajectory and context for future health, but thereafter nutrition in the womb and throughout life, together with overall lifestyle, influences the impact of our genetic inheritance. Furthermore, time continuously pushes the pendulum towards ill health and disability. The Task Force adopted a life-course approach to the study of ageing, considering how each organ system ages over time and the evidence for nutrition and/or lifestyle having the potential to hold back the effects of time. Chapters in the report (Stanner, Thompson and Buttriss 2009) cover teeth and the oral cavity, bones, joints, skeletal muscle, skin, the brain, the cardiovascular system, the immune system, the gut and the endocrine system. The Task Force found evidence of protection against chronic disease; preservation of immune function, digestive health, cardiovascular health, functional ability, bone health, oral health and vision; benefits for cognitive function, mental health and well-being; ability to minimise risk of weight loss, undernutrition, low nutrient status and deficiency diseases; and capacity to aid recovery from illness.

Once the science had been established, the Task Force moved on to consider the public health implications and all the nutritional information was drawn together, by

Table 20.2 Examples of the impact of global folic acid fortification on neural tube defect (NTD) prevalence.

Country	Year of introduction	Fortification	Decrease in NTDs
Canada	1998	150µg/100 wheat flour	46% by 2002
Chile	2000	220µg/100 wheat flour	40% by 2002
South Africa	2003	150µg/100 wheat flour 221µg/100 maize flour	31% by 2005
USA	1998	140µg/100 wheat flour	27% by 2000

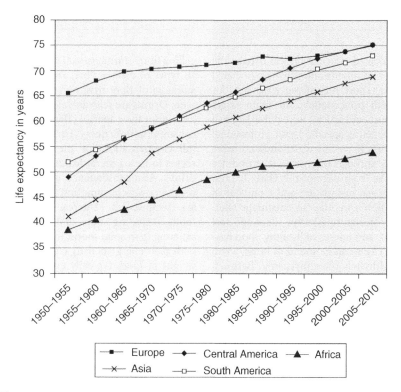

Figure 20.5 Global life expectancy at birth by demographic region, 1950–2010. Data from Population Division of the Department of Economic and Social Affairs of the United Nations Secretariat.

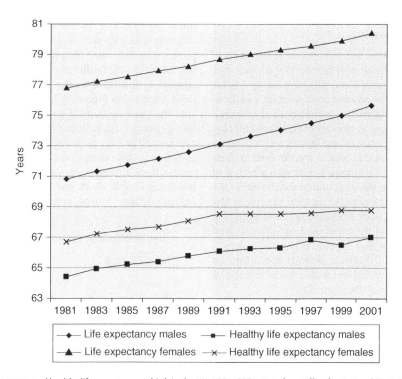

Figure 20.6 Life expectancy and healthy life expectancy at birth in the UK, 1981–2001. Data from Office for National Statistics licensed under the Open Government Licence v.1.0 (http://www.ons.gov.uk/ons/rel/disability-and-health-measurement/health-expectancies-at-birth-and-age-65-in-the-united-kingdom/index.html).

organ system. This collated information was used as the basis of the consumer communications work associated with the launch of the report. A conference was held for researchers and health professionals, the main target audiences for the report, and articles were published in a variety of journals targeting specific heath professional groups, although efforts to reach a wider audience were undertaken primarily through the media (the findings were published on the front page of the *Daily Express* and in five other national newspapers and a number of magazines) and via BNF's website. To encourage take-up of the messages a poster, tips, recipe ideas and fact sheets were produced, and images of 'healthy' food baskets were provided. These can be found at http://www.nutrition.org.uk/healthyliving/healthyageing. Between January 2010 and April 2013, the poster attracted 6019 hits, the top tips for healthy ageing 17 512 hits and the recipes 7813 hits. Of course, the national media coverage of the messages reached far greater numbers. Articles were also produced for a range of consumer magazines with different key audiences and talks were given to specific groups such as those running care homes. These targeted activities enabled the information to be presented in an appropriate format for different groups.

Communicating the concepts of satiation and satiety

Satiation is the condition that prompts the termination of eating and satiety is the sense of fullness that persists after eating. Both are important in controlling energy intake: satiation influences the amount consumed on a particular occasion and satiety influences the length of time until the next eating occasion. A number of organ systems (e.g. gut, adipose tissue, pancreas and brain) and hormones (e.g. insulin, gut hormones, leptin) are involved in these mechanisms. Work on this topic began with a review of the available evidence, this time undertaken by one of the BNF team with input from international experts in this field of research. A BNF Briefing Paper emerged that included definitions of the terms used and discussion of the mechanisms by which appetite is controlled, measurement techniques, the effects of foods and drinks on satiety and satiation, behavioural effects and the role of satiety in weight control (Benelam 2009).

The impact of macronutrients on satiety varies: protein has a greater effect than carbohydrate, and carbohydrate a greater effect than fat. Studies have shown that in free-living situations, higher-protein diets tend to be more satiating than those with a lower protein content. An implication of this is the need to maintain protein intakes on energy-reduced slimming diets. Some dietary fibre components, in particular viscous fibres and novel

gelling fibres, influence satiety, but this does not apply to all types of dietary fibre. Dose is also important: large amounts of fibre may be required for an effect to be seen. Drinks are relevant: alcohol-containing drinks are known for their aperitif effect and support passive over-consumption of energy. Furthermore, there is a lack of full compensation for the energy consumed, which seems to be a general feature for all energy-containing drinks. As a consequence, drinks have the potential to result in over-consumption of energy, although the data are inconsistent. Interestingly, though, high-water foods, including soups and stews, appear to be more satiating than solid foods; this is presumed to be linked with their energy density (the energy provided per unit weight of food, typically expressed as kcal/g or kJ/g), hence the volume consumed to achieve a particular energy intake. Energy density is influenced by the water content of a food, in particular, and also by the food's fat and fibre content.

It was important to draw out key strands of information that could be used as the basis for communications activities aimed at health professionals, schools and the general public. The decision was taken to focus on the concept of energy density. Studies have shown that people typically consume a relatively constant weight of food, although total energy intake may vary to a greater degree. This raises the possibility of reducing energy intake by reducing the energy density of foods, while ensuring that emphasis is placed on those dietary components, in particular the protein, fibre and water content of foods, that influence satiation and satiety. This concept is illustrated by the work of Professor Barbara Rolls, depicted in Figure 20.7. Both displays of food provide the same amount of energy – 1575 kcal – but the energy density determines the volume of food available: the lower the energy density, the more food can be consumed. This concept was used as the basis of a communications strategy with health professionals and the public. A simple chart was produced illustrating how energy density varies across commonly consumed

Two strategies for eating 1575 kcal during a day

Food ED = 2.3

Food ED = 0.52

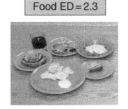
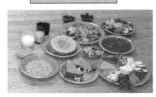

Figure 20.7 The effect of energy density (ED, kcal/g) on quantity of food. By courtesy of Dr B. Rolls and based on Rolls, B. and Hermann, M. (2012) The Ultimate Volumetrics Diet, William Morrow, New York.

foods and some recipes were included. A leaflet was subsequently produced for slimmers and those wishing to maintain a healthy weight (see http://www.nutrition. org.uk/healthyliving/fuller/eat-more-lose-weight). Between June 2010 and April 2013, the chart attracted 12 834 hits, the recipes 7328 hits and the weight-loss leaflet 33 134 hits. A podcast for use in schools, explaining the concepts in simpler terms, was also produced (http://www.nutrition.org.uk/healthyliving/fuller/ introduction-to-satiation-and-satiety).

Despite the emerging science in this area and the potential for energy density and satiation to be used as tools by those wishing to manage their weight and/or control appetite, by mid-2014 no health claims had been cleared by the European Food Safety Authority (EFSA) for use on foods. A suggested reason for this is that EFSA has required evidence of weight loss rather than appetite control per se.

Hydration

The BNF receives many enquiries about fluid intake – how much should be drunk each day? Which drinks count? Is it possible to drink too much fluid? To get to the facts, a thorough review of the evidence was undertaken, with the support of an advisory group including experts in physiology, sports nutrition, dental health, paediatrics and dietetics. The review covered the physiology of hydration, health effects of different dietary water sources, and current recommendations, and provided the basis for a series of communications: a conference for health professionals and researchers as well as website-based resources for the public and for use in schools (see http://www.nutrition.org.uk/healthyliving/ hydration). This approach was supplemented by press releases, a day of radio interviews and articles in health professional publications.

The main messages emerging from the review emphasised that water is essential for life and constitutes the greater part of an individual's body weight (on average around 60%). Body water content is closely monitored and maintained within narrow limits, through stimulation of thirst or increased urinary output. However, if losses are not sufficiently replaced, dehydration occurs and extreme dehydration can be fatal, with even mild dehydration (about 2% loss of body weight) resulting in headaches, fatigue and reduced physical and mental performance. Excessive water consumption, though rare, is also dangerous as it can result in hyponatraemia (low blood sodium levels). Food provides about 20% of total water intake, on average, and almost all drinks contribute positively to water balance, the exceptions being stronger alcoholic drinks such as wine, spirits and strong beers. Individual fluid needs vary widely depending on factors including body size and composition, the environment and physical activity levels, but current recommendations in the UK are to drink the equivalent of 6–8 glasses of fluids per day (about 1.2 litres), in addition to the water acquired through foods. Though water is a good choice, many other drinks count too, such as milk, juices, low-calorie and other soft drinks, tea and coffee. Clearly, some of these choices bring with them a calorific value, as a result of the sugars and sometimes fat that they contain, some are acidic and so have the potential to erode tooth enamel, and some provide caffeine.

The information on suitable choices was communicated by a poster (http://www.nutrition.org.uk/healthyliving/ hydration/healthy-hydration-guide), supported by tips and hints (http://www.nutrition.org.uk/healthyliving/ hydration/getting-the-balance-right-everyday-examples) that provided more detail and tailored the advice, for example stressing the recommendation to limit caffeine consumption during pregnancy. The aim of this poster was to correct the many misperceptions currently held on the topic of hydration through its use directly by the general public or by health professionals during consultations with clients. Between February 2010 and April 2013, it received 27 190 000 hits. In 2013, a poster specifically targeting parents and carers with information about fluid intake for children was also published (http://www.nutrition.org.uk/attachments/591_ Childrens%20hydration%20guide_final.pdf).

Back to basics with healthy eating

The 'eatwell plate' is the UK's principal public health tool for communicating information about healthy eating and is a pictorial representation of how different groups of foods contribute to a varied and healthy diet. Nevertheless, research such as the UK's Family Food survey, conducted annually by the government, shows that many people have difficulty putting this guidance into practice and may benefit from additional information. To investigate this further, BNF conducted a poll to understand how the resource is currently used and whether the provision of additional materials would enhance its communication. The results and subsequent discussions indicated that supplementary information on each of the five food groups, portion-size guidance, a recommended number of servings from each of the groups, a menu plan and the use of different and targeted communication channels may aid in the dissemination and application of the messages conveyed by the eatwell plate. A working group was established to take this forward, resulting in new web-based resources including 'Putting it into practice', which provides examples of meals and snacks that, over the course of a day, are in line with the eatwell plate, with Government guidelines on energy intake at different meal occasions and meeting dietary reference values (http://www.nutrition.org.uk/healthyliving/healthyeating).

The eatwell plate also has a pivotal role in BNF's *Food – a fact of life* resources for schools and was featured in the Foundation's Healthy Eating Weeks (3-7 June 2013 and 2 – 6 June 2014), a national campaign for primary and secondary schools throughout the UK that focuses on healthy eating, being active, knowing where food comes from and cooking. Registered schools were able to access specially developed free resources, watch podcasts delivered by nutrition experts and take part in a number of events. Resources were available to download after the week itself was over. In its first year, Healthy Eating Week attracted registration from over 3000 schools, enabling over 1.2 million children to be involved in school-based activities linked to the week, and 27 500 pupils also participated in a survey about attitudes and knowledge on food and healthy eating. In 2014, 4,400 schools participated (1.75 million pupils) and the pupils' survey again proved popular (the results of both surveys can be found at www.healthyeatingweek.org.uk).

Determining content and language for schools resources

The final example concerns the importance that BNF attaches to determining the content of and the language used in resources for schools. The nutrition information conveyed of course has to be accurate and up to date, but it also needs to be written and presented in a way that is appropriate and understood by the target age group. It is very important that the content is relevant to the school curriculum and essential that it engages young people's interest and enthusiasm. To ensure curriculum relevance, the Foundation has four regional Education Working Groups in England, Northern Ireland, Scotland and Wales; the groups critically appraise the work that is underway aimed at schools, discuss regional educational issues (e.g. the need to translate resources into Welsh and Gaelic) and help define future priorities.

BNF has developed a dedicated website (www.food afactoflife.org.uk) for its schools resources, all of which are free to download. Website visits and downloads have been increasing progressively, as illustrated in Figure 20.8, which compares the month of January over the period 2006–14. In the period June 2013 – May 2014, the site attracted 1 907 612 visitors, an increase of 25% compared to the previous 12 months, and they collectively downloaded 3 536 998 resources, an increase of 8.5%. The resources available have recently been extended to support school curriculum developments in England. From September 2014, lessons on healthy eating, food provenance and cooking (food preparation) will be compulsory for all aged 5–14 years.

The *Food – a fact of life* website provides a progressive approach to teaching young people aged 3–16 years about healthy eating, cooking, food provenance and farming. The site provides a wealth of free resources to stimulate learning, ensuring that consistent and up-to-date messages are delivered. The website is a unique resource in the UK in delivering accurate and current information to schools.

Prior to its launch, the *Food – a fact of life* programme was piloted with users. This involved gathering teacher feedback on pedagogy and students' comments on the design, layout and content of the resources. BNF education

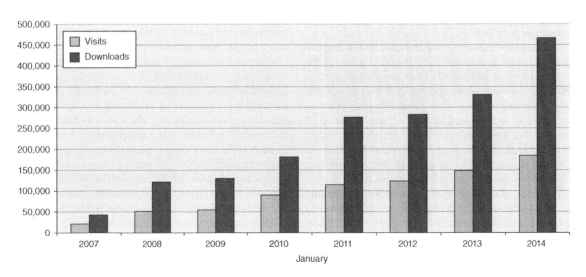

Figure 20.8 *Food – a fact of life* visits and downloads during the month of January, 2006–2014.

staff also visited schools to observe pupils using the resources in the classroom. Audit and evaluation are features of the provision and there are regular teacher surveys, which have revealed that the programme is well positioned to support good-quality food and nutrition teaching and learning in schools.

The BNF aspires to use new technologies to support effective teaching and learning. In response to demand from teachers for continuing professional development, and acknowledging the difficulties teachers encounter in being released from school, eSeminars are provided on a range of nutrition topics. These are live seminars offered over the internet with the opportunity for teachers to ask questions in real time. The format also gives the opportunity for GCSE/Standard Grade and A-level/Advanced Higher students to participate. In addition there is a video podcast series that has proved popular in schools: during the period May 2009–April 2013 there were 137 067 views. These internet-delivered resources have been extended to support a series of face-to-face BNF events designed to help teachers in England prepare for delivery of the new curriculum in September.

A development during 2012 was to pilot interactive textbooks (on iPads) to ascertain the future potential of this technology in schools. Two interactive textbooks were developed, one for primary schools and one for secondary schools. Both books included text, photographs, video, interactive charts and questions. The books were created in-house using Apple's iBook Author software. A limitation currently is the lack of iPads in schools, but the feedback from those schools that were able to participate was generally very positive and some useful pointers for the future were provided.

As well as continuing to develop resources under BNF's *Food – a fact of life* banner, support is also given to the work in schools undertaken by a range of other organisations, including the government. For example, working with the Food Standards Agency (FSA), Food Competencies for young people were developed. These competences have recently been updated to bring them in line with the new curriculum for England (more details can be found at http://www.nutrition.org.uk/foodinschools/competences/competences). The competences set out a framework of core skills and knowledge on diet and heath, shopping (consumer awareness), food safety and cooking. They are for use by teachers and have been designed to be applicable in schools across the UK, despite differences in curricula. There was a consultation phase during which teacher input was collated and utilised. Building on this work, a series of Food Route resources were produced for the FSA, interpreting the Food Competencies for use by children themselves. Pupils were directly involved in the development of the resources, which employ different formats depending on the intended age group – cartoons, tick boxes and minimal words for younger children and a self-complete diary style for older children. A series of focus groups (for children in the age group 5–16 years) were arranged throughout the UK. This exercise provided powerful insight into reading abilities and concept understanding at different ages. The voices of young people helped to shape the design and content of the final resource.

Subsequent work has continued to build on this approach, also embracing physical activity and energy balance as well as diet and nutrition, and a European Food Framework has been published (http://www.europeanfoodframework.eu). The opinions of experts working in the fields of education, nutrition and lifestyle helped shape the framework through a series of project advisory groups and wider consultation. An online survey for young people (translated into a number of languages) was used to gather the opinions of young people across Europe.

20.3 How legislation shapes the information that can be communicated

Nutrition and Health Claims Regulation

Introduction

The Nutrition and Health Claims (NHC) Regulation (EC No 1924/2006) came into force in July 2007, with the aims of protecting consumers and encouraging innovation in the food industry. Prior to its introduction there were voluntary schemes in some European countries (such as the Joint Health Claims Initiative in the UK), but no specific regulations relating to health claims other than Council Directive 2000/13/EC, which banned medicinal claims on foodstuffs (i.e. foodstuffs cannot claim to treat, cure or prevent disease).

The NHC Regulation applies to all food, drinks and dietary supplements sold within the European Union (EU) and any supporting materials, including websites, labels, promotional goods and advertorials. It ensures that all nutrition and health claims used are scientifically substantiated and communicated in a clear, understandable way. To this end, the European Commission (EC) has published a list of permitted claims for food, drinks and dietary supplements sold in Europe (http://ec.europa.eu/nuhclaims). The Regulation covers various types of claim and for a claim to be permitted it stipulates that the product has to comply with rules linked to a particular nutrient profile that takes account of the amounts of fat, salt and sugars present. However, detail about the nutrient profile has yet to be published despite plans in the legislation for it to be in place by 2009. A claim must refer to the product as consumed, prepared according to the manufacturer's instructions, and must not call into question the safety or nutritional content of other foods or the adequacy of a balanced diet. Claims will not be permitted if they:

- Relate to preventing, treating or curing a disease.
- Relate to alcoholic beverages other than low/reduced alcohol or energy.
- Suggest that health could be affected by *not* consuming the product.
- Make reference to a rate or amount of weight loss.
- Make reference to recommendations of individual doctors and health professionals.

Types of claim

The Regulation covers both nutrition and health claims, for which there are different authorisation processes.

Nutrition claims are those that refer to what a product does or does not contain, for example being a source of vitamin C, low in fat and, high in fibre. A list of permitted claims and criteria are available on the EC website: http://ec.europa.eu/food/food/labellingnutrition/claims/community_register/nutrition_claims_en.htm

Health claims are those that state, suggest or imply that a relationship exists between a food category, a food or one of its constituents and health. There are different categories of health claims (see Figure 20.9), but it is always the European Food Safety Authority's (EFSA) Dietetic Products, Nutrition and Allergy (NDA) panel that provides a scientific opinion on the claim. For each submission, the NDA panel considers three questions, to which the answers must all be yes:

- Is the food constituent sufficiently defined or characterised?
- Is the claimed health effect sufficiently defined and is there a beneficial nutritional or physiological effect?
- Has a cause-and-effect relationship been established between consumption of the food/constituent and the claimed health effect?

The EC uses EFSA's opinion, alongside considerations of consumer understanding of the wording of the claim, to

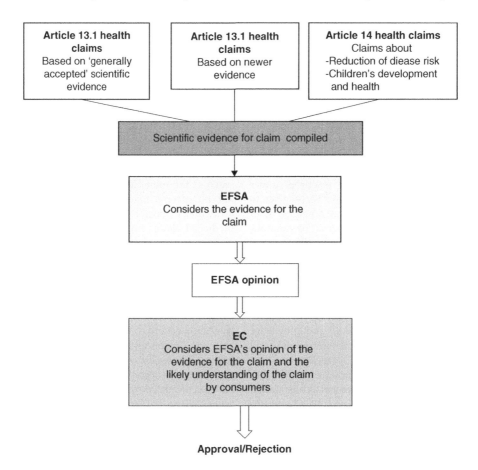

Figure 20.9 The approval process for the different categories of health claims.

make the final decision as to whether the claim should be approved or rejected. All claims assessed to date (rejected and authorised) are listed on the EC website: http://ec.europa.eu/nuhclaims.

Article 13.1 claims are supported by 'generally accepted scientific evidence'. Although there has been some confusion as to what exactly this means, the claims accepted onto the list have generally been those that are supported by substantial scientific evidence in the public domain and already appear in standard nutrition science textbooks, for instance that vitamin D contributes to the maintenance of normal bones, or iron contributes to normal oxygen transport in the body. The approval process began in 2007 when the legislation was introduced and 40 000 claims were submitted via member states; this number fell to about 4000 once duplications and ineligible claims were removed. Assessment by EFSA followed, and the list of accepted claims was published in May 2012 and came into force in December 2012.

Article 13.5 covers the procedure for claims that are based on more recent scientific evidence than that used to support Article 13.1 claims. For a claim to be authorised, a detailed dossier of evidence must be submitted, which is considered by EFSA on behalf of the EC. By mid-2014, five claims had been approved under this Article.

Article 14 health claims concern reduction of disease risk (14a) or children's health and development (14b). Again, a detailed dossier of evidence must be submitted and is considered by EFSA to establish whether there is a causal relationship, as described earlier. The claim is then either rejected or approved by the EC. For claims on disease risk reduction, the claim must refer to reduction of a risk factor, for instance raised blood cholesterol, rather than the disease (cardiovascular disease) itself. Examples include 'Oat beta-glucan has been shown to reduce blood cholesterol. High cholesterol is a risk factor for the development of coronary heart disease' and 'Plant sterols [or stanols] have been shown to lower blood cholesterol. High cholesterol is a risk factor for the development of coronary heart disease.' An example of a 14b claim is 'Protein is needed for normal growth and development of bone in children.'

Wording and communication

Dossiers submitted to EFSA should contain a suggested wording for the health claim. If the NDA panel decides that a cause-and-effect relationship has been established, it will consider the proposed wording of the claim and may suggest an alternative for the EC to consider. Once the EC has authorised a claim it is recommended that, where possible, food companies stick to the authorised wording, although the Regulation stipulates that there is some flexibility, so long as any changes made are to help in consumer understanding.

Problems with the Regulation

Since the Regulation came into force in 2007, there have been a number of problems with its implementation. As mentioned earlier, a very large number of claims were submitted under Article 13.1 and these took far longer to process than anticipated. Furthermore, there was initially limited guidance on the expected content of Article 13.5 and Article 14 dossiers, so many claims that were submitted did not meet EFSA's requirements and were rejected even before the science was considered, as the food or constituent to which the claim related had not been adequately defined. Examples here are some of the dietary fibre claims and the group of claims concerning probiotics. Since that time, however, more guidance has been published.

Regarding fibre, current intakes fall well below the recommendation of at least 18 g non-starch polysaccharides a day and dietary fibre is widely recognised as a feature of a healthy diet. Despite the authorisation of the nutrition claim 'high in dietary fibre' (if the product contains at least 6 g of fibre per 100 g), the majority of health claims relating to dietary fibre have not been successful, as the food constituent had not been sufficiently characterised. So a loaf of wholemeal bread can carry a 'high in dietary fibre' claim, but currently it is not legal to say why this is beneficial to health as no relevant general fibre claims are on the permitted list. Beta glucan, pectin and arabinoxylan, all types of fibre, have received positive opinions, but claims such as 'consumption of arabinoxylan contributes to a reduction of the glucose rise after a meal' are probably unlikely to aid in communicating the importance of eating more fibre in general.

There remains uncertainty about the applicability of permitted claims to particular products in the absence of the overdue nutrient profile referred to in the legislation, as mentioned earlier.

It is important that issues such as these are addressed to ensure that the Regulation does not stifle scientific research related to diet and health or the product innovation that is needed if improvements in diet and food security are to be assured; and, indeed, that it does not hinder the communication of messages that are in line with government recommendations for a healthy diet, such as the need for dietary fibre.

Regulation on provision of food information to consumers

In the UK, food labelling has been regulated in the past by a number of pieces of legislation. Underpinning this has been the General Food Labelling legislation (http://www.legislation.gov.uk/uksi/1970/400/contents/made)

and the nutrition labelling legislation (http://www.legislation.gov.uk/uksi/1996/1499/made). Over the years the legislation has been added to, updated and amended. European Regulation on Provision of Food Information to Consumers (FIC) 1169/2011 was introduced in 2011 to consolidate EU rules on general and nutrition labelling into one piece of European legislation, with the aim of making it easier to follow and to improve compliance. Food and drink companies may implement the rules at any stage during the transition periods included in the legislation. The majority of the rules will be mandatory from December 2014, after a three-year transition period, but companies are not legally obliged to provide back-of-pack nutrition information until December 2016.

The Regulation specifies certain information that must by law be clearly communicated on labels for pre-packed food. To ensure the clarity of the information, the Regulation stipulates a minimum font size and states that all information should be easily visible and clearly legible. Apart from a couple of exceptions discussed below that are new, the list of mandatory particulars is not drastically changed from previous legislation and includes:

- Product name
- Product description
- Ingredient list
- Allergen information
- Genetically modified ingredients
- Weight/volume of product
- Date marks
- Beverages containing > 1.2% by volume of alcohol and > 150 mg/l of caffeine (except coffee and tea) must state so
- Weight or volume of food/drink (if a product > 5 g/5 ml)
- Storage and preparation conditions
- Name or business name and address of the food manufacturer
- Country of origin and place of provenance.

There are nevertheless a couple of changes to the list that are worthy of comment. One concerns allergen labelling. Over recent years, allergen warning boxes on packaged products have become familiar, but these are no longer included in the legislation. Instead, the requirement is for allergens to be highlighted in the ingredients list using a distinctive font, style or background colour. For foods that are not pre-packed, all allergens must be stated at the point of sale using the word 'contains' followed by the name of the substance or product as listed in the regulation, for example 'contains nuts'. Some useful guidance on this has been developed by the British Retail Consortium (http://www.brc.org.uk/downloads/Guidance%20on%20Allergen%20Labelling.pdf).

	Per 100 g
Energy	1500 kJ/356 kcal
Fat	7.4 g
of which saturates	1.1 g
Carbohydrates	58.1 g
of which sugars	16.8 g
Protein	9.9 g
Salt	Below 0.1 g

Figure 20.10 Example of a back-of-pack nutrient declaration, which will be mandatory from 2016.

Another change concerns the provision of nutrition information, which until now has been voluntary unless a claim is made about the content of a particular nutrient. From 2016, the FIR requires all pre-packed products to be clearly labelled with back-of-pack nutrition information, presented per 100 g or 100 ml; it can additionally be presented per portion or consumption unit. The law requires the listing of the particular nutrients shown in Figure 20.10 (with energy provided as kcal and kJ and the other nutrients listed as g). Monounsaturates, polyunsaturates, starch, fibre, vitamins or minerals can be listed, but this is not obligatory unless a nutrition or health claim is made for the nutrient.

Front-of-pack labelling

The UK has been a pioneer in establishing access to 'at a glance' front-of-pack nutrition information as the norm. Over the past few years two distinct approaches have become widespread. One is characterised by so-called traffic lights and dates back to 2006, when the FSA recommended that businesses adopt voluntary front-of-pack nutrition labelling using the traffic light colours of red, amber and green to interpret nutrient levels for fat, saturated fat, sugars and salt on seven categories of food: sandwiches and similar products; ready meals (hot and cold); burgers and sausages; pies, pastries and quiches; breaded, coated or formed meat/poultry/fish; pizzas; and breakfast cereals (http://www.food.gov.uk/news/newsarchive/2006/mar/signpostnewsmarch). The scheme was subsequently applied more extensively and was characterised by four aspects: separate information on fat, saturated fat, sugars and salt; red, amber or green colour coding to provide 'at a glance' information on the level (i.e. whether high, medium or low) of individual nutrients in the product; provision of additional information on the levels of nutrients present in a portion of the product; and use of nutritional criteria to determine the colour banding. The cut-offs for green/amber were set at levels consistent with nutrition claims legislation and the amber/red (medium/high) boundaries were based on existing advice for fat, saturated fat, sugars and salt, using 25% of recommended intake levels per 100 g and 30% (40% for salt) per portion (www.food.gov.uk/multimedia/pdfs/frontofpackguidance2.pdf). Different sets of criteria were established for foods and drinks.

The second approach uses comparisons with guideline daily amounts (GDAs) to steer consumer choice. GDAs are derived from UK dietary reference values and very similar values have been established by the EFSA, known as labelling reference values. (Under the FIC regulation, the term reference intake, RI, replaces GDA.)

The two approaches have polarised opinion and it should be noted that no studies have seriously grappled with assessing the ability of either scheme to effect long-term change in food-consumption behaviour. Meanwhile, interest has grown in a hybrid approach. In 2009, the FSA commissioned research that focused primarily on three key content-related signposting elements: traffic light colours, interpretative text (high, medium, low) and nutrients presented as % of GDA. The aim of the research was to establish which front-of-pack labelling format or combination of elements best facilitated consumers' accurate interpretation of key nutritional information so that they were assisted in making informed choices about the foods they purchase. The research addressed three key questions (http://www.food.gov.uk/multimedia/pdfs/pmpreport.pdf):

- How well do individual schemes (or elements of schemes) enable consumers to interpret levels of key nutrients correctly?
- How do consumers use front-of-pack labels in real-life contexts in the retail environment and at home?
- How does the coexistence of a range of front-of-pack label formats affect the accurate interpretation of the labels?

The research found that levels of comprehension of the different formats tested were generally high (ranging from 58% to 71% when looking at labels on single products), but that the balance of evidence favoured the combination of GDAs, traffic light colours and text. This hybrid format has been used by several major retail chains for some years.

Additional and voluntary front-of-pack nutrition labelling is allowed in the FIC, but only in one of two specific formats: energy (presented as both kcal and kJ) alone; or energy in combination with fat, saturates, sugars and salt (that is, just energy and fat, for example, is not allowed). It has been suggested that the requirement to display both kcal and kJ on labels may deter food companies from providing front-of-pack nutrition information, as it could lead to consumer confusion or 'messy labels'; similar concerns have been raised with regard to labelling in the out-of-home sector. In 2012, health ministers announced that they would work with food companies to establish a consistent scheme based on a hybrid approach combining GDAs (% GDA) and colour coding, details of which were published in 2013 (https://www.gov.uk/government/uploads/system/uploads/attachment_data/file/300886/2902158_FoP_Nutrition_2014.pdf).

Other food legislation

Regulations also exist covering supplements (Directive 2002/46/EC), the voluntary addition of vitamins and minerals to foods (Regulation (EC) No 1925/2006) and herbal remedies. For example, the European Traditional Herbal Medicinal Products Directive (THMPD) came into effect at the end of April 2011 and established an EU regulatory approval process for herbal medicines (http://ec.europa.eu/health/human-use/herbal-medicines/index_en.htm). The legislation defines herbal medicinal products as 'any medicinal product, exclusively containing as active ingredients one or more herbal substances, or one or more herbal preparations, or one or more such herbal substances in combination with one or more such herbal preparations'. Compliance with 'traditional use' requires evidence of the medicinal use of the product throughout a period of at least 30 years, including at least 15 years in the EU. In September 2012, the EC published a discussion paper that considered whether health claims on botanicals in foods should be assessed via the 'traditional use route' or via the approach used by EFSA for other health claims, which requires evidence from clinical studies (see earlier in this chapter).

20.4 How research and policy shape public health communications

There are many examples of how evidence linking nutrition and health has resulted in policies and initiatives that have shaped public health communications and dietary advice, including the following:

- Research on folate status and NTD risk resulted in advice about peri-conceptional use of folic acid supplements (see earlier in this chapter).
- Concerns about the prevalence of obesity (25% among UK adults) and the impact of this on risk of disease and chronic ill health resulted in the Department of Health's Public Health Responsibility Deal (PHRD) initiative (https://responsibilitydeal.dh.gov.uk/category/food-network/), whereby food producers and retailers are encouraged to provide calorie information on foods consumed out of home and voluntarily to reduce the energy provided by the foods and drinks they produce.

- Evidence that oil-rich fish, a major source of long-chain n-3 fatty acids, can benefit heart health resulted in recommendations to consume two servings of fish a week.
- Recognition of the link between sodium intake and blood pressure and hence cardiovascular disease risk led to recommendations to reduce salt intake to below 6 g/day (see later in this chapter).
- Dietary advice was produced stimulated by associations between saturates intake and LDL cholesterol and hence risk of cardiovascular disease.
- Inverse associations between intake of fruit and vegetables and health resulted in the 5-a-day advice.
- Concerns about vitamin D status and the re-emergence of rickets led to the reaffirmation of advice on supplementation.

The process of determining public health advice from the available research often involves advisory committees that assess the available evidence and generate risk assessments, which are taken into account by governments when determining the need for advice to manage these risks and promote health. Alongside epidemiology, randomised controlled trials and mechanistic studies, there is an important role for diet and nutrition surveys and accurate food composition data (Chapter 5) in making these decisions.

Sodium

In 2004 the Food Standards Agency in the UK launched a salt campaign, in which it raised awareness of the harm that a high salt intake can cause and worked with the food industry to reduce the sodium content of foods (http://www.food.gov.uk/multimedia/pdfs/saltreductioninitiatives.pdf). The message was simplified to grab attention and encourage action. Over the last decade sodium intake in the UK, as determined by urinary sodium, has been declining steadily. Salt levels in many staple foods have fallen by 40–50% and since 2007, according to the Department of Health, more than 11 million kg of salt have been removed from foods covered by the government's salt-reduction targets. In 2011, average salt consumption among adults was 8.1 g/day (6.8 g in women and 9.3 g in men), having fallen from 9.5 g/day in 2001, but it remains much higher than the 6 g target for adults.

Salt policy has shaped the public messages around salt and salt reduction has been a key feature of the PHRD. To maintain momentum, the PHRD's Food Network developed a salt strategy for action beyond 2012, based around four themes: reformulation, further activity by the catering sector, behaviour change, and broadening the sign-up to salt reduction; new UK salt reduction targets for 2017 have been set (https://responsibilitydeal.dh.gov.uk/responsibility-deal-food-network-new-salt-targets-f9-salt-reduction-2017-pledge-f10-out-of-home-salt-reduction-pledge/). The World Health Organisation has mapped salt-reduction initiatives in Europe and noted how the UK's initiative paved the way for action in other countries.

Vitamin D

The main source of vitamin D for most people is via the action of sunlight on skin; there is relatively little present naturally in the diet. The need of some population groups, such as pregnant and breastfeeding women, infants and housebound elderly people, for vitamin D supplements has been recognised for some time; more recently, the low vitamin D status of some ethnic groups living in the UK and elsewhere in Europe has also been recognised. Yet supplement use was not widely promoted by health professionals until recently, when it became evident that rickets was returning to the UK and that many age groups have low vitamin D status, according to the National Diet and Nutrition Survey (Figure 20.11). This prompted a campaign to increase the uptake of vitamin D supplements during pregnancy and early childhood. The government's Scientific Advisory Committee on Nutrition is also reviewing the evidence on vitamin D and health, partly because since the current intake recommendations were published in 1991, a number of functions of vitamin D beyond its role in bone health have been proposed.

20.5 How research shapes the agenda for the food industry

As is evident from the example of salt, research and public health policy can shape the agenda for the food industry. Decades ago the adverse effect of excessive intakes of saturates on CVD risk was recognised and pressure was placed on the milk and meat industries to reduce the saturates (and total fat) content of these foods. More recently there has been recognition of the detrimental effect of *trans* fatty acids produced during the hardening of vegetable oils in the manufacture of spreads.

Saturates

In the 1980s, following a report on CVD from a government advisory committee, the UK government called for a reduction in the fat content of meat and a move towards reduced-fat milk because of the evidence linking saturates with CVD risk. In the mid-1980s saturates contributed about 17% of the energy from food in the average

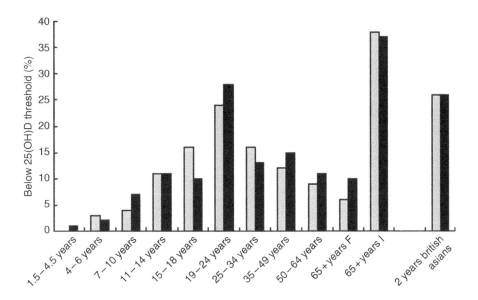

Figure 20.11 Prevalence of vitamin D deficiency in individuals in the UK (25(OH)D < 25 nmol/L). Reproduced from Lanham-New, S.A., Buttriss, J.L., Miles, L.M. *et al.* (2011). Proceedings of the Rank Forum on Vitamin D. *British Journal of Nutrition*, **105**, 1, 144–156.

UK diet and policy dictated a reduction to 11% of food energy. Following action by farmers and processors, saturates intake fell to 13% in 2000, but has since plateaued (12.6% in the 2014 report of the National Diet and Nutrition Survey, adults aged 19–64). In February 2009 the FSA launched a campaign to tackle 'saturated fat' intakes, but levels remained resistant to change; further action through the PHRD was initiated in 2013 (https://responsibilitydeal.dh.gov.uk/new-saturated-fat-pledge/).

Trans *fatty acids*

There are two sources of *trans* fatty acids in the diet, those produced in the processing of oils and those naturally produced in the digestive system of ruminant animals and hence present in milk and the meat of ruminants. It has been the *trans* fatty acids produced during oil processing that have been targeted for reduction. Research demonstrating the detrimental effect on CVD risk was acknowledged by the major spread manufacturers and they took action to change the way spreads were manufactured so as to avoid the generation of *trans* fatty acids. As a consequence, during the period 1986–2011 *trans* fatty acid intake in the UK fell from 2.2% energy to 0.7–0.8% energy, against a population recommendation of 2% energy. The small residual amount of *trans* fatty acids in the UK diet derived from the processing of oils has been the target of PHRD pledges.

20.6 Conclusions

This chapter has provided examples of how nutrition research can be translated and communicated to various audiences, and how legislation, research and policy shape the information that is communicated and the agenda for the food industry. Ultimately, a major purpose of nutrition science communication is behaviour change, which in many situations remains elusive and in nearly all cases challenging. Ipsos Mori (2013) poses the question: 'How do we change behaviour?' The report discusses how, in recent years, governments around the world have looked for alternatives to 'heavy-handed' legislation, choosing softer interventions – sometimes called 'nudges' – that draw on understanding of human behaviour to inform, persuade or influence, helping people make better decisions for themselves. This change has in part come about because of the global economic crisis of 2007/08 resulting in there being less money for large government-funded public health programmes (e.g. the campaign on salt in the UK).

The behaviour change wheel (Figure 20.12), developed by Professor Susan Michie and colleagues (2011), draws on the features of 19 frameworks relevant to behaviour change and provides a structured way of thinking about behaviour as a system that can be a stimulus for appropriate interventions and policies considering behaviour in context. Central to the wheel is the idea that behaviour change requires consideration of capability, motivation and opportunity. It provides a framework

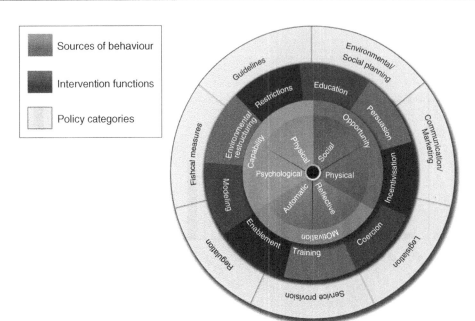

Figure 20.12 The behaviour change wheel. Reprinted from Michie, S., van Stralen, M. and West, R. (2011) The behaviour change wheel: A new method for characterising and designing behaviour change interventions. *Implementation Science*, **6**, 42. © BioMed Central.

for thinking systematically about the barriers and enablers of a specific behaviour.

Models such as this, coupled with so-called nutrition economics, can be expected to be of increasing importance in the future. Nutrition economics first assesses the impact of diet on health and disease prevention and then evaluates options for changing dietary choices, including regulatory measures including taxation, social marketing, differential pricing, direct service provision and dialogue with the food industry. This approach can be used to tackle under-nutrition, over-nutrition, enhance the nutritional contribution of conventional foods and develop policy in relation to 'functional' foods. To be effective it needs to incorporate an understanding of the potential consequences of dietary change, such as the impact of the food substitutions that people may make, and in this context will be a useful tool in discussions around global food security.

Acknowledgements

Bethany Hooper helped collate some of the information used within this chapter.

References and further reading

Adamson, A.J. (2013) Behaviour change in relation to healthier lifestyles. *Nutrition Bulletin*, **38**, 1 (special issue), 1–124.

Atkins, L. and Mitchie, S. (2013) Changing eating behaviour: What can we learn from behavioural science? *Nutrition Bulletin*, **38**, 1, 30–35.

Benelam, B. (2009) Satiation, satiety and their effects on eating behaviour. *Nutrition Bulletin*, **34**, 2, 126–173.

Benelam, B. and Wyness, L. (2010) Hydration and health: A review. *Nutrition Bulletin*, **35**, 1, 3–25.

British Nutrition Foundation (2013) *Nutrition and Development – Short and Long Term Consequences for Health*. Wiley-Blackwell, Oxford.

Buttriss, J.L. (2013) Food security through the lens of nutrition. *Nutrition Bulletin*, **38**, 2, 254–261.

Department of Health (1991) *Dietary Reference Values for Food Energy and Nutrients for the United Kingdom. Report of the Panel on Dietary Reference Values of the Committee on Medical Aspects of Food Policy*. HSMO, London.

Department of Health (2013) *National Diet and Nutrition Survey*. Available at http://transparency.dh.gov.uk/category/statistics/ndns/ (accessed May 2013).

Department for Environment, Food & Rural Affairs (2011) *Family Food Survey*. Available at https://www.gov.uk/government/publications/family-food-2011 (accessed May 2013).

Global Food Security Programme. Available at http://www.foodsecurity.ac.uk/programme/index.html (accessed June 2014).

Harland, J., Buttriss, J. and Gibson, S. (2012) Achieving eatwell plate recommendations: Is this a route to improving both sustainability and healthy eating? *Nutrition Bulletin*, **37**, 324–343.

Ipsos Mori Social Research Institute (2013) *How Do We Change Behaviour? Understanding Society*. Ipsos Mori, London. Available at http://www.ipsos-mori.com/DownloadPublication/1552_sri-understanding-society-april-2013.pdf (accessed June 2014).

Lenoir-Wijnkoop, I., Jones, P.J., Uauy, R. *et al.* (2013) Nutrition economics – food as an ally of public health. *British Journal of Nutrition*, **109**, 777–784.

Macdiarmid, J., Kyle, J., Horgan, G.W. *et al.* (2012) Sustainable diets for the future: Can we contribute to reducing greenhouse gas emissions by eating a healthy diet? *American Journal of Clinical Nutrition*, **96**, 3, 632–639.

Michie, S., van Stralen, M. and West, R. (2011) The behaviour change wheel: A new method for characterising and designing behaviour change interventions. *Implementation Science*, **6**, 42.

Stanner, S., Thompson, R. and Buttriss, J.L. (eds) (2009) *Healthy Ageing: The Role of Nutrition and Lifestyle. The Report of a British Nutrition Foundation Task Force.* Wiley-Blackwell, Oxford.

Stubbs, R.J. and Lavin, J.H. (2013) The challenges of implementing behaviour changes that lead to sustained weight management. *Nutrition Bulletin*, **38**, 5–22.

Vollset, S.E., Clarke, R., Lewington, S. et al. (2013) Effects of folic acid supplementation on overall and site-specific cancer incidence during the randomised trials: Meta-analyses of data on 50,000 individuals. *Lancet*, **381**, 1029–1036.

Which? (2013) *The Future of Food – Giving Consumers a Say.* Which?, London. Available at http://press.which.co.uk/wp-content/uploads/2013/04/Future-of-Food-Report-2013_Final.pdf (accessed June 2014).

World Health Organisation (2013) *Mapping Salt Reduction Initiatives in the WHO European Region.* WHO Regional Office for Europe, Copenhagen. Available at http://www.euro.who.int/__data/assets/pdf_file/0009/186462/Mapping-salt-reduction-initiatives-in-the-WHO-European-Region.pdf (accessed April 2013).

Wyness, L.A., Buttriss, J.L. and Stanner, S.A. (2012) Reducing the population's sodium intake: The UK Food Standards Agency's salt reduction programme. *Public Health Nutrition*, **15**, 254–261.

Glossary

Fariba Kolahdooz

University of Alberta

Accelerometer A device used to measure or detect acceleration.

Active transport The movement of molecules against their concentration gradient, from low to high, passing across a membrane with the assistance of enzymes and/or energy input.

Acute phase response Immune responses that occur soon after the onset of infection, trauma, inflammation and some malignant conditions.

Acute postprandial effects Brief and severe effects after consuming a meal.

Ad libitum diet Diet in which an individual only eats based on his/her appetite and desires.

Adenomatous colon polyps Abnormal growth arising from the mucous lining of the colon that is associated with changes in the DNA. Usually benign or non-cancerous growths, but may be precursors to the development of colorectal cancer over time.

Adiabatic A thermodynamic process resulting in no heat gain or loss within a system.

Adiposity Composed of fat or being fatty.

Adverse event An undesired or unintentional result or effect associated with an intervention, supplementation or drug; a side effect.

Aetiology The study of disease causes or origins.

Agglomerative clustering A bottom-up clustering analysis method, which begins with single variables and then repeatedly condenses them into pairs of similar groups until all of the data are in one cluster, used to form a hierarchy within a cluster.

Agouti gene The gene responsible for the appearance (colour and pattern) of a mammal's coat.

Agro-biodiversity The variation of food sources as a result of natural selection and other agricultural selection processes.

Air displacement plethysmography Use of air displacement in an enclosed chamber to measure the body's composition of fat and lean muscle.

Algorithms A set of defined steps to solve a problem or carry out a procedure.

Aliquot A smaller sample or portion of a larger population.

Alkylresorcinols Potential biomarkers of wholegrain consumption; phenolic lipids are found exclusively in the external layer of grains.

Allostasis Homeostasis by means of physical and behavioural changes in organisms.

Ameliorating To improve or make better.

Ampholytes A molecule that possesses both a positive charge and a negative charge; it has both an acidic group and a basic group and therefore has the ability to react as either.

Amplification A mechanism that involves the replication of a chromosome region in a chromosome arm.

Anaemia A condition in which one has low numbers of red blood cells or haemoglobin in the blood.

Analysis of covariance A statistical method used to evaluate the strength of the relationship between two variables.

Anchorage dependence The need for a cell to be attached to a solid surface in order to grow, divide and function.

Angiogenesis The formation or growth of new blood vessels.

Antenatal clinic A medical clinic for pregnant women.

Anthocyanins Water-soluble plant pigments that appear red, blue or purple.

Anthropometric Measurements of the size and comparative physiological proportions of the human body.

Anthropometric indicators Using certain anthropometric measures to help determine the health status of an individual.

Anti-nutrients Compounds that obstruct the absorption of nutrients from foods.

Antioxidant defence A defence strategy of antioxidants to neutralise free radicals and protect the body cells from harm.

Aperitif effect An alcoholic drink consumed before a meal to promote appetite.

Apoptotic Apoptosis is a natural process of cell self-destruction to eliminate damaged or unwanted cells. It can be triggered by environmental factors, like irradiation or toxic substances, or by removal of repressor agents.

Ascites The excessive accumulation of fluid between the abdomen and the abdominal cavity.

Association A relationship of any kind observed between two variables.

Atherosclerotic cardiovascular disease The build-up of fatty plaques on the interior walls of arteries.

Basal energy needs The amount of energy that one needs to maintain life.

Basal metabolic rate The amount of energy expended by organisms at rest.

Bayesian statistics A form of statistics in which the conclusions of a study are expressed in terms of beliefs and probabilities rather than fixed truths.

Beadchip technologies A form of DNA microarray used to analyse chromosomal variation relevant to disease, whereby nucleotide probes are positioned on small beads to allow for the production of increased information.

Bilateral trade Trade involving only two countries.

Binary data Data that are demonstrated in the binary numeral system.

Bioassay data Data collected from a study where a substance is tested in a living organism or tissue.

Bioactive effects Cells, tissues and/or living organisms' responses to substances or processes.

Nutrition Research Methodologies, First Edition. Edited by Julie A Lovegrove, Leanne Hodson, Sangita Sharma and Susan A Lanham-New.
© 2015 John Wiley & Sons, Ltd. Published 2015 by John Wiley & Sons, Ltd.
Companion Website: www.wiley.com/go/nutritionsociety

Bioactive non-nutrient   A chemical compound present in plants that is non-essential for the human body, although many have some benefits.

Bioavailability   The degree to which a micronutrient or drug can be absorbed into the bloodstream and used for its intended purpose in the body.

Biobank   Storage of biological samples for research purposes.

Biodiversity   The variation of plants and animals and other living things in a particular area or region.

Bioelectrical impedance analysis   The measurement of body composition based on the degree of conduction when an electric current is passed through the body.

Biological variation   Diverse range of biological or genetic characteristics.

Biomarkers   Indicators (an event, characteristic or molecule) that help provide information about an individual's health status or exposure to environmental factors.

Blood vessel cannulation   Inserting a cannula, or small tube, into a blood vessel for the drainage of fluid or the administration of medication.

Brown adipose tissue   One of the two types of adipose tissue that generates body heat and contains high amounts of iron, which give it a brown colour.

Buffy coat   The fraction of a blood sample that contains the white blood cells and platelets. Visible after centrifuging as a whitish (or 'buff') coloured layer between the red blood cells and plasma.

Calibration factor   A factor that converts between the value of the measured parameter and the actual parameter.

Calibration studies   Studies that ensure the accuracy of the measurement/evaluation process by relating it to other information.

Calorimetry   The science of measuring the amount of heat exerted or the heat transfer as a proxy for the calorie expenditure.

Candidate gene approach   Focusing on just one or a few genes of interest, when conducting an investigation on genetic associations.

Canonical correlation analysis   A method for identifying correlations between two different variables.

Carotenoids   Fat-soluble plant pigments that appear yellow, orange or red.

Case study   An in-depth investigation of an individual unit (person, illness, event, activity etc.).

Case-control studies   A comparison study between individuals with a disease or outcome of interest (cases) and individuals without a disease or outcome (controls), which retrospectively compares frequency/amount of exposure to a risk factor.

Catecholamine   Hormones originating from the adrenal gland that are derived from the amino acid tyrosine.

Categorical variable   A variable that can adopt a number of different possible values.

Ceruloplasmin   A copper-carrying protein made in the liver, which aids with iron metabolism.

Chi-squared tests   Statistical hypothesis tests that have chi-squared sampling distribution. This occurs when the null hypothesis is true.

Chick chorioallantoic membrane   The vascular membrane found in eggs, comprising the fused mesodermal layers, allantois and chorion. In mammals, this is the placenta.

Chip-on-chip   A technique that analyses the relations of proteins and DNA using chromatin immunoprecipitation and microarray technology.

Cholesteryl esters   An ester of cholesterol associated with atherosclerosis.

Chondrocyte   A cartilage cell that occupies a lacuna within the cartilage matrix.

Chromatin   Genetic (DNA or RNA) material found in the nucleus of eukaryotic cells that condenses to form chromosomes during cell division.

Chromatin immunoprecipitation   A process that aims to investigate whether certain proteins are associated with a specific location of a chromosome.

Chylomicrons   Transport lipoproteins that facilitate the movement of triglycerides and cholesterol from the small intestine to other tissues in the body.

Circadian rhythm   The body's natural sleep and wake cycles.

Cluster sampling   'Cluster units' are selected from a population based on homogenous properties and then random samples are selected from these units.

Clustering   The gathering of many populations based on a common factor.

Coeliac disease   An autoimmune disease in which the absorptive walls of the small intestine are damaged by gluten causing a decrease in the absorption of nutrients.

Co-expressed genes   Genes that have been found by cluster analysis to share similar expression patterns.

Co-morbidities   The presence of two or more coexisting diseases.

Cohort study   A longitudinal study designed to analyse risk factors for the development of certain conditions by observing a population over a long period of time (usually more than ten years).

Collagen substratum   An underlying layer of collagen.

Colonic microbiome   The microorganisms populated in the colon.

Compliance   The extent of accuracy with which a patient/research participant follows an assigned regimen.

Computed axial tomography (CAT)   Also known as the computerised tomography (CT) scan. The CT scanner takes multiple x-rays and combines them to give a 3D image of the body or organs.

Concomitantly   An event or situation that happens simultaneously, or is connected to another.

Concurrent mixed methods   Collection of both qualitative and quantitative data at the same time.

Conditional logistic regression model   Investigates the relationship between the case and the control based on a set of factors.

Confluence   Convergence at a point or junction.

Confocal microscopy   A microscopy technique used to increase the optical resolution and the contrast of the magnified image by using distinct spotlighting and a spatial pinhole.

Confounder   An extraneous variable that distorts the association between observed exposure and outcome.

Contingency table   A table in which data is recorded and analysed to show the relationship between two or more variables.

Continuous variable   An infinite variable that can take any value between its minimum value and maximum value, for example time, length or weight.

Convenience sampling   Collecting data from a group that is easily accessible.

Copy number variants   Alterations in a genome that result in multiple copies of DNA sequences for a given trait.

Cori cycle   The metabolic pathway whereby lactic acid in the muscles, produced through anaerobic glycolysis, is transported to the liver and converted to glucose.

Coronary heart disease (CHD)   A disease in which plaque (fat and cholesterol) is deposited within the walls of the coronary arteries.

Correlation coefficient   A statistic that evaluates how well a straight line describes the relationship between a pair of variables.

Covariate   A variable that is related to the dependent variable and therefore possibly predictive of the outcome.

CPG islands   Promoter regions of DNA with many cytosines – guanine dinucleotides.

Craniocaudal direction   The entry of the x-ray beam from the cranial end of the part being tested, moving towards the caudal end.

Creatinine   A breakdown product resulting from the metabolism of creatine phosphate in muscle during normal muscle contraction.

Crohn's disease　A chronic disease involving inflammation of the gastrointestinal tract.

Cross-sectional study　A type of observational study that records data from a given population at a specific point in time.

Cruciferous vegetables　Vegetables that belong to the cabbage family, such as broccoli and cauliflower.

Cultivar　A variety of plant that has been intentionally maintained through production because of desirable properties (nutrition, taste, palatability).

Cycle-ergometer　A stationary bike used to measure health-related variables such as energy expenditure.

Cytobands　The pattern of bands that form on chromosomes as they undergo metaphase.

Cytosolic proteins　Proteins that are present in the cytoplasm in cells.

De novo synthesis　Use of simple molecules to synthesise complex molecules.

Deamination　To remove an amine group from a compound.

Dedifferentiation　The reversal of differentiated cells or tissues into an unspecialised form.

Degrees of freedom　The amount by which a statistical value can vary without violating any stated constraints.

Dendrogram　A tree diagram that branches into different categories depending on the degree of similarity.

Deuterated water　Also known as heavy water; water that contains mostly deuterium oxide.

Deuterium　A stable isotope of hydrogen containing a neutron in the nucleus that is not present in the hydrogen nucleus.

Deuterium dilution　A technique used to measure total body water by evaluating the concentration of deuterium excreted in urine.

Dichotomous outcome　An outcome that is divided into two sharply distinguished parts.

Dietary acculturation　The process of adopting the dietary habits of another culture, most often as a result of immigration and/or prolonged exposure to a new culture.

Differential distribution　Varying prevalence of disease among populations depending on differing circumstances and risk factors.

Differential expression analysis　Microarray experiments carried out in an effort to find genes that are uniquely expressed between multiple cells.

Diffusion　A process in which molecules move from highly concentrated to less concentrated regions.

Discriminant analysis　A statistical procedure used to predict or categorise responding variables to whichever group or variable is most likely to be the cause.

Distal determinants of health　Large-scale background factors that may predispose certain populations to specific health outcomes, i.e. social structure, demographics, political systems and cultural structures.

Diurnal variation　Fluctuations that happen daily.

Divalent cations　Positively charged ions with a valence of +2.

Divisive clustering　Dividing a large data set into separate clusters or variables.

DNA acetylation　The addition of acetyl groups to lysine residues on the histone protein of DNA.

DNA microarrays　This technology facilitates the high-throughput study of genetic variation and gene expression; the analysis evaluates the hybridisation of nucleotides within an experimental sample to probe nucleotides present on particular, known microarray regions.

Dose–response relationship　A relationship between the amount of exposure to a substance or variable and the degree or severity of the outcome.

Dossier　A collection of documents or information on a particular person or subject.

Double-blind study　An experimental procedure in which neither the participant nor the experiment administrator knows which treatment the participant will receive.

Doubly labelled water　A method of measuring metabolic rate of the hydrogen and oxygen molecules in water are replaced by stable isotopes of hydrogen and oxygen before it is administered to subjects. The rates of elimination of these isotopes are then measured.

Dual-energy x-ray absorptiometry (DEXA)　A method used to quantify fat, lean and bone mass, offering both whole-body and regional analyses.

Dual isotope method　A technique used to determine the absorption of a molecule or element through a specific pathway by administering distinguishable tracers simultaneously via separate pathways, and then measuring the concentrations of each tracer at the end.

Dynamometer　A device used to measure mechanical force.

Echogenicity　The echo that the organs or tissues in the body bounce back when ultrasound is conducted.

Ecological fallacy　An error in making an assumption about an individual based on misinterpretation of a group of people.

Ectopic fat distribution　Fat located in regions where it should not be, i.e. the liver, skeletal muscle, heart muscles and pancreas.

Ectopically　An organ or tissue occurring in an abnormal place.

Electron microscopy　A microscopy technique used to produce extremely high magnifications by using beams of electrons focused by magnetic lenses.

Electrophoresis　A method in which proteins and macromolecules are separated based on size and charge.

Electrospray ionisation　A procedure used in mass spectrometry in order to produce ions from macromolecules.

Enantiomer　Mirror-image stereoisomer.

Endogenous　Originating or being produced within an organism.

Energy cost of arousal　The amount of energy used when engaged in sexual activity.

Energy-dense convenience food　Food high in calories per gram, low in nutrition and easily accessible.

Enterocyte　Cells found in the lining of the intestinal mucosa, responsible for absorption of nutrients.

Enzymatic activity　The activity of an enzyme on its target.

Epidemiological transitions　Changing patterns of population age distributions, mortality, disease, life expectancy and causes of death.

Epidemiology　The study of the allocation and causes of health-related conditions in defined populations, and the employment of that knowledge to help control disease and improve health.

Epigastrium　The upper-middle region of the abdomen that covers the stomach and the liver.

Epigenetics　The study of how environmental factors affect how a gene is expressed.

Equipoise　An equal or fair distribution.

Erythrocyte protoporphyrin　A type of porphyrin that forms the haem group in haemoglobin and myoglobin when combined with iron.

Erythrocytes　Red blood cells.

Essential polyunsaturated fatty acids (PUFA)　Fatty acids that contain more than one double bond in their backbone structure and must be provided through diet.

Ethos　The characteristic beliefs, spirit and disposition of a culture or community.

Euchromatin　The loosely packed portion of chromatin, the active portion allowing for transcription.

Euglycaemic hyperglycaemic clamp　A technique used to quantify beta-cell sensitivity to glucose.

Euglycaemic low-dose hyperinsulinaemic clamp A method used to determine sensitivity to insulin by continuous administration of a low dose of insulin.

Exogenous Not originating from or produced within an organism.

Exon Coding nucleotide that provides sequencing information for protein synthesis.

Explant Biopsy or tissue sample taken from an animal or human tissue.

Extrapolation Making an estimation or calculation outside of the range of known events, but based on those events.

Factor analysis A method used to identify groups or variables that are related.

Fetal origin Relating to a fetus.

First trimester The first 12 weeks of a pregnancy.

Fisher's exact probability test A statistical test used to determine the level of association between two variables.

Flatulence An accumulation of gas in the gastrinal intestinal tract.

Flavonoids Plant pigments having a structure similar to that of flavones.

Flow cytometry A method of counting, sorting and identifying cells by passing them by an electron detection apparatus as they are suspended in a fluid stream.

Fluorescence microscopy A light microscope that uses fluorescence to generate an image by exciting fluorochromes under ultraviolet light.

Fluorophores Fluorescent compounds that can re-emit light on excitation.

Fold change The quantity of difference from an initial value to a final value.

Food fortification Increasing the amount of a micronutrient (vitamins or minerals) in a food item whether the nutrients are naturally occurring in the food or not.

Food frequency questionnaire (FFQ) A questionnaire assessing portion size and frequency of consumption of foods during a specific time period; these data help assess an individual's dietary patterns.

Food taboos Food that people abstain from consuming due to religious or cultural laws.

Fractional polynominal regression A method for demonstrating curved relationships between variables.

Gastrointestinal Relating to the stomach or intestines.

Gene ontology A major initiative in bioinformatics to standardise information and knowledge regarding genes and gene products.

Gene set enrichment An evaluation of microarray data of gene sets that have previously been identified based on biological knowledge.

Genetic polymorphism Two or more forms of the same allele present in a single population at a frequency of ≥ 1%.

Glucocorticoid A corticosteroid that is involved in metabolism and anti-inflammatory effects.

Glycaemic response The response of blood sugar after the consumption of meals.

Glycated haemoglobin A form of haemoglobin in which glucose is bound as a result of elevated blood glucose. It is useful to identify the average concentration of plasma glucose in the blood over an extended period of time.

Glycoside A simple sugar that has had one of its hydroxyl groups replaced with another compound.

Glycosylation The process by which a carbohydrate attaches to another molecule.

Green fluorescent protein A protein found naturally in some marine organisms that fluoresces bright green when excited by blue to ultraviolet wavelengths.

Grounded theory A research practice aimed at generating a theory or hypothesis.

Gut microbiome A complex of microorganisms that live in the digestive tract.

Haematocrit A ratio representing the volume of red blood cells in relation to the total blood volume.

Haemodynamics The study of blood flow and circulation.

Haemostatic response The body's response to blood loss.

Haplotype A combination of alleles in close proximity to the same chromosome, resulting in them frequently being inherited together.

Haptocorrin A protein that protects vitamin B12 from acids in the stomach.

Hayflick limit The number of times a human cell will divide before it reaches senescence and stops dividing.

Health claims Claims that imply or suggest a relationship between the contents in a food product and a health outcome.

Hemicellulose A compound that is present in plant cell walls.

Hepatocyte A cell of the liver.

Heterochromatin The highly condensed portion of a chromosome, genetically inactive.

Heterogeneity The state of being diverse.

Heterotrophic organisms Organisms that obtain nutrition for their growth and development from organic food sources and are unable to synthesise it on their own.

Heuristic Problem-solving or discovery techniques based on previous experience.

Hierarchical clustering A method of cluster analysis that builds clusters based on hierarchy, or levels, either from a 'bottom-up' or a 'top-down' approach.

High-penetrance single-gene defects Disorders that result from a single gene defect on an autosome. The inheritance of these disorders follows Mendelian's Law.

Histochemistry The study and identification of chemical compounds in tissues and biological samples.

Histones Structural proteins around which DNA wind to form organised genetic units called nucleosomes.

Homeothermic organism An organism that has a constant body temperature, independent of its surroundings.

Homocysteine An amino acid produced naturally in the body as a by-product of metabolism.

Homology The study of the similarities or variances of a specific organ between different species.

Hybridoma A hybrid cell comprising lymphocyte and tumour cell fusion.

Hydrolysis The breakage of chemical bonds in the presence of water.

Hypergeometric A probability distribution that describes the probability of an outcome without replacement to the sample population.

Hyperglycaemia High levels of blood glucose.

Hypothalamo-pituitary-adrenal system A feedback-control mechanism responsible for the body's response to stress.

Idiosyncrasies A unique behavioural or structural characteristic of a group or an individual.

Ileostomy A type of surgery where an opening in the abdominal wall is made and the lowest part of the small intestine is brought to the skin's surface, usually on the lower-right region of the abdomen. The waste (or stool) from the body no longer leaves the anus but leaves through the small intestine that has been relocated to the skin's surface.

Iliac crest The long top curved part of the ilium, the biggest bone in the pelvic area, which gives an individual's hips their shape.

Immortalised cell lines Cells that have circumvented normal senescence as a result of mutation and can therefore continue to replicate.

Immune surveillance   The recognition and destruction, by the immune system, of tumour cells that arise constantly throughout the life of an individual.

Immunoblotting   A method used for the identification of proteins in a mixture whereby separation of proteins is performed by electrophoresis followed by staining with antibodies.

Immunocytochemistry   A technique that uses antibodies to identify specific proteins or antigens in a cell. The antibodies help make the proteins or antigens visible under a microscope.

Immunohistochemistry   The use of antibodies to detect specific protein molecules in a biological sample.

Impedance jumps   Generated by boundaries between tissues of different impedance to acoustic waves.

In vitro **studies**   Studies conducted in a controlled environment, in which components of an organism are isolated and studied.

Incident cases   A person (a participant of a study) who has newly developed a disease of interest.

Infrared carbon dioxide analyser   A method of measuring trace gas (in this case, carbon dioxide) amounts by investigating the amount of absorption of an infrared light source in a given sample of gas.

Insensible loss   An immeasurable amount of fluid lost from the body through respiration, perspiration etc.

Insulin resistance   A state in which body cells do not respond properly to insulin, therefore cannot easily absorb glucose from the blood.

Intention to treat analyses   Data analysis in which all participants of an experiment are included.

Intermediate determinants of health   Factors that act as buffers between proximal and distal determinants of health in an effort to minimise their potential impact, i.e. healthcare systems, educational systems, community infrastructure and resources.

Interoperability   The ability to make processes or organisations work together.

Intra-myocellular fat   Small droplets of fats located in the cytoplasm of muscle cells.

Intragenic methylation   Methylation within genes, which regulates important genetic functions such as RNA splicing.

Intrinsic factors   A glycoprotein found in the stomach that aids in the absorption of vitamin B12.

Intron   A DNA sequence that is non-coding and therefore does not translate into protein synthesis.

Ionising radiation   Radiation that has an ample amount of energy to knock an atom's tightly bound electron out of orbit, causing the atom to become charged.

Ischaemia   A restriction of blood flow to a particular part of the body (i.e. brain or heart), which causes shortage of oxygen and glucose needed for metabolism.

Isoelectric point   The pH point at which a molecule has no electrical charge.

Isoelectric focusing   A technique used to separate proteins by altering the pH environment and taking advantage of variances in their isoelectric points.

Isoschizomers   Pairs of restriction enzymes that share the same genetic sequence.

Isothermal   A thermodynamic process in which there can be heat gain or loss as long as the temperature remains constant in the system.

Isotope dilution   A technique used for analysing chemical substances whereby a known amount of an isotope is added to a sample, and then, by comparison to the natural isotopic ratio, the amount of an element in the original sample can be calculated.

Isotopic probes   A group of atoms or molecules used to examine the properties of other molecules or structures.

K-means   A clustering algorithm aimed at minimising the average squared Euclidean distance from the mean.

Kruskal–Wallis one-way analysis of variance   A non-parametric method used to determine whether samples arise from the same distribution.

Ligand binding   The process in which a ligand (signal-triggering molecule) binds to a receptor site to initiate a process.

Lignans   Oestrogen-like compounds found in plants.

Linea alba   The white fibrous tissue that divides the muscles of the body and helps facilitate movement.

Linkage disequilibrium   When genes at two different loci are dependent on one another.

Lipodystrophy   A disorder in fat metabolism characterised by fat loss in selective parts of the body.

Lipophilicity   The ability of a compound to integrate and dissolve lipids and fats.

Liquid chromatography   A technique in organic chemistry using a liquid solvent to separate molecules in a mixture and quantify its components.

Log transform   A method used to help make highly skewed data less skewed, improving the interpretability of the data.

Logistic regression analysis   A statistical classification model that is used in estimating the values of qualitative parameters.

Longitudinal study   A correlation research study that follows the same cohort over a period of time, involving observation and recording of the same variable.

Lower limit of quantification   The lowest quantifiable presence of a biomarker that can be reproduced with relative certainty.

Magnetic activated cell sorting (MACS™)   A method of separating cell populations based on their unique surface antigens.

Magnetic resonance imaging (MRI)   A medical imaging technique used to generate computerised images of internal organs with the use of radio waves and a strong magnetic field.

Malnutrition   Poor nutrition caused by an imbalanced diet in which certain nutrients are lacking.

Mann–Whitney U test   A non-parametric test used to determine the difference between two independent variables when the dependent variable is not normally distributed.

Mass spectrometry   A method for analysing the components of a sample based on their molecular mass, useful in determining the isotopic signature of a sample.

Mean corpuscular volume (MCV)   The average volume of red blood cells in a complete blood count.

Measurement variation   When different results are produced after measuring the same object or variable multiple times. Differences can be minimal or substantial.

Megaloblastic anaemia   A type of anaemia characterised by the presence of large, immature red blood cells that do not function like healthy blood cells.

Meta-analysis   A statistical technique used to gather and combine information from various independent studies.

Metabolic disequillibrium   The flow of materials in and out of cells that ensures that metabolic pathways never reach equilibrium; a defining feature of life.

Metabolic suites   Enclosed rooms in which an individual's metabolic energy can be measured.

Metabolic syndrome   A group of medical conditions that, when occurring simultaneously, increase the risk of developing type 2 diabetes and cardiovascular disease.

Metabolome   The total number of metabolites (components involved in metabolism) present within an organism, cell or tissue.

Metabolomic profile   A quantitative measure of metabolites involved in the metabolic response to stimuli.

Metabolomics   A discipline that studies metabolites and their chemical processes.

Methodological limitations Characteristics of a study design in which lack of validity or bias may be present.

Microarray Placing microscopic gene sequences together on a hard surface, such as a glass slide, in order to study gene expression.

Microarray hybridisation A method used to identify the organism in a sample by hybridising DNA.

Microbiological assay An analysis of compounds that have an effect on microorganisms.

Microbiome A specific microorganism population present in an environment.

Microcarrier beads Small spheres that allow for the attachment and growth of adherent cells. The specific material used for the microcarrier beads can influence cellular behaviour.

MicroRNA (miRNA) MicroRNA are non-coding RNA molecules that function as post-transcriptional regulators of gene expression.

Miscible When two substances can be mixed together to form a homogenous solution.

Missense change A genetic mutation that occurs when a single nucleotide is changed and codes for a different amino acid, resulting in a non-functional protein.

Mixed-methods approach Research that utilises multiple methods of obtaining data and an end result (i.e. quantitative, qualitative, predetermined or emerging methods).

Monetisation The selling of donated food or items to generate cash to implement projects or programmes.

Monoclonal antibodies Manufactured antibodies that are all clones of one unique parent cell, and therefore bind to only one substance.

Monogenic A phenotype determined by one gene.

Monogenic autosomal-dominant disorders Disorders that result from the inheritance of a single copy of a defective gene, sufficient to override the normal gene.

Monogenic autosomal-recessive disorders Disorders that only occur if both genes are defective.

Monovalent cations Positively charged ions with a valence of +1.

Morbidity The prevalence of a particular disease in a population.

Multilateral trade Trade involving more than two countries.

Multimodality When data produce more than one peak when graphed or plotted.

Multiple linear regression Modelling the relationship of a dependent variable compared to an independent variable in order to predict the outcome of the dependent variable.

Multivariate analyses A statistical analysis in which one or more statistical variables are being observed at the same time.

Myokines Muscle-derived cytokines that provide cell communication for immune responses in situations such as infection or inflammation.

Narrative research A research method involving the use of written or spoken accounts, or visual representations of individuals' lives.

Necrotic cell A dead cell.

Nested case-control study A variation on a case-control study in which only a portion of the controls are compared to the outcome.

Nitrogen balance The difference between nitrogen intake and nitrogen excretion.

Nitrosylation A reaction that occurs between nitric oxide and a biological compound.

Non-parametric methods A method to model and analyse data that do not require the data to follow a normal distribution or an assumption about the distribution.

Non-nutrients Compounds found in foods that are not essential nutrients like vitamins and minerals (e.g. fibre), but help to promote health if consumed.

Normal (Gaussian) distribution Data that produce a symmetrical, bell-shaped curve when graphed or plotted.

Nuclear magnetic resonance The absorption of specific frequencies of electromagnetic radiation when an atom is placed in a strong magnetic field.

Nuisance variable A variable that is important to the probability model but not of interest.

Null hypothesis Hypothesis that opposes the suggested relationship between two variables.

Nutrients tolerable upper limits The highest level of nutrient intake that could be ingested by almost any individual in the population without any risk.

Nutrigenomics The study of the effect of food on gene expression.

Nutrition security Adequate availability and variety of food, nutrition and health services in order to ensure adequate nutrition for the population to achieve an active and healthy life at all times for all members of society.

Nutrition transition Shift away from traditional diets and towards Western diets.

Nutritional epidemiology The study of how diet and nutritional status affect the prevalence and distribution of disease and health conditions.

Odds ratio (OR) Quantifies the odds of a group of people being exposed to or having a disease and those who do not.

Oedema Excessive fluid accumulation within a region of the body.

Oligonucleotide microarrays A study of genetic variation and gene expression using microarrays of oligonucleotides where each gene is represented by multiple probes, called a probe set.

Ontologies A representation of something that we know about or that can be observed.

Ordinal scale Ranking of something on a scale of the lowest to the highest magnitude. For example, dislike very much to like very much.

Orthogonal partial least squares discriminant analysis A multivariate model that condenses dimensions and improves visualisation to produce an easy-to-interpret linear relationship.

Orthogonal vectors Two vectors that are perpendicular to each other.

Oxidative stress The result of an imbalance in reactive oxygen species compared to antioxidants, producing free radicals and peroxides that are damaging to cells.

P-systems A computer science inspired by biological processes, in particular the movement of chemicals across membranes.

P-value The estimated likelihood of rejecting the null hypothesis of a study question when that hypothesis is true.

Palatability Being acceptable by the mouth in terms of taste and texture.

Paramagnetic oxygen analyser A device used to determine the concentration of oxygen in an environment or sample by using a focused magnetic field and taking advantage of oxygen's paramagnetic nature.

Parametric method Statistical method based on assumptions of the approximate normal distribution of the population. Theoretical distribution described by parameters is estimated from the data.

Partial least squares A method for predicting relationships between single variables or variable sets.

Pathogenesis The origin and mechanism of a disease or pathogen.

Pathophysiology The physical functional changes associated with a medical condition or injury.

Pathway topology The study of specific gene pathways or how genetic expressions are associated between genes.

Penetrance The proportion of individuals in a population who carry a gene that has an associated trait expression.

Performance-oriented mobility The ability to perform balance-related activities.

Perfused Supplying fluid into an organ, tissue or body through blood vessels.

Perfused organs Organs to which blood or fluid is flowing.

Periconceptual period The period from just before conception to embryo development.

Peripheral blood mononuclear cells Blood cells with a round nucleus.

Permutation distribution An unknown distribution of test statistics.

Pernicious anaemia A type of megaloblastic anaemia that results from the lack of intrinsic factor in the small intestine for the absorption of vitamin B12.

Perturbations Deviations from normal state or path.

Pharmacokinetic The interaction of drugs in the human body, such as absorption or elimination.

Phase contrast microscopy A type of light microscopy in which light is passed through a transparent specimen to reveal its phase via brightness variations.

Phenolic lipids Lipids that contain phenols and aliphatic chains found in plants, fungi and bacteria.

Phenome The set of all phenotypical traits expressed by a cell, tissue, organ, organism or species.

Phenomenological research The study of the human mind, experience and consciousness.

Phenylketonuric (PKU) patients Patients who suffer from phenylketonuria, which is an inherited genetic disorder where the person is missing an enzyme that metabolises the essential amino acid phenylalanine.

Photometric test Measurement of the relative or perceived luminous intensity of light.

Photonic scanning A technique used to estimate regional and total body volumes by taking a three-dimensional scan of the body using numerous data points.

Phyto-nutrients Nutrients from plant origins believed to be beneficial to human health.

Pi-calculus A mathematical process used to describe and analyse properties of concurrent computation.

Piezoelectric transducer A device used to detect mechanical or acoustic signals and convert them to electrical signals or vice versa.

Polycythaemia A condition in which there is an increased concentration in blood cells in the blood.

Polygenic A phenotype determined by more than one gene.

Polymerise To undergo the process of combining one product with others to form a product of higher molecular weight.

Polymorphic allele Variations or mutations in an allele or DNA sequence that cause different phenotypical traits within a given population.

Polyphenols A complex variety of compounds containing multiple phenolic groups found naturally in many foods and potentially having effects on health.

Population stratification Differences in allele frequencies observed in different subpopulations, possibly related to ancestry.

Population-based studies A type of study used to answer a research question regarding a population where the participant sample is selected randomly from the general population with at least 50% participation rate.

Positional cloning A method used to locate and identify specific areas of interest on a genome.

Positively correlated A relationship between two variables in which one variable follows the direction of the other variable (i.e. if one variable increases, the other one also increases).

Positron emission tomography A technique used to measure the functional and metabolic processes of the body.

Post-translational modifications Modifications that occur in proteins after translation from mRNA to become functional proteins in cells.

Posteriori technique Exploratory non-hypothesis methods based on observations.

Postprandial period Period of time following eating a meal.

Pragmatic Being concerned more with practical results than theories.

Pre-clinical phase A control test of a new drug or procedure, conducted to gather evidence in a clinical trial.

Precursor-product method A method used to measure macromolecule synthesis or degradation based on a known amount of a precursor and subsequent measuring of its product(s) generated.

Predictive biomarker Biomarkers that indicate the intake of a substance with a consistent and time-dependent relationship; however, there is incomplete recovery.

Pre-eclampsia A condition during pregnancy that causes elevated blood pressure, fluid retention and protein excretion in the urine.

Pre-protocol analysis Data analysis in which only data from participants that met the protocol are used and participants who have deviated from the protocol are excluded.

Principal component analysis A statistical method used to reduce the number of variables in a data set containing a large number of variables, while retaining most of the information in the large data set.

Prions A misfolded protein that forms an infectious agent that causes many neurological diseases, such as Alzheimer's and bovine spongiform encephalopathy.

Priori technique Research based on information known or assumed.

Probing Asking non-specific questions to gain further detail in an interview. For example, in a 24-hour recall a respondent may say that they have eaten toast for breakfast. To get more information the interviewer may ask the respondent if they had anything with their toast instead of asking them if they had jam or butter on the toast.

Proportional hazards regression Survival models in statistics to analyse the effect of several factors up to the time a specific event occurs.

Protease inhibitors Antiviral drugs that prevent the replication of viruses by selectively binding to viral proteases.

Protein homogenate A mixture of protein molecules and tissues that have been ground together.

Proteolysis The process of protein breakdown into polypeptides.

Proteomic profile An evaluation of the proteins found in a sample (i.e. blood or urine).

Proteomics A discipline that studies the proteins in an organism and their structures.

Proximates Major constituents of food products as they would be used in human metabolism. Categories include moisture, lipid, protein, ash and carbohydrates.

Proxy A representative for individuals not fit to represent themselves.

Psychometric score A psychological score that indicates an individual's knowledge, abilities, attitudes, personality traits and intelligence.

Public health policies Policies or programmes implemented with the goal of having some effect on the health status of a population.

Putative factors Assumed or reputable factors.

Pyrolysed Organic material that has been irreversibly decomposed using heat in the absence of oxygen.

Qualitative research methods Research methods that involve the observation and recording of a variable that cannot be quantified.

Quantitative research methods Research involving quantifiable variables and outcome.

Quantum dots Nanoparticles of semiconducting material that fluoresce when excited and can be embedded in cells for various purposes, such as protein labelling.

Quartiles Three points that divide data into four equal groups, each group being a quarter of the data.

Quiescent state The state of rest or inactivity.

Quota sampling A non-probability sampling technique in which a sample population is separated into smaller subgroups based on similarities. From the subgroups, individuals are then selected or targeted for specific qualities based on inclusion/exclusion criteria for the study.

Radioisotope Radioactive isotopes of an element.

Random variation Unpredictable variability subject to change; value cannot be accurately predicted using a model.

Randomised controlled trial (RCT) Scientific experiment in which a group of people selected randomly from a population receive a clinical intervention, which is then compared to other clinical interventions tested on other groups of people.

Recall bias Inaccuracy in response regarding recollections, particularly in a retrospective study; may be intentional or unintentional (e.g. forgotten).

Recovery biomarker Biomarkers that are present in known amounts, over a given period of time, based on the input (consumption) of a given substance; there is a strong dose–response relationship. Often measured using 24-hour urine samples.

Reductant The element that donates an electron to another element in an oxidation/reduction reaction.

Refection Ingesting food or drink for refreshment.

Relative risk ratios The ratio of the probability of an event occurring in a group exposed to a risk compared to that event happening in a group not exposed to that risk.

Repository of nutrient data A database in which nutrition data are stored.

Residual confounding The distribution that remains after taking into account confounding as much as possible.

Residuals The difference between the observed value and the theoretical value.

Respiratory quotient The volume of carbon dioxide produced or eliminated from the body compared to the amount of oxygen inhaled.

Respirometry Techniques that estimate metabolic rate through indirect measures of heat production.

Retinoids Chemical compounds related to vitamin A and having a similar effect in the body.

Retinol equivalents A comparison of the bioavailable quantities of retinol present in different carotenoids.

Retrospective recall A method in which participants recall information from past events.

Revealedness The degree of disclosure of the details of the study to participants.

Reverse engineering algorithms The process of determining the mechanism of function through analysis and observations.

Ridge regression A method used to analyse multicollinear regression data.

RNA integrity number An assigned value (from 1–10) given to an RNA sample to represent its quality.

Robust multiarray average An algorithm used to create an expression matrix.

Sampling frame A population from which samples can be randomly drawn.

Satiation The state of feeling satisfactorily full and, in response, terminating eating.

Satiety The sense of fullness that continues after eating a meal.

Scatter diagram A diagram used to determine the relationship between two variables.

Scintillation counter A device used to detect and measure radioactive emissions (from radioisotopes).

Selection bias When an error exists in deciding on the individuals or groups to participate in a study.

Senescent Describes cells that can no longer divide but can maintain metabolic functioning.

Sensible loss Fluid loss by a means that is apparent to an individual (i.e. urine, feces, blood loss etc.).

Sequelae Any abnormal health-related conditions that follow after a disease, attack or injury.

Sequential mixed methods When a researcher seeks to expand on the findings of existing data by utilising another method of data collection.

Serum ferritin A protein found in the blood that stores iron and releases it in a controlled fashion.

Serum triglycerides Fat molecules found in the blood.

Short-chain fatty acids A group of fatty acids that has aliphatic tails with carbon atoms ranging from two to six.

Shotgun lipidomics The use of electrospray ionisation with mass spectrometry to investigate the biological function, significance and make-up of lipids.

Sieverts A measure of the effect of low amounts of radiation on human health.

Signal transduction A process in which extracellular molecules activate a cell surface receptor.

Single nucleotide polymorphisms A common form of genetic variation whereby a single nucleotide in a genetic sequence is different (e.g. CAGGTTA to CAAGTTA)

Single-arm study Everyone in the study group is treated in the same way and the outcome is observed.

Skewness Asymmetry observed when data are graphed or plotted.

Snowball sampling Having existing study participants suggest or recruit new participants via their own personal connections.

Solid-phase extraction A technique used to separate solids in which these compounds, depending on their physical and chemical properties, may dissolve in a liquid and separate.

Solubilise To make a substance more soluble or dissolvable, particularly in water.

Spirometer A device that measures the volumes of air inhaled and expired from the lungs.

Spurious associations False associations made due to error or bias during sampling.

Stadiometer A device used to measure height.

Steatosis The excessive collection of fat in the liver.

Stereomicroscope A relatively low-magnifying binocular microscope that utilises light reflecting off the surface of an object rather than through it.

Stigmatisation Disapproval or condemning associations with a specific group or defining feature.

Stratification When a population is grouped into different categories.

Subscapular The region of an individual's shoulder blade.

Subcutaneous fat Fat located under the skin.

Sum of squares A method for determining the dispersion of data points.

Supine position When an individual lies down on his/her back (facing up).

Supra-iliac The front region of the iliac crest, the hip bone.

Surrogate markers Indirect markers that are used in the place of clinical endpoints.

Survival data Data in a study where the outcome variable is the occurrence of an event (death, disease etc.)

Survival function   The probability that a participant will survive a given amount of time after entering a study.

Synergy   The combination of different elements to create an effect that is greater than the sum of the element's effects when produced separately.

Systematic reviews   A literature review, collected from all high-quality research evidence, to answer a research question.

Tandem mass spectrometry   A machine that analyses the composition of a sample. Tandem mass spectrometry uses two different stages of mass analysis.

Taxonomic level   Different classifications of organisms based on similar features, evolutionary similarities and hierarchy.

Telomerase transfection   The act of deliberately inserting a gene for the catalyst, telomerase, into normal, ageing cells resulting in extended telomeres and, consequently, extended cell life.

Telomeres   Repetitive nucleotide sequences located at the end of a chromosome.

Terminal differentiation   Exit from the cell cycle; a cell that is no longer dividing by mitosis.

Terminal ileum   The most distal part of the small intestine.

Thalassaemia   A blood disease in which the body produces abnormal haemoglobin. This leads to the production of irregular red blood cells, which can lead to anaemia.

Thermoneutral zone   The range of temperatures that an endotherm can tolerate.

Throughput   The rate or amount of a product or process that can be completed in a certain period of time.

Thyrotoxicosis   A condition in which there are high levels of thyroid hormone in the blood, increasing the rate of body functions and causing conditions such as weight loss, increased heart rate or sweating. Also known as hyperthyroidism.

Tracer dilution   A technique used to quantitatively investigate substrates within the human body by introducing a tracer to a particular body pool (extra-cellular fluid) and then calculating the rate of change in concentration of the tracer.

Transamination   Transfer of an amino group from one chemical compound to another.

Transcobalamin   Carrier proteins that bind to different chemical forms of vitamin B12.

Transcriptomic signature   A cell's particular collection of RNA transcripts.

Transcriptomics   The study of all RNA molecules in an organism.

Transesterification   The process in which the R group is interchanged from an ester to an alcohol.

Transfection techniques   Techniques by which nucleic acids are inserted into mammalian cells.

Transformative mixed methods   A research method in which the researcher uses both qualitative and quantitative data collection to focus on specific topics of interest or outcomes anticipated in the study.

Transgenerational epigenetic inheritance   When a phenotypical trait caused by environmental factors is passed down to multiple generations.

Transgenic   An organism that contains a gene that has been transferred from another species.

True reference value   A widely known value that can be used for reference.

Ubiquitination   A process whereby a protein is inactivated by the attachment of ubiquitin.

Ubiquitous   Describes a substance or object that appears everywhere.

Ulna length   The measurement of the distance between the prominent bones of the wrist to the tip of the prominent bone on the elbow to estimate an individual's height. The measurement is usually done on the left arm and when the arm is bent up and towards the body.

Univariate analysis   A type of analysis in which only one dependent variable is used to assess a hypothesis and/or to draw a conclusion about a population.

Urinary nitrogen excretion   The nitrogen that is found in the urine as a result of protein metabolism.

Validation studies   Studies conducted to ensure the accuracy of the measurement/evaluation process.

Venepuncture   To puncture a vein in order to administer drugs, draw blood or perform another medical procedure.

Visceral fat   Fat present around the organs in the abdominal region.

Washout period   A period in a study during which no treatment or drugs are used.

Wild-type allele   An allele that produces the typical phenotypical traits seen in the wild.

X-linked disorders   Disorders in which the defective gene lies on the X chromosome. These disorders are more common in men, as they only have one X chromosome and no possibility of overriding a defect.

Xenobiotics   A chemical substance found within a biological system but that is foreign to that system (not naturally produced).

Xenografts   The transplant of a tissue or organ from one species to another.

Xerophthalmia   Abnormal dryness of the eyes as a result of the inability to produce tears; it may be caused by vitamin A deficiency.

Z-scores   Values that quantify how far a value is from the mean; always zero for values equal to the mean, positive for values greater than the mean and negative for values less than the mean.

Index

Note: Page numbers in *italics* refer to Figures; those in **bold** to Tables.

Nutrition Research Methodologies, First Edition. Edited by Julie A Lovegrove, Leanne Hodson, Sangita Sharma and Susan A Lanham-New.
© 2015 John Wiley & Sons, Ltd. Published 2015 by John Wiley & Sons, Ltd.
Companion Website: www.wiley.com/go/nutritionsociety

Printed and bound by CPI Group (UK) Ltd, Croydon, CR0 4YY

27/10/2024

14580204-0001